INSTRUCTOR'S RESOURCE MANUAL

Tony Crystal, ScD, EMT-P, RPhT

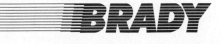

Prehospital Emergency Care

EIGHTH EDITION

Joseph J. Mistovich, MEd, NREMT-P

Chairperson and Professor
Department of Health Professions
Youngstown State University
Youngstown, Ohio

Keith J. Karren, PhD

Professor, Department of Health Sciences
Brigham Young University
Provo, Utah

Medical Editor
Howard A. Werman, MD

Legacy Author
Brent Q. Hafen, PhD

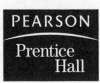

PEARSON

Prentice Hall

Upper Saddle River, New Jersey 07458

O9-BTZ-135

Publisher: Julie Levin Alexander
Publisher's Assistant: Regina Bruno
Executive Editor: Marlene McHugh Pratt
Senior Managing Editor for Development: Lois Berlowitz
Development Editor: Triple SSS Press Media Development
Assistant Editor: Matthew Sirinides
Director of Marketing: Karen Allman
Executive Marketing Manager: Katrin Beacom
Marketing Specialist: Michael Sirinides
Managing Editor for Production: Patrick Walsh
Production Liaison: Faye Gemmellaro
Production Editor: Jessica Balch, Pine Tree Composition
Manufacturing Manager: Ilene Sanford
Manufacturing Buyer: Pat Brown
Cover Designer: Amanda Kavanagh
Cover Photography: Nathan Eldridge
Composition: Pine Tree Composition, Inc.
Printer/Binder: Bind-Rite Graphics
Cover Printer: Phoenix Color Corp.

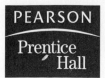

10 9 8 7 6 5 4 3 2 1
ISBN-13 978-0-13-174156-0
ISBN-10   0-13-174156-X

Notice on Care Procedures

This Instructor's Resource Manual (IRM) reflects current EMS practices based on the 1994 U.S. Department of Transportation's EMT-Basic National Standard Curriculum. It is the intent of the authors and publisher that this IRM be used as part of a formal Emergency Medical Technician education program taught by qualified instructors and supervised by a licensed physician. The procedures described in the textbook and this IRM are based upon consultation with EMS and medical authorities. The authors and publisher have taken care to make certain that these procedures reflect currently accepted clinical practice; however, they cannot be considered absolute recommendations.

The material in this IRM contains the most current information available at the time of publication. However, federal, state, and local guidelines concerning clinical practices, including, without limitation, those governing infection control and universal precautions, change rapidly. The reader should note, therefore, that new regulations may require changes in some procedures.

It is the responsibility of the reader to familiarize himself or herself with the policies and procedures set by federal, state, and local agencies as well as the institution or agency where the reader is employed. The authors and the publisher of this workbook disclaim any liability, loss, or risk resulting directly or indirectly from the suggested procedures and theory, from any undetected errors, or from the reader's misunderstanding of the text. It is the reader's responsibility to stay informed of any new changes or recommendations made by any federal, state, and local agency as well as by his or her employing institution or agency.

Notice on Gender Usage

The English language has historically given preference to the male gender. Among many words, the pronouns "he" and "his" are commonly used to describe both genders. Society evolves faster than language, and the male pronouns still predominate in our speech. The authors have made great effort to treat the two genders equally, recognizing that a significant percentage of EMTs are female. However, in some instances, male pronouns may be used to describe both males and females solely for the purpose of brevity. This is not intended to offend any readers of the female gender.

Notice on CPR and ECC

The national standards for Cardiopulmonary Resuscitation (CPR) and Emergency Cardiovascular Care (ECC) are reviewed and revised on a regular basis and may change slightly after this manual is printed. It is important that you know the most current procedures for CPR and ECC, both for the classroom and your patients. The most current information may always be downloaded from www.bradybooks.com or obtained from the appropriate credentialing agency.

Notice on "Case Studies"

The names used and situations depicted in the case studies throughout this workbook are fictitious.

Notice on Medications

The authors and the publisher of this manual have taken care to make certain that the equipment, doses of drugs, and schedules of treatment are correct and compatible with the standards generally accepted at the time of publication. Nevertheless, as new information becomes available, changes in treatment and in the use of equipment and drugs become necessary. The reader is advised to carefully consult the instruction and information material included in the page insert of each drug or therapeutic agent, piece of equipment, or device before administration. This advice is especially important when using new or infrequently used drugs. Prehospital care providers are warned that use of any drugs or techniques must be authorized by their medical director, in accord with local laws and regulations. The publisher disclaims any liability, loss, injury, or damage incurred as a consequence, directly or indirectly, of the use and application of any of the contents of this manual.

Dedication

This Instructor's Resource Manual is dedicated to all the hard-working EMS educators making a difference in the improvement of prehospital care.

CONTENTS

As we enter the 21st Century, dynamic changes will be taking place in Emergency Medical Services and health care in general. With shorter hospital stays, an increase in home care activities, and the general changes in society, the number and types of patients receiving pre-hospital care are increasing. We have come a long way from "The White Paper" of 1966 (*Accidental Death and Disability: The Neglected Disease of Modern Society*) to the present, and we still have a long way to go. The skills needed and types of treatment rendered by EMS personnel have changed in recent years and will continue to change. Skills and treatment modalities once reserved for physicians and other specialists are now being performed by Paramedics, Advanced EMTs and EMTs.

The National Highway Traffic Safety Administration has developed a series of documents to help guide our path. The *EMS Agenda for the Future* serves as a guideline for EMS providers, health care organizations and institutions, governmental agencies, and policymakers committed to improving health care in their communities and to ensure that EMS efficiently contributes to that goal. The *EMS Education Agenda for the Future* serves as a guideline that provides EMS educational outcomes designed to meet the needs of the public. This system also emphasizes the integration of EMS within the overall healthcare system. The *National EMS Research Agenda* serves as a guideline for EMS research and for elevating the science of EMS and prehospital care to the next level. The *Trauma System Agenda for the Future* documents the importance of full implementation of quality trauma systems across the United States to provide optimal care for injured patients and to enhance the country's readiness to respond to future acts of terrorism. The *National EMS Scope of Practice Model* project will help take the *EMS Agenda for the Future* into the streets.

This *Instructor's Resource Manual* has been developed to provide you with resources needed to effectively present the materials related to emergency medical care. It not only covers the materials in the National Standard Curriculum, but incorporates numerous references to a variety of Brady/Prentice Hall Health products to enhance student education, evaluate student progress, and provide for remediation of materials, as needed. These materials have been developed by a team of EMS educators and production professionals to bring you state-of-the-art resources for today's EMS educational programs.

Tony Crystal
EMS Education Coordinator
St. Mary's Hospital
Decatur, Illinois

ACKNOWLEDGMENTS

Introductory material and many of the ideas for the organization of this Instructor's Resource Manual were provided by:

George Angus, Jr., A.A.S., NREMT-P
President and Paramedic Program Director
Aurora North Emergency Services Academy
Anchorage, Alaska

The following instructors contributed hand-out exercises to this Instructor's Resource Manual. We thank them for their creativity, skill, and dedication to excellence.

Brenda M. Beasley, R.N., B.S., EMT-P
EMS Program Director
Calhoun Community College
Decatur, Alabama

David M. Habben, NREMT-P
EMS Instructor/Consultant
Boise, Idaho

Eric W. Heckerson, R.N., M.A.
EMS Coordinator Mesa Fire Department
Mesa, Arizona

Deborah Kufs, B.S., R.N., NREMT-P
Clinical Instructor
Hudson Valley Community College
Institute of Prehospital Emergency Medicine
Troy, New York

James B. Miller, EMT-P
EMS Coordinator Fire & Emergency Services
Fort Sam Houston, Texas

Jarrod Taylor, NREMT-P
EMS Instructor Calhoun Community College
Decatur, Alabama

OVERVIEW OF TEXTBOOK CONTENTS

This edition of *Prehospital Emergency Care* is based on the 1994 DOT EMT-Basic Curriculum. Everything in the curriculum is contained within the textbook, although the order in which some material is presented has been rearranged to provide a better development of ideas and to enhance student understanding. Some additional material has been introduced to give students a fuller picture of certain topics. Each module in the textbook corresponds to a module in the 1994 curriculum. Chapters in the textbook correspond to lessons in the curriculum. The content of *Prehospital Emergency Care*, Eighth Edition is summarized below.

Module 1, Preparatory: Chapters 1–6
This first module sets a framework for all the modules that follow by introducing some essential concepts, information, and skills. The Emergency Medical Services system and the role of the EMT within the system are introduced. Issues of the EMT's safety and well-being and legal and ethical issues are covered. Students are introduced to the basics of anatomy and physiology. Finally, they learn the basic techniques for safe lifting and moving of patients that they will employ throughout this program and throughout their EMS careers.

Module 2, Airway: Chapter 7
There is only one chapter in Module 2, but it may be considered the most important module in the text because no patient will survive without an open airway. Basic airway management techniques are covered in detail.

Module 3, Patient Assessment: Chapters 8–11
Module 3 holds the key to the 1994 assessment-based curriculum. The ability to perform a rapid but accurate assessment, treat for life-threatening conditions, and initiate transport to the hospital within optimum time limits is the essence of the EMT's job. In this module, students learn how to perform a scene size-up and an initial assessment and how to obtain vital signs and a SAMPLE history. The arrangement of material in this edition makes all the steps of the assessment of trauma and medical patients easier for students to track and comprehend. A separate chapter treats special assessment considerations that arise with geriatric patients. Finally, the skills of communication and documentation are explained and illustrated.

Module 4, Medical Emergencies: Chapters 12–25
The medical emergencies module begins with a chapter on pharmacology in which the medications the EMT can administer or assist with administering under the 1994 curriculum are introduced. The module continues with chapters on respiratory, cardiac, diabetic, seizure, allergy, poisoning and overdose, environmental, behavioral, and obstetric/gynecological emergencies.

Module 5, Trauma: Chapters 26–35
The trauma module begins with a chapter on bleeding and shock, then continues with chapters on soft tissue injuries, burns, musculoskeletal injuries, injuries to the head and spine, and other specific body regions. A chapter on special considerations with agricultural and industrial emergencies is also included.

Module 6, Pediatrics and Geriatrics: Chapters 36-37
This module explores the special aspects of pediatric care by detailing medical conditions and injury patterns that are especially common to or critical for pediatric and geriatric patients.

Module 7, Operations: Chapters 38-42
This module deals with nonmedical operations and special situations, including ambulance operations, access and extrication in motor vehicle collisions, and multiple-casualty and hazardous materials incidents. A new chapter has been added on EMS response to weapons of mass destruction.

Module 8, Advanced Airway Management Elective: Chapter 43
In some states and regions, EMTs will be trained to perform invasive airway management procedures, including orotracheal intubation, and in children, nasogastric intubation. Module 8 is included as an elective to cover these advanced airway management skills.

Appendices
There are two appendices to this program, covering basic life support skills and advanced life support (ALS) assist skills.

INSTRUCTOR RESPONSIBILITIES

Many of us can remember a favorite teacher or instructor. Think back to what made that person special. Chances are, the memorable instructor was a dynamic, knowledgeable person who took the job seriously yet was able to interject a sense of informality and fun that made learning the material easy and enjoyable.

Instructors who fit this description (and who probably became role models for many of their students) didn't get that way by accident. In addition to countless hours behind a desk or podium and in front of a keyboard learning about or presenting information on their chosen subjects, they also worked to develop a solid foundation of knowledge about the needs of student learners.

For the most part, students in EMT courses are adult learners. This is significant because adults learn differently than children do. Adults also have very different needs and motivational factors. Understanding these needs and motivations is the key to being a successful EMT instructor.

So what do adult learners need? Simply put, adult learners want to have a reason for being in the classroom. In other words, when adult learners sit down in the classroom, they expect to find out how the information being presented is pertinent to their needs.

Sometimes, the relevance of the learning is obvious and does not need to be clarified—for example, that direct pressure stops most bleeding. The reasons for learning other things may take more explanation on the part of the instructor—for example, why learning and using correct terminology is important. The relevance of learning to student needs can sometimes be emphasized through textbook case studies or through the relation of personal experiences by the instructor.

This leads to another important aspect of adult learners. They have life experiences that are important to them. The life experiences that adult learners bring to the classroom can be a tremendous motivational tool for the student as well as the instructor. Perhaps a student is taking the EMT course because he or she was first on scene at an accident and felt helpless at being unable to assist the victim. It is easy to see that this student will be highly motivated and will understand the reason for learning the material presented in class.

For another example, a group of students might be in class because they plan to volunteer together with their local ambulance service. Their motivation will likely be quite high. Students such as the ones described above are some of the easiest for an instructor to teach.

Unfortunately, few EMT classes will be so straightforward. EMT classes usually contain a mix of students with a wide variety of motivations and life experiences. Reaching out to and making the class meaningful for such a range of students is a real challenge for the instructor. In order to do so, the instructor must employ a variety of educational techniques. The following sections will be helpful to instructors in making the EMT class a valuable experience.

Basic Course Coordination

The following section may be one of the most important for first-time instructors to read. Experienced instructors may also pick up some tips to help make teaching their EMT courses a little easier.

Teaching an EMT course involves much more than just preparing a lecture and presenting the material in class. Course coordination is the essential framework that holds the class together and can determine how successful the learning experience will be for students.

Depending on where the course is taught, much of the course coordination work may be done for the instructor. For example, an EMT instructor who teaches a program at a community college may have the schedule pre-set, books available at the campus bookstore, and access to audiovisual needs at a moment's notice. Other instructors may be asked to hold classes for a community agency and will be responsible for everything from site selection to equipment rental. Although the amount of work that goes into coordinating the course will vary, there are some basic components of course coordination that should be considered in any setting.

Regulations. The first areas to look at when coordinating an EMT course are state and local regulations. Many states have requirements that must be met before teaching of the course can begin. These requirements can range from applying for course approval to designating a physician sponsor for the course.

One of the easiest ways to get into serious trouble as an instructor is to ignore or not comply with applicable state and local regulations. Take the time to learn which regulations apply to teaching in your specific area.

Schedule. A great deal of time should be invested in developing a course schedule that works for the students as well as for the instructor. An EMT course contains a lot of information. Any course schedule should be paced to allow proper absorption and retention of the material.

Generally, an 8-hour-a-day, 5-day-a-week course for 3 weeks should not be considered. Exceptions can be made when a specific group of students being trained has a demonstrated history of EMS experience, such as a group of First Responders. But most adult learners have other obligations that would not permit them to take such a full-time course.

Many instructors will schedule an EMT class for 3- to 4-hour blocks. These blocks for the most part work well in terms of teaching specific sections or chapters of the text. When scheduling the time for each class session, remember to build in enough time at the beginning of each class to give the quiz or to handle any administrative details.

The suggested amount of time it takes to teach a full EMT course is 110–120 hours. Given the amount of material to be covered, there is little to no extra time in the course. When setting the schedule, pay attention to the suggested teaching time listed in the front of each chapter of this manual.

Facility Selection. Forethought and planning in selecting the site where the course will be taught will save an instructor from approximately 120 hours of headache. A comfortable, complete facility can have a profound effect on the students' ability to learn and on the instructor's ability to present the material. When selecting a facility for the course, a number of factors need to be considered.

The site needs to be large enough to hold the number of students enrolled in the course comfortably. If the space available is limited, it can be maximized through proper arrangement of the tables and chairs or desks. Experiment with various set-ups to find the best placements for the size of the room. Keep in mind that the students need to be able to see the instructor and any audio-visual materials that are used.

The students also need room to move around as well as adequate space to sit comfortably. There also needs to be room for the instructor to move around in the front of the class. Some instructors are roamers and need a lot of space, whereas others are more home oriented and tend to stay at the podium or front table. Evaluate your own style and factor that into the site selection.

Remember also that an EMT class is very much skills oriented. There must be plenty of room to break the students up into small groups to practice skills. A facility with access to more than one classroom is ideal.

An appropriate facility is one that is relatively free from distractions. Trying to hold an entire EMT class in the kitchen of the fire hall will more than likely prove a frustrating experience for the instructor. More importantly, an environment with too many distractions detracts from the learning process for the students.

Make sure the heating and/or ventilation systems for the facility are appropriate and working. If the classroom temperature is too hot or too cold, the students will pay more attention to trying to get comfortable and less attention to the instructor. Also avoid sites where the ventilation system is too noisy.

Other site selection factors to be considered include availability of restrooms, water fountains, and adequate parking for the students.

Course Materials and Resources. Not having required course materials in place for the class reflects poorly on the instructor. Planning far enough in advance can prevent most of the problems related to course materials. Some materials such as textbooks or workbooks can be ordered well ahead of time. Remember that it never hurts to order a few more texts than you think you'll need. It's more expensive to have to order just one or two books at a time.

Access to a copy machine is an absolute necessity. Everything from handouts to quizzes to CPR cards must be copied. It's probably best to do the copying of materials for the course every few class sessions instead of trying to make all of the copies for the entire course in one sitting. Sometimes schedules and topics change slightly, and smaller and more frequent copy jobs will prevent having to re-do a quiz or handout.

Leave yourself plenty of time to do the copying. It's inappropriate to take the first 30 minutes of the class time making copies.

Also, think about materials you'll need for skills demonstrations and practices and for role-playing scenarios. The lesson plans in this manual list the resources you'll need for such activities on the first page of each lesson.

If you are teaching in a dedicated classroom with equipment storage on site, equipment availability is generally not a problem. There may be times, however, when it is necessary to obtain extra pieces of equipment. Reserve such equipment far in advance to keep from being caught short when the equipment is actually needed.

Additional Instructors. There will be times at which another instructor may be invited to class, either to help with skills or to serve as guest lecturer. Guest lecturers can be valuable in several ways. They can give a new slant to required information and provide useful supplementary knowledge. They can spark student interest by providing a break in the routine. They can also give students the opportunity to observe different teaching styles and techniques—something that can be valuable for the regular instructor as well.

When a guest instructor is invited, he or she should be provided with both lesson objectives and a lesson plan. Plan on observing a first-time guest lecturer to get a sense of his or her instructional abilities and success in covering the objectives. Be alert for tendencies to deviate from the topic excessively.

When additional instructors are used for skills practice sessions, a ratio of one instructor for every four to five students is probably most appropriate.

Final Considerations. In terms of coordinating a course, the instructor's best friend and worst enemy is time. If there is enough time, almost anything can be accomplished. If there isn't any time, nothing can be accomplished. The bottom line is that in order to make your course a truly successful one, take care of as many details as far in advance of the course as possible.

PREPARATION FOR STATE AND/OR NATIONAL CERTIFICATION

The successful end of an EMT course will be the completion by students of all requirements for state and/or national certification as EMTs. Instructors should have a very clear understanding of what those requirements are.

There are some other things that can be done to help increase the student's chances of passing the written and practical examinations for certification.

Written Exams

Most of the state certification exams as well as the National Registry written exam use the multiple-choice format. There are definite keys to successfully passing multiple-choice examinations. These are discussed later in the section titled, "Assisting Student Learning."

One of the best ways to prepare students for taking certification exams is to make multiple-choice examinations a part of the course from the very beginning. Doing so will hone students' test-taking skills and will prepare them for the format they are most likely to see. Each chapter in this manual contains a multiple-choice quiz to build student familiarity with the format. In addition, *Prentice Hall Test Manager for Prehospital Emergency Care,* Eighth Edition, allows you to easily prepare multiple-choice tests custom-tailored to your students' needs.

If multiple-choice testing reveals some deficiencies in student understanding of chapter material, you might assign some of the reinforcement handouts available with each lesson. The Chapter Review provides a fill-in-the-blank format, while other handouts offer a variety of approaches for reviewing chapter content.

Practical Exams

Students fear practical examinations from the first day of the EMT course right up through test day. Nothing an instructor can do will completely eliminate this apprehension. The fear is generally of performance, not ability.

One of the best techniques to help relieve some of their anxiety is to have the students practice their skills at every opportunity. This will build their confidence and provide an opportunity for the instructor to stress some of the finer points of the more detailed skills.

It will be helpful to discuss the state and national examination process with the students at the first class session. Allow them to ask questions and give them frank answers.

Instructional media are the tools that can help make lectures more colorful, informative, and interesting. An EMT course will contain over 60 hours of lecture time. Proper use of slides, overheads, videos, and whiteboards will enhance student learning and retention of the material presented.

The instructional media an instructor will use in the classroom will vary with equipment and resource materials available. The instructor's comfort level with a particular medium also affects what resources are used in the classroom. Experimenting with different media is strongly encouraged; this will increase the instructor's familiarity with other media and enlarge the pool of resources he or she is likely to draw on.

Remember also that it is important to not saturate students through overuse of one type of audio-visual material. There may be an entire slide set for the course, but it may not be the soundest educational policy to use nothing but those slides as you teach the course.

Think of audio-visual aids as the spice that enhances the flavor of your lectures. The following tips and techniques will guide you through the audio-visual maze.

POWERPOINT® SLIDES

A set of PowerPoint® slides is available to support *Prehospital Emergency Care,* Eighth Edition, and this Instructor's Resource Manual. The 43 slide presentations follow the chapters of the text.

PowerPoint® slides are a wonderful tool to help teach topics in an EMT course, and there are a number of advantages to using them. First, many are developed specifically for a particular textbook and work extremely well with that text and other ancillary materials associated with it, such as the Instructor's Manual and the Workbook. The slides are consistent with what the student learns in his or her reading. Additionally, the use of such slide programs can decrease preparation time for the instructor.

If an instructor doesn't wish to be completely tied to a slide program prepared by someone else, PowerPoint® allows for easy alteration of slides to personalize programs for lectures; new slides may be added, sequence may be altered, text and pho-

tographs may be changed, deleted, or inserted. This allows the instructor the freedom to include information particularly pertinent to the way he or she teaches the course.

Whether slides used are prepackaged or self-prepared, 35mm or electronic, the medium is one that the students are familiar with. They should feel fairly comfortable with a slide presentation.

Disadvantages in using slides are usually related to equipment problems and a tendency to overuse the medium. In order for the slide presentation to be successful, the projector has to be working, the computer must be capable of showing PowerPoint® slides, and there has to be a screen for showing the slides. Also remember that lighting conditions in the room must be appropriate for the projection of the slides. If there are no shades for the windows and class is held during daylight hours, students may have trouble seeing the images.

Here are some tips for using slides:

- Use slides sparingly.
- Review all slides well in advance.
- Have a backup plan in case of equipment failure.
- Don't use a whiteboard as a screen.

OVERHEAD TRANSPARENCIES

Overhead transparencies are among the most versatile tools instructors can use to present material. They are easy to work with, readily available, and not too expensive. The equipment needed to show overhead transparencies includes an overhead projector, the transparencies, and a surface on which to view the images. The projected images can easily be seen by students even with minimal darkening of the room.

Overhead projectors can be had for as little as $300 and a box of transparencies is in the $20 to $30 range. The transparencies are easy to store, as they are letter size and can go into a topic file with other lesson plan material.

Overheads are available in a wide variety of commercially produced formats that are both colorful and informative. They can be written on with a dry-erase marker and used over and over again. Also, hard copy from almost any source can be made into an overhead by using transparencies that can run through a copier. Some presentation software currently available actually includes formatting for black-and-white overheads. Color overheads can be reproduced at most print shops but at a significant cost.

The disadvantages of overhead transparencies are few. Sometimes transitions between images can be a little awkward. Practice with using overheads will take care of this problem in a short amount of time. Like slide projectors, the overhead projectors can fail. Keeping a spare bulb on hand is recommended.

Here are some other tips and techniques for using overhead transparencies:

- Tape a 3 × 5 index card over the head of the projector. Flip the card down when changing overheads, but remember to flip the card back up afterward.

- Use a progressive disclosure technique. Use a sheet of paper to cover the sections of the overhead that you are not yet speaking about. This stops the students from getting ahead of you in the lecture.

- Commercially produced overheads are available for anatomy topics. They work especially well for those instructors who don't feel comfortable creating their own artwork.

- Use an overlay technique. Laying one overhead on top of another allows you to build on a graphic or a concept.

- Use a simplified version of your lesson outline in overhead format and fill in the appropriate words, phrases, or information as you speak about it. See the Lecture Masters that accompany each chapter of this manual for models.

- Remember to check the focus on the projector occasionally.

VIDEOTAPES

The age of video has not left EMS instruction untouched. The sheer volume and range of subjects available in commercial training tapes today is tremendous. The many timely topics available in the format lend a state-of-the-art feel to the classroom. Also, students are extremely comfortable with the medium, probably more so than with any other.

Videotapes offer vivid, dynamic images and sounds that excite and stimulate most students—and instructors. Real-life footage conveys the nature of EMS work in a way that other audio-visual aids cannot. Videos can be an excellent choice for dramatizing a specific point an instruc-

tor wants to make. Perhaps most important, difficult procedures can be shown on tape over and over until students understand the concept or skill.

The disadvantages of videotape use include heavy reliance on the equipment. The TV has to be operating correctly, as do the VCR and the videotape cassette. If any one component fails, the entire presentation fails. Initial outlay to purchase the equipment can be expensive. Also, in a large class setting it may be difficult to position the video monitor so that all students have a good view of it. Finally, the fact that so many topics are available on tape may tempt instructors to overuse this audio-visual aid in the classroom.

Tips for using videotapes include:

- Always preview the tape for quality and appropriateness of the material.

- Never put in a video and then just leave the classroom. Videos should not be used to "babysit" the students.

- Have a backup plan in case of equipment failure.

- Preset the video for the appropriate starting point before class.

- Use short, pertinent video segments instead of always running entire tapes. The shorter segments can have a more profound impact.

- Be prepared to pause the tape and ask or answer pertinent questions.

- Set up the TV/VCR before class so that you can check to ensure sight and sound quality throughout the room.

Using videotapes in the classroom can add a dynamic boost to your lectures. Sprinkle them liberally throughout the course and watch the impact they have on students.

WHITEBOARDS

This modern-day relative of the chalkboard can be found in nearly every classroom setting. Students expect to see a writing surface of one type or another in a classroom, and the simplicity, spontaneity, and versatility that whiteboards make possible can hardly be matched.

The major limitation on the use of the whiteboard is the instructor's imagination. Even if a lesson plan calls for a class to be lecture based, a particular point that needs to be emphasized or explained can be written on the board. The variety of colors available for use on the whiteboard enlivens presentations. Complicated or detailed drawings or formulas can be written on the board before class, allowing more time for discussion during the lesson. Finally, with no bulbs to burn out or other electronics to fail, whiteboards are extremely reliable.

The disadvantages of whiteboards are relatively few and often instructor related. Poor penmanship on the part of the instructor can leave students frustrated. The dry-erase markers used on whiteboards can dry up, leaving the instructor with few options. In very large classroom settings, it may be difficult for all students to see the board. Lastly, inadvertent use of a permanent marker may ruin a whiteboard.

Here are some tips for using whiteboards:

- Use blue or black for the main color, and use a bright color like red or green to highlight key words or concepts.
- Never use the yellow marker, as yellow will be nearly invisible to most students sitting any distance away.
- Don't talk to the board while you are writing—your listeners are in the seats.
- Draw complex images before the class starts.
- Print legibly.
- Use letters large enough for all to see.
- Do not allow permanent markers in the classroom, especially in the marker tray.
- Watch for spelling and grammatical errors.
- Give students ample time to write material down in their notebooks before erasing it.

Whiteboards are a wonderful visual aid that when used appropriately can make the instructor's job easier, while providing students with a familiar and colorful visual stimulus.

COMPUTERS

Every year that goes by brings us further along the technological highway. In many respects, technology can make the instructor's job much easier. This section focuses on some ways to take advantage of the new technology.

Are Computers Really Necessary?
The answer to this question is an emphatic "Absolutely!" Sometimes it is difficult to imagine how instructors got along before computers. The type, availability, and cost of computers today allow most instructors to have access to this essential tool.

Instructors can use computers in myriad ways. From course recordkeeping to research to lecture preparation, a computer is an instructor's best friend. Computers allow you to manage your time appropriately and free you up to concentrate on important matters. Also, industry software has become much more intuitive and user friendly. This allows first-time users of word processing or database programs to load the software and start working with the programs almost immediately, with very little extra training.

Let's look a little closer at some of the specific areas of EMT instruction that can benefit from the use of a computer.

Course Recordkeeping
Instructors are obligated to keep accurate records of all aspects of the course. These administrative details such as rosters, grades, and attendance are much easier to keep track of when a computer is used. There are programs designed for tracking just these types of training data. Some of this specialty software is extremely expensive, so consider instead purchasing a simple word processing and database program. With a little time, practice, and patience you can use such a program to develop forms and databases that can be adapted to every course that you teach.

Using a computer for course recordkeeping provides greater accuracy and consistency. In addition, once the initial work is completed, it is relatively easy to update the data or forms that you use most.

Use of the computer can also aid your professional image. Producing consistent, accurate, and professional-looking records enhances your credibility as an instructor.

Research
The computer's use as a research tool has been well documented. If you have a computer with a modem and access to the Internet, you have access to millions of computers around the world. In addition to the obvious volumes of material that are available through the Internet, the computer can put you in touch with thousands of instructors who have many of the same questions and concerns that you do. More importantly, they may have answers to many of the questions and problems that you are facing in your class. A list of EMS Websites and other Internet resources can be found below in Resources for the Instructor.

A computer allows you to research topics and gain more insight into a given subject area. You may also find the answer to that stumper question that a student asked in the last class session. Either way, a computer allows an EMT instructor to remain current on the latest trends and controversies in the ever-changing world of EMS.

Lecture Preparation

This is an area that will be one of the most helpful to instructors. Preparing lectures on a computer has several distinct advantages over handwriting your lesson plans or typing them out on a standard typewriter. Lectures developed and printed with a word processor are generally neater and easier to interpret. This could be of value if guest lecturers or substitute instructors come in to teach.

Most word processors also have templates or they allow you to develop your own. Using such templates permits you to apply a consistent format in the preparation of your lectures; this can help you become more alert to the organization and structure of your lectures. Templates may also allow you to create an outline of a lecture to give to your students for note-taking purposes.

Having the lectures for an EMT class stashed on your hard drive also makes updating any information a doable task, one that doesn't require the scrapping of an entire set of lecture notes.

One of the most exciting reasons for developing your lectures on a computer is the presentation software currently available. Presentation software such as Microsoft PowerPoint® allows a degree of versatility and creativity that is not feasible with written lesson plans.

Presentation software allows you to put together dynamic lectures using a variety of type fonts and graphic designs. These programs also allow you to insert clip art images, which can be used to illustrate a point or just make a presentation more interesting. Lectures that are developed for multimedia presentations can also include everything from sound bites to video clips. Finally, presentation software lets the instructor print the lecture in a number of formats including slides, overhead transparencies, and lecture notes.

What Kind of Computer Do You Need?

Selecting a computer is a very personal decision. Friends, family, and coworkers are generally eager to give their recommendations, but the best advice is to research the choices based on how much you can afford to pay.

The good news is that a vast majority of the work that you do with a computer can be accomplished with a simple model that has a word processing program. New computers can be purchased in most parts of the country for around $1,000 and usually include most applicable software and other necessary components.

Instructors in it for the long haul will probably benefit most by purchasing a computer that not only meets their needs of today but also will be adaptable to their needs of tomorrow.

Improvements and enhancements to computer processors, operating systems, features, peripherals, and software are introduced at a rapid rate. There are always new bells and whistles that can add to the functions—and the price—of a computer. You should consult with a technology specialist at an office supply or electronics retailer to find the hardware and software that best meet your needs.

A good computer system is an invaluable tool for the EMS instructor. Whether you use Power-Point® presentations, websites and Internet video clips, or interative computer programs, the variety of materials available will help enrich your students' learning experience.

Multimedia and the Classroom

The most intriguing option in the world of high-tech training today is the use of multimedia presentations in the classroom. Multimedia presentations involve the use of a special projector and a computer with presentation software when delivering a lecture. These presentations are impressive in their complexity and dynamics. More importantly, they seem to help students better retain information from the lecture.

When this technology first became available, its was seen largely at national or regional conferences and in large corporate training facilities. This was mainly due to the extremely high cost of the equipment—above $10,000 for even the most basic models. Prices have fallen significantly, and this technology is now becoming more prominent in classroom settings across the country. As an EMT instructor, you will have access to this excellent teaching tool more and more often in classrooms. For those who are freelance instructors, the cost reductions may enable you to add this useful tool to your store of audio-visual aids.

Today, it is not unusual to find multimedia projectors for under $1,500. While such prices are still high for many, they represent an investment that will pay off handsomely. Use of such equipment in your presentations will add luster to your professional image. In addition, once the presentation has been developed, it can be used again for other classes.

Students, too, can benefit from multimedia presentations in the classroom. The dynamic "nearly video" format piques their interest and holds their attention for longer periods of time. This results in greater retention of the material presented. Multimedia presentations allow for progressive disclosure techniques. The medium is limited only by the instructor's imagination.

One disadvantage of this type of presentation is that it is absolutely equipment dependent. If the projector or the computer fails, the entire lecture fails. The instructor planning a multimedia presentation should always have a back-up plan in place.

Multimedia presentations are a tool that instructors should consider incorporating into their classrooms. As prices continue to drop and as instructors become more comfortable with the hardware and software, this medium will take hold of people and quite possibly change the way EMT instructors teach their classes.

SKILL INSTRUCTION

The work that EMTs do is very skills oriented. These skills are based upon a sound foundation of knowledge and the understanding of when and how to apply that knowledge in appropriate settings. At least 50 percent of the EMT course will be spent teaching, demonstrating, and performing skills. The time, effort, and energy you put into the teaching of skills in the classroom will directly affect the future success of your students as competent EMTs.

There are many ways of teaching the necessary skills in an EMT class. No one way is correct for all instructors at all times. The appropriateness of methods used will depend on factors such as the number of students in the class, their motivations for being in the class, and the individual differences among students in a particular class.

To be most effective at teaching skills in an EMT class, instructors must be competent in and fully aware of the skills criteria used locally. Some states or localities use a packet of skill sheets containing separate skill sheets for each discrete skill. Other areas may use the skill sheets developed by the National Registry of EMTs. Still other areas use both. Take the time to review and study such materials prior to the start of the course and before each class session in which skills will be taught.

SKILL DEMONSTRATIONS

Demonstrating a skill for EMT students can be one of the most difficult and challenging responsibilities for an instructor. The pressure to perform is enormous because so much is riding on the outcome. Even an instructor who is very comfortable with his or her EMT skills may suffer from intimidation or performance anxiety.

The first time a skill is demonstrated for the students is critical to the student's performance of that skill in the future. The first time most students see a skill performed leaves a strong impression; if a part of the skill was demonstrated incorrectly, the students are likely to repeat the mistake. It is easy to see why this first demonstration of a skill is so crucial and why it can produce anxiety for the instructor.

There are things that you as an instructor can do to help alleviate this anxiety. First and fore-most, have faith in your ability. Many instructors have been EMTs for years and have the background and experience to support their textbook knowledge. Also, EMT instructors are EMTs who have been through the class before and, in many cases, have helped with skills training even before becoming instructors themselves. Have the confidence to realize that you know the skills and are more than capable of presenting them to the class.

It may be helpful to practice certain skills prior to the class session. Review the materials found in the textbook as well as the instructor manual.

You might also consider videotaping a demonstration of the skill before the class. This allows for greater control of any possible mistakes; the taped demonstration can also then be used with other classes.

The disadvantage to videotaping is that, if the production quality is poor, it can distract students who will pay more attention to inadequacies of the lighting, script, or sound than the skill being demonstrated. Also, remember that the best way to become comfortable with demonstrating skills in front of the class is demonstrating skills. As with public speaking, the only thing that makes it any easier is doing it often.

When demonstrating a skill to your students, remember that as adult learners they bring a multitude of life experiences with them. They may also have some experience with a particular skill and may offer comments, feedback, or suggestions. Do not discount such input. Instructors have a tendency to teach something the way they themselves were taught and too often fail to keep an open mind to other ways a skill might be performed or taught. The most important thing to remember is that different is not necessarily wrong. The best instructors are flexible and adapt to new information or circumstances and to the needs of their students.

SCENARIOS FOR LEARNING

One of the best ways for instructors to integrate cognitive knowledge with practical skills is through the use of scenarios. Throughout this Instructor's Resource Manual, there are a wide variety of scenarios pertinent to the chapters.

Scenarios are beneficial to the students in a number of ways. They can add a sense of realism to the course. They also can give students a hint of the pressures they will face in the real world. Scenarios promote interaction among the students and can go far in terms of enhancing student bonding and camaraderie. Student performance in the scenarios will provide instructors with an opportunity to evaluate how well the students have grasped both the skill and the ideas in the textbook that are behind it.

There are some basic points that instructors should keep in mind when running patient care scenarios in the classroom setting:

- The scenario has to be doable. Giving students impossible scenarios sets them up for failure and can destroy their confidence.

- The scenario has to be winnable. A winnable scenario is one in which students have the opportunity to see an improvement in patient outcome based on their care.

- Keep the scenario simple. The "bus load of hypochondriacs that goes off the cliff into a toxic waste dump" scenario may be fun, but it's complicated, uses up too much precious time, and probably involves so many considerations that students actually learn very little.

- Start using scenarios early in the course. Even on the first night of class, an appropriate scenario can be run. Consider a simple CPR call or a call for choking.

- Use scenarios often. Many instructors will use a scenario in every class session.

Like most things, scenarios work most effectively and smoothly when you take the time to plan them out in advance. There are detailed instructions for scenarios in this manual that make such planning easier. There are also collections of ready-to-go scenarios available from publishers.

Your own experiences as an EMT, however, may make the best, most effective scenarios for your class. There are many benefits to using personal experiences as a basis for scenarios. Real calls that you have been on have a different flavor from generic scripts borrowed from books. This heightens the sense of their realism. In addition, after the students have played out the scenario, you can tell them what actually happened and compare notes. By objectively evaluating your responses to the call with the students, you can demonstrate to them that there is no such thing as a "perfect" call. This will help remind them that there is always room for improvement, even for the instructor.

One key to running successful scenarios is the use of an appropriate evaluation tool. A proper evaluation tool need not be fancy—in fact, the simpler the better. An evaluation tool can consist of nothing more than a sheet of paper containing appropriate information about the call and room to write notes and comments about student performance. The evaluation tool can even be incorporated into the scenario planning sheet.

When developing your own classroom scenarios, always use a scenario planning sheet. A well-prepared planning sheet should ensure similar learning outcomes for students even if other instructors use the sheet to run the scenario. The planning sheet should contain the following:

- Description of the call
- Environmental factors that might affect the call
- Pertinent findings in the scene size-up, initial assessment, focused history and physical exam, and baseline and follow-up vital signs
- An area for information about such things as interventions performed and time they were done
- A list of the objectives for the call—what you are trying to teach the students with this scenario
- A list of equipment needed to run the call
- Moulage instructions if pertinent
- Instructions to the "patient"
- A space for any additional comments in which you can evaluate student performance (Leaving enough space to write comments probably works better than trying to develop a complicated checklist of things the students should have done in the scenario.)

One of the easiest ways to incorporate scenarios into the classroom is to pair the students up into responder teams and place a different team on call for each class session. This gives the students both a feel for what it's like to be on duty and an opportunity to apply their skills in a fairly realistic setting. The on-call crew should check at the beginning of the class to ensure that the jump kits to be used are complete and operational. It's also a good idea to assign a second crew as backup in case the first crew needs additional help.

There are many ways to make scenarios an everyday part of the class. Evaluate the characteristics of your facility and your students to determine the best way to use scenarios in your classes.

MAKING IT REAL—MOULAGE TIPS

In the earlier section on using scenarios, moulage was mentioned. Moulage is the application of materials to a volunteer "patient" to simulate injuries and other significant clinical signs. EMS instructors have used moulage techniques for years to enhance the realism of scenarios for their students. A well-done job of moulage creates an impressively real patient, while a poorly handled job detracts from the scenario and from student learning.

The application of makeup and other objects to simulate injuries has long been a staple in Hollywood films. However, EMT instructors do not need access to the movie industry's makeup artists to learn to create effects that are believable and accurate in "patients." Some great moulage techniques can be achieved with minimal amounts of material and training. Contrary to what some may think, applying good moulage does not have to be a time-consuming ordeal. The benefit of moulage is lost if it takes an hour to apply the makeup.

Basic Moulage Techniques

Injuries are not perfect, so it's difficult to make a "bad" injury. Here are some basic rules that will allow the instructor to create realistic injuries and skin signs simply:

- First and foremost, remember that "less is more." A light application of whites, blues, and grays will have a more profound impact than a heavily applied layer of clown white when simulating paleness or cyanosis.

- Simplicity is the key in creating realistic "injuries" in a short period of time. Most injuries can be simulated with a few commonly available items. A basic list of supplies for moulage can be found below.

- Always apply a light application of cold cream under any injuries or skin signs that you apply. Cold cream helps the makeup stay on the skin and makes the removal of the makeup much easier for the "patient."

- Accuracy is important in creating believable injuries. Placing a giant bruise over the entire area of the chest to simulate a pneumothorax probably does more to detract from the scenario than illustrate it.

- To simulate cyanosis, try a light application of blue to the nail beds, ear lobes, and around the lips after applying a basic underlay of white or light gray.

- Use a mixture of water with a small amount of glycerin to simulate diaphoresis. Keep the mixture in a small spray bottle and apply immediately prior to the arrival of the "rescuers."

- To simulate burns, apply a layer of cold cream followed by a base coat of red to the entire area. Lay some tissue over the area and then apply some water-soluble lubricant such as K-Y® jelly over the tissue. Gently break the tissue by rolling it from the center of the "burned" area towards the edges. This will create a remarkably realistic looking second-degree burn.

- Use activated charcoal applied with a cotton swab around the edges of the nares and the mouth and tongue to simulate a respiratory burn.

- Place a small amount of effervescent tablet in a simulated chest wound. Just prior to "rescuer" arrival, place a few drops of water on the tablet to help simulate a sucking chest wound. The bubbling action is usually quite impressive.

- Whenever there is a chance that the "patient" may "bleed" or "ooze," be sure to place a tarp under the patient to avoid staining the carpet or flooring underneath the patient.

The best way to become comfortable with moulage is to use it often. Experiment with different materials and household items. Remember that because real injuries are not perfect, it's difficult to go wrong.

Resources for Moulage

Putting together a useful moulage kit does not have to be expensive or complicated. One of the biggest decisions to make is whether to build your own kit or purchase one of the commercially available injury simulation kits. There are advantages and disadvantages to each approach.

Commercially available kits usually contain a variety of fake injuries made from rubber or plastic that can be either strapped on or held in place by spirit gum. They also contain a variety of colored makeup. The advantage to this type of moulage kit is its completeness.

The biggest drawback to such kits is the price. Some of the more elaborate kits can cost hundreds of dollars. Also, many of the injuries included are not very realistic, and the time that it takes an instructor to develop a level of expertise using the kits may be unreasonable for most EMT instructors.

Another drawback is that using a single source for moulage materials and techniques limits the development of the instructor's skill in using moulage as a resource. An instructor forced by circumstances to use a kit other than his or her own may have difficulty using moulage patients.

An alternative to purchasing a ready-made kit is putting together a kit of your own. Most of the materials are inexpensive, and this will also give you the flexibility to be creative. Experiment with different items and find the things that work the best for you. Some items that such a kit might contain include the following:

- Cold cream—for applying under makeup
- Plumber's putty—to use as a modeling clay when building injuries
- Eye shadow—a variety of shades of eye shadow to simulate cyanosis and bruises
- Dirt—A container of dirt is handy to help make realistic road rashes and other injuries.
- Halloween makeup—Search the costume aisles of your local store in October. A wide variety of makeup colors and simulated injuries are available. Hint: Shop the day after Halloween to get bargain prices.

- Chicken bones—for use in the simulation of open fractures. Place them in a bag and lightly crush them to obtain realistic bone fragments.
- Clear plastic cups—crushed, they provide pieces of very good looking "glass" for use in an injury
- Fake blood—one of those items that can be purchased commercially. Many instructors have also come up with their own recipes that work well. Try to avoid any red dyes that stain too easily.
- Knife handles—Use just the handle of a knife and build putty around the knife end to simulate an impaled object.
- Effervescent tablets—to help simulate chest wounds
- Condoms—filled with a little water or K-Y jelly for creating simulated evisceration
- Brushes—variety of makeup brushes for applying colors for cyanosis and bruising
- Activated charcoal—for burn moulage

The type and amount of information covered in EMT classes can be overwhelming for students if they are not prepared to study effectively. Unfortunately, many adult learners lack the tools and background for efficient study. For a large percentage of your students, the EMT class represents a first return to the classroom in many years. Much has changed since they were in school, and tools and resources taken for granted today were often unavailable then and are thus unfamiliar to these students. Anything that you can do as an instructor to help such students study more effectively is an investment that will pay off handsomely for both the students, in terms of their future employment prospects, and for your EMS system, in terms of better-trained, more capable EMTs.

It would be extremely difficult for most EMT students to make it through the course without spending a substantial amount of time in study outside the classroom. It is not unusual for students to spend three to four hours outside the class for each class hour. To help students get the most from their study time, you might consider suggesting some of the following strategies for success that have worked for others in the past:

- Encourage the formation of study groups. Students in a study group can benefit from each other. Often a member of the study group can explain a concept in a way that allows another student to understand something that wasn't grasped in class. One problem with study groups, however, is that if students misunderstand something, the misinformation will be more widely circulated. If your students do form study groups, pay attention to what your evaluation tools reveal about student understanding of key concepts and ideas.
- Use the student workbooks that accompany textbook. Workbooks include many different types of activities that will reinforce what students have read in the text.
- Use computer resources if available. There are some excellent computer programs that can enhance student understanding of key ideas, things like test banks for reviewing course knowledge or anatomy models for illustrating how the body works. If a classroom computer is available, consider purchasing one or more

of these programs for student use at appropriate times.

- Make yourself available for questions before and after class as well as during breaks. Some students are shy about classroom participation and will hesitate to bring up what they may see as "silly" questions.
- Pace yourself when delivering lectures. Give students enough time to write their notes. When pencils stop moving, then pick up the topic and carry on with the lecture.
- Give students outlines of your lecture with plenty of spaces for them to write notes. Most of today's computer presentation software can generate such simplified outlines from the more detailed lecture preparations.
- Finally, encourage the students to balance study, work, and play in their lives. Retention of course material will be enhanced if students are relatively relaxed and not overloading any one area of their lives.

By applying some or all of the ideas above, you really can help students with their studies. Remember that instructors are responsible not just for lecturing and teaching skills but also for doing what it takes—within reason—to help students through the course.

See pages xxvii–xxx for "Advice to Students." These pages, which can be copied and distributed to students, contain ideas that will help students organize their study with the goal of preparing for their written and practical examinations.

INSTRUCTING STUDENTS WITH LEARNING DISABILITIES

Each adult learner who enrolls in an EMS course possesses a unique personality and a unique ability to learn. Factors such as learning ability and style, preexisting knowledge, life experience, and motivation will contribute to the level of achievement of each student. Very few, if any, adult education classes will contain a truly homogeneous group of students. Competent educators realize this and use the strengths of each learner to achieve the desired educational outcomes. As a result, instructors have a responsibility to identify students who may be deficient in learning skills and to provide appropriate remediation and support.

Learning disabilities do not mean a lack of intelligence. Many famous people have overcome learning disabilities to contribute their talents to all walks of life—Albert Einstein, Winston Churchill, Cher, Walt Disney, Whoopi Goldberg, Bruce Jenner, Woodrow Wilson, just to name a few. Although not all people with learning disabilities will achieve success, even in modest terms, many can complete training programs in a wide variety of fields such as EMS. The message is this: Students with learning disabilities of any age *can* learn.

In recent decades, state and federal governments have extended protection to learning disabled students through a wide variety of court decisions and laws such as the Americans With Disabilities Act (ADA) of 1990. Today educational institutions must have operational plans aimed at identifying and assisting learning disabled students. Adult learners who have benefited from these programs in their primary and secondary educations are aware of these laws and are entering EMS programs in greater numbers than in the past. They will request—and rightly so—the educational accommodations and compensatory mechanism that have helped them achieve prior learning success. EMS educators, therefore, will be asked to develop a wide variety of instructional strategies—diverse methods of presentation that will not only enrich the educational experience of learning disabled students, but of all the students in the class.

Of the many types of learning disabilities, the ones that an EMS instructor can expect to encounter most frequently are "academic skills disorders." Of particular concern are developmental reading disorders, such as dyslexia. It may be necessary for a reading impaired student to go over a paragraph many times to reach an understanding. The assignment of a complex chapter on anatomy, for example, can seem like an impossible task.

If a student with a reading disorder (or any other learning disability) appears in an EMT-B class, an instructor has a legal and/or ethical responsibility to seek appropriate remediation. For example, assistance for a dyslexic student may include referral to a reading skills program or to a service that provides "audio books." In most cases, however, moderate assistance on the part of the instructor can help adult learners deficient in one or more skills—especially if they have received remediation during their earlier education.

In deciding upon a course of action for learning disabled students, an EMS educator must be careful not to confuse the educational process with certification. The educational component is designed to facilitate the acquisition of cognitive knowledge and psychomotor skills necessary to obtain a certificate or license to practice EMS. Although many EMS educational institutions work closely with the entities that certify and license EMS providers, the two processes—education and certification—must remain separate. the EMS educator's only concern should be that of preparing the student for the credentialization process. In the case of the learning disabled students, the educator should focus on strategies that will help each student accomplish the instructional objectives, while providing "reasonable" remediation and compensation measures.

Point out this distinction to learning disabled students. It would not be ethical to have learning disabled students—or any other students for that matter—assume the completion of an EMT-B course assures success in the certification or licensure process. As a result, an EMS educator should urge learning disabled students to initiate early contact with the certifying or licensing agency to determine what accommodations will be accepted or made for them.

All EMS instructors in the 21st century should investigate the programs, laws, and regulations related to learning disabilities specified by local, state, and federal governments. Some sources of information are listed in "Resources for the EMT Instructor at the end of the introductory material. Most important, keep in mind that the majority of learning disabled adults function as normal, productive members of society. They aspire to the same educational goals as people without learning disabilities—and, in many cases, with a higher motivation. Far too often, however, they become frustrated by an inability to learn using the same method or at the same rate as other students.

An astute EMS educator must seek to create new opportunities for the learning disabled students. One of the best resources is a caring educator willing to take the time to recognize learning disabilities and then to provide the additional assistance—videos, audiotapes, and teamwork with other students—that can mean the difference between success and failure.

There are probably as many motivations for being an EMT instructor as there are EMT instructors. Many instructors feel a sense of obligation to contribute something to their EMS service. Some instructors end up teaching almost by accident and then find that they really enjoy it and would prefer to do more of it. Some instructors are almost forced into the role because of their job descriptions or other factors.

Regardless of the motivation, the job of EMS instructor is a demanding one that creates unique stresses. Teaching an EMT class is a tremendous amount of work. The amount of time and energy that goes into preparing even a single class session may be lost on the students or others who are not in a teaching role. This can cause stress for instructors. Teaching is also stressful because there is so much riding on how well the instructor conveys information to the students. In addition, students often directly reflect the instructor's approaches and ideas about EMS; living up to this role model image can be difficult at times for instructors.

To succeed as an EMT instructor, you must be aware of the things that cause stress in your day-to-day activities. Awareness of the issues generally makes them easier to deal with. Focus on the rewards of teaching EMTs. The good points of teaching far outweigh the bad and with the proper perspective, an EMT instructor can look forward to many years of passing his or her knowledge on to fellow EMS providers.

Here are some other ideas to increase your longevity as an instructor:

- Strive for balance in your life. Most of us lead busy lives. The dedication that so many people in EMS have often leads them to place work ahead of their personal lives. Make time to do the things that you find personally rewarding every day. All work and no play is unhealthy and will greatly decrease your effectiveness as an instructor.

- Avoid doing all of the prep work for a course at the last minute. While most of us work well under pressure, we shouldn't work under pressure when we don't have to. Remember that time is your best friend.

- Sometimes you have to learn to "just say no." Good instructors will be asked to teach frequently. Most of us love to teach, and it may be difficult to turn down an opportunity. But if teaching that extra class means ignoring your personal needs and relationships, pass up the chance. There will always be other opportunities.

- Make the time to exercise a little before each class session. Even a brisk walk around the parking lot will help to clear your mind and allow you to focus on the task at hand.

- Get plenty of rest. This is for the students' benefit as well as your own. Exhaustion is reflected in lectures and your overall demeanor.

- Don't be afraid to ask for help. There will be times when you are psychologically just not able to face going to class. When this happens, rely on another instructor whom you trust and who understands what it means to need a break. You and your students will be glad you did.

- Understand that flexibility is one of the keys to success as an EMT instructor. Keeping your mind open to new ideas and new ways of doing things will benefit both you and your students in the long run.

- Teaching EMTs is serious business, but that doesn't mean there's no room for fun. Try using some learning games in the classroom. Make the learning experience an enjoyable one for the students and your teaching experience will be enjoyable as well.

INSTRUCTOR RESOURCES

Below are lists of various types of resources that instructors might find valuable. The lists are not all inclusive, and instructors should add to them and create a file that suits their needs. Although all information has been checked and is current at time of publication, contact and website information may change.

PROFESSIONAL ORGANIZATIONS

NOTE: Access to some areas of organizational websites may be limited to members only.

American Ambulance Association
1255 Twenty-Third Street
Washington, D.C. 20037-1174
202-452-8888
www.the-aaa.org

American College of Emergency Physicians
P.O. Box 619911
Dallas, TX 75261-9911
800-798-1822
www.acep.org

American Heart Association
7272 Greenville Ave.
Dallas, TX 75231
800-242-8721
www.americanheart.org

Association of Air Medical Services
526 King Street, Suite 415
Alexandria, VA 22314-3143
703-836-8732
www.aams.org

Citizen CPR Foundation
PO Box 15945-314
Lenexa, KS 66285-5945
913-495-9816
www.citizencpr.com

Emergency Nurses Association
915 Lee Street
Des Plaines, IL 60016-6569
800-900-9659
www.ena.org

National Association of EMS Educators
Foster Plaza 6
681 Andersen Drive
Pittsburgh, PA 15220-2766
412-920-4775
www.naemse.org

National Association of EMS Physicians
P.O. Box 15945-281
Lenexa, KS 66285-5945
800-228-3677
www.naemsp.org

National Association of EMTs
PO Box 1400
Clinton, MS 39060-1400
800-34-NAEMT
www.naemt.org

National Association for Search and Rescue
4500 Southgate Place, Suite 100
Chantilly, VA 20151-1714
703-222-6277
www.nasar.org

National Association of State EMS Directors
111 Park Place
Falls Church, VA 22046-4513
703-538-1799
www.nasemsd.org

National Council of State EMS Training Coordinators
201 Park Washington Court
Falls Church, VA 22046-4513
703-538-1794
www.ncsemstc.org

National Emergency Medical Services Alliance
1947 Camino Vida Roble
Carlsbad, CA 92008
619-431-7054

National Registry of EMTs
6610 Busch Blvd.
P.O. Box 29233
Columbus, OH 43229
614-888-4484
www.nremt.org

EMS WEBSITES

One of the big advantages of owning a computer today is the availability of information through the Internet. To steer a course through this electronic maze, we've compiled a list of websites at which instructors can find information they can use in developing lectures or enhancing student knowledge of emergency medicine. These sites have the potential to provide access to a whole new realm of information and entertainment for you and your students.

Each of these EMS websites has been visited and reviewed for appropriateness and content. Remember to bookmark the sites for easy access to them the next time you are surfing.

News Groups

emsvillage.com

prehospitalperspective.net

These news groups are excellent places to learn about the latest trends in EMS. They also offer the opportunity to ask questions and gain insights into what other EMS providers across the country are doing.

In addition, many EMS organizations support list servers where members can ask questions and interact with other EMS professionals.

Websites

www.bennye.com

Make up and kits for applying moulage

www.bradybooks.com

The home page of the publisher of *Prehospital Emergency Care.*

www.cdc.gov

The home page for the Centers for Disease Control and Prevention. An excellent source of information on infectious diseases.

www.cpem.org

Teaching resource for instructors in prehospital pediatrics.

www.fire-ems.net

The fire and EMS information network. A site that features everything from chat areas to web site development for fire and EMS services.

www.jems.com/

JEMS online. *The Journal of Emergency Medical Services* home page.

www.LessStress.com

This site contains a prehospital care simulator.

www.lifeart.com

A source for medical clip art that can be useful for overheads and handouts.

www.merck.com

The famous Merck manual on-line.

www.ncemsf.org/

The National EMS Collegiate Foundation. This home page contains information about EMS educational programs around the country.

www.nhtsa.dot.gov/portal/site/nhtsa/menuitem

The home page for the National Highway Traffic Safety Administration. Download curricula for all of the EMT levels.

www.osha.gov

The home page for the Occupational Safety and Health Administration. Information from ergonomics to OSHA documents.

www.pcrf.mednet.ucla.edu/

The Prehospital Care Research Forum is dedicated to the promotion, education, and dissemination of prehospital research.

www.shrs.pitt.edu/emergency/index.html

The Center for Emergency Medicine's site with information about the revision of the EMT-Intermediate and EMT-Paramedic Curricula.

www.ptialaska.net/~bearmt/

Information on an inexpensive AED Trainer.

www.trauma.org/prehospital/ph-images.html

Prehospital images of accident scenes and the like.

Books

Brown, C. *Square Pegs and Round Holes.* Lake Worth, FL: EES Publications, 1990.

An easy-to-use text designed specifically for EMS instructors. Not quite as meaty as the McClincy text listed below, but it still contains some good information.

Hoff, R. *I Can See You Naked.* Kansas City, MO: Andrews and McMeel, 1992.

Once you get past the title, you will find a text that contains pertinent information on public speaking.

Martini, F.H., Bartholomew, E.F., and Bledsoe, B.E., *Anatomy and Physiology for Emergency Care,.* 2nd ed. Upper Saddle River, NJ: Brady-Prentice Hall, 2006

Anatomy and physiology text for students in emergency care and allied health programs requiring an overview of the human body's systems.

McClincy, W. *Instructional Methods in Emergency Services*. 2nd ed. Upper Saddle River, NJ: Brady-Prentice Hall, 2002

This text is the most comprehensive manual to date on methods of instruction for EMS personnel. Experienced and new instructors alike will find this book to be a valuable source of information.

Oosterhof, A. *Classroom Applications of Educational Measurement*. Columbus, OH: Merrill, 2000.

This text is directed towards theory and makes a nice addition to the libraries of those instructors who want more information on evaluation tools.

Simmons, S. *How to Be the Life of the Podium*. New York: AMACOM, 1993.

This book contains quips, quotes, and stories that can be used to spice up almost any presentation.

U.S. Department of Transportation. *Paramedic and EMT-Intermediate National Standard Curricula*. Washington, D.C.: GPO, 1999.

Journals
ACLS Alert
3525 Piedmont Rd. NE
Six Piedmont Center
Suite 400
Atlanta, GA 30305

Annals of Emergency Medicine
P.O. Box 619911
Dallas, TX 75261

EMS Insider
Jems Communications
1947 Camino Vida Roble
Carlsbad, CA 92008
619-431-9797

Emergency
6200 Yarrow Drive
P.O. Box 159
Carlsbad, CA 92008
1-800-854-6449

Emergency Medical Services
Creative Age Publications
7628 Densmore Ave.
Van Nuys, CA 91406
818-782-7328

Emergency Training
Miller Landing
Building 200
150 N. Miller Road
Akron, OH 44333
216-836-0600

Journal of Emergency Medical Services
P.O. Box 370
Escondido, CA 92033
1-800-334-8152

Journal of Emergency Medicine
Pergamon Press
660 White Plains Road
Tarrytown, NY 10591

911 Magazine
18201 Weston Pl.
Tustin, CA 92680
714-544-7776

Prehospital Emergency Care
Hanley & Belfus, Inc., Medical Publishers
210 South 13th Street
Philadelphia, PA 19107
800-962-1892
215-546-7293
Fax 215-790-9330
www.hanleybelfus.com

Rescue
Jems Communications
P.O. Box 370
Escondido, CA 92033
1-800-334-8152

Topics in Emergency Medicine
200 Orchard Ridge Dr.
Gaithersburg, MD 2087
1-800-638-8437

Video Producers
Pulse/Emergency Medical Update
P.O. Box 11380
Winslow, WA 98110
1-800-327-3841

For Students with Learning Disabilities

This partial listing has been compiled from sources available at the time of the publication of the Instructor's Resource Manual. Changes in laws, regulations, and/or technology may have an affect on the resources available in the future.

Alliance for Technology Access (ATA)
2175 East Francisco Blvd., Suite L
San Rafael, CA 94901
415-455-4575
FAX: 415-455-0491
www.atacess.org
   Provides access to supportive technology for people with disabilities.

Association on Higher Education and Disability (AHEAD)
P.O. Box 21192
Columbus, OH 43221
614-488-4972
FAX: 614-488-1174
www.ahead.org
   Provides information about full participation in higher education for people with disabilities.

Council for Learning Disabilities (CLD)
P.O. Box 40303
Overland Park, KS 66204
913-492-8755
FAX: 913-942-2546
www.cldinternational.org
   Offers enhancement for the education and development of the learning disabled.

Division of Adult Education and Literacy
Clearinghouse
U.S. Department of Education
Office of Vocational and Adult Education
400 Maryland Avenue, SW
Washington, DC 20202
202-205-9996
FAX: 202-205-8873
www.ed.gov
   Links the adult education community with existing resources in adult education available through the Adults in Education Act.

HEATH Resource Center
National Clearinghouse on Postsecondary Education for Individuals with Disabilities
American Council on Education
One Dupont Circle, NW, Suite 800
Washington, DC 20036
202-939-9320
FAX: 202-833-4760
www.ACENET.edu

Collects and disseminates information about postsecondary education for individuals with disabilities.

National Association for Adults With Special Learning Needs (NAASLN)
P.O. Box 716
Bryn Mawr, PA 19010
610-525-8336
FAX: 610-525-8337
www.naasln.org/
   Provides information for helping adults with special learning needs.

National Center for Learning Disabilities (NCDL)
381 Park Avenue South, Suite 1420
New York, NY 10016
212-545-7510
FAX: 212-545-9665
www.ncld.org
   Provides programs and services to promote a better understanding and acceptance of learning disabilities.

Rebus Institute
1499 Bayshore Blvd., Suite 146
Burlingame, CA 94010
415-697-7424
FAX: 415-697-3734
   Disseminates information on adult issues related to specific learning disabilities and Adult Attention Deficit Disorders (AADD)

Recording for the Blind and Dyslexic (RFBD)
20 Roszel Road
Princeton, NY 20542
609-452-0606
800-221-4792
www.rfbd.org
   Offers free recordings and speech software versions of books for the blind and dyslexic.

U.S. Department of Education
National Library of Education
Office of Educational Resource and Improvement
Institute of Education Sciences
455 New Jersey Ave., NW
Washington, DC 20208
202-219-2221
www.ed.gov
   Houses the Educational Resources Information Center (ERIC)—the source of a wide variety of educational literature and resources.

ADVICE TO STUDENTS

The following pages contain ideas that will help students organize their study with the goal of preparing for their written and practical examinations.

TAKING WRITTEN EXAMINATIONS

Passing a written examination is a matter of choices made. To have the absolute best chance of making the right choices, you have to have a plan. Having a plan for taking the test can significantly decrease anxiety. A plan will help reinforce good test-taking habits so that testing skills and scores improve with each exam. The plan also should be in place well before the day of the examination and cover what needs to be done before, during, and after the test.

Before the Examination
This period is the main focus of your plan. How you prepare for the exam is at least as important as taking the exam. You should start preparing for the exam on the first day of class.

Take clear, concise notes during each lecture. Keep your notes, any handouts, and any reference materials organized and easily accessible. For your notes to be meaningful, they must be organized. If they are easily accessible, you will be more inclined to study them.

Your notes are a record of the important issues that have been emphasized in classroom discussions. Use them for study, to jog your memory, and as flash cards.

Transferring your notes to audiotape is a good idea. Reading them onto the tape will reinforce the material in your memory. The completed tape will then give you another study method that you can use while commuting, exercising, or relaxing.

Flash cards can be a helpful tool. They aid in the retention of material through repetition. Write questions or terms on the front of a card and your answers or definitions on the back. For each subject, prepare a separate pile of cards. The cards will be easier to manage, and you can use specific sets to study any weak areas. Flash cards can be used in a group or on your own. They are a great way to get a spouse or significant other involved in your learning.

Consider spending time each day to review the highlights from class lessons. This will keep you on top of the material. Reviewing material on a daily basis can help to relieve some of the pressure to cram at the end of the course.

Some thoughts about cramming: Cramming defeats the purpose of education. What you learn through cramming is rarely retained long enough to be of any real benefit. You owe it to yourself and your future patients to be truly familiar and comfortable with the material.

Develop a schedule for study time and stick to it. Schedule study for a time when you are alert and rested and for a time that fits in with your day-to-day activities. If the time isn't convenient for you to study, then you probably won't. Always try to study in the same place. Your study place should be comfortable, free of distraction, well lit, and easy to access.

Study groups can be helpful if the members are serious about studying. The group should consist of about five people who are close in ability and motivation. Comparing notes and discussing concepts with others often leads to a better understanding of the material.

In the last few weeks before the exam, review all important material and put some extra time into studying your weak areas. Spend the last week before the exam in a general review of all material from the course.

The Day Before the Examination
The day before the examination is your free day. A light review of the material is all that you should need. Stick to your normal schedule and do an activity that you enjoy and that is relaxing. Here is a list of suggestions that may be helpful as you face the final 24 hours before the exam:

- Get a good night's sleep. Do not cram. If you don't know the material by this point, you won't be able to learn it adequately before tomorrow's exam.

- Avoid alcohol, caffeine, or anything else that may alter your judgment. You need to be at the peak of performance for the exam.

- Take a brisk walk or exercise lightly immediately prior to the exam.

- Eat a normal, well-balanced breakfast the morning of the exam.
- Engage in an enjoyable, relaxing activity.
- Finally, the 24 hours before the examination belong to you. Use them to do things that take your mind off the exam or to mentally prepare and focus your thoughts.

Entering the Examination

As you mentally prepare to take the exam, believe in yourself. You have studied hard to earn the right to take this test. A positive attitude will help you do well on the test and will help you avoid the problem of second- and third-guessing a question that you answered correctly.

Select a seat in a well-lit area that is free from distractions. All of your energy and thoughts should be focused on the exam.

Read and/or listen to all instructions the test proctor gives you. Important questions you should have about the exam will be answered for you in the instructions. Is this a timed exam? How many questions are there? Are stretch or bathroom breaks allowed? Is a #2 pencil needed? May the test be written on? These are a few of the questions you should be thinking of when you sit down to take the examination.

Multiple-Choice Examinations

Many exams for certification use the multiple-choice format. The standard multiple choice is little more than an extended true-or-false question. You must carefully read the question and then validate the truthfulness of each possible response. For every question with four possible responses, three of the options must be wrong. This means that over the whole multiple-choice field, an intimidating majority (75 percent) of the material is deliberately misleading. Because you must sort through all of that information, it is to your advantage to know as much as possible about multiple-choice examinations.

In a multiple-choice question, the question or problem is called a stem. Four or five alternatives follow the stem and include the correct answer and the wrong ones, or distracters. Your job is to separate the correct or most correct answer from the distracters. The stem deserves as much attention as the distracters. Find out what the stem is asking for and you're half way to the correct answer. It's important to thoroughly read and understand what the stem is asking or looking for before you select an answer. Careless mistakes made on examinations are most often the result of not taking the time to read the question or stem completely.

Understanding how a multiple-choice exam is written allows you to take a logical approach to selecting the correct response. Here are some general guidelines that test writers use when developing multiple-choice examinations:

- Alternatives should be chosen so that they seem likely.
- Alternatives should be grammatically consistent with the stem.
- Alternatives should be about the same length.
- Alternatives should avoid absolutes and *all of the above* or *none of the above*.

As a test taker, you need to be aware of:

- Specific words that can serve as clues. For example, *not, always, except,* and *never.*
- Alternatives not consistent in length.
- Alternatives that are illogical or have no basis in fact.

Start by reading the question carefully, making mental note of words such as *except, never, always, most,* and *not*. Always suspect questions with the word *always* and never be fooled by those that include the word *never*. Before you read any of the alternatives, try to formulate the answer in your head. This may make the correct answer easier to recognize, but before you mark the answer on the answer sheet, be sure to read all of the alternatives. There may be an answer more correct than the one you first chose.

If you have read the entire question and all of the alternatives and you are completely stumped, go with your initial response to the question. More often than not this will be the correct answer. Many times people will answer the question correctly only to talk themselves out of the answer. Be cautious about changing your mind after answering a question.

The process of elimination can be used with questions that have you stumped. Get rid of as many wrong alternatives as you can. By narrowing your choices, you increase your chances of guessing correctly. In most cases, you can be faced with a 50/50 chance of guessing the correct answer by eliminating obviously incorrect answers. If you are still in doubt, move on. Trying too long on one question can ruin your confidence. It's not a wise idea in a timed exam.

Don't read too much into the question. The test writer has ensured that the question has enough information in it to be answered correctly. "What if-ing" the question will cause you more grief and frustration than you need, so take the question at face value.

If you have enough time, recheck all of your answers. This is both beneficial and dangerous. You may find obvious blundering errors. If so, great! But beware of second-guessing and "what if-ing." Avoid their temptations, remain confident in your original answers, and turn in your test and answer sheet.

After the Examination
When you have turned in your test and answer sheet, remember that others are still taking the test, so be sure to leave the room quietly. Put the exam out of your mind until you receive the results. Comparing answers out in the hall with the other examinees is guaranteed to give you an ulcer and will not improve your score.

Now is the time to give yourself a big pat on the back. Do something special for yourself. You deserve a reward for all of the studying and dedication over the last few months. Do not wait for the results before you congratulate yourself. No matter what the results say, you get an "A" for developing and sticking to your study plan.

PASSING PRACTICAL EXAMINATIONS

The word *test* causes physiological changes within the body. Test taking or even the knowledge of a future examination causes stress and anxiety. The body responds to this anxiety as a threat to its calm, equal state. Although each of us may have mechanisms for coping with stress and anxiety, the body always reacts, in varying degrees, by preparing for "fight or flight." This reaction is known as the general adaptation syndrome and is actually caused by the dominance of the sympathetic over the parasympathetic nervous system. Norepinephrine is secreted and the blood pressure rises. Epinephrine is secreted and the central nervous system is activated; cardiac output increases; oxygen exchange is enhanced; and pupils dilate.

This type of reaction can be beneficial, if harnessed, and can be used to a person's advantage. Preparation is the best way to harness this powerful system.

Throughout your EMS career, you will be faced with this situation. Be it state or national certification, ACLS, PHTLS, or even basic CPR, you will be required to adequately perform the skills for which you have been trained in a practical examination.

The ultimate objective of every practical examination is that the candidate demonstrates for evaluation some sample of what he or she will be doing on the job.

Let's look at that a little closer. "Perform for evaluation" This, more than anything else, describes the job every student has at a practical exam. *Knowing* how to do the skill isn't the problem; *performing* it is. The nervousness described above is not unique to new EMTs. It affects providers at all levels, from First Responder through physician.

There are some things you can do before, during, and after the practical exam to help make it a success for you.

Before the Practical
A practical exam is no different from a written exam when it comes to preparation. The most important thing you can do to prepare yourself is to study and become familiar with the material beforehand.

If at all possible, find out which skills you will be tested on, and work on them. You would be surprised how many skills can be practiced with little or no equipment. Buddy up with someone in the class or with someone who has recently been through the course and has successfully completed the skills. Knowing what to expect can help to alleviate some of the anxiety.

For most continuing education programs—for example, PHTLS and ACLS—textbooks are mailed to the students at least 30 days in advance. Take advantage of this opportunity to become familiar with and practice the skills that you will be tested on in class. If possible, obtain a schedule of the class from the course coordinator. This will give you an idea of the skills that are involved and the length of time allotted for them.

If the practical exam is for certification at one of the EMT levels, study the materials previously given to you by the instructor of the class. Studying EMT texts, skill manuals, and practice scenarios will all be a big help on the day of the exam.

Note that the night before the exam is not the time to practice skills. A good night's rest will do far more to improve your chances of passing than an all-night cram session.

The Day of the Practical
If you've followed your plan of preparation, you should have the energy and confidence to do what you have to do when the day of the practical examination arrives. As you go through the test

stations at the exam, there are some important things to remember.

First and foremost, you should relax. Being relaxed allows you to focus your energy on what you need to do, and not on how well you are performing. Remind yourself that these skills are nothing new. You have studied and practiced them, and you are ready to perform the skill.

If you know that you are not ready to perform the skill, then if at all possible delay going into the station. Stage fright overcomes everyone at one time or another. Take a breather, try to put things back in perspective, and steady yourself for your successful completion of the skill.

The skill stations themselves are straightforward. They are not designed to trick you. They are, however, designed to allow your performance of the skill to be evaluated accurately. Try to keep in mind that the people rating you now once stood in the same spot themselves. A good proctor will remember what it was like and do what he or she can to help reduce some of the anxiety.

Before you go into the station, the proctor may give you directions or information about that particular station. Make sure to pay attention to what the proctor is saying. That information may prove useful as you perform the skill.

Don't hesitate to ask pertinent questions about the skill stations or available equipment. Try to be comfortable before you begin. When you first go into the station, take the time to check the equipment. Make sure that every piece of equipment needed is available to you. If you don't see a piece of equipment that you may need, be sure to ask. If a piece of equipment is not functioning properly, point this out to the proctor as soon as you notice the malfunction. Don't wait until after you've completed the station to point out such problems. By then, it may be too late to affect the outcome.

If the station is for CPR, ask if you can give the mannequin a few test breaths and compressions. This allows you to get the feel for the mannequin, as each one is a little different.

One of the most important things to do when performing any skill is to verbalize. If you verbalize every single thing that you do, see, palpate, or hear, you will have greatly increased your chances of passing the skill station. Verbalizing accomplishes several important things, so don't be afraid to speak up. It helps you keep track of where you are. More importantly, it helps the proctor know where you are. If you see that the victim's skin is pale and that fluid is coming from the left ear, verbalize that so the proctor will know that these two significant findings have caught your eye. As far as the proctor is concerned, if you don't say something about it, then it hasn't been checked.

While you are in the station, don't be in a rush. Mistakes are most often made from not taking the time to do the skill correctly. You won't earn extra points for completing the spinal immobilization station in two minutes flat. Generally, there is more than enough time allotted for the station, so use the extra time to your advantage.

Sometimes your train of thought will derail right in the middle of performing a skill. If this happens, don't panic. Stop, sit back for a second, and think about what it is you are doing as well as what you have already done. Go through a mental checklist of all the steps involved in the skill. Generally speaking, there is enough time within the station to do this. The alternative is fumbling your way through the skill until you get back on track. That period of fumbling is where you are most likely to make costly mistakes.

After the Examination

When the testing is over, if given the opportunity to evaluate the exam, take advantage of it. This is the chance to express what you liked and disliked about the exam process. Quality improvement is a big issue, and most administrators enjoy getting some kind of feedback, positive or negative. Evaluations give the administrator the tools needed to make the most objective, least stressful, and most appropriate exam possible.

Practical exams will never be completely stress free. However, there are steps that can be taken to help relieve the anxiety. If you prepare yourself, get a good night's rest before the exam, relax and verbalize, chances are you will pass that practical with flying colors!

The information above on passing practical exams was adapted from an article by George Angus, Jr., that originally appeared in the August 1992 issue of the Journal of Emergency Medical Services.

TRANSITION GUIDES

TRANSITION GUIDE 1

FROM: BRADY, *PREHOSPITAL EMERGENCY CARE*, SEVENTH EDITION
TO: BRADY, *PREHOSPITAL EMERGENCY CARE*, EIGHTH EDITION

The following *Transition Guide* will help you coordinate course materials for Brady, *Prehospital Emergency Care*, Eighth Edition if you previously used Brady, *Prehospital Emergency Care*, Seventh Edition for EMT class instruction.

Transition Guide 1	Brady Seventh Edition	Brady Eighth Edition
Introduction to Emergency Medical Care	Chap 1, pp. 1-11	Chap 1, pp. 2-17
The Emergency Medical Services System	Chap 1, pp. 2-5	Chap 1, pp. 3-8
The EMT-Basic	Chap 1, pp. 5-10	
The EMT		Chap 1, pp. 8-14
The Well-Being of the EMT-Basic	Chap 2, pp. 12-28	
The Well-Being of the EMT		Chap 2, pp. 18-40
Emotional Aspects of Emergency Care	Chap 2, pp. 13-19	Chap 2, pp. 20-26
Scene Safety	Chap 2, pp. 19-26	Chap 2, pp. 26-35
Enrichment	Chap 2, 26-28	Chap 2, pp. 35-38
Medical, Legal, and Ethical Issues	Chap 3, pp. 29-39	Chap 3, pp. 41-56
The Scope of Practice	Chap 3, pp. 30-32	Chap 3, pp. 42-44
Issues of Patient Consent and Refusal	Chap 3, pp. 32-35	Chap 3, pp. 44-49
Other Legal Aspects of Emergency Care	Chap 3, pp. 35-38	Chap 3, pp. 49-54
The Human Body	Chap 4, pp. 40-71	Chap 4, pp. 57-100
Anatomical Terms	Chap 4, pp. 41-45	Chap 4, pp. 58-63
Body Systems	Chap 4, pp. 45-64	Chap 4, pp. 63-87
Enrichment	Chap 4, pp. 64-67	Chap 4, pp. 87-89
Medical Terminology		Chap 4, pp. 89-95
Baseline Vital Signs and SAMPLE History	Chap 5, pp. 72-85	
Baseline Vital Signs and History Taking		Chap 5, pp. 101-122
Gathering Patient Information	Chap 5, pp. 73-74	Chap 5, p. 103
Baseline Vital Signs	Chap 5, pp. 74-83	Chap 5, pp. 103-119
The Sample History	Chap 5, pp. 83-84	Chap 5, pp. 119-120
Preparing to Lift and Move Patients	Chap 6, pp. 86-94	
Lifting and Moving Patients		Chap 6, pp. 123-149
Body Mechanics	Chap 6, pp. 87-89	Chap 6, pp. 124-127
General Guidelines for Lifting and Moving	Chap 6, pp. 89-93	Chap 6, pp. 127-130
Lifting and Moving Patients		Chap 6, pp. 130-135
Packaging for Transportation		Chap 6, pp. 135-147
Enrichment		Chap 6, pp. 147-148

TRANSITION GUIDE 1: From Brady, Prehospital Emergency Care, Seventh Edition

TRANSITION GUIDE 1: From Brady, *Prehospital Emergency Care, Seventh Edition*

TRANSITION GUIDE 1: *From Brady, Prehospital Emergency Care, Seventh Edition*

TRANSITION GUIDE 2

FROM: AAOS, *EMERGENCY CARE AND TRANSPORTATION OF THE SICK AND INJURED,* NINTH EDITION
TO: BRADY, *PREHOSPITAL EMERGENCY CARE,* EIGHTH EDITION

The following *Transition Guide* will help you coordinate course materials for Brady, *Prehospital Emergency Care,* Eighth Edition if you previously used AAOS, *Emergency Care and Transportation of the Sick and Injured,* Ninth Edition for EMT class instruction.

Transition Guide 2	AAOS Ninth Edition	Brady Eighth Edition
Introduction to Emergency Medical Care	Chap 1, pp. 2-21	Chap 1, pp. 2-17
The Emergency Medical Services System		Chap 1, pp. 3-8
Introduction to Emergency Medical Care	Chap 1, p. 4	
Course Description		Chap 1, pp. 4-5
Current Standards	Chap 1, pp. 4-5	
EMT-B Training: Focus and Requirements	Chap 1, pp. 5-6	Chap 1, p. 6
Certification Requirements	Chap 1, pp. 6-7	Chap 1, p. 6-7
Overview of the Emergency Medical Services System	Chap 1, pp. 7-8	Chap 1, pp. 3-4
Levels of Training	Chap 1, pp. 8-10	Chap 1, pp. 6-7
Components of the EMS System	Chap 1, pp. 11-16	Chap 1, pp. 5-8
Roles and Responsibilities of the EMT-B	Chap 1, pp. 16-18	Chap 1, pp. 8-14
Continuing Education	Chap 1, p. 18	
The Well-Being of the EMT-B	Chap 2, pp. 22-69	
The Well-Being of the EMT		Chap 2, pp. 18-40
The Well-Being of the EMT-B	Chap 2, p. 24	
Emotional Aspects of Emergency Care	Chap 2, p. 24	Chap 2, pp. 20-26
Death and Dying	Chap 2, pp. 25-29	Chap 2, pp. 20-21
Caring for Critically Ill and Injured Patients	Chap 2, pp. 29-31	
Stressful Situations	Chap 2, pp. 31-32	Chap 2, pp. 21-25
Stress Warning Signs and the Work Environment	Chap 2, pp. 32-38	Chap 2, p. 25
Workplace Issues	Chap 2, pp. 38-41	
Scene Safety and Personal Protection	Chap 2, pp. 41-42	Chap 2, pp. 26-33
Communicable Diseases	Chap 2, p. 42	Chap 2, pp. 35-38
Risk Reduction and Prevention	Chap 2, pp. 43-48	Chap 2, pp. 26-33
Immunity	Chap 2, pp. 48-50	Chap 2, p. 33
Duty to Act	Chap 2, pp. 50-51	
Some Diseases of Special Concern	Chap 2, pp. 51-55	Chap 2, pp. 35-38
General Postexposure Management	Chap 2, p. 55	Chap 2, p. 33
Establishing an Infection Control Routine	Chap 2, pp. 55-56	Chap 2, pp. 26-33
Scene Hazards	Chap 2, pp. 56-60	
Protective Clothing: Preventing Injury	Chap 2, pp. 60-63	Chap 2, pp. 27-32
Violent Situations	Chap 2, pp. 63-64	Chap 2, p. 34
Behavioral Emergencies	Chap 2, pp. 64-65	Chap 24, pp. 673-682
Medical, Legal, and Ethical Issues	Chap 3, pp. 70-89	Chap 3, pp. 41-56
Medical, Legal and Ethical Issues	Chap 3, p. 72	
The Scope of Practice	Chap 3, p. 72	Chap 3, pp. 42-44
Standards of Care	Chap 3, pp. 72-74	Chap 3, p. 43
Duty to Act	Chap 3, p. 74	Chap 3, pp. 43-44
Negligence	Chap 3, pp. 74-75	Chap 3, p. 49
Abandonment	Chap 3, p. 75	Chap 3, p. 50
Consent	Chap 3, pp. 75-77	Chap 3, pp. 44-45
Assault and Battery	Chap 3, p. 77	Chap 3, p. 50

TRANSITION GUIDE 2: From AAOS, Emergency Care and Transportation of the Sick and Injured, Ninth Edition

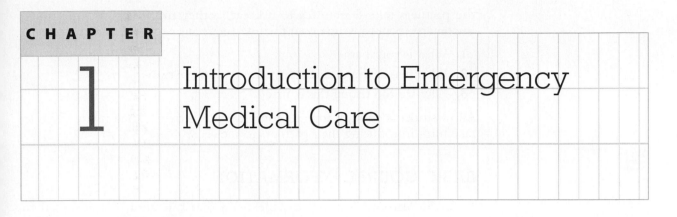

CHAPTER 1

Introduction to Emergency Medical Care

This chapter covers Lesson 1-1 and portions of Lesson 1-7 of the U.S. Department of Transportation's EMT-Basic National Standard Curriculum.

OBJECTIVES

Numbered objectives are from the U.S. Department of Transportation's EMT-Basic National Standard Curriculum. Asterisked objectives, if any, pertain to material that is supplemental to the DOT curriculum. Page numbers refer to pages in the textbook.

Cognitive

1-1.1 Define Emergency Medical Services (EMS) systems. (pp. 3–4)
1-1.2 Differentiate the roles and responsibilities of the EMT-Basic from other prehospital care providers. (pp. 6–7)
1-1.3 Describe the roles and responsibilities related to personal safety. (pp. 9–10)
1-1.4 Discuss the roles and responsibilities of the EMT-Basic toward the safety of the crew, the patient, and bystanders. (pp. 9–10)
1-1.5 Define quality improvement and discuss the EMT-Basic's role in the process. (p. 14)
1-1.6 Define medical direction and discuss the EMT-Basic's role in the process. (p. 13)
1-1.7 State the specific statutes and regulations in your state regarding the EMS system. (pp. 4, 9, 11)

Affective

1-1.8 Assess areas of personal attitude and conduct of the EMT-Basic. (pp. 12–13)
1-1.9 Characterize the various methods used to access the EMS system in your community. (pp. 5–6)

INTRODUCTION TO THE COURSE

Welcome students to the Emergency Medical Technician course and introduce yourself to them, giving your name, title, and affiliation. Introduce the following ice-breaking exercise to give the students—and yourself—a chance to get to know one another.

Divide the class in half. Have students in each half count off "1, 2, 3, etc.," and ask each student to remember his or her number. If there is an odd number of students, you should take the leftover student. Tell students to find the other person in the class who has the same number. Then have

Total Teaching Time
95 minutes

Additional Resources
Larmon/Davis, *Basic Life Support Skills*

Elling, *EMT Achieve: Basic Test Preparation*

Limmer/Mistovich/O'Keefe, *Audio Lecture and Study Guide: EMT*

the partners take 5 minutes to ask each other the following questions. Encourage them to write down their partner's answers to all the questions.

1. What is your name?
2. What makes you different from every other person?
3. Why are you taking this course?

Allow students enough time to complete this activity. Then invite them to take turns introducing their partners to the class.

BASIC COURSE INFORMATION

After the introductions are over, explain that this course is designed to instruct students to become competent, productive Emergency Medical Technicians (EMTs). Note that the majority of prehospital emergency medical care in this country is provided by EMTs. The course will cover all the skills necessary for an EMT to provide emergency medical care at a basic life support level with an ambulance service or other specialized service.

Have students turn to the table of contents in the text. Point out that this course is divided into 43 chapters, grouped into seven modules and an elective element. Briefly paraphrase for students what will be learned in each module.

Distribute a schedule of classes that lists the dates of future classes, the assignments that should be completed before coming to class, and what will be covered in class.

If you are using *Brady's Prehospital Emergency Care, Eighth Edition, Workbook,* explain to students that they are to complete the assigned portions of the workbook before each class. Clarify this policy and answer any questions students may have regarding assignments. Tell students that they are expected to master all the objectives in the text by the end of the course. Emphasize that mastery of the objectives is essential to their effectiveness as EMTs.

Distribute copies of the Chapter 1 Objectives Checklist. Mention to students that they will be given an Objectives Checklist at the beginning of each lesson. These checklists will help them keep track of which objectives they have mastered and which ones they still need to learn. Explain any additional procedures you have developed for tracking student performance and allowing students access to your records of their performance. At this time, explain your policy concerning chapter quizzes and/or tests. This *Instructor's Resource Manual* offers a quiz for every text chapter. In addition, you may wish to create tests specifically suited to the needs of your students using Prentice Hall *TestGen for Prehospital Emergency Care, Eighth Edition.*

At the end of each chapter, there is a quiz that covers many of the chapter objectives. Rather than assigning grades for the quizzes, it is recommended that the quizzes be used as learning tools by the students. The quizzes are designed to help students identify how well they have learned the objectives in any given chapter. Suggest that students who miss any items on a quiz go back to the chapter and find the correct answer.

If end-of-module exams and a final exam are to be given, describe what they will involve.

Spell out your procedures for remediation and reexamination of students who do not master 100 percent of each module's objectives. Advise students that you might use the handout "Chapter Review" as an alternative type of quiz for students whose performance on the initial quiz indicates failure to understand key objectives.

Point of Interest
Acquaint students with local EMS opportunities in the growing health-care market.

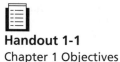

Teaching Tip
Walk students through their text, pointing out how the table of contents, chapter headings, and index can help them learn as they read and study for a quiz.

Handout 1-1
Chapter 1 Objectives Checklist

Describe your course's requirements for student interaction with patients in a clinical setting. Also, inform students about any required or available immunizations.

Describe your state's procedures for becoming a certified/licensed EMT. Also describe the certification requirement of the National Registry of Emergency Medical Technicians.

INTRODUCTION TO MODULE 1

When the basic course expectations and procedures have been explained, introduce Module 1: Preparatory. In this module, students will learn some basics about the emergency medical services system and about being an EMT; about how to protect themselves from injury and illness; about medical, legal, and ethical issues; about how the human body is organized; about how to take vital signs and obtain a patient's medical history; and about how to lift and move patients.

INTRODUCTION TO CHAPTER 1

Chapter 1, "Introduction to Emergency Medical Care," is the first lesson in Module 1. Among the most critical health problems in the United States today are the sudden loss of life and the disabilities caused by catastrophic injuries and illnesses. Every year thousands of people in this country die or suffer permanent harm because of the lack of adequate and available emergency medical services. An Emergency Medical Technician (EMT) can make a positive difference. Give students a few minutes to look over the Chapter 1 Objective Checklist that you distributed earlier. Briefly paraphrase the objectives for this lesson in your own words.

LECTURE

The following suggested lecture outline is based on the Department of Transportation's EMT-Basic National Standard Curriculum. In some places, the DOT curriculum has been rearranged or expanded upon so that it is more complete or easier for the student to understand. The page numbers in parentheses refer to pages in the textbook. The parenthetical references in bold type are to figures, tables, and scans in the textbook.

● ➤

Lecture Master
You may wish to display Lecture Master 1 when presenting the lecture to the class.

INTRODUCTION TO EMERGENCY MEDICAL CARE

I. **The Emergency Medical Services System** (pp. 3–8)
  A. A brief history (pp. 3–4)
    1. The National Highway Safety Act (1966)
    2. The Emergency Medical Services System Act (1973)
    3. The American Heart Association
    4. The National Registry's 1993 National Emergency Medical Services Education and Practice Blueprint
    5. EMS Agenda for the Future (1996)
    6. NHTSA National EMS Scope of Practice Model (2005)
  B. Current standards (pp. 4–8)
    1. National Highway Traffic Safety Administration's Technical Assistance Program Assessment Standards
      a. Regulation and policy
      b. Resource management

On the Net
NHTSA has a website at:
http://www.nhtsa.dot.gov

c. Human resources and training
d. Transportation
e. Facilities
f. Communications
g. Public information and education
h. Medical direction
i. Trauma systems
j. Evaluation
2. Access to the system (**Fig. 1-1, p. 5**)
   a. Public service answering point (PSAP)
   b. 9-1-1
   c. Non 9-1-1
3. Levels of training (**Fig. 1-2, p. 6**)
   a. First Responder (FR)
   b. Emergency Medical Technician (EMT)
   c. Advanced EMT (AEMT)
   d. Paramedic
   e. National EMS Scope of Practice Model (**Fig. 1-3, p. 7**)
     (1) Emergency Medical Responder (EMR)
     (2) Emergency Medical Technician (EMT)
     (3) Advanced Emergency Medical Technician (AEMT)
     (4) Paramedic
4. The health-care system
   a. Emergency departments
   b. Specialty facilities
     (1) Trauma center (**Fig. 1-4, p. 8**)
     (2) Burn center
     (3) Obstetrical center
     (4) Pediatric center
     (5) Poison center
     (6) Stroke center
     (7) Cardiac center
     (8) Hyperbaric center
     (9) Spine injury center
     (10) Psychiatric center
     (11) Other specialty centers
5. Hospital personnel
   a. Physicians
   b. Nurses
   c. Other health professionals
6. Liaison with other public safety personnel (**Fig. 1-5, p. 8 and Fig. 1-6, p. 9**)
   a. Fire service
   b. Law enforcement
7. Overview of the local EMS system

II. Emergency Medical Technician (pp. 8–13)
  A. Roles and responsibilities of the EMT (pp. 8–11) (**Table 1-1, p. 9**)
    1. Personal safety (**Fig. 1-7, p. 10**)
    2. Safety of crew, patient, and bystanders
    3. Patient assessment
    4. Emergency care (**Fig. 1-8, p. 10; Fig. 1-9 and 1-10, p. 11**)
    5. Safe lifting and moving
    6. Transport of the patient
    7. Transfer of patient care (**Fig. 1-11, p. 11**)
    8. Record keeping and data collection
    9. Patient advocacy

B. Professional attributes (pp. 12–13)
  1. Appearance
      a. Neat
      b. Clean
      c. Positive image
  2. Knowledge and skills
      a. Continuing education
      b. Refresher courses
      c. Use and maintenance of common emergency equipment
      d. Assistance with the administration of approved medications
      e. Cleaning, disinfection, and sterilization of nondisposable equipment
      f. Safety and security measures
      g. Territory and terrain
      h. State and local traffic laws and ordinances
      i. Maintains current knowledge of local, state, and national issues affecting EMS
  3. Physical demands
      a. Lift and carry up to 125 pounds
      b. Good eyesight
      c. Good color vision
      d. Good hearing
      e. Effective oral and written communications
      f. Puts patient's needs as a priority without endangering self
  4. Personal traits
      a. Calm and reassuring personality
      b. Leadership ability
      c. Good judgment
      d. Good moral character
      e. Stability and adaptability
      f. Ability to listen
      g. Resourcefulness and improvisation
      h. Cooperativeness
C. Medical direction/medical oversight (p. 13)
  1. Medical director
      a. A physician responsible for the clinical and patient care aspects of an EMS system
      b. Every ambulance service/rescue squad must have physician medical direction
  2. Medical oversight
      a. Comprehensive term that includes all of the clinical and administrative functions and activities performed by the medical director
  3. Types of medical direction
      a. On-line (Fig. 1-9, p. 11)
          (1) Telephone
          (2) Radio
      b. Off-line
          (1) Protocols
          (2) Standing orders
  4. Responsible for reviewing quality improvement
  5. The relationship of the EMT to medical direction
      a. Designated agent of the physician

Teaching Tip
If possible, arrange for the Medical Director of the local EMS system to visit the class and speak to students on his or her philosophy of EMS.

On the Net
Explanations and guidelines of EMS medical direction.
www.acep.org/1,617,0.htm

Teaching Tip
Review with students how your local QI process works.

Point to Emphasize
The aim of QI is to improve patient care, *not* to find fault with EMT performance.

    b. Care rendered is considered an extension of the medical director's authority (varies by state law)

  D. Specific statutes and regulations regarding EMS in your state (p. 13)

III. Quality improvement (p. 14)

  A. Definition (p. 14)

    1. A system of internal/external reviews and audits of all aspects of an EMS system so as to identify those aspects needing improvement to ensure that the public receives the highest quality of prehospital care

    2. Should not be used as a penalty tool but as an evaluation system geared toward overall system improvement

  B. The role of the EMT in quality improvement (p. 14) **(Fig. 1-12, p. 14)**

    1. Document carefully

    2. Perform run reviews and audits

    3. Obtain feedback

    4. Maintain equipment

    5. Participate in continuing education

    6. Maintain skills

CASE STUDY FOLLOW-UP

Ask a student volunteer to read the Case Study that begins on page 3 of the textbook. You may wish to use the following questions to engage students in a discussion of the Case Study Follow-up that begins on page 15. Provide missing information and clarify ideas as needed.

Q1. Why was the information that the rescue squad members had Emergency Medical Responder training important?

A1. *Without Emergency Medical Responder training, the rescue squad might have aggravated the patient's injuries.*

Q2. Under what circumstances would it have been acceptable for an EMT to go down to the patient with the rescue squad?

A2. *Such a move would have been acceptable only if the EMT had been trained and qualified in that type of rescue.*

Q3. What did you learn about the patient from the Emergency Medical Responder?

A3. *She said that the patient's chief complaint is of pain to his right wrist and right thigh and that the patient has warm and dry skin, his airway is patent with respirations of 24 per minute, and pulse at 90 and strong.*

Q4. What did your physical exam and focused history reveal?

A4. *The physical exam revealed abrasions to the arms, with pain and a slight deformity to the right wrist. There were also superficial abrasions to the right leg, with deformity, swelling, and pain to the right thigh. The patient could not feel or move the toes of his right foot. The focused history confirmed sharp pain to the right wrist and thigh, which started immediately after he landed at the bottom of the embankment. The patient also reported that he did not lose consciousness. He denies any other complaints, but says that he is allergic to sulfa drugs and takes medication for high blood pressure.*

Q5. What did you do en route to the hospital and upon arrival there?

A5. *En route, a detailed head-to-toe physical exam was performed to ensure that no injuries were overlooked. The hospital is notified that the ambulance is en route, and details of the patient's condition are given. An ongoing assessment is performed every 5 minutes to monitor the patient's condition until arrival at the hospital. Upon arrival, care of the patient is transferred without incident to the emergency department staff and the staff are given a verbal report. The written prehospital care report is completed and the unit prepared for the next call.*

IN REVIEW

Assess student's ability to apply what they have learned by discussing the Review Questions on page 17 of the textbook.

Q1. Describe the purpose of the modern EMS system.

A1. *The purpose of the modern EMS system is to allow those who need it easy access, a prompt response, and high-quality prehospital emergency care from trained professionals. (p. 4)*

Q2. Name two ways the public accesses the EMS system. Explain advantages or disadvantages of each.

A2. *The public can access the EMS system by way of the universal telephone number 9-1-1 or by using a non 9-1-1 number—a seven-digit number—to call a dispatch center or to call the emergency service needed directly. The advantages of a universal number are that central dispatch is generally staffed by trained technicians and the number is easy to remember. Probably the most serious drawback to using a seven-digit number is the delay in reaching the appropriate services. (pp. 5–6)*

Q3. List the four levels of prehospital emergency care training.

A3. *The four levels of emergency medical technician training are Emergency Medical Responder (EMR) (formerly First Responder), Emergency Medical Technician (EMT) (formerly EMT-Basic), Advanced Emergency Medical Technician (AEMT) (formerly EMT-Intermediate), and Paramedic (formerly EMT-Paramedic). (pp. 6–7)*

Q4. List six types of special facilities, other than a hospital emergency department, to which some patients may have to be transported.

A4. *Six types of special facilities to which patients may be transported include: trauma center, burn center, obstetrical center, pediatric center, poison center, and stroke center. (p. 8)*

Q5. List the general responsibilities of an EMT.

A5. *The general responsibilities of the EMT include personal safety and the safety of others, patient assessment and emergency medical care, safe lifting and moving, transport and transfer, record keeping and data collection, and patient advocacy. (pp. 8–9)*

Q6. Describe at least five steps you can take to protect your own safety as an EMT.

A6. *Among the ways you can protect your own safety as an EMT are: drive safely; use seatbelts; do not enter potentially hazardous sites; never enter a volatile crowd situation until it has been controlled by law enforcement; take extra precautions with patients, relatives, and bystanders who are under the influence of drugs or alcohol, have a behavioral disorder, or are emotionally charged; follow direction from police, fire, utility, and other expert personnel; create a safe area in which patients can be treated; redirect traffic for the safety of all; wear reflective emblems or clothing at night; provide adequate lighting at an accident scene; wear personal protective equipment, including BSI equipment, appropriate for scene hazards. (pp. 9–10)*

Q7. Describe at least three ways you might act as the patient's advocate.

A7. *Among the ways you can act as a patient's advocate are: collect and safeguard a patient's valuables, transport them with the patient, document what was given to emergency department personnel; answer the patient's questions truthfully; conceal from curious onlookers the body of a patient who has died; make sure the patient's relatives or friends at the scene know how to get to the hospital; make certain you provide necessary information to hospital personnel; honor any patient requests that you reasonably can; protect the patient's privacy and confidentiality. (p. 11)*

Q8. Describe the EMS physician medical director's primary responsibility.

A8. *The EMS system physician medical director's primary responsibility is to oversee the clinical and patient-care aspects of the system. (p. 13)*

Q9. List the goals of quality improvement.

A9. *The goals of quality improvement are to identify those aspects of the system that can be improved and to implement plans and programs that will remedy any shortcomings. (p. 14)*

Q10. Describe the EMT's role in quality improvement.

A10. *The EMT's role in quality improvement includes documenting each call; performing reviews and audits as requested; gathering feedback from patients, other EMS personnel, and hospital staff; conducting preventive maintenance on vehicles and equipment; participating in refresher courses and continuing education; and maintaining skills in all aspects of patient care and equipment operation. (p. 14)*

CRITICAL THINKING

Assess students' ability to respond to real-life emergency situations by discussing the Critical Thinking questions on page 17 in the textbook.

Q1. What are your responsibilities while on this call?

A1. *While on this call you should ensure the safety of all individuals present (including yourself), properly assess the patient (and provide any necessary emergency care), safely move the patient to the ambulance* *and transport him to an appropriate facility. Once at the receiving hospital, you should transfer the patient's care to the facility staff and complete all documentation.*

Q2. How can you serve as the patient's advocate?

A2. *Many answers are possible, but the following should be included: documenting and safeguarding any valuables transported with the patient, shielding the patient from curious neighbors, explaining to the niece that the stroke center would be better able to care for her uncle than the local hospital, ensuring that the niece knows how to get to the receiving facility, and providing all necessary information to the receiving facility staff.*

Q3. How can you use medical direction in this situation?

A3. *In at least two important ways: the first is to utilize the local standing orders to properly care for the stroke patient and the second is to seek advice from the on-line physician as to which receiving facility the patient should be transported to.*

ASSIGNMENTS

Assign students to read Chapter 2, "The Well-Being of the EMT," before the next class. Also ask them to complete Chapter 1 of the Workbook.

EVALUATION

Chapter Quiz Distribute copies of the Chapter Quiz provided in Handout 1-2 to evaluate student understanding of this chapter. Remind students not to refer to their textbooks or notes while taking the quiz.

Test Manager You may wish to create a custom-tailored test using Prentice Hall *TestGen for Prehospital Emergency Care, Eighth Edition* to evaluate student understanding of this chapter.

Online Test Preparation (for students and instructors) Additional test preparation is available through *EMT Achieve: Basic Test Preparation* at http://www.prenhall.com/EMTAchieve. Instructors can also monitor student mastery online.

REINFORCEMENT

Handouts If classroom discussions or performance on the quiz indicates that some students have not fully mastered the chapter content, you may wish to assign some or all of the Reinforcement Handouts for this chapter.

Reading/Reference
Textbook, pp. 18–40

Workbook
Chapter 1 Activities

Chapter Quiz
Handout 1-2

TestGen
Chapter 1 Test

Online Test Preparation
Send your students to
http://www.prenhall.com/
EMTAchieve

Handouts 1-3 to 1-6
Reinforcement Activities

**Brady Skills Series
EMT-B Videos/CD**
Visual Reinforcement

**PowerPoint
Presentation**
Chapter 1

Student CD
Chapter 1

Companion Website
http://www.prenhall.com/
mistovich

TECH EXTRAS

Brady Skills Series EMT-B Videos/CD Have your students watch the skills come to life on either VHS or CD-ROM.

PowerPoint Presentation (for instructors) The PowerPoint material developed for this chapter offers useful reinforcement of chapter content.

Student CD A wide variety of material on this CD-ROM will reinforce and also expand student knowledge and skills.

Companion Website (for students) Additional review quizzes and links to EMS resources will contribute to further reinforcement of this chapter. Please visit http://www.prenhall.com/mistovich.

OBJECTIVES CHECKLIST

Cognitive		Date Mastered
1-1.1	Define Emergency Medical Services (EMS) systems.	
1-1.2	Differentiate the roles and responsibilities of the EMT-Basic from other prehospital care providers.	
1-1.3	Describe the roles and responsibilities related to personal safety.	
1-1.4	Discuss the roles and responsibilities of the EMT-Basic toward the safety of the crew, the patient, and bystanders.	
1-1.5	Define quality improvement and discuss the EMT-Basic's role in the process.	
1-1.6	Define medical direction and discuss the EMT-Basic's role in the process.	
1-1.7	State the specific statutes and regulations in your state regarding the EMS system.	

Affective		Date Mastered
1-1.8	Assess areas of personal attitude and conduct of the EMT-Basic.	
1-1.9	Characterize the various methods used to access the EMS system in your community.	

CHAPTER 1 QUIZ

Write the letter of the best answer in the space provided.

_____ **1.** The first priority of the EMT on the emergency scene is to
   A. manage a hostile crowd.
   B. secure the patient.
   C. ensure personal safety.
   D. provide a situation update to dispatch.

_____ **2.** An EMT is operating as a designated agent of the
   A. EMT-Intermediate.   **C.** medical director.
   B. ER nurse.   **D.** shift commander.

_____ **3.** The _____ is legally responsible for the clinical and patient-care aspects of an EMS system.
   A. paramedic   **C.** Advance EMT
   B. shift commander   **D.** medical director

_____ **4.** The first concern of an EMT always must be _____ safety.
   A. patient   **C.** vehicle
   B. bystander   **D.** personal

_____ **5.** A policy set by an EMS Medical Director that allows EMTs to administer glucose to patients in certain circumstances without speaking to the physician is an example of a(n)
   A. direct order.   **C.** standing order.
   B. on-line order.   **D.** QI order.

_____ **6.** An order from an EMS system's on-duty physician given by radio or phone is an example of
   A. off-line medical control.   **C.** designated direction.
   B. on-line medical direction.   **D.** standing orders.

_____ **7.** The level of EMS that involves medical training for those who are usually first on the scene of an emergency is
   A. Emergency Medical Responder.   **C.** Advanced EMT.
   B. EMT.   **D.** Paramedic.

_____ **8.** Most EMT courses today are based on models developed by the
   A. AHA.   **C.** DOT.
   B. ARC.   **D.** NST.

_____ **9.** The system of internal and external reviews and audits for all aspects of an emergency medical system is known as
   A. quality improvement.   **C.** EMDs.
   B. protocols.   **D.** standing ORs.

_____ **10.** The aspect of the EMT's job that involves protecting the patient's rights is
   A. assessment.   **C.** advocacy.
   B. transfer.   **D.** protocol.

IN THE FIELD

Review the following real-life situation. Then answer the questions that follow.

You and an EMT partner are assigned to EMS Unit 5 one morning in September. At 1035, the emergency dispatcher directs you to an accident on Mesa Drive. A woman driving her car along that road called 9-1-1 on her cell phone to report that the car ahead of her had swerved to avoid a dog, gone off the road, plunged into a ditch, and hit a tree.

Your unit pulls up at the scene 6 minutes later. As you don your personal protective equipment, you note that a county sheriff's car is already on-scene. A deputy is kneeling beside a male in his early 20s who is lying on the ground. Even from the top of the ditch, you can see that the young man's shirt and pants are blood soaked. The deputy is applying direct pressure to the patient's right wrist. As you approach, the deputy tells you that after the crash, the patient, who had been wearing a seatbelt, did not believe himself injured. However, before the deputy arrived, the patient attempted to get out of the car. In doing so, he sliced his wrist on jagged metal.

Your partner takes over holding direct pressure to the wound. Meanwhile, you introduce yourself to the patient as you begin your assessment of his condition. The patient seems anxious and restless, and as you assess him, you talk to him, explaining what you are doing, and try to calm him.

Because of the circumstances of the accident, you are especially alert during the assessment to the possibility that the patient may have received internal and/or spinal injuries. In fact, you determine that the patient is showing signs and symptoms of internal bleeding and shock (hypoperfusion). Shock is a life-threatening condition, so you decide that he needs immediate transport to the hospital, some 20 minutes away.

You have provided the patient with high-flow oxygen. Now, as you prepare him for transport, you ask the police officer to call in a request for a rendezvous with paramedics of the Advanced Life Support (ALS) unit. When he has done so, he joins you and your partner in moving the patient, now immobilized to a long spine board, to the ambulance. You remain with the patient, holding direct pressure on the wrist wound, while your partner drives. You also monitor the patient's airway, breathing, and circulation and reassess his vital signs.

Seven minutes later, you meet the paramedics of the ALS unit at the parking lot of a farm produce stand. You provide the paramedics with a concise report of the patient's condition and your interventions. The paramedics assume care of the patient. They contact medical direction and report on their findings and expected time of arrival at the hospital as transport continues.

At 1105, the ambulance reaches County General Hospital. The emergency room staff is briefed on the patient's status and vital signs and on the care he has received. The hospital crew takes over, and wheels the patient off to surgery.

1. Which components of the EMS system were involved in this scenario?

2. What roles and responsibilities of an EMT were demonstrated in this scenario?

CHAPTER 1 REVIEW

Write the word or words that best complete each sentence in the space provided.

1. The modern Emergency Medical Services (EMS) system began in the

_____.

2. The National Highway Safety Act charged the United States _____

_____ _____ with developing an EMS system.

3. The emergency medical treatment given by EMTs to patients before they are transported to a

facility is called _____ _____.

4. The type of facility that provides specialized treatment for injuries that exceed normal hospital

emergency department capabilities is a(n) _____

_____.

5. The system of answering emergency telephone calls that uses specially trained EMS personnel who

obtain information about emergency situations from callers and also provide instructions for

emergency care to callers is _____ _____

_____.

6. The 9-1-1 telephone number used to access emergency services in many parts of the nation is often

referred to as the _____ _____.

7. A(n) _____ _____ is a basic-level EMS provider

who has passed specific additional training programs and is authorized to provide some level of

advanced life support such as intravenous therapy and advanced defibrillation.

8. The system of internal and external reviews and audits of all aspects of an emergency medical system

is known as _____ _____.

9. Standing orders that allow EMTs to give certain medications or perform certain procedures without

speaking directly to a physician are examples of _____ -

_____ medical direction.

10. An EMT has responsibility for a patient until the _____

_____ _____ to hospital personnel has been

properly completed.

EMT: LISTING

1. List five of the categories in which the National Highway Traffic Safety Administration Technical Assistance Program sets standards for EMS systems.

2. List three types of specialty hospitals.

3. List three responsibilities of Emergency Medical Dispatchers.

4. List the four general levels of EMS training and certification.

5. List at least four responsibilities of the EMT.

EMT: True or False

Indicate if the following statements are true or false by writing T or F in the space provided.

_____ **1.** As an EMT, your authority to give medications and provide emergency care is an extension of the Medical Director's license to practice medicine.

_____ **2.** As an EMT, you will be one of the many persons and professions that come together to form an EMS system.

_____ **3.** Trauma centers are not yet considered "specialty" hospitals.

_____ **4.** Certification as an EMT requires only that a person successfully complete the DOT EMT-National Standard Training Program.

_____ **5.** Keeping yourself safe is your second priority after patient safety when providing medical care.

_____ **6.** The care an individual patient requires may range from simple emotional support to life-saving CPR.

_____ **7.** You must never abandon care of the patient at the hospital until transfer to hospital personnel has been properly completed.

_____ **8.** Good personality traits are really not very important to the EMT.

_____ **9.** Good quality continuing education can often take the place of an original EMT training course.

_____ **10.** Quality improvement is designed and performed to ensure that the public receives the highest quality prehospital care.

_____ **11.** The EMT has no direct role in the quality improvement process.

_____ **12.** Striving for quality in the care you personally give to patients and as a collective part of an ambulance squad is to uphold the highest standards of the EMS system.

LECTURE MASTER 1

Introduction to Emergency Medical Care

EMS Systems
Brief History

9-1-1

Other Health Care Components

Roles and Responsibilities
Personal Safety

Lifting and Moving Patients, Transport, and Transfer of Care

Record Keeping

Personal Attributes

Medical Direction
On-Line

Off-Line

Physician Relationship

Quality Improvement
EMT's Role in QI

HANDOUT 1-2: Chapter 1 Quiz

1. C	4. D	7. A	9. A
2. C	5. C	8. C	10. C
3. D	6. B		

HANDOUT 1-3: In the Field

1. The emergency dispatcher; an Emergency Medical Responder (the deputy); the EMT on Unit 5; the Paramedics from the ALS unit; the emergency room personnel at the hospital
2. Personal safety; safety of patient; patient assessment; patient care; lifting and moving; transport; transfer of care

HANDOUT 1-4: Chapter 1 Review

1. 1960s
2. Department of Transportation
3. prehospital care
4. trauma center
5. Emergency Medical Dispatching
6. universal number
7. Advanced EMT
8. quality improvement
9. off-line
10. transfer of care

HANDOUT 1-5: EMT: Listing

1. Any five: Regulation and Policy, Resource Management, Human Resources and Training, Transportation, Facilities, Communications, Public Information and Education, Medical Direction, Trauma Systems, Evaluation.
2. Any three: trauma centers, burn centers, pediatric centers, poison centers, stroke centers
3. To obtain appropriate information from callers; to facilitate dispatch of emergency services; to provide medical instructions for emergency care.
4. Emergency Medical Responder, EMT, Advanced EMT, Paramedic.
5. Responsibilities include preparation for response, safe response, safe transportation, patient assessment, patient care, proper transfer of the patient to hospital personnel for continuity of care.

HANDOUT 1-6: EMT: True or False

1. T	4. F	7. T	10. T
2. T	5. F	8. F	11. F
3. F	6. T	9. F	12. T

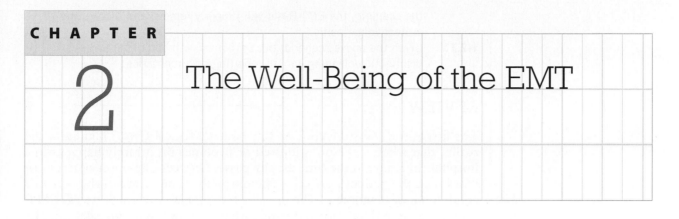

CHAPTER

2

The Well-Being of the EMT

This chapter covers Lesson 1-2 and portions of Lesson 1-7 of the U.S. Department of Transportation's EMT-Basic National Standard Curriculum.

OBJECTIVES

Numbered objectives are from the U.S. Department of Transportation's EMT-Basic National Standard Curriculum. Asterisked objectives, if any, pertain to material that is supplemental to the DOT curriculum. Page numbers refer to pages in the textbook.

Cognitive

1-2.1 List possible emotional reactions that the EMT-Basic may experience when faced with trauma, illness, death, and dying. (p. 23)

1-2.2 Discuss the possible reactions that a family member may exhibit when confronted with death and dying. (p. 20)

1-2.3 State the steps in the EMT-Basic's approach to the family confronted with death and dying. (pp. 20–21)

1-2.4 State the possible reactions that the family of the EMT-Basic may exhibit due to their outside involvement in EMS. (p. 24–25)

1-2.5 Recognize the signs and symptoms of critical incident stress. (pp. 23–25)

1-2.6 State possible steps that the EMT-Basic may take to help reduce/alleviate stress. (pp. 23–25)

1-2.7 Explain the need to determine scene safety. (p. 20)

1-2.8 Discuss the importance of body substance isolation (BSI). (pp. 26–27)

1-2.9 Describe the steps the EMT-Basic should take for personal protection from airborne and bloodborne pathogens. (pp. 26–33)

1-2.10 List the personal protective equipment necessary for each of the following situations:
— Hazardous materials (p. 33)
— Rescue operations (pp. 33–34)
— Violent scenes (pp. 34–35)
— Crime scenes (pp. 33–35)
— Exposure to bloodborne pathogens (pp. 26–33)
— Exposure to airborne pathogens (pp. 26–33)

Affective

1-2.11 Explain the rationale for serving as an advocate for the use of appropriate protective equipment. (p. 26)

Psychomotor

1-2.12 Given a scenario with potential infectious exposure, the EMT-Basic will use appropriate personal protective equipment. At the completion of

Total Teaching Time
95 minutes

Resources Needed
- Scored Chapter 1 Quizzes
- Latex gloves
- Pairs of goggles, side protectors, or protective glasses
- Surgical masks
- Surgical gowns
- Paper cutout of a gun
- Trauma jump kit

Additional Resources
Larmon/Davis, *Basic Life Support Skills*

Elling, *EMT Achieve: Basic Test Preparation*

Limmer/Mistovich/ O'Keefe, *Audio Lecture & Study Guide: EMT*

Mistovich/Kuvlesky, *SUCCESS! for the EMT, Second Edition*

the scenario, the EMT-Basic will properly remove and discard the protective garments.

1-2.13 Given the above scenario, the EMT-Basic will complete disinfection/cleaning and all reporting documentation.

REVIEW

The first lesson, "Introduction to Emergency Medical Care," highlights the reality that when a person is injured or becomes ill, it rarely happens in a hospital. In reality, some time usually passes between the onset of injury or illness and the patient's arrival at the hospital—time in which the patient's condition may deteriorate. The modern Emergency Medical Services (EMS) system has been developed to provide what is known as prehospital care. Its purpose is to get trained personnel to the patient as quickly as possible to provide emergency care. The EMT is a key member of the EMS team.

Distribute the scored quizzes from the last class. Go over each question on the quiz and handle any concerns students may have about the answers.

INTRODUCTION TO CHAPTER 2

Chapter 2, "The Well-Being of the EMT," is the second lesson in Module 1. Tell students that as an EMT they will encounter high-stress circumstances as well as dangerous life-threatening situations. This chapter will help them learn to recognize and deal with the stress that normally accompanies emergency work, to practice all appropriate body substance isolation precautions, and to wear the appropriate personal protective equipment at the scenes of injuries and illnesses. Distribute the Chapter 2 Objectives Checklist and give students a few minutes to look it over. Then briefly paraphrase the objectives for this lesson in your own words.

LECTURE

The following suggested lecture outline is based on the Department of Transportation's EMT-Basic National Standard Curriculum. In some places, the DOT curriculum has been rearranged or expanded upon so that it is more complete or easier for the student to understand. The page numbers in parentheses refer to pages in the textbook. The parenthetical references in dark, heavy type are to figures, tables, and scans in the textbook.

THE WELL-BEING OF THE EMT

I. Emotional aspects of emergency care (pp. 20–26)
    A. Death and dying (pp. 20–21)
        1. Five emotional stages
            a. Denial ("Not me")
                (1) Defense mechanism creating a buffer between shock of dying and dealing with the illness or injury
            b. Anger ("Why me?")
                (1) EMTs may be the target of the anger
                (2) Don't take anger or insults personally
                    (a) Be tolerant
                    (b) Do not become defensive
                (3) Employ good listening and communication skills

---

Handout 2-1
Chapter 2 Objectives Checklist

Lecture Master
You may wish to display Lecture Master 2 when presenting the lecture to the class.

Teaching Tip
Invite any students who would like to share a loss they experienced and how they felt about it.

    (4) Be empathetic
   c. Bargaining ("OK, but first let me . . .")
    (1) Agreement that, in the patient's mind, will postpone death for a short time
   d. Depression ("OK, but I haven't . . .")
    (1) Characterized by sadness and despair
    (2) Patient is usually silent and retreats into own world
   e. Acceptance ("OK, I am not afraid")
    (1) Does not mean the patient will be happy about dying
    (2) The family will usually require more support during this stage than the patient
  2. Dealing with the dying patient, family, and bystanders
   a. Maintain the patient's dignity
   b. Show the greatest possible respect
   c. Communicate
   d. Allow family members to express themselves
   e. Listen empathetically
   f. Do not give false assurances
   g. Use a gentle tone of voice
   h. Use a reassuring touch, if appropriate
   i. Do what you can to comfort the family
   j. Do not allow the family to enter a crime scene or touch the body until permission is given by law enforcement, coroner, or medical examiner

B. High-stress situations (p. 21) **(Fig. 2-1, p. 22)**
 1. Multiple-casualty incidents
 2. Abuse and neglect of infants, children, adults, and the elderly
 3. Emergencies involving infants and children
 4. Injury or death of a coworker
 5. Responding and providing emergency care to a relative or bystander
 6. Severe traumatic injuries such as amputations

C. Stress reactions (pp. 21–23)
 1. Acute stress reaction
 2. Delayed stress reaction
  a. Posttraumatic stress disorder (PTSD)
 3. Cumulative stress reaction
  a. Burnout

D. Common signs and symptoms (p. 23) **(Fig. 2-2, p. 23)**
 1. Irritability to coworkers, patients, family, and friends
 2. Inability to concentrate
 3. Difficulty sleeping and nightmares
 4. Anxiety
 5. Indecisiveness
 6. Guilt
 7. Loss of appetite
 8. Loss of interest in sexual activities
 9. Isolation
 10. Loss of interest in work

E. General categories of signs and symptoms (p. 23)
 1. Thinking
  a. Confusion
  b. Inability to make judgments or decisions
  c. Loss of motivation

Reading/Reference
"Check Your Fabric. Beyond the Books," *EMS Magazine,* Jan. 2005.

Reading/Reference
Dernocoeur, K. "Sweet Dreams? Sleep Deprivation and Shift Work in EMS," *EMS Magazine,* Feb. 2003.

         d. Chronic forgetfulness

         e. Loss of objectivity

    2. Psychological

         a. Depression

         b. Excessive anger

         c. Negativism

         d. Hostility

         e. Defensiveness

         f. Mood swings

         g. Feelings of worthlessness

    3. Physical

         a. Persistent exhaustion

         b. Headaches

         c. Gastrointestinal distress

         d. Dizziness

         e. Pounding heart

    4. Behavioral

         a. Overeating

         b. Increased alcohol or drug use

         c. Grinding teeth

         d. Hyperactivity

         e. Lack of energy

    5. Social

         a. Increased interpersonal conflicts

         b. Decreased ability to relate to patients as individuals

F. Stress management (pp. 23–25)

    1. Maintaining health

         a. Physical

         b. Emotional

         c. Social

         d. Behavioral

         e. Psychological

    2. Recognize the signs and symptoms

    3. Manage the stress before it progresses

    4. Lifestyle changes

         a. Change diet

             (1) Reduce sugar, caffeine, and alcohol intake

             (2) Avoid fatty foods

             (3) Increase protein and carbohydrates

         b. Exercise more often

         c. Learn to relax

         d. Avoid self-medication

    5. Keep balance in life

    6. Recognize the responses of your family and friends

         a. Lack of understanding

         b. Fear of separation and of being ignored

         c. Worry about on-call situations

         d. Inability to plan

         e. Frustrated desire to share

    7. Work environment changes may include:

         a. Develop a "buddy system" with a coworker

         b. Encourage and support coworkers

         c. Take an exercise break (**Fig. 2-3, p. 25**)

         d. Request work shifts that allow more time with family and friends

         e. Request a rotation to a less busy area

◉

Point to Emphasize

Our bodies strive for physiological balance. Encourage students to strive for balance in their lives by mixing work with recreational activities.

8. Seek professional help

G. Critical incident stress management (CISM) (pp. 25–26)
    1. Critical incident stress debriefing (CISD)
        a. Designed to accelerate the normal recovery process of experiencing a critical incident
        b. Held within 24 to 72 hours of incident
        c. Phases
            (1) Review facts of the event
            (2) Share feelings
            (3) Identify signs and symptoms
            (4) Sort through feelings with the assistance of a mental health professional
            (5) Receive suggestions for overcoming the stress
            (6) Develop a plan of action for returning to the job
            (7) Obtain the ability to follow up if lingering issues are present
            (8) Open discussion of feelings, fears, and reactions
        d. Not an investigation or interrogation
        e. All information is confidential
    2. Defusing
        a. Less structured version of a CISD
        b. Held within 1 to 4 hours of incident
    3. Comprehensive CISM
        a. Preincident stress education
        b. On-scene peer support
        c. One-on-one support
        d. Disaster support services
        e. Defusing
        f. CISD
        g. Follow-up services
        h. Spouse and family support
        i. Community outreach programs
        j. Other health and welfare programs
    4. Accessing CISM in your EMS system

II. Scene safety (pp. 26–35)
    A. Protecting yourself from disease (pp. 26–33)
        1. How diseases spread (**Table 2-1, p. 27; Fig. 2-4, p. 27**)
            a. Pathogens
            b. Directly
                (1) Contact with contaminated blood or other body fluids
            c. Indirectly
                (1) Contaminated objects
        2. Body substance isolation (BSI) precautions
            a. Hand washing (**Fig. 2-6, p. 29**)
                (1) Soap and water
                (2) Alcohol-based sanitizer
            b. Personal protective equipment (PPE)
                (1) Eye protection (**Figs. 2-7, 2-8, p. 29**)
                (2) Gloves (**Fig. 2-9, pp. 30–31**)
                    (a) Vinyl
                    (b) Latex
                    (c) Other synthetic
                (3) Gowns

On the Net

Data on critical incident stress debriefing is available at: http://www.fire-ems.net

On the Net

A general overview of the CISD process. http://www.ncptsd.org/publications/cq/v4/n2/hiley-yo.html

On the Net

Information and techniques to help reduce stress levels. http://www.mentalhealth.com/mag1/p51-str.html

On the Net

The Centers for Disease Control and Prevention's home page is at: http://www.cdc.gov

Slides/Videos

"Infectious Diseases," *Pulse,* Feb. 1999.

Point to Emphasize

Gloves are for the protection of the patient as well as the rescuer.

On the Net

OSHA has a website at: http://www.osha.gov

Slides/Videos

Brady Skill Series: EMT-B, "Body Substance Isolation (BSI) Precautions"

   (4) Masks (**Figs. 2-10, 2-11, p. 32**)
    (a) Surgical type
    (b) HEPA or N-95
  c. Proper cleaning or disposal of contaminated equipment (**Figs. 2-12, 2-13, p. 32**)
 3. Immunizations
  a. Purified protein derivative (PD) test for TB (annually)
  b. Tetanus prophylaxis (every 10 years)
  c. Hepatitis B vaccine
  d. Influenza vaccine (annually)
  e. Polio immunization (if needed)
  f. Rubella (German measles) vaccine
  g. Measles vaccine (if needed)
  h. Mumps vaccine (if needed)
 4. Reporting exposure incidents (**Fig. 2-5, p. 28**)
B. Protecting yourself from accidental injury (pp. 33–35)
 1. Hazardous materials
  a. Identify materials before approaching
   (1) Binoculars
   (2) Signs and placards (**Fig. 2-14, p. 34**)
   (3) Emergency Response Guidebook (**Fig. 2-15, p. 34**)
  b. Specially trained teams wear protective clothing (**Figs. 2-16, 2-17, p. 35**)
  c. EMTs provide emergency care only after scene is safe and patients have been decontaminated
 2. Rescue situations
  a. EMTs identify life threats and call for specialized teams
   (1) Electricity (**Fig. 2-18, p. 35**)
   (2) Fire
   (3) Explosion
   (4) Hazardous materials
   (5) Structural collapse potential
   (6) Low oxygen levels in confined spaces
   (7) Trenches not properly secured
   (8) Biological, nuclear, or chemical weapons
  b. Wear clothing appropriate to the situation (**Fig. 2-19, p. 36**)
   (1) Type of rescue
   (2) Location of rescue
   (3) Time of day
   (4) Weather
 3. Violence and crime
  a. Before entering the scene, it should always be controlled by law enforcement, including:
   (1) Perpetrator of the crime
   (2) Bystanders
   (3) Family members
  b. Behavior at crime scene (covered in greater detail in Chapter 3, "Medical, Legal, and Ethical Issues")
   (1) Do not disturb the scene unless required for medical care
   (2) Maintain chain of evidence

Point to Emphasize

An injured EMT is part of the problem, not part of the solution. Training and proper use of equipment beat out heroics any time.

Reading/Reference

Johnson, J. et al. "Close to the Vest: Body Armor Changes the Face of Penetrating Trauma," *JEMS,* Aug. 2000.

The following sections contain information that is valuable as background for the EMT, but that goes substantially beyond the U.S. Department of Transportation's EMT-Basic National Standard Curriculum.

I. Diseases of concern (pp. 35–38)**(Table 2-1, p. 00)**
    A. Hepatitis B (pp. 35–36)
        1. Transmission
            a. Blood
            b. Body fluids
        2. Signs and symptoms
            a. Fatigue
            b. Nausea and loss of appetite
            c. Abdominal pain
            d. Headache
            e. Fever
            f. Yellowish color of skin and whites of eyes (jaundice)
        3. Protection recommendations
            a. Hepatitis B vaccination
            b. Wear disposable gloves
            c. Wash hands thoroughly
            d. Double-bag and seal all soiled refuse
            e. Disinfect or sterilize nondisposable equipment
            f. Report any exposure
    B. Hepatitis C (p. 36)
        1. Most common bloodborne infection in the United States
        2. Transmission
            a. Blood
            b. Body fluids
         3. Signs and symptoms
            a. Approximately 80 percent no signs and symptoms
            b. Jaundice (yellow color to skin and eyes)
            c. Fatigue
            d. Abdominal pain (may be located in right upper quadrant)
            e. Nausea
            f. Dark urine
            g. Loss of appetite
        4. Protection recommendations
            a. There is no Hepatitis C vaccine
            b. Wear disposable gloves
            c. Wash hands thoroughly
            d. Double-bag and seal all soiled refuse
            e. Disinfect or sterilize nondisposable equipment
            f. Report any exposure
    C. Tuberculosis (pp. 36–37)
        1. Transmission
            a. Droplet
            b. Sputum
        2. Signs and symptoms
            a. Fever
            b. Cough (often coughing up blood)
            c. Night sweats
            d. Weight loss
        3. Protection recommendations
            a. Wear disposable gloves

  b. Wear a HEPA or N-95 (respirator) mask

  c. Perform artificial ventilation with OSHA-approved equipment

  d. Wash hands thoroughly

  e. Disinfect all nondisposable equipment

  f. Report any exposure

D. Acquired immunodeficiency syndrome (AIDS)/human immunodeficiency virus (HIV) (p. 37)

 1. Transmission

  a. Blood and blood products

  b. Semen

  c. Vaginal or cervical secretions

  d. Infected needles

  e. Mother-to-fetus

 2. Signs and symptoms

  a. Persistent, low-grade fever

  b. Night sweats

  c. Swollen lymph glands

  d. Loss of appetite

  e. Nausea

  f. Persistent diarrhea

  g. Headache

  h. Sore throat

  i. Fatigue

  j. Weight loss

  k. Shortness of breath

  l. Mental status changes

  m. Muscle and joint aches

  n. Rash

  o. Various opportunistic infections

 3. Protection recommendations

  a. Not all patients infected with HIV will develop AIDS

  b. Wear disposable gloves

  c. Wash hands thoroughly

  d. Double-bag and seal all soiled refuse

  e. Disinfect or sterilize nondisposable equipment

  f. Report any exposure

E. Severe acute respiratory syndrome (SARS) (pp. 37–38)

 1. Mode of transmission

  a. Respiratory droplets

 2. Signs and symptoms

  a. A high fever (usually greater than 100°F [38°C])

  b. Headache and body ache

  c. General feeling of discomfort

  d. Respiratory symptoms

  e. Diarrhea

  f. Dry cough

  g. Most patients will develop pneumonia

 3. Protection recommendations

  a. Wear a surgical mask

  b. Avoid inhaling respiratory droplets

  c. Wear eye protection

  d. Wear disposable gloves

  e. Avoid touching your eyes, nose, or mouth with your gloved hands

  f. Wash hands thoroughly

      g. Report any exposure

      h. Look for signs of fever and respiratory symptoms for 10 days after the exposure

F. West Nile virus (p. 38)

  1. Mode of transmission

      a. Bite of an infected mosquito

  2. Signs and symptoms

      a. Approximately 80 percent will not show any signs or symptoms

      b. Severe signs and symptoms

          (1) High fever

          (2) Headache and stiff neck

          (3) Confusion and disorientation to coma

          (4) Seizures

          (5) Muscle weakness

          (6) Numbness

          (7) Paralysis

          (8) Vision loss

          (9) Signs and symptoms in severe cases may last for several weeks

      c. Mild signs and symptoms

          (1) Fever

          (2) Headache and body ache

          (3) Nausea and vomiting

          (4) Skin rash to chest, stomach, and back

          (5) Soreness to neck from swollen lymph glands

          (6) Some signs and symptoms may be permanent

          (7) In mild cases, the signs and symptoms can last for only a few days to several weeks

  3. Protection recommendations

      a. Standard body substance isolation procedures

      b. More likely to contract the virus from a mosquito bite than through occupational exposure

G. Multidrug-resistant organisms (p. 38)

  1. Pathogens that have adapted to and have developed the ability to resist antimicrobial drugs

  2. Transmission

      a. Usually through direct person-to-person contact

  3. Most common types of pathogens

      a. Methicillin/oxacillin-resistant *Staphylococcus aureus* (MRSA)

      b. Vancomycin-resistant enterococci (VRE)

      c. Penicillin-resistant *Streptococcus pneumoniae* (PRSP)

      d. Drug-resistant *Streptococcus pneumoniae* (DRSP)

  4. Can produce many different types of infections resistant to standard antibiotic therapy

  5. Patients may develop

      a. Pneumonia

      b. Blood infections

      c. Ear infections

      d. Sinus infections

      e. Infections of the lining of the abdomen (peritonitis)

  6. Protection recommendations

      a. Standard body substance isolation procedures

CASE STUDY FOLLOW-UP

Ask a student volunteer to read the Case Study on page 19 of the textbook. You may wish to use the following questions to engage students in a discussion of the Case Study Follow-up that begins on page 39 of the textbook. Provide missing information and clarify ideas as needed.

Q1. How did you protect yourself from harm before the scene was secured by the police?

A1. *By keeping down and back as ordered by the police officer.*

Q2. How did you protect yourself from disease?

A2. *By approaching the scene after taking full BSI precautions.*

Q3. How could you tell that your partner was emotionally troubled by the call?

A3. *He was very quiet and tense. When he spoke, it was in anger. When you tried to get him to discuss the call, he responded angrily and said he was going to quit EMS.*

Q4. What did you and your partner do to handle the adverse emotional effects of this call?

A4. *The EMTs alerted their supervisor, who initiated the procedure for a critical incident stress debriefing (CISD) session in which feelings about the incident could be expressed. Your partner also received additional counseling.*

IN REVIEW

Assess students' ability to apply what they have just learned by discussing the In Review questions on page 00 in the textbook.

Q1. List the five stages through which a dying patient may pass.

A1. *The five stages through which a dying patient may pass are: denial— "Not me."; anger—"Why me?"; bargaining—"Okay, but first let me"; depression—"Okay, but I haven't"; and acceptance—"Okay, I am not afraid." (p. 20)*

Q2. Describe several things you can do—other than provide emergency medical care—to help dying patients.

A2. *Things you can do to help the dying patient may include: Maintain the patient's dignity; show respect for the patient; communicate who you are and what you are doing; allow family members to express themselves; listen empathetically; do not give false assurances, but allow for some hope; use a gentle tone of voice; let the patient know that everything that can be done to help will be done; use a reassuring touch if appropriate; do what you can to comfort the family. (pp. 20–21)*

Q3. List five of the signs and symptoms of chronic stress and burnout.

A3. *Signs and symptoms of chronic stress and burnout may include irritability with coworkers, family, and friends; inability to concentrate; difficulty sleeping and nightmares; anxiety; indecisiveness; guilt; loss of appetite; loss of sexual desire or interest; isolation; loss of interest in work. Also, problems in thinking—confusion, inability to make judgments or decisions, loss of motivation, chronic forgetfulness,* and loss of objectivity; psychological problems—depression, excessive anger, negativism, hostility, defensiveness, mood swings, and feelings of worthlessness; physical problems—persistent exhaustion, headaches, gastrointestinal distress, dizziness, and pounding heart; behavioral problems—overeating, increased alcohol or drug use, grinding teeth, hyperactivity, and lack of energy; social problems—increased interpersonal conflicts; decreased ability to relate to patients as individuals. (p. 23)

Q4. List four ways you can help deal with the stress in your life.

A4. *Ways to help deal with stress may include making lifestyle changes, such as improving diet, exercising, learning to relax, and avoiding self-medication of any kind; making changes to the work environment, such as developing a "buddy" system with a coworker, encouraging and supporting coworkers, taking periodic breaks for exercise, requesting work shifts that allow more time with family and friends, and requesting a rotation of duty assignment. (pp. 23–24)*

Q5. Identify some of the negative feelings families of EMTs may have in response to the job. Describe some of the ways you can help.

A5. *Negative feelings families of EMTs may have include lack of understanding, fear of separation or of being ignored, worry about on-call situations, inability to plan, frustrated desire to help and support. Ways to help include explaining the nature of your work and what you do for patients and how you feel about what you do; answering their questions and easing their anxieties; and encouraging them to join you in staying fit. (p. 24)*

Q6. Describe the safety precautions an EMT can take to prevent the spread of infectious disease.

A6. *Safety precautions to prevent the spread of infectious disease include body substance isolation (BSI) precautions taken at all times, including hand washing; use of personal protective equipment such as protective eyewear, protective gloves, gowns, and masks; cleaning, disinfecting, and sterilizing clothing and equipment; vaccinations; and reporting exposures as required by state law. (pp. 24–25)*

Q7. Discuss the responsibilities employers have, under OSHA guidelines, to protect emergency care personnel from transmission of infectious diseases.

A7. *Under OSHA guidelines, employers have the responsibility for developing a written exposure control plan and providing training, certain immunizations, and the proper equipment for protection against disease transmission. The employer is also responsible for developing and enforcing a written policy to be used in the case of an exposure of an employee to an infectious substance. (pp. 26–27)*

Q8. Discuss the responsibilities emergency care employees have, under OSHA guidelines, for their own protection against transmission of infectious diseases.

A8. *Employees share—along with employers—the responsibility of ensuring that the necessary equipment and procedures are in place for protection against exposure to infectious disease. In addition, employees must complete proper training and follow the procedures outlined in their exposure control plan. (pp. 27–33)*

Q9. List the personal protective equipment necessary for hazardous materials situations, rescue operations, and scenes of violence or crime.

A9. *Personal protective equipment for special situations includes the following: in a hazardous materials situation, a self-contained breathing apparatus and specialized "HAZMAT" suit; in a rescue operation, turnout gear, puncture-proof gloves, impact-resistant protective helmet, protective eyewear, and additional equipment dictated by local protocol, such as reflective clothing, rubber boots and slip-resistant gloves, or dust respirator. For violent scenes or crime scenes, rescuers may also wear body armor. (pp. 33–35)*

CRITICAL THINKING

Assess students' ability to respond to real-life emergency situations by discussing the Critical Thinking questions on page 40 in the textbook.

Q1. What would you do to ensure scene safety?

A1. *Make sure that law enforcement has secured the scene and deemed it safe for entry by ambulance personnel—and always stay alert for possible further violence. Another important aspect of ensuring scene safety would be to take standard (BSI) precautions and utilize appropriate personal protective equipment (PPE).*

Q2. What other resources should be requested?

A2. *Law enforcement should always be requested for calls involving crimes and/or violence. As for patient care resources, the EMTs should consider calling for ALS assistance.*

Q3. Why is this a potential high-stress situation?

A3. *This situation could be considered high-stress for two reasons; it involves a violent crime and a critically injured child.*

Q4. What can be done to reduce your stress associated with the call?

A4. *In preparation for calls such as this, the EMT should maintain good physical, emotional, social, behavioral, and psychological health. Following this call, the EMT should consider utilizing their agency's psychological resources—whether professional or peer-based.*

SKILLS DEMONSTRATION AND PRACTICE

Provide each student with a pair of latex gloves; pair of goggles, side protectors, or protective glasses; surgical mask; and surgical gown. Explain and demonstrate the correct technique for putting on each item. Emphasize again the purpose of each item and when each should be used.

Together as a group, direct students to put on each item. Encourage students to help one another, if necessary. Observe and correct errors.

ROLE PLAY

Provide students with the opportunity to apply what they have learned to a real-life situation encountered by EMS personnel. Ask two volunteers to play the role of EMT who are responding to a 9-1-1 call. Invite three other volunteers to be members of the public at the scene. Take the two EMT

©2008 by Pearson Education, Inc.
Prehospital Emergency Care, 8th ed.

players outside of the classroom and provide them with a jump kit containing two sets of latex gloves, goggles or protective glasses, surgical masks, and surgical gowns. Describe the following situation to them:

You are called to an unknown emergency at a tavern. You should act appropriately on what you find there. The emphasis of the scene is on your well-being. Do not worry about actually administering patient care. We will call you to the scene in just a minute.

Have the three "members of the public" come to the front of the classroom. Determine which of them will act as the patient, the patient's friend, and the stranger. Give the stranger a paper cutout of a gun. Describe the following situation to them and the class: All three of you are customers at a local tavern. Two of you are friends who have gotten into an argument (make up your own reason) with a stranger. You go outside to fight. The stranger pulls a small revolver from his waistband and shoots one of the friends in the abdomen. The other friend jumps on the stranger and they scuffle over the gun. Meanwhile, the bartender has called 9-1-1. When the EMTs arrive, behave as you would if you really were these people. Whoever has the gun should feel free to shoot the EMTs if he or she feels threatened. Tell the members of the public to take their places and to start acting. Call the "EMTs" back into the classroom. Allow the role play to progress naturally. Intervene only if the players seem to be at a loss for what to do.

If the EMTs call for police backup, say: "OK, the police have arrived and disarmed the person with the gun. The scene is now safe from violence."

Once the EMTs have put on the proper BSI equipment, end the role play. (The EMTs should not be asked to treat the "patient," since they have not yet reached this point in training.)

With the entire class, discuss the following:

- What did the EMTs do correctly to secure the scene from violence? What might have been done differently?

- What did the EMTs do correctly to protect themselves from biohazards? What might have been done differently?

ASSIGNMENTS

Assign students to read Chapter 3, "Medical, Legal, and Ethical Issues," before the next class. Also ask them to complete Chapter 2 of the Workbook.

EVALUATION

Chapter Quiz Distribute copies of the Chapter Quiz provided in Handout 2-2 to evaluate student understanding of this chapter. Remind students not to refer to their textbooks or notes while taking the quiz.

Test Manager You may wish to create a custom-tailored test using Prentice Hall *TestGen for Prehospital Emergency Care, Eighth Edition* to evaluate student understanding of this chapter.

Online Test Preparation (for students and instructors) Additional test preparation is available through *EMT Achieve: Basic Test Preparation* at http://www.prenhall.com/EMTAchieve. Instructors can also monitor student mastery online.

Reading/Reference
Textbook, pp. 41–56

Workbook
Chapter 2 Activities

Chapter Quiz
Handout 2-2

TestGen
Chapter 2 Test

Online Test Preparation
Send your students to
http://www.prenhall.com/
EMT Achieve

Handouts 2-3 to 2-6
Reinforcement Activities

**Brady Skills Series
EMT-B Videos/CD**
Visual Reinforcement

**PowerPoint
Presentation**
Chapter 2

Student CD
Chapter 2

Companion Website
http://www.prenhall.com/
mistovich

REINFORCEMENT

Handouts If classroom discussions or performance on the quiz indicates that some students have not fully mastered the chapter content, you may wish to assign some or all of the Reinforcement Handouts for this chapter.

TECH EXTRAS

Brady Skills Series EMT-B Videos/CD Have your students watch the skills come to life on either VHS or CD-ROM.

PowerPoint Presentation (for instructors) The PowerPoint material developed for this chapter offers useful reinforcement of chapter content.

Student CD A wide variety of material on this CD-ROM will reinforce and also expand student knowledge and skills.

Companion Website (for students) Additional review quizzes and links to EMS resources will contribute to further reinforcement of this chapter. Please visit http://www.prenhall.com/mistovich.

OBJECTIVES CHECKLIST

Cognitive	Date Mastered
1-2.1 List possible emotional reactions that the EMT-Basic may experience when faced with trauma, illness, death, and dying.	
1-2.2 Discuss the possible reactions that a family member may exhibit when confronted with death and dying.	
1-2.3 State the steps in the EMT-Basic's approach to the family confronted with death and dying.	
1-2.4 State the possible reactions that the family of the EMT-Basic may exhibit due to their outside involvement in EMS.	
1-2.5 Recognize the signs and symptoms of critical incident stress.	
1-2.6 State possible steps that the EMT-Basic may take to help reduce/alleviate stress.	
1-2.7 Explain the need to determine scene safety.	
1-2.8 Discuss the importance of body substance isolation (BSI).	
1-2.9 Describe the steps the EMT-Basic should take for personal protection from airborne and bloodborne pathogens.	
1-2.10 List the personal protective equipment necessary for each of the following situations: —Hazardous materials —Rescue operations —Violent scenes —Crime scenes —Exposure to bloodborne pathogens —Exposure to airborne pathogens	

Affective	Date Mastered
1-2.11 Explain the rationale for serving as an advocate for the use of appropriate protective equipment.	

Psychomotor	Date Mastered
1-2.12 Given a scenario with potential infectious exposure, the EMT-Basic will use appropriate personal protective equipment. At the completion of the scenario, the EMT-Basic will properly remove and discard the protective garments.	
1-2.13 Given the above scenario, the EMT-Basic will complete disinfection/cleaning and all reporting documentation.	

CHAPTER 2 QUIZ

Write the letter of the best answer in the space provided.

_____ 1. The stage of the dying process that can be characterized by the words "Why me?" is
  A. denial.   **C.** anger.
  B. acceptance.   **D.** depression.

_____ 2. A type of emergency call likely to produce extreme levels of stress is one involving
  A. a patient with a communicable disease.
  B. injury or death of a coworker.
  C. a geriatric patient.
  D. narcotics.

_____ 3. The goal of the CISD is to
  A. assign blame for the incident.
  B. assist patients in their recovery.
  C. assist emergency care workers in dealing with stress.
  D. allocate funds for ambulance services.

_____ 4. A less structured version of the CISD, which may be held from 1 to 4 hours after an incident and before the formal debriefing, is called a(n)
  A. resolution.   **C.** escape mechanism.
  B. defusing.   **D.** R&R process.

_____ 5. The stage of grieving in which a patient seeks to postpone death, even for a short time, is
  A. anger.   **C.** acceptance.
  B. bargaining.   **D.** denial.

_____ 6. Organisms that cause infection, such as viruses and bacteria, are
  A. toxins.   **C.** venoms.
  B. pathogens.   **D.** poisons.

_____ 7. The standard that assumes all blood and body fluids are infectious and requires emergency personnel to follow strict procedures to protect themselves from them is referred to as
  A. infective body fluid measures.
  B. isolated infection controls.
  C. preventive control substance standards.
  D. body substance isolation.

_____ 8. Gloves, masks, and gowns are examples of
  A. turnout gear.
  B. optional field equipment.
  C. personal protective equipment.
  D. "red bag" gear.

_____ 9. If a patient is suspected of having tuberculosis, an EMT should wear a _____ respirator.
  A. PPD   **C.** HEPA
  B. CISD   **D.** BSI

_____ **10.** Lifestyle changes that can help an EMT deal with stress include all of the following *except*
   A. cut down on sugar, fat, and caffeine.
   B. avoid exercise in your daily routine.
   C. avoid self-medication.
   D. keep balance in your life.

_____ **11.** Which of the following materials is *not* recommended for gloves to be used when there is the potential for contact with blood and other body fluids?
   A. latex   **C.** cotton
   B. vinyl   **D.** synthetics

_____ **12.** Equipment used as a BSI precaution includes all of the following *except*
   A. a HEPA respirator.   **C.** cotton scrub pants.
   B. vinyl gloves.   **D.** goggles.

_____ **13.** The process by which an object is subject to a chemical or physical substance that kills all microorganisms on the surface is
   A. sterilization.   **C.** disinfection.
   B. OR cleaning.   **D.** scouring.

_____ **14.** A situation that would usually call for the use of a gown as protection would be one involving a
   A. drug-overdose patient.   **C.** suspected TB patient.
   B. childbirth.   **D.** patient with a fractured leg.

_____ **15.** Dispose of all needles immediately after use in a(n)
   A. "green bag."   **C.** "OSHA jar."
   B. "HAZMAT box."   **D.** "sharps container."

_____ **16.** The single most important way an EMT can prevent the spread of infection is
   A. up-to-date immunizations.   **C.** wearing a jumpsuit.
   B. hand washing.   **D.** using a mask.

_____ **17.** In general, before entering a hazardous materials scene, EMTs should
   A. call for an ambulance.   **C.** put on a mask.
   B. put on goggles.   **D.** call for a specialized HAZMAT team.

_____ **18.** The test that can detect exposure to tuberculosis is the _____ test.
   A. PSA   **C.** SAT
   B. Mantoux   **D.** Rubella

_____ **19.** If you suspect the potential for violence at a scene, before entering it, you should
   A. call law enforcement.   **C.** put on body armor.
   B. turn on all lights and sirens. **D.** approach on foot.

_____ **20.** Vehicles, structures, and storage containers holding hazardous materials should be identified by
   A. signs or placards.   **C.** reflectors.
   B. strobe lights.   **D.** warning flags.

IN THE FIELD

Review the following real-life situation. Then answer the questions that follow.

You and your partner are dispatched to the scene of a motor-vehicle collision. As you approach the scene, you note that a large tanker truck has overturned in the middle of the road. The truck's driver is trapped in the cab. You are also informed by dispatch that a bystander has reported that the truck has placards displayed on its exterior.

1. What should you do at this point?

2. If you determine that the truck carries hazardous materials, what should you do next?

CHAPTER 2 REVIEW

Write the word or words that best complete each sentence in the space provided.

1. Dying patients experience five emotional stages—denial, anger, _____,

_____, and _____.

2. A(n) _____ _____

_____ is a single incident in which there are multiple patients.

3. Chronic _____ brought about by work-related problems in an emotionally

charged environment can lead to burnout.

4. _____ _____, which include deep-breathing

exercises and meditation, are valuable stress reducers.

5. Held within 24 to 72 hours of a critical incident, a(n) _____

_____ _____ _____ is a

process in which a team of trained peer counselors and mental health professionals meet with

rescuers and health care providers who have been involved in the incident.

6. The state of emotional exhaustion and irritability that can markedly decrease an EMT's effectiveness

in delivering medical care is called _____.

7. According to the U.S. Public Health Service, most contaminants can be removed from the skin with

_____ to _____ seconds of vigorous

_____.

8. Airborne _____ are spread by tiny droplets sprayed during breathing,

coughing, or sneezing.

9. The strict form of infection control for emergency personnel is known as

_____ _____ _____.

10. In addition to eye protection, gloves, and a mask, another item of personal protective equipment

that should be worn when there may be significant contact with blood or other body fluids is a(n)

_____.

11. As an advance safety precaution, an EMT should have a _____

_____ test for TB every year.

12. The level of cleaning for items such as backboards and cervical collars, which come in contact with

the intact skin of patients, is _____.

13. EMS personnel treating a patient suspected of having TB should use a(n)

_____ respirator.

14. Before entering scenes involving domestic disputes, gang fights, or bar fights, an EMT should first

_____ _____ _____

_____.

15. When approaching a wrecked vehicle that may be carrying hazardous materials, use binoculars to try

to find _____ or _____ that can identify the

material as hazardous.

WELL-BEING BASICS: LISTING

1. List at least five signs and/or symptoms of stress.

2. List four types of calls that have a higher-than-normal potential for causing stress in EMS personnel.

3. List and define five emotional stages a dying patient may go through.

4. List the basic types of personal protective equipment that EMTs can be expected to use on a regular basis.

REINFORCEMENT

WELL-BEING BASICS: TRUE OR FALSE

Indicate if the following statements are true or false by writing T or F in the space provided.

_____ **1.** Emergencies are rarely stressful.

_____ **2.** All seriously ill patients pass through a five-stage grieving process.

_____ **3.** The main purpose of a CISD is to affix responsibility for the events that took place during an incident.

_____ **4.** If a CISD is thorough, follow-up is not essential.

_____ **5.** Keeping yourself safe is your first priority when providing medical care as an EMT.

_____ **6.** Diseases are caused by pathogens, which may be spread through the air or by contact with blood and/or body fluids.

_____ **7.** In the practice of prehospital emergency care, all body fluids must be considered infectious.

_____ **8.** It is imperative that the EMT changes gloves between every patient contact.

_____ **9.** Because EMTs wear protective gloves while with patients, hand washing is not essential immediately after each call.

_____ **10.** A HEPA or N-95 respirator should be worn after contact with an HIV-positive patient.

_____ **11.** In some jurisdictions, when a patient is suspected of having an infection spread by droplets, a surgical-type mask may be placed on the patient if he or she is alert and cooperative.

_____ **12.** An EMT called to a scene of suspected violence should treat any life-threatening emergencies before calling law enforcement.

_____ **13.** A copy of the *Emergency Response Guidebook* should be on board every emergency vehicle.

_____ **14.** An EMT exposed to bloodborne pathogens should seek medical attention within 4 weeks after the exposure.

_____ **15.** An EMT should make preservation of evidence at a crime scene the highest priority.

LECTURE MASTER 2

The Well-Being of the EMT

Emotional Aspects of Emergency Care
Death and Dying
- Stages
- Family Members

Stress
- High-Stress Situations
- Stress Management
- Warning Signs
- Lifestyle Changes
- Balance
- Family and Friends
- Work Environment
- Professional Help

Critical Incident Stress Management

Scene Safety
Protection from Disease
Body Substance Isolation (BSI)
Advance Safety Precautions

Protection from Accidental Injury
Hazardous Materials
Rescue Situations
Violence and Crime

HANDOUT 2-2: Chapter 2 Quiz

1. C	**6.** B	**11.** C	**16.** B
2. B	**7.** D	**12.** C	**17.** D
3. C	**8.** C	**13.** A	**18.** B
4. B	**9.** C	**14.** B	**19.** A
5. B	**10.** B	**15.** D	**20.** A

HANDOUT 2-3: In the Field

1. Before approaching the truck, you should, from a safe distance, use binoculars to try to identify the placards on the truck. Check in the DOT's *Emergency Response Guidebook* to see what the placards indicate.

2. If the placards indicate the truck carries hazardous materials, call for assistance from appropriate specialized teams before attempting to assist the driver. Provide basic emergency care only after the scene is secured and patient contamination is limited. Follow your local protocols in regard to protective clothing.

HANDOUT 2-4: Chapter 2 Review

1. bargaining, depression, acceptance
2. multiple-casualty incident
3. Stress
4. Relaxation techniques
5. critical incident stress debriefing
6. burnout
7. 10, 15, hand washing
8. pathogens
9. body substance isolation
10. gown
11. Purified Protein Derivative (PPD)
12. disinfection
13. HEPA (or N-95)
14. call law enforcement
15. placards, signs

HANDOUT 2-5: Well-Being Basics: Listing

1. Any five: irritability with family, friends, or coworkers; inability to concentrate; difficulty in sleeping; nightmares; loss of appetite; loss of interest in sexual activity; anxiety; indecisiveness; guilt; isolation; loss of interest in work

2. Any four: multiple-casualty incidents; calls involving infants or children; severe injuries; abuse and neglect; death of a coworker

3. Denial ("Not me."); anger ("Why me?"); bargaining ("OK, but first let me . . ."); depression (OK, but I haven't . . ."); acceptance ("OK, I'm not afraid.")

4. Protective eyewear (safety glasses, goggles, side shields); gloves; gown; mask (surgical type for blood or other body fluids, HEPA or N-95 respirator for patient with suspected TB)

HANDOUT 2-6: Well-Being Basics: True or False

1. F	**5.** T	**9.** F	**13.** T
2. F	**6.** T	**10.** F	**14.** F
3. F	**7.** T	**11.** T	**15.** F
4. F	**8.** T	**12.** F	

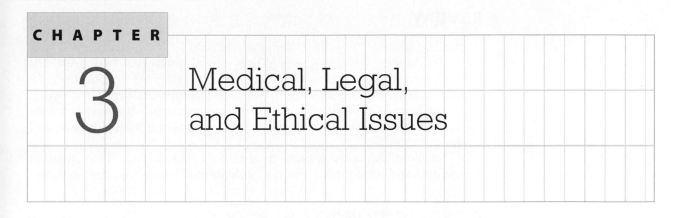

CHAPTER

3 Medical, Legal, and Ethical Issues

This chapter covers Lesson 1-3 and portions of Lesson 1-7 of the U.S. Department of Transportation's EMT-Basic National Standard Curriculum.

OBJECTIVES

Numbered objectives are from the U.S. Department of Transportation's EMT-Basic National Standard Curriculum. Asterisked objectives, if any, pertain to material that is supplemental to the DOT curriculum. Page numbers refer to pages in the textbook.

Cognitive

1-3.1 Define the EMT-Basic scope of practice. (pp. 42–44)

1-3.2 Discuss the importance of Do Not Resuscitate (DNR) (advanced directives) and local or state provisions regarding EMS application. (pp. 45–46)

1-3.3 Define consent and discuss the methods of obtaining consent. (pp. 44–46)

1-3.4 Differentiate between expressed and implied consent. (p. 45)

1-3.5 Explain the role of consent of minors in providing care. (p. 45)

1-3.6 Discuss the implications for the EMT-Basic in patient refusal of transport. (pp. 46, 49)

1-3.7 Discuss the issues of abandonment, negligence, and battery and their implications to the EMT-Basic. (pp. 49–50)

1-3.8 State the conditions necessary for the EMT-Basic to have a duty to act. (pp. 43–44)

1-3.9 Explain the importance, necessity, and legality of patient confidentiality. (p. 51)

1-3.10 Discuss the considerations of the EMT-Basic in issues of organ retrieval. (p. 52)

1-3.11 Differentiate the actions that an EMT-Basic should take to assist in the preservation of a crime scene. (p. 53)

1-3.12 State the conditions that require an EMT-Basic to notify local law enforcement officials. (p. 54)

Affective

1-3.13 Explain the role of EMS and the EMT-Basic regarding patients with DNR orders. (pp. 45–46)

1-3.14 Explain the rationale for the needs, benefits, and usage of advanced directives. (pp. 45–46)

1-3.15 Explain the rationale for the concept of varying degrees of DNR. (p. 46)

Total Teaching Time
125 minutes

Resources Needed
- Scored Chapter 2 Quizzes
- Medical jump kit with BSI equipment

Additional Resources
Larmon/Davis, *Basic Life Support Skills*

Elling, *EMT Achieve: Basic Test Preparation*

Limmer/Mistovich/ O'Keefe, *Audio Lecture & Study Guide: EMT*

Mistovich/Kuvlesky, *SUCCESS! for the EMT, Second Edition*

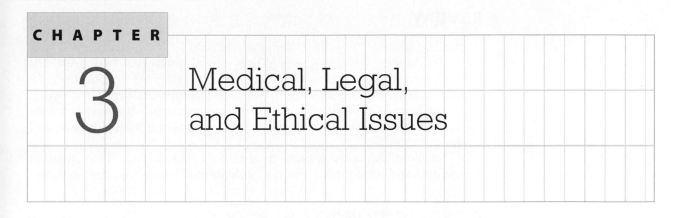

REVIEW

In the last lesson, "The Well-Being of the EMT," students learned why safeguarding their well-being as EMTs is critical. Strategies were presented that will help students cope with all kinds of stress they will encounter—job-related or otherwise—including that which accompanies death and dying. They also learned about equipment to use in dangerous situations and ways to approach such situations that will keep them physically safe and emotionally well.

Distribute the scored quizzes from the last class. Go over each question on the quiz and handle any concerns students may have about the answers.

INTRODUCTION TO CHAPTER 3

Chapter 3, "Medical, Legal, and Ethical Issues," is the third lesson in Module 1. Point out that medical, legal, and ethical issues are vital elements of the EMT's life, both on and off duty. Your students may already have questions, such as: "Should I stop to treat an accident victim when I'm off duty?", "Should patient information be released to an attorney over the phone?", "May a child be treated without parents being present?" Students may begin to wonder if they can provide emergency care at all without being sued! To arrive at answers to questions like those above, they will have to consider their scope of practice, advance directives, the issues surrounding patient consent, their duty to act, and other factors.

Distribute the Chapter 3 Objectives Checklist and give students a few minutes to look it over. Then briefly paraphrase the objectives for this lesson in your own words.

LECTURE

The following suggested lecture outline is based on the Department of Transportation's EMT-Basic National Standard Curriculum. In some places, the DOT curriculum has been rearranged or expanded upon so that it is more complete or easier for the student to understand. The page numbers in parentheses refer to pages in the textbook. The parenthetical references in dark, heavy type are to figures, tables, and scans in the textbook.

MEDICAL, LEGAL, AND ETHICAL ISSUES

- **I. Legal responsibilities** (pp. 42–44)
  - **A.** Scope of practice (pp. 42–43)
    - **1.** Actions and care that are legally allowed by the state in which he or she is providing emergency medical care
    - **2.** National EMS Scope of Practice
  - **B.** Standard of care (pp. 42–43)
    - **1.** Right assessment and care
    - **2.** Properly performed assessment and care
    - **3.** Sources
      - **a.** Recognized and accepted EMT textbooks
      - **b.** Expected care in community or region
      - **c.** Local and state protocols
      - **d.** USDOT National Standard Curriculum
      - **e.** EMS system's polices and procedures
  - **C.** Duty to Act (pp. 43–44)
    - **1.** A contractual or legal obligation to provide care

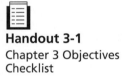

Handout 3-1
Chapter 3 Objectives Checklist

Lecture Master
You may wish to display Lecture Master 3 when presenting the lecture to the class.

Teaching Tip
Be prepared to answer a lot of questions when teaching this chapter. New EMTs are naturally curious and concerned about the issues covered in this chapter.

Reading/Reference
Barishansky, R.M. "An Interview with Doug Wolfberg on EMS legal Issues," *EMS Magazine,* Jan. 2005.

      a. Implied

        (1) Patient calls for an ambulance and the dispatcher confirms that an ambulance will be sent

        (2) Treatment is begun on a patient

      b. Formal

        (1) Ambulance service has a written contract with a municipality

        (2) Specific clauses within the contract should indicate when service can be refused to a patient

  2. Legal duty to act may not exist. May be moral/ethical considerations

      a. In some states, while off duty, if the EMT comes upon an accident while driving

      b. When driving the ambulance not in the company's service area and EMT observes an accident

        (1) Moral/ethical duty to act

        (2) Risk management

        (3) Documentation

      c. Specific state regulations regarding duty to act

  3. Responsibilities

      a. Duty to self

      b. Duty to your patient

      c. Duty to your partner

      d. Duty to take care of equipment

D. Good Samaritan laws (p. 44)

  1. Protection from liability

  2. Performed in good faith

  3. Willful or wanton harm

E. Sovereign immunity (p. 44)

  1. Protection for government

F. Medical direction (p. 44)

  1. Follow approved standing orders and protocols

  2. Establish communications with medical direction

  3. Consult medical direction with patient care questions

II. Ethical responsibilities (p. 44)

A. Patient priority (p. 44)

  1. Place patient welfare above all else, except personal safety

  2. Respect human dignity, without regard to nationality, race, gender, creed, or status

B. Knowledge and skills (p. 44)

  1. Maintain skills mastery

  2. Keep current on changes in EMS

C. Professionalism (p. 44)

  1. Uphold professional standards

  2. Critically review performances for areas of improvement

  3. Report with honesty

  4. Maintain confidentiality

  5. Work harmoniously with other responders and health care personnel

III. Issues of patient consent and refusal (pp. 44–45)

A. Types of consent (p. 45)

  1. Informed consent

      a. Informed of the care to be provided and associated risks

  2. Expressed consent

      a. Patient must be of legal age

      b. Patient must be able to make a rational decision

On the Net

Explanation of Good Samaritan Laws with state-by-state listing. http://www.medicalreserve corps.gov/appendixc.htm

c. Patient must be informed of the steps of the procedures and all related risks

d. Consent must be obtained from every conscious, mentally competent adult before rendering treatment

3. Implied consent

   a. Consent assumed from the unconscious patient requiring emergency intervention

   b. Based on the assumption that the unconscious patient would consent to lifesaving interventions

4. Children and mentally incompetent adults

   a. Consent for treatment must be obtained from the parent or legal guardian

     (1) Emancipation issues

     (2) State regulations regarding age of minors

   b. When life-threatening situations exist and the parent or legal guardian is not available for consent, emergency treatment should be rendered based on implied consent

IV. **Advanced directives** (pp. 45–46)

  A. Do Not Resuscitate (DNR) orders (pp. 45–46) **(Fig. 3-1, p. 47)**

   1. May also be called Do Not Attempt Resuscitation (DNAR) order

   2. Patient has the right to refuse resuscitative efforts

   3. In general, requires written order from physician

   4. Review state and local legislation/protocols relative to DNR orders and advance directives

   5. When in doubt or when written orders are not present, the EMT should begin resuscitation efforts

  B. Living will (p. 46)

   1. General health care issue outlining patient's requests

  C. Health care proxy (p. 46)

   1. Also called Durable Power of Attorney for Health Care

   2. Appoints a surrogate to make medical decision when patient is not able

V. **Refusals** (pp. 46–49)

  A. The competent patient has the right to refuse treatment (p. 46)

  B. The patient may withdraw from treatment at any time (p. 46)

  C. Refusals must be made by mentally competent adults following the rules of expressed consent (p. 46)

  D. The patient must be informed of and fully understand all the risks and consequences associated with refusal of treatment/transport (p. 46)

  E. Patient must sign a "release from liability" form (p. 46) **(Fig. 3-2, p. 48)**

  F. When in doubt, err in favor of providing care (p. 46)

  G. Protecting yourself (pp. 46–49)

   1. Try again to persuade the patient to go to a hospital

   2. Ensure that the patient is able to make a rational, informed decision, for example, not under the influence of alcohol or other drugs, or illness/injury effects

   3. Consult medical direction as directed by local protocol

   4. Consider assistance of law enforcement

     a. Document any assessment findings and emergency medical care given; if the patient still refuses, then have the patient sign a refusal form

On the Net

Overview of advanced directives and DNR orders. http://familydoctor.org/handouts/003.html

On the Net

What an EMT can do to help the patient without dishonoring advanced directives. http://www.fix.net/~sloemsa/policy/117.html

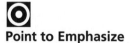

Point to Emphasize

Stress that run reports may be called into court as evidence years after the incidents they document.

Point to Emphasize

Most lawsuits against EMS systems arise over acts of commission, not of omission.

5. Encourage the patient to seek assistance if symptoms develop
6. The EMT should never make an independent decision not to transport

VI. Other legal aspects of emergency care (pp. 49–51)
    A. Negligence (p. 49)
        1. Act of deviating from an accepted standard of care through carelessness, inattention, disregard, inadvertence, or oversight, which results in further injury to the patient
        2. Simple negligence
            a. Deviation from the standard of care
        3. Gross negligence
            a. Care that is dangerous to the patient
        4. Plaintiff must prove:
            a. EMT had a duty to act
            b. EMT breached that duty
            c. Patient suffered a compensable injury (damages)
                (1) Injuries that are real, demonstrable, and recognizable by law
            d. Proximate cause
                (1) Injuries suffered by the patient were the direct result of (caused by) the EMT's negligence
    B. Intentional tort (pp. 49–51)
        1. Action knowingly committed by an individual that is considered to be civilly wrong according to law
        2. Abandonment
            a. Termination of patient care without ensuring continuation of care at the same level or higher **(Fig. 3-3, p. 50)**
        3. Assault
            a. Threat to inflict harm
         4. Battery
            a. Unlawfully touching a patient without his or her consent
        5. False imprisonment
            a. Intentionally transporting a competent patient without his consent
        6. Defamation
            a. Damaging a person's character, reputation, or standing within the community
            b. Slander
                (1) Spoken defamation
            c. Libel
                (1) Written defamation

VII. Confidentiality (p. 51)
    A. Confidential information (p. 51)
        1. Patient history gained through interview
        2. Assessment findings
        3. Treatment rendered
    B. Releasing confidential information (p. 51)
        1. Requires a written release form signed by the patient
            a. Do not release on request, written or verbal, unless legal guardianship has been established
        2. When a release is not required
            a. Other health care providers need to know information to continue care

Point to Emphasize
Issues of confidentiality should be guarded at all times by the EMT.

    b. State law requires reporting incidents such as rape, abuse, or gunshot wounds

    c. Third-party payment billing forms

    d. Legal subpoena

  C. Health Insurance Portability and Accountability Act (HIPAA) (p. 51)

    1. Protects the privacy of patient health care information

    2. Provides the patient with control over how the information is distributed and used

    3. Policies and procedures regarding record-keeping storage, access, release, and discussion

    4. Discussing patient-specific information only with individuals with whom it is medically necessary

    5. Training on specific policies and procedures regarding privacy issue by your EMS agency

    6. EMT and patient provided with the policies and procedures

    7. Obtain patient signature acknowledging receipt (usually part of the insurance/release form)

    8. EMS agency will designate a Privacy Officer to oversee HIPAA regulations

VIII. **Consolidated Omnibus Budget Reconciliation Act (COBRA) and Emergency Medical Treatment and Active Labor Act (EMTALA)** (pp. 51–52)

  A. Federal regulations to ensure public's access to emergency health care (p. 51)

  B. EMTALA also known as "anti-dumping statute" (p. 51)

  C. Affects ambulance services, especially if hospital owned (p. 52)

  D. Transferring facility must ensure patient stability to the extent of their capabilities (p. 52)

  E. Ensure transferring crew is capable of care needed during transport (p. 52)

  F. Hospital-based ambulance must avoid bypass due to insurance/financial reasons (p. 52)

  G. Initial transport to a medical facility (p. 52)

    1. Do not base transport to a specific facility on ability to pay

    2. Never report ability to pay over the radio

    3. Do not bypass a medical facility able to treat the patient unless directed by medical direction or the patient

    4. Clearly document the reason for bypassing a specific medical facility

  H. Transport between medical facilities (pp. 52)

    1. Get a full and clear report about the patient's condition

    2. Ensure appropriate level of care within the scope of practice

    3. Obtain patient consent form

    4. Obtain written certification of transfer including sending and receiving physician information

    5. Know where you are going and take the quickest possible route

IX. **Special situations** (pp. 52–53)

  A. Donor/organ harvesting consideration (p. 52)

    1. Requires a signed legal permission document

      a. Separate donor card

      b. Intent to be a donor on the reverse of patient's driver's license

2. A potential organ donor should not be treated differently from any other patient requesting treatment
3. The EMT's role in organ harvesting
   a. Identify the patient as a potential donor
   b. Establish communication with medical direction
   c. Provide care to maintain viable organs

B. Medical identification insignia (p. 52)
1. Bracelet, necklace, card, sticker on driver's license (**Fig. 3-4, p. 53**)
2. Indicates a serious medical condition of the patient
   a. Allergies
   b. Diabetes
   c. Epilepsy
   d. Others

C. Recognizing death in the field (pp. 52–53)
1. Presumptive signs of death
   a. Absence of a pulse, breathing, and breath sounds
   b. Complete unresponsiveness to any stimuli
   c. No eye movement or pupil response
   d. Absence of a blood pressure
   e. No reflexes
   f. Dependent lividity
2. Obvious signs of death
   a. Decapitation
   b. Rigor mortis
   c. Decomposition
   d. Dependent lividity
3. Cases of death usually requiring investigation by medical examiner or coroner
   a. Homicides
   b. Suicides
   c. Violent deaths
   d. Crash-related deaths
   e. Unusual scene characteristics
   f. Sudden infant death syndrome (SIDS)
   g. Dead on arrival (depending on protocol)

X. Potential crime scene/evidence preservation (pp. 53–54)
A. Dispatch should notify police personnel (p. 53)
B. Responsibility of the EMT (pp. 53–54)
1. Touch only what you need to touch
2. Move only what you need to move to protect the patient and to provide proper emergency care
3. Do not use the telephone unless the police give you permission to do so
4. In the absence of police permission, move the patient only if the patient is in danger or must be moved in order for you to provide care
5. Observe and document anything unusual
6. If possible, do not cut through holes in clothing possibly caused by bullets or stabbing
7. Do not cut through any knot in a rope or tie (a possible clue); cut away from the knot; do not cover the patient with a sheet
8. If the crime is rape, do not wash the patient or allow the patient to wash; ask the patient not to change clothing, use

Slides/Videos
Medic Alert Slides. Medic Alert Foundation, PO Box 381009, Turlock, CA 95381-9009.

the bathroom, or take anything by mouth, because doing so may destroy evidence

XI. Special reporting situations (p. 54)

    A. Established by state legislation and may vary from state to state (p. 54)

    B. Commonly required reporting situations (p. 54)

        1. Abuse

            a. Child

            b. Elderly

            c. Spouse

        2. Crime

            a. Wounds obtained by violent crime

            b. Sexual assault

        3. Drug-related injuries

    C. Infectious disease exposure (p. 54)

    D. Patient restraint laws, for example, forcing someone to be transported against his or her will (p. 54)

    E. Mentally incompetent, for example, intoxication with injuries

    F. Attempted suicide (p. 54)

    G. Dog bites (p. 54)

CASE STUDY FOLLOW-UP

Ask a student volunteer to read the Case Study that begins on page 42 of the textbook. You may wish to use the following questions to engage students in a discussion of the Case Study Follow-up that begins on page 55 of the textbook. Provide missing information and clarify ideas as needed.

Q1. What signs alerted you to the possibility that neglect or abuse was involved in this scene?

A1. *Mrs. Schuman was wearing only a nightgown even though the temperature was only 38°F. She said, "It's my husband, I just can't handle him anymore." The house was in shambles. The rooms were so cluttered that you and your partner could barely pass through. Schuman's bedsheets and undergarments were stained with dried urine. The odor was very strong and the temperature inside the room was very low.*

Q2. What was your legal and ethical responsibility in this situation?

A2. *To report the situation in order to ensure the Schumans' safety after discharge from the hospital.*

Q3. What action did you take regarding this situation?

A3. *Contacting the hospital's social service department.*

Q4. What was the result of your action?

A4. *Mr. Schuman was diagnosed with a gastric ulcer and organic brain syndrome. Additionally, Mrs. Schuman was diagnosed with Alzheimer's disease. Both became residents of a local extended-care nursing home, under 24-hour supervision.*

Assess students' ability to apply what they have just learned by discussing the Review Questions on page 56 in the textbook.

Q1. Define a "Do Not Resuscitate (DNR)" order, and explain how an EMT should respond if presented with such an order.

A1. *A DNR order is an order, written in advance, signed by the patient and usually by a doctor, refusing attempts to resuscitate the patient. The EMT must be familiar with local protocols regarding DNRs and should consult medical direction before following a DNR. If in doubt, the EMT must provide resuscitation. (pp. 45–46)*

Q2. Define the three types of consent that must be obtained before emergency care is provided.

A2. *The three types of consent are as follows: Expressed consent must be obtained from every conscious, mentally competent adult before treatment is started and after necessary procedures and related risks have been explained in terms the patient can understand. Implied consent is understood when an unresponsive patient requires life-saving emergency treatment. Consent to provide emergency treatment to a minor or to a mentally incompetent adult must be obtained from a parent or legal guardian. (p. 45)*

Q3. Explain how to handle a refusal of treatment.

A3. *A patient must be informed of and fully understand all risks and consequences involved in refusing treatment or transport. Then the patient must sign an official "release from liability" form—or a patient's witnessed refusal to sign the form must be obtained—and must be part of the documentation of the case. (pp. 46–49)*

Q4. Describe what must happen for the EMT to be liable for abandonment or negligence.

A4. *An EMT can be charged with abandonment if he or she discontinues treatment of a patient (unless so ordered by law enforcement personnel) or if treatment is discontinued without ensuring that another health care professional with at least as much expertise has taken over treatment. An EMT can be charged with negligence if the emergency care provided to a patient deviates from the accepted standard of care and results in further injury. (p. 50)*

Q5. Describe what it means for an EMT to have a duty to act.

A5. *An EMT while on the job has a duty to act, or a legal obligation to provide necessary emergency care to the best of his or her ability and training to a patient who needs it. (pp. 43–44)*

Q6. List the conditions under which an EMT may release confidential patient information.

A6. *In general, releasing confidential patient information requires a written release form signed by the patient or a legal guardian. An EMT may also be allowed to release confidential patient information when another health care provider needs it in order to continue medical care, when requested to by the police as part of a criminal investigation, when the information is required on a third-party billing form, and when required by legal subpoena to provide the information in court. (p. 51)*

Q7. List some ways in which an EMT can preserve evidence at a crime scene.

A7. *An EMT can preserve evidence at a crime scene by not touching or moving anything that is not needed to provide proper emergency care to the patient; by using the telephone only if the police have given permission; by moving the patient only if the patient is in danger or must be moved in order to provide care; by observing and documenting anything unusual at the scene; by not cutting through holes in the patient's clothing that may have been caused by bullets or stabbing weapons, if possible; and by asking the rape patient not to change clothing, use the bathroom, or take anything by mouth. (pp. 53–54)*

Q8. List situations that an EMT may be required to report.

A8. *The types of situations an EMT may be required to report include suspected abuse of children or the elderly; injuries that may have resulted from a crime, including sexual assault; drug-related injuries; suspected infectious disease exposure; use of patient restraints; cases in which a patient appears mentally incompetent or intoxicated; attempted suicides; and dog bites. (p. 54)*

CRITICAL THINKING

Assess students' ability to respond to real-life emergency situations by discussing the Critical Thinking questions on page 56 in the textbook.

Q1. How would you initially gain consent in this patient?

A1. *Since the patient is alert, the EMT would seek expressed consent by simply asking for permission to treat her. The patient could then give consent in three ways; verbal, physical (such as a nod), or by not protesting or pulling away as the care is initiated.*

Q2. How would you manage the patient's refusal to be transported?

A2. *The EMT should begin by explaining in detail the potential consequences of refusing care. The patient should then be asked to repeat those consequences back so it is clear that she understands them and is competent to make personal care decisions. The EMT should seek consent several more times that to allow for continuation of treatment and transport. If the patient continues to refuse and is deemed competent and able to make a rationale decision, document in detail what was told to the patient, including the consequences of not allowing for further treatment or transport, read back to the patient what was documented, and then secure a patient signature on the appropriate refusal of care form and fully document the incident. Have a witness, preferably a family member or neutral person, sign the report.*

Q3. What legal issues may you face if you continue with treatment and transport?

A3. *Since the patient is of legal age, and if she has been found competent to make personal care decisions, forcing treatment or transport following her refusal of care could result in charges of assault, battery, and/or false imprisonment.*

ROLE PLAY

Provide students with the opportunity to apply what they have learned to a real-life situation encountered by EMS personnel. Ask two volunteers to play the role of EMTs who are responding to a 9-1-1 call, one volunteer to be the patient, and two volunteers to be the patient's mother and father.

Take the two EMT players outside of the classroom and provide them with a jump kit containing BSI equipment. Describe this situation to them:

You are called to the home of an AIDS patient who may be near death. You should act appropriately on what you find there. The focus of the scene is its medical, ethical, and legal considerations. However, you should also act to protect your well-being, as you learned in the last lesson. Do not worry about administering patient care. We will call you to the scene in just a minute.

Have the patient and two family members come to the front of the classroom. Determine which of them will act as the patient and which as the patient's parents. Describe the following situation to them and the class:

The patient is a young adult male who is living at his parent's home. He is in the end stages of AIDS and is near death. He is suffering from dementia but is conscious. He says he does not want to die and has not signed an advance directive. The patient's parents have been caring for him for a year. They love their son and are tired of seeing him suffer.

They ask the EMTs to let the patient "go in peace."

Tell the patient and his parents to take their places and to start acting. Call the EMTs back into the classroom. Allow the role play to progress naturally. Intervene only if the players seem to be at a loss for what to do.

If the EMTs fail to put on the proper BSI equipment, remind them to do so. If the EMTs decide to phone their medical director, play that part and direct them to transport the patient.

End the play when a decision has been made about whether the patient will be treated. (The EMTs should not be asked to treat the patient since they have not yet reached this point in training.)

With the entire class, discuss the following: Did the EMTs make the proper decision about treating this patient? Why or why not? What, if anything, could they have done differently?

ASSIGNMENTS

Assign students to read Chapter 4, "The Human Body," before the next class. Also ask them to complete Chapter 3 of the Workbook.

EVALUATION

Chapter Quiz Distribute copies of the Chapter Quiz provided in Handout 3-2 to evaluate student understanding of this chapter. Remind students not to refer to their textbooks or notes while taking the quiz.

Test Manager You may wish to create a custom-tailored test using Prentice Hall *TestGen for Prehospital Emergency Care, Eighth Edition* to evaluate student understanding of this chapter.

Reading/Reference
Textbook, pp. 57–100

Workbook
Chapter 3 Activities

Chapter Quiz
Handout 3-2

TestGen
Chapter 3 Test

Online Test Preparation
Send your students to
http://www.prenhall.com/
EMTAchieve

Handouts 3-3 to 3-6
Reinforcement Activities

**Brady Skills Series
EMT-B Videos/CD**
Visual Reinforcement

**PowerPoint
Presentation**
Chapter 3

Student CD
Chapter 3

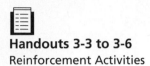

Companion Website
http://www.prenhall.com/
mistovich

Online Test Preparation (for students and instructors) Additional test preparation is available through *EMT Achieve: Basic Test Preparation* at http://www.prenhall.com/EMTAchieve. Instructors can also monitor student mastery online.

REINFORCEMENT

Handouts If classroom discussions or performance on the quiz indicates that some students have not fully mastered the chapter content, you may wish to assign some or all of the Reinforcement Handouts for this chapter.

TECH EXTRAS

Brady Skills Series EMT-B Videos/CD Have your students watch the skills come to life on either VHS or CD-ROM.

PowerPoint Presentation (for instructors)   The PowerPoint material developed for this chapter offers useful reinforcement of chapter content.

Student CD A wide variety of material on this CD-ROM will reinforce and also expand student knowledge and skills.

Companion Website (for students)   Additional review quizzes and links to EMS resources will contribute to further reinforcement of this chapter. Please visit http://www.prenhall.com/mistovich.

OBJECTIVES CHECKLIST

Cognitive		Date Mastered
1-3.1	Define the EMT-Basic scope of practice.	
1-3.2	Discuss the importance of Do Not Resuscitate (DNR) (advance directives) and local or state provisions regarding EMS application.	
1-3.3	Define consent and discuss the methods of obtaining consent.	
1-3.4	Differentiate between expressed and implied consent.	
1-3.5	Explain the role of consent of minors in providing care.	
1-3.6	Discuss the implications for the EMT-Basic in patient refusal of transport.	
1-3.7	Discuss the issues of abandonment, negligence, and battery and their implications to the EMT-Basic.	
1-3.8	State the conditions necessary for the EMT-Basic to have a duty to act.	
1-3.9	Explain the importance, necessity, and legality of patient confidentiality.	
1-3.10	Discuss the considerations of the EMT-Basic in issues of organ retrieval.	
1-3.11	Differentiate the actions that an EMT-Basic should take to assist in the preservation of a crime scene.	
1-3.12	State the conditions that require an EMT-Basic to notify local law enforcement officials.	

Affective		Date Mastered
1-3.13	Explain the role of EMS and the EMT-Basic regarding patients with DNR orders.	
1-3.14	Explain the rationale for the needs, benefits, and usage of advanced directives.	
1-3.15	Explain the rationale for the concept of varying degrees of DNR.	

OBJECTIVES

CHAPTER 3 QUIZ

Write the letter of the best answer in the space provided.

_____ 1. Mentally competent adults of legal age who accept care from an EMS crew are said to give _____ consent.
    A. guardian   **C.** partial
    B. implied   **D.** expressed

_____ 2. EMS personnel can treat unconscious patients because the law holds that rational patients would consent to treatment if they were conscious. This principle is known as _____ consent.
    A. expressed   **C.** emergency
    B. implied   **D.** actual

_____ 3. Minors who are married or of a certain age and who are legally able to give consent for medical care are known as
    A. emancipated.   **C.** released.
    B. practiced.   **D.** responsible.

_____ 4. When a patient refuses care, he or she must sign a(n)
    A. codicil.   **C.** DNR order.
    B. insurance rider.   **D.** release from liability form.

_____ 5. A legal document, usually signed by the patient and his physician, which states that the patient has a terminal illness and does not wish to prolong life through resuscitative efforts, is called a(n)
    A. surrogate statement.   **C.** codicil.
    B. DNR order.   **D.** unspecified treatment order.

_____ 6. A person whom the signer of a document names to make health care decisions for her in case the signer is unable to make such decisions for herself is called a(n)
    A. proxy.   **C.** designated agent.
    B. assistant.   **D.** heir.

_____ 7. Legislative measures intended to provide legal protection for citizens and some health care personnel who administer emergency care are known as
    A. First Responder laws.   **C.** Helping Hands legislation.
    B. EMS Acts.   **D.** Good Samaritan laws.

_____ 8. An EMT's obligation in certain situations to provide care to a patient is referred to as a(n)
    A. agency.   **C.** proxy.
    B. surrogate's role.   **D.** duty to act.

_____ 9. If a jury finds that an EMT had a duty to a patient, that he failed to carry out that duty properly, and that his action caused harm to the patient, the EMT could be convicted of
    A. failure to act.   **C.** fraud.
    B. libel.   **D.** negligence.

_____ 10. A living will is one example of a(n)
    A. Good Samaritan law.   **C.** warrant.
    B. confidentiality agreement.   **D.** advance directive.

©2008 by Pearson Education, Inc.
Prehospital Emergency Care, 8th ed.

_____11. The principle that information about a patient's history, condition, or treatment must not be shared with unauthorized parties is called
A. duty to withhold.
B. breach of duty.
C. confidentiality.
D. disclosure.

_____12. If you discover that a critically injured patient is an organ donor, as an EMT, you should
A. not provide further care.
B. contact medical direction.
C. notify the trauma team.
D. notify the police.

_____13. Once police have made the scene safe, the priority of the EMT at a crime scene is to
A. preserve evidence.
B. provide patient care.
C. contact dispatch.
D. assist the investigation.

_____14. Leaving a patient after care has been initiated and before the patient has been transferred to someone with equal or greater medical training is known as
A. assault.
B. abandonment.
C. false imprisonment.
D. proximate cause.

_____15. The actions and care that an EMT is legally allowed to perform are referred to as
A. duty to act.
B. professional practice.
C. limits of liability.
D. scope of practice.

IN THE FIELD

Review the following real-life situation. Then answer the questions that follow.

You are dispatched to 44 Crescent Drive for a "difficulty breathing" call. There is something familiar about the address, which is in a neighborhood of fashionable homes, but you can't quite place it.

Pulling up at the residence, you quickly make sure the scene is quiet and safe. You and your partner grab the jump kit and head for the front door. Before you can ring the bell, a man swings the door open and motions you inside. Now you know why the address is familiar. The man is James Sherman, a prominent figure in city politics.

He leads you upstairs, explaining as you go that his son has long suffered from cystic fibrosis. Right now, he's having extreme difficulty in breathing, and Mr. Sherman would like you to transport him to Samaritan Hospital.

In the bedroom to which he leads you, you find the son, Jared, lying in bed. He appears to be in his early 20s and is obviously struggling to breathe. Yet as you approach the bed, he manages to gasp out, "Go 'way . . . no doctors . . . want to die."

His father turns to you and says, "Don't pay him any mind. Just get him on oxygen and to the hospital."

1. What should you do in this situation?

2. Later that day, you return to base. As you're getting out of your vehicle, a woman walks up. She identifies herself as a reporter for the local paper and says, "I hear there was a tough call at Jim Sherman's house with his son, Jared. You know, you can help protect yourself if you get the straight facts into the paper. I won't have to mention your name, and I won't reveal who my sources are." What should you do in this situation?

CHAPTER 3 REVIEW

Write the word or words that best complete each sentence in the space provided.

1. In the case of a(n) _____ patient, consent to treat may be assumed.

2. When dealing with children and mentally incompetent adults, the _____ or _____ have the legal authority to give consent.

3. _____ minors are those who are married or of a certain age to provide consent.

4. Failure to provide the standard of care is one of the elements that must be proved in a case involving a charge of _____ against an EMT.

5. If all efforts fail and the patient does not accept your care or transportation, you must have the patient sign a(n) _____ form.

6. To refuse care, a patient must be _____ and understand the risks of rejecting treatment.

7. A legal _____ _____ is an advance directive that prevents unwanted resuscitation.

8. An EMT who is on an ambulance and is dispatched to a call clearly has a(n) _____ _____ _____.

9. In many states, an off-duty EMT has no legal obligation to provide emergency _____.

10. If the EMT is off duty and begins care, then leaves the patient before other trained personnel arrive, he or she may be considered to have _____ the patient.

11. _____ _____ laws have been developed in most states to provide immunity to individuals trying to help others in emergencies.

12. The only time that confidential information about a patient may be disclosed is when the patient has signed a(n) _____ _____.

13. A(n) _____ _____ is a patient who has completed a legal document that allows for that patient's organs and tissues to be used by others in the event of death.

14. A(n) _____ _____ is a place where a crime has

been committed or any place that evidence relating to a crime may be found.

15. Obvious signs of death, with which resuscitative efforts do not have to be made, include

decomposition of the body, dependent lividity, _____, and

_____ _____.

MEDICAL, LEGAL, AND ETHICAL ISSUES: LISTING

1. List three types of consent.

2. List five actions you should take if a patient refuses treatment.

3. List the four specific elements of a malpractice case against an EMT.

4. List three types of incidents that most states require health care professionals to report to authorities.

5. List six presumptive signs of death that should be identified when dealing with a patient who has a Do Not Resuscitate order.

REINFORCEMENT

MEDICAL, LEGAL, AND ETHICAL ISSUES: TRUE OR FALSE

Indicate if the following statements are true or false by writing T or F in the space provided.

_____ 1. Consent, or permission from the patient, is required for any treatment or action by the EMT.

_____ 2. An unconscious patient must regain consciousness before consent can be granted and treatment can begin.

_____ 3. Expressed consent must be obtained from patients who are able to give it.

_____ 4. It is not legally necessary to explain all procedures and risks of treatment to the rational, conscious patient.

_____ 5. Emergency care for a patient identified as an organ donor should not differ from the care provided to any other patient.

_____ 6. Children and mentally incompetent adults are legally allowed to provide consent for their treatment.

_____ 7. Patients who are mentally competent have the right to refuse medical care.

_____ 8. A release form is designed to protect health care providers from liability arising from the patient's informed refusal of treatment and transport.

_____ 9. In all cases of refusal, the EMT should advise the patient to feel free to seek help if certain symptoms develop.

_____ 10. A DNR order is an actual legal document.

_____ 11. In most cases, the oral requests of a family member are a sufficient reason to withhold care from a patient.

_____ 12. An EMT's duty to act continues throughout the call or until care is transferred to someone with equal or greater expertise.

_____ 13. Good Samaritan laws do not prevent someone from initiating a lawsuit, nor will they protect the rescuer from being found liable for acts of gross negligence and other violations of the law.

_____ 14. Basically, an EMT who places the patient's welfare above all else when providing medical care will rarely commit an unethical act on the job.

_____ 15. An EMT is legally responsible for any of the patient's property he or she picks up at the emergency scene.

Medical, Legal, and Ethical Issues

Scope of Practice
Definition
Standard of Care
Duty to Act
Good Samaritan Laws
Ethical Responsibilities
Advanced Directives
Consent
Expressed
Implied
Minor or Mentally Incompetent
  Adult
Refusal of Care
Patient's Rights
Competency
Documentation
Abandonment and Neglect
Confidentiality
Special Situations
Organ Donors
Recognizing Death in the Field
Crime Scenes
Special Reporting Requirements
  • Abuse
  • Crime
  • Drug-related Incidents

HANDOUT 3-2: Chapter 3 Quiz

1. D	**5.** B	**9.** D	**13.** B
2. B	**6.** A	**10.** D	**14.** B
3. A	**7.** D	**11.** C	**15.** D
4. D	**8.** D	**12.** B	

HANDOUT 3-3: In the Field

1. Jared is an adult and if he is competent, he should make his own health care decisions unless he named his father as his health care proxy. Attempt to determine if Jared is competent. Contact medical direction for guidance. Discuss the consequences of refusing treatment with Jared. Be sure that he signs a refusal of care if treatment is refused.

2. Patient confidentiality is the controlling factor. Say "No comment" and walk away.

HANDOUT 3-4: Chapter 3 Review

1. unconscious
2. parents, guardians
3. Emancipated
4. negligence
5. refusal of treatment
6. competent
7. DNR order
8. duty to act
9. care
10. abandoned
11. Good Samaritan
12. written release
13. organ donor
14. crime scene
15. decapitation, rigor mortis

HANDOUT 3-5: Medical, Legal, and Ethical Issues: Listing

1. Expressed; implied; consent to treat minors or incompetents

2. Try again to persuade the patient to accept treatment or transport; make sure the patient is competent to make a rational, informed decision; consult medical direction; have the patient sign a refusal of treatment form; encourage the patient to seek help if the problem persists or gets worse.

3. Findings must be made that (1) the EMT had a duty act; (2) the EMT breached that duty; (3) the patient suffered a compensable injury; (4) injuries were the result of the EMT's negligence.

4. Any three: abuse (usually child, but sometimes spousal or elderly); injuries that have resulted from a crime; drug-related injuries; cases of exposure to certain infectious diseases; dog bites; cases of transportation against a patient's will

5. Absence of pulse, breathing, and breath sounds; complete unresponsiveness to any stimuli; no eye movement or pupil response; absence of blood pressure; no reflexes; dependent lividity

HANDOUT 3-6: Medical, Legal, and Ethical Issues: True or False

1. T	**5.** T	**9.** T	**13.** T
2. F	**6.** F	**10.** T	**14.** T
3. T	**7.** T	**11.** F	**15.** T
4. F	**8.** T	**12.** T	

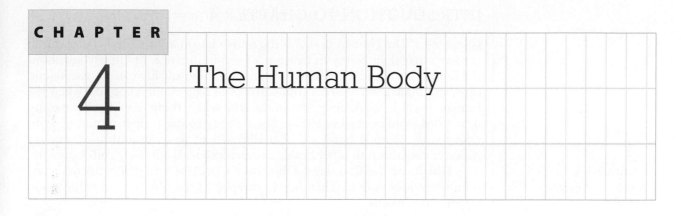

CHAPTER

4   The Human Body

This chapter covers Lesson 1-4 of the U.S. Department of Transportation's EMT-Basic National Standard Curriculum.

OBJECTIVES

Numbered objectives are from the U.S. Department of Transportation EMT-Basic National Standard Curriculum. Asterisked objectives, if any, pertain to material that is supplemental to the DOT curriculum. Page numbers in parentheses refer to pages in the textbook.

Cognitive

1-4.1   Identify the following topographic terms: medial, lateral, proximal, distal, superior, inferior, anterior, posterior, midline, right and left, midclavicular, bilateral, and midaxillary. (pp. 60,62)

1-4.2   Describe the anatomy and function of the following major body systems: respiratory (pp. 69, 71–76), circulatory (pp. 76–82), musculoskeletal (pp. 63–69), nervous (pp. 83–85), and endocrine (pp. 85–89).
— Identify and define other common descriptive anatomical terms. (pp. 58–62)
— Describe the anatomy and function of the skin. (p. 87)

REVIEW

In Chapter 3, "Medical, Legal, and Ethical Issues," your students learned that every time they respond to a call, they will face some type of medical, legal, or ethical issue. The issue may be as simple as making sure that the patient will accept help or be as complex as dealing with a terminally ill patient who refuses all care. Students learned that they may also be faced with decisions such as: "Should I stop and help even though I am off duty?", or "Can I get sued if I stop to help outside of my ambulance district?" Students gained an understanding of the medical, legal, and ethical issues that are an essential foundation for all EMS care. This knowledge can help reduce or prevent the legal liability that they may face.

     Distribute the scored quizzes from the last class. Go over each question on the quiz and handle any concerns students may have about the answers.

Resources Needed
- Scored Chapter 3 Quizzes
- List of 20 preselected terms with their definitions
- Inexpensive items for EMS Bowl winners (self-stick notes, pens, etc.)

Total Teaching Time
200 minutes

Additional Resources
Larmon/Davis, *Basic Life Support Skills*

Elling, *EMT Achieve: Basic Test Preparation*

Limmer/Mistovich/O'Keefe, *Audio Lecture & Study Guide: EMT*

Mistovich/Kuvlesky, *SUCCESS! for the EMT, Second Edition*

Handout 4-1

Chapter 4 Objectives
Checklist

Lecture Master

You may wish to display
Lecture Master 4 when
presenting this lecture to
the class.

✓

Teaching Tip

Stress to students the
importance of obtaining
and using a good medical
dictionary.

On the Net

A great source for medical
clip art that can be used
for overheads and
handouts is Lifeart's web
site at: http://www.
lifeart.com

On the Net

BodyWorlds: An
Anatomical Exhibition
of Real Human Bodies,
http://www.bodyworlds
.com/index.html

INTRODUCTION TO CHAPTER 4

Chapter 4, "The Human Body," is the fourth lesson in Module 1. Point out to students that their ability to develop a solid foundation of knowledge about the human body and its systems is essential to high-quality patient assessment, care, and management. That foundation will help them recognize when the human body is working as it should and when there are life-threatening deviations from normal function. Their ability to use proper terminology to describe the human body will also allow them to communicate necessary patient information to other health care professionals concisely and accurately.

Distribute the Chapter 4 Objectives Checklist and give students a few minutes to look it over. Then briefly paraphrase the objectives for this lesson in your own words.

LECTURE

The following suggested lecture outline is based on the Department of Transportation's EMT-Basic National Standard Curriculum. In some places, the DOT curriculum has been rearranged or expanded upon so that it is more complete or easier for the student to understand. The page numbers in parentheses refer to pages in the textbook. The parenthetical references in dark, heavy type are to figures, tables, and scans in the textbook.

THE HUMAN BODY

I. Anatomical terms (pp. 58–64)
  A. Terms of position (pp. 58–60) **(Fig. 4-1, p. 59)**
    1. Normal anatomical position
    2. Supine
    3. Prone
    4. Lateral recumbent (recovery) position
    5. Fowler's position
    6. Semi-Fowler's position
    7. Trendelenburg position
  B. Anatomical regions of the body and related parts (pp. 60–61) **(Figs. 4-2 to 4-8, pp. 60–64)**
  C. Terms related to anatomical planes (pp. 60–62) **(Fig. 4-2, p. 60; Fig. 4-4, p. 61; Fig. 4-6, p. 62)**
    1. Midline
    2. Midaxillary line
    3. Transverse line
  D. Other descriptive terms (pp. 62–63) **(Fig. 4-2, p. 60; Fig. 4-4, p. 61; Fig. 4-6, p. 62)**
    1. Anterior and posterior
    2. Superior and inferior
    3. Dorsal and ventral
    4. Medial and lateral
        a. Bilateral
        b. Unilateral
        c. Ipsilateral
        d. Contralateral
    5. Proximal and distal
    6. Right and left
    7. Midclavicular
    8. Plantar and palmar
    9. Abdominal quadrants **(Fig. 4-9, p. 65)**

II. **Body systems** (pp. 64–87)

    A. Musculoskeletal system (pp. 63–69)

        1. Skeletal system (**Fig. 4-10, p. 66**)

            a. Skull

                (1) Cranium

                (2) Face

                (3) Orbits

                (4) Nasal bones

                (5) Maxillae

                (6) Mandible (lower jaw)

                (7) Zygomatic (cheek) bones

            b. Spinal column

                (1) Cervical (neck), 7

                (2) Thoracic (upper back), 12

                (3) Lumbar (lower back), 5

                (4) Sacral (back wall of pelvis), 5

                (5) Coccyx (tailbone), 4

            c. Thorax

                (1) Ribs

                (2) 12 pair

                (3) Sternum

                (4) Manubrium

                    (a) Superior portion of sternum

                (5) Body

                    (a) Middle

                (6) Xiphoid process

                    (a) Inferior portion of sternum

            d. Pelvis

                (1) Iliac crest

                (2) Wings of pelvis

                (3) Pubis

                (4) Anterior portion of pelvis

                (5) Ischium

                (6) Inferior portion of pelvis

            e. Lower extremities

                (1) Hip joint

                (2) Greater trochanter (ball)

                (3) Acetabulum (socket)

                (4) Femur (thigh)

                (5) Patella (kneecap)

                (6) Tibia (shin, lower leg)

                (7) Fibula (lower leg)

                (8) Medial and lateral malleolus

                (9) Surface landmarks of ankle joint

                (10) Tarsals and metatarsals (foot)

                (11) Calcaneus (heel)

                (12) Phalanges (toes)

            f. Upper extremities

                (1) Clavicle (collarbone)

                (2) Scapula (shoulder blade)

                (3) Acromion (tip of shoulder)

                (4) Humerus (superior portion of upper extremity)

                    (a) Olecranon (elbow)

                    (b) Radius (lateral bone of forearm)

                    (c) Ulna (medial bone of forearm)

                    (d) Carpals (wrist) and metacarpals (hand)

                    (e) Phalanges (fingers)

---

g. Joints (**Fig. 4-11, p. 67; Fig. 4-12, p. 68**)
  (1) Movement
  (2) Flexion
  (3) Extension
  (4) Abduction
  (5) Adduction
  (6) Circumduction
  (7) Pronation
  (8) Supination
  (9) Types
  (10) Ball and socket
  (11) Hinged
  (12) Pivot
  (13) Glicing
  (14) Saddle
  (15) Condyloid
  (16) Bone injury (**Fig. 4-13, p. 69**)
2. Muscular system (pp. 00–00) (**Fig. 4-14, p. 70; Fig. 4-15, p. 71**)
  a. Voluntary (skeletal)
    (1) Is attached to bones
    (2) Forms the major muscle mass of body
    (3) Contracts and relaxes by will of individual
    (4) Responsible for movement
  b. Involuntary (smooth) (**Fig. 4-16, p. 71**)
    (1) Found in walls of tubular structures of gastrointestinal tract and urinary system, as well as blood vessels and bronchi
    (2) Controls flow of blood in those structures
      (a) Vasodilation
      (b) Vasoconstriction
    (3) Carries out automatic muscular functions of body
    (4) Individuals have no control over it
    (5) Responds to stimuli such as stretching, heat, and cold
  c. Cardiac
    (1) Found only in heart
    (2) Involuntary; has its own supply of blood through coronary artery system
    (3) Can tolerate interruption of blood supply for only very short periods
    (4) Individuals have no control over it
    (5) Automaticity, or the ability to contract on its own
B. Respiratory system (pp. 69–76) (**Fig. 4-17, p. 72**)
  1. Ventilation
    a. Mechanical process of moving air in and out of the lungs
  2. Respiration
    a. Process of exchanging oxygen and carbon dioxide in the cells and tissues
  3. Nose and mouth
  4. Pharynx
    a. Oropharynx
    b. Nasopharynx
  5. Epiglottis
    a. Leaf-shaped structure that prevents food and liquid from entering trachea during swallowing

On the Net
Interactive information on the human body.
http://www.innerbody.com /htm/body.html

6. Trachea (windpipe)
7. Cricoid cartilage
    a. Firm cartilage ring forming the lower portion of larynx
8. Larynx (voice box)
9. Bronchi
    a. Two major branches of the trachea to the lungs, each subdividing into smaller air passages, ending at the alveoli
10. Lungs
11. Diaphragm **(Fig. 4-18, p. 73; Fig. 4-19, p. 74)**
    a. Inhalation (active)
        (1) Diaphragm and intercostal muscles contract, increasing the size of the thoracic cavity
            (a) Diaphragm moves slightly downward, flares lower portion of rib cage
            (b) Ribs move upward/outward
            (c) Air flows into the lungs
    b. Exhalation
        (1) Diaphragm and intercostal muscles relax, decreasing the size of the thoracic cavity
            (a) Diaphragm moves upward
            (b) Ribs move downward/inward
            (c) Air flows out of the lungs
12. Respiratory physiology
    a. Alveolar/capillary exchange **(Fig. 4-21, p. 75)**
        (1) Oxygen-rich air enters the alveoli during each inspiration
        (2) Oxygen-poor blood in the capillaries passes into the alveoli
        (3) Oxygen enters the capillaries as carbon dioxide enters the alveoli
    b. Capillary/cellular exchange **(Fig. 4-22, p. 76)**
        (1) Cells give up carbon dioxide to the capillaries
            (a) Capillaries give up oxygen to the cells
    c. Adequate breathing
        (1) Normal rate
            (a) Adult
                (i) 12–20/minute
            (b) Child
                (i) 15–30/minute
            (c) Infant
                (i) 25–50/minute
        (2) Rhythm
        (3) Regular
        (4) Quality
        (5) Breath sounds
            (a) Present and equal
        (6) Chest expansion
            (a) Adequate and equal
        (7) Effort of breathing
            (a) Use of accessory muscles, predominantly in infants and children
        (8) Depth (tidal volume)
    d. Inadequate breathing
        (1) Rate
            (a) Too slow
            (b) Too fast

(2) Rhythm
    (a) Irregular
(3) Quality
(4) Breath sounds
    (a) Diminished or absent
(5) Chest expansion
    (a) Unequal or inadequate
(6) Increased effort of breathing
    (a) Use of accessory muscles, predominantly in infants and children
(7) Depth (tidal volume)
    (a) Deep
    (b) Shallow
(8) The skin may be pale or cyanotic (blue) and cool and clammy
(9) There may be retractions above the clavicles, between the ribs and below the rib cage, especially in children
(10) Nasal flaring may be present, especially in children
(11) In infants, there may be "seesaw" breathing, where the abdomen and chest move in opposite directions
(12) Head bobbing
(13) Agonal respirations (occasional gasping breaths) may be seen just before death
13. Infant and child anatomy considerations **(Fig. 4-20, p. 75)**
  a. Mouth and nose
    (1) In general, all structures are smaller and more easily obstructed than in adults
  b. Pharynx
    (1) Infants' and children's tongues take up proportionally more space in the mouth than adults
  c. Trachea (windpipe)
    (1) Infants and children have narrower tracheas that are obstructed more easily by swelling
    (2) The trachea is softer and more flexible in infants and children
  d. Cricoid cartilage
    (1) Like other cartilage in the infant and child, the cricoid cartilage is less developed and less rigid
  e. Diaphragm
    (1) Chest wall is softer; infants and children tend to depend more heavily on the diaphragm for breathing
C. Circulatory (pp. 76–82) **(Fig. 4-23a, p. 77)**
  1. Heart **(Fig. 4-23b, p. 78)**
    a. Structure/function
      (1) Atrium
      (2) Right
        (a) Receives blood from the veins of the body and the heart, pumps oxygen-poor blood to the right ventricle
      (3) Left
        (a) Receives blood from the pulmonary veins (lungs), pumps oxygen-rich blood to left ventricle

Teaching Tip
Bring in several cattle or pig hearts and point out the appropriate structures. Check with your local butcher shop or meat-packing plant.

(4) Ventricle

(5) Right

  (a) Pumps blood to the lungs

(6) Left

  (a) Pumps blood to the body

(7) Valves prevent backflow of blood

(8) Tricuspid valve

(9) Pulmonary valve

(10) Mitral valve

(11) Aortic valve

b. Cardiac conduction system

  (1) Heart is more than a muscle

  (2) Specialized contractile and conductive tissue in the heart

    (a) Electrical impulses

2. Arteries

  a. Function

    (1) Carry blood away from the heart to the rest of the body

  b. Major arteries

    (1) Aorta

    (2) Major artery originating from the heart, lying in front of the spine in the thoracic and abdominal cavities

    (3) Divides at the level of the navel into the iliac arteries

    (4) Supplies all other vessels with blood

    (5) Coronary arteries

    (6) Vessels that supply the heart with blood

    (7) Carotid

    (8) Major artery of the neck

    (9) Supplies the head with blood

    (10) Pulsations can be palpated on either side of the neck

    (11) Femoral

    (12) The major artery of the thigh

    (13) Supplies the groin and the lower extremities with blood

    (14) Pulsations can be palpated in the groin area (the crease between the abdomen and thigh)

    (15) Dorsalis pedis

    (16) An artery in the foot

    (17) Pulsations can be palpated on the anterior surface of the foot

    (18) Posterior tibial

    (19) Pulsations can be palpated on the posterior surface of the medial malleolus

    (20) Brachial

    (21) An artery of the upper arm

    (22) Pulsations can be palpated on the inside of the arm between the elbow and the shoulder

    (23) Used when determining a blood pressure (BP) using a BP cuff (sphygmomanometer) and a stethoscope

    (24) Radial

On the Net

Directory of links to detailed anatomy sites. http://dir.yahoo.com/ Science/Biology/Anatomy/

        (25) Major artery of the lower arm

        (26) Pulsations can be palpated at the wrist thumbside

        (27) Pulmonary

        (28) Artery originating at the right ventricle

        (29) Carries oxygen-poor blood to the lungs

3. Arterioles

    a. Smallest branch of an artery leading to the capillaries

4. Capillaries

    a. Tiny blood vessels that connect arterioles to venules

    b. Found in all parts of the body

    c. Allow for the exchange of nutrients and waste at the cellular level

5. Venules

    a. Smallest branch of the veins leading from the capillaries

6. Veins

    a. Function

        (1) Vessels that carry blood back to the heart

    b. Major veins

        (1) Pulmonary vein

            (a) Carries oxygen-rich blood from the lungs to the left atrium

        (2) Venae cavae

        (3) Superior

        (4) Inferior

            (a) Carries oxygen-poor blood back to the right atrium

7. Blood composition

    a. Red blood cells

        (1) Give the blood its color

        (2) Carry oxygen to organs

        (3) Hemoglobin

        (4) Carry carbon dioxide away from organs

    b. White blood cells

        (1) Part of the body's defense against infections

    c. Plasma

        (1) Fluid that carries the blood cells and nutrients

    d. Platelets

        (1) Essential for the formation of blood clots

8. Physiology

    a. Pulse

        (1) Left ventricle contracts, sending a wave of blood through the arteries

        (2) Can be palpated anywhere an artery simultaneously passes near the skin surface and over a bone

            (a) Peripheral

            (b) Radial

            (c) Brachial

            (d) Posterior tibial

            (e) Dorsalis pedia

            (f) Central

            (g) Carotid

            (h) Femoral

            (i) Apical pulse

    b. Blood pressure

        (1) Systolic

Teaching Tip

Point out that, as with a hydraulic system, the pump must function properly, there can't be any leaks in the pipes, and there must be a proper amount of fluid for the system to function properly.

                (a) Pressure exerted against the walls of the
                    artery when the left ventricle contracts
            (2) Diastolic
                (a) Pressure exerted against the walls of the
                    artery when the left ventricle is at rest
            (3) Hydrostatic (**Fig. 4-24, p. 80**)
            (4) Edema
            (5) Pulse pressure
    9. Perfusion (**Fig. 4-25, p. 81**)
        a. Delivery of oxygen and other nutrients to the cells of all
           organ systems and the removal of waste products
        b. Hypoperfusion
            (1) Inadequate circulation of blood through an organ
        c. Transport of gases in the blood (**Fig. 4-26, p. 82**)
        d. Oxygen
        e. Carbon dioxide
    10. Cell metabolism
        a. Aerobic
        b. Anaerobic
    11. Inadequate circulation
        a. Shock (hypoperfusion)
            (1) State of profound depression of the vital processes
                of the body
            (2) Signs and symptoms
                (a) Pale
                (b) Cyanotic (blue-gray color)
                (c) Cool
                (d) Clammy skin
                (e) Rapid, weak pulse
                (f) Rapid and shallow breathing
                (g) Restlessness
                (h) Anxiety or mental dullness
                (i) Nausea and vomiting
                (j) Reduction in total blood volume
                (k) Low or decreasing blood pressure
                (l) Subnormal temperature
D. Nervous system (pp. 83–85) (**Fig. 4-27, p. 83**)
    1. Function
        a. Controls the voluntary and involuntary activity of the
           body
    2. Components
        a. Central nervous system (**Fig. 4-28, p. 84**)
            (1) Brain
            (2) Located within the cranium
            (3) Cerebrum
            (4) Cerebellum
            (5) Brain stem
            (6) Spinal cord
            (7) Located within the spinal column from the brain
                through the lumbar vertebrae
        b. Peripheral nervous system
            (1) Voluntary nervous system
            (2) Autonomic nervous system (**Fig. 4-29, p. 86**)
                • Sympathetic
                • Parasympathetic
            (3) Sensory

          (a) Carry information from the body to the brain and spinal cord

      (4) Motor

          (a) Carry information from the brain and spinal cord to the body

E. Endocrine system function (pp. 85–87) **(Fig. 4-30, p. 87)**

  1. Secretes chemicals, such as insulin and adrenaline; responsible for regulating body activities and functions

  2. Components

    a. Pituitary gland

    b. Thyroid gland

    c. Parathyroid glands

    d. Adrenal glands

    e. Pancreas

      (1) Islets of Langerhaus

    f. Gonads

  3. Receptors

    a. Alpha 1

      (1) Vasoconstriction

    b. Alpha 2

      (1) Regulate release of Alpha 1

    c. Beta 1

      (1) Increases heart rate

      (2) Increases cardiac contraction

      (3) Increases cardiac conduction

    d. Beta 2

      (1) Bronchodilation

  4. Epinephrine

    a. Affects Alpha 1, Alpha 2, Beta 1, and Beta 2

  5. Norepinephrine

    a. Primarily affects Alpha 1 and Alpha 2

    b. Minimal effects on Beta 1 and Beta 2

F. Skin (p. 87) **(Fig. 4-31, p. 88)**

  1. Function

    a. Protects the body from the environment, bacteria, and other organisms

    b. Helps regulate the temperature of the body

    c. Senses heat, cold, touch, pressure, and pain; transmits this information to the brain and spinal cord

  2. Layers

    a. Epidermis

      (1) Outermost layer of skin

    b. Dermis

      (1) Deeper layer of skin containing sweat and sebaceous glands, hair follicles, blood vessels, and nerve endings

    c. Subcutaneous layer

  3. Accessory structures

    a. Nails

    b. Hair

    c. Sweat glands

    d. Oil glands

ENRICHMENT (OPTIONAL)

The following sections contain information that is valuable as background for the EMT, but that goes substantially beyond the U.S. Department of Transportation's EMT-Basic National Standard Curriculum.

G. Digestive system (pp. 87–88)
1. Basic anatomy
    a. Stomach
    b. Pancreas
    c. Liver
    d. Spleen
    e. Gallbladder
    f. Small intestine
    g. Large intestine
2. Processes
    a. Mechanical
        (1) Chewing
        (2) Swallowing
        (3) Peristalsis
        (4) Defecation
    b. Chemical process
        (1) Breakdown
        (2) Enzymes
        (3) Carbohydrares to glucose
        (4) Fats to fatty acids
        (5) Proteins to amino acids
        (6) Absorption

H. Urinary system (p. 89) **(Fig. 4-32, p. 89)**
1. Basic Anatomy
    a. Kidneys
    b. Ureters
    c. Urinary bladder
    d. Urethra
2. Processes
    a. Maintain balance of water and chemicals
    b. Filtration
        (1) Wastes eliminated
        (2) Useful products returned to circulation

I. Reproductive system (p. 89) **(Fig. 4-33, p. 90)**
1. Basic anatomy—female
    a. Ovum
    b. Ovaries
    c. Uterine (Fallopian) tubes
    d. Uterus
    e. Cervix
    f. Vagina
    g. External genitalia
2. Basic anatomy—male
    a. Sperm
    b. Testes
    c. Ducts
    d. Prostrate
    e. Urethra
    f. Penis

3. Processes
   a. Ovulation
   b. Fertilization
   c. Implantation
      (1) Embryo
      (2) Fetus
      (3) Newborn
   d. Menstruation
III. **Medical words and word parts** (pp. 90–95) **(Table 4-1, pp. 92–93; Table 4-2, p. 94; Table 4-3, p. 95)**

CASE STUDY FOLLOW-UP

Ask a student volunteer to read the Case Study that begins on page 58 of the textbook. You may wish to use the following questions to engage students in a discussion of the Case Study Follow-up that begins on page 96 of the textbook. Provide missing information and clarify ideas as needed.

Q1. How might a nonmedical person describe the patient's injuries?

A1. *Her entire right arm from the elbow to the fingertips has been severely charred. The burns to her head are minor and cover the right side of her face.*

Q2. How might a medical professional describe the patient's burns?

A2. *There is a full-thickness burn originating at the right elbow joint, which proceeds inferiorly and circumferentially to the distal fingers. The burn to the skull appears to be a superficial burn that involves the right cranium and face. The facial burn involves the lateral aspect of the right mandible, maxilla, and zygomatic arch.*

Q3. What are the two major advantages of using medical rather than nonmedical terms to describe the body?

A3. *(1) The ability to communicate clearly with emergency department staff, and (2) to document injuries and illnesses accurately in the prehospital care report.*

IN REVIEW

Assess students' ability to apply what they have just learned by discussing the Review Questions on page 100 in the textbook.

Q1. Describe the following six positions: normal anatomical position, supine, prone, lateral recumbent, Fowler's, and Trendelenburg.

A1. *Normal anatomical position—erect, face forward, with arms down at the sides and palms forward. Supine—on the back. Prone—on the stomach. Lateral recumbent—lying horizontally on the left or right side. Fowler's—lying on the back with upper body elevated at a 45° to 60° angle. Trendelenburg—lying on the back with the lower part of the body elevated approximately 12 inches. (pp. 58–60)*

Q2. Define the following five descriptive terms: midline, midclavicular line, midaxillary line, plantar, and palmar. Also define the following five terms and name and define the opposite of each term: anterior, superior, dorsal, lateral, and distal.

A2. *Midline—an imaginary line drawn vertically through the middle of the body, dividing it into the right and left planes. Midclavicular line—the* *imaginary line from the center of either clavicle down the anterior thorax. Midaxillary line—an imaginary line from the middle of the armpit to the ankle that divides the body into anterior and posterior planes. Plantar—refers to the sole of the foot. Palmar—refers to the palm of the hand. Anterior—toward the front; opposite: posterior—toward the back. Superior—above or toward the head; opposite: inferior—below, away from the head. Dorsal—toward the back or spine; opposite: ventral—toward the front. Lateral—refers to the left or right of the midline or away from the midline of the body; opposite: medial—toward the midline. Distal—distant, or far from the point of reference; opposite: proximal—near the point of reference. (pp. 60–62)*

Q3. Briefly describe the anatomy and physiology of the musculoskeletal system.

A3. *The musculoskeletal system consists of the bones of the skeleton held together by layers of muscles and other connective tissues. The skeletal system consists of skull, face, spinal column, thorax, pelvis, and extremities, and it gives the body its shape, protects the vital internal organs, and provides for movement. Movement of the body is the result of work performed by the muscles, which have the ability to contract when stimulated by nerve impulses. (pp. 63–69)*

Q4. Briefly describe the anatomy and physiology of the respiratory system.

A4. *In the respiratory system, oxygen from the air is made available to the blood through the respiratory system, which includes the nose and mouth, pharynx, epiglottis, trachea and larynx, bronchi, lungs, and diaphragm. (pp. 69–76)*

Q5. Briefly describe the anatomy and physiology of the circulatory system.

A5. *The circulatory system includes the heart; blood vessels—arteries, arterioles, capillaries, venules, and veins; and blood. The blood brings oxygen, nutrients, and other essential elements to all the cells of the body and removes carbon dioxide and other waste products resulting from cell activity. (pp. 76–82)*

Q6. Identify the central and peripheral pulse points and their locations.

A6. *The central pulse points are the carotid artery at either side of the neck and the femoral artery in the crease between the abdomen and the groin. The peripheral pulse points include the radial artery at the point proximal to the thumb on the wrist; the brachial artery on the medial aspect of the arm, midway between the shoulder and the elbow; the posterior tibial artery on the posterior surface of the medial malleolus or ankle bone; and the dorsalis pedis artery on the anterior surface of the foot. (p. 80)*

Q7. Define shock (hypoperfusion).

A7. *Shock, or hypoperfusion, is the insufficient supply of oxygen and other nutrients to some of the body's cells and the inadequate elimination of carbon dioxide and other wastes that result from inadequate circulation of blood. (p. 81)*

Q8. Briefly describe the anatomy and physiology of the nervous system.

A8. *The nervous system controls the voluntary and involuntary activity of the human body. It is divided into two main systems: the central* *nervous system, which includes the brain and spinal cord, and the peripheral nervous system, which includes the sensory and motor nerves. (pp. 83–85)*

Q9. Briefly describe the anatomy and physiology of the endocrine system.

A9. *The endocrine system is made up of ductless glands that secrete hormones, which affect body functions such as growth and mental, emotional, physical, and sexual behavior. The endocrine glands include the thyroid, parathyroids, adrenals, gonads, islets of Langerhans, and pituitary. (pp. 85–87)*

Q10. Briefly describe the anatomy and physiology of the skin.

A10. *The skin is the largest organ in the body. It has three basic layers—the epidermis, the dermis, and a subcutaneous layer. The four accessory structures of the skin are the nails, hair, sweat glands, and oil glands. The skin protects the human body from the environment, bacteria, and other organisms. The skin helps regulate body temperature, and it serves as a receptor organ. (p. 87)*

CRITICAL THINKING

Assess students' ability to respond to real-life emergency situations by discussing the Critical Thinking questions on page 100 in the textbook.

Q1. What body systems do you suspect could be injured by the knife wounds?

A1. *Based on the locations of the wounds, an EMT should anticipate injuries to the musculoskeletal system, the respiratory system, the circulatory system, the nervous system, the endocrine system, and the digestive system.*

Q2. Pick a knife wound location on this patient's body and provide a brief description of the injury using medical terminology and anatomical terms as you would use them in your written EMS report.

A2. *Using a little creative license, the neck wounds might be described as "penetrating trauma to the anterior neck, approximately three centimeters left lateral of the trachea, just inferior to the mandible." The chest wounds might be written as "penetrating trauma to the right anterior chest, on the midclavicular line just superior to the nipple." The abdominal wounds could be "a knife wound 4 cm from the umbilicus at a ten o'clock position."*

Q3. What is causing the elevated heart rate?

A3. *The patient's heart rate is elevated because his circulatory system is attempting to compensate for blood loss and maintain an appropriate blood pressure.*

Q4. What is causing the skin to be pale, cool, and clammy?

A4. *The patient's skin is pale, cool, and clammy because he is hypoperfusing due to the loss of blood volume. His circulatory system is redirecting blood to the core of his body by constricting the vessels in the skin. This shunts the warm, red blood away from the skin making it appear pale and feel cool. The alpha stimulation from the circulating epinephrine*

©2008 by Pearson Education, Inc.
Prehospital Emergency Care, 8th ed.

and norepinephrine cause stimulate the sweat glands to release sweat causing to patient to feel clammy.

Q5. What is the significance of the systolic and diastolic blood pressure?

A5. *The systolic blood pressure measures the pressure created by the blood being ejected out of the left ventricle. A fall in the systolic blood pressure would indicate a decrease in the amount of blood being ejected by the left ventricle. The diastolic blood pressure measures the pressure in the arteries between contractions. This pressure is related directly to the resistance in the vessel. Vessel resistance is determined by the vessel size. As the diameter of the vessel increases (vasodilation), the pressure inside the vessel will decrease. Likewise, as the diameter of the vessel decreases (vasoconstriction), the pressure inside will increase. In the case of this patient, the systolic blood pressure and diastolic blood pressure values are coming closer together. This is known as a narrow pulse pressure. This is an indication that the systolic blood pressure is falling, most likely from blood loss, and the diastolic is either being maintained or increasing, as a result of significant vasoconstriction. As the body loses more blood, the vessels will continue to constrict to maintain a pressure. The narrow pulse pressure reflects the decreasing volume and increasing vasoconstriction to make up for the low blood volume.*

EMS BOWL

Provide students with an opportunity to review what they just learned about the human body and its systems by playing a game called "EMS Bowl." Divide the class into two teams. The members of each team should arrange their chairs so that they can easily talk to one another. Ask one student to be the timekeeper/scorekeeper. The score should be recorded on a blackboard, flip chart, or overhead transparency. Each team should choose a captain. The captain will give the official answers for each team.

Have students close their textbooks and put away their class notes. Then read 20 definitions—one at a time—related to the anatomy and physiology of the human body. After reading each definition, allow both teams 30 seconds to confer and choose a term that matches the definition. The captain of team A will state his or her team's answer, and then team B must decide whether team A's answer is correct. If team B judges team A's answer to be incorrect, it must offer an answer of its own. Scoring will be as follows:

- If team A is correct and team B agrees that they are correct, then team A receives two points and team B receives one point.

- If team A is correct and team B disagrees, A gets two points and B gets none.

- If team A is incorrect and team B is correct, A gets no points and B gets one point.

- If both teams are incorrect, neither team gets any points.

Play will then pass to team B and continue in turn until all questions have been considered. The textbook will be used to settle any dispute about correct or incorrect answers.

Flip a coin to determine which team gets to answer first.

Elaborate on student answers, if necessary, and provide the correct term if neither team provides it.

Provide each member of the winning team with a prize.

Reading/Reference
Textbook, pp. 101–122

Workbook
Chapter 4 Activities

Chapter Quiz
Handout 4-2

TestGen
Chapter 4 Test

Online Test Preparation
Send your students to
http://www.prenhall.com/
EMTAchieve

Handouts 4-3 to 4-6
Reinforcement Activities

**Brady Skills Series
EMT-B Videos/CD**
Visual Reinforcement

**PowerPoint
Presentation**
Chapter 4

Student CD
Chapter 4

Companion Website
http://www.prenhall.com/
mistovich

ASSIGNMENTS

Assign students to read Chapter 5, "Baseline Vital Signs and History Taking," before the next class. Also ask them to complete Chapter 4 of the Workbook.

EVALUATION

Chapter Quiz Distribute copies of the Chapter Quiz provided in Handout 4-2 to evaluate student understanding of this chapter. Remind students not to refer to their textbooks or notes while taking the quiz.

Test Manager You may wish to create a custom-tailored test using Prentice Hall *TestGen for Prehospital Emergency Care, Eighth Edition* to evaluate student understanding of this chapter.

Online Test Preparation (for students and instructors) Additional test preparation is available through *EMT Achieve: Basic Test Preparation* at http://www.prenhall.com/EMTAchieve. Instructors can also monitor student mastery online.

REINFORCEMENT

Handouts If classroom discussions or performance on the quiz indicates that some students have not fully mastered the chapter content, you may wish to assign some or all of the Reinforcement Handouts for this chapter.

TECH EXTRAS

Brady Skills Series EMT-B Videos/CD Have your students watch the skills come to life on either VHS or CD-ROM.

PowerPoint Presentation (for instructors) The PowerPoint material developed for this chapter offers useful reinforcement of chapter content.

Student CD A wide variety of material on this CD-ROM will reinforce and also expand student knowledge and skills.

Companion Website (for students) Additional review quizzes and links to EMS resources will contribute to further reinforcement of this chapter. Please visit http://www.prenhall.com/mistovich.

OBJECTIVES CHECKLIST

Cognitive	Date Mastered
1-4.1 Identify the following topographic terms: medial, lateral, proximal, distal, superior, inferior, anterior, posterior, midline, right and left, midclavicular, bilateral, and midaxillary.	
1-4.2 Describe the anatomy and function of the following major body systems: respiratory, circulatory, musculoskeletal, nervous, and endocrine. —Identify and define other common descriptive anatomical terms. —Describe the anatomy and function of the skin.	

CHAPTER 4 QUIZ

Write the letter of the best answer in the space provided.

_____ 1. The functions of the body are called its
- A. physiology.
- B. kinesiology
- C. pathology.
- D. microbiology.

_____ 2. The structure of the body is referred to as its
- A. analogy.
- B. anatomy.
- C. kinesiology.
- D. pathology.

_____ 3. The normal anatomical position is best described as a person
- A. standing, facing forward, palms forward.
- B. lying on his back, palms facing down.
- C. standing, facing sideways, palms facing thighs.
- D. lying on his stomach, palms up.

_____ 4. An imaginary line down the center of the body that passes between the eyes and extends down through the navel is the
- A. plane.
- B. outline.
- C. midline.
- D. quadrant.

_____ 5. The term that refers to a position closer to the midline is
- A. medial.
- B. lateral.
- C. posterior.
- D. anterior.

_____ 6. An opposite of anterior is
- A. posterior.
- B. superior.
- C. exterior.
- D. proximal.

_____ 7. The lateral recumbent position is also known as the _____ position.
- A. Fowler's
- B. supine
- C. recovery
- D. Trendelenburg

_____ 8. The Fowler's position is usually achieved by elevating the patient's upper body to a _____ angle.
- A. 60° to 90°
- B. 45° to 60°
- C. 50° to 70°
- D. 55° to 90°

_____ 9. The spinal region that is most prone to injury is the
- A. thoracic.
- B. cervical.
- C. sacral.
- D. coccyxal.

_____ 10. The clavicle is commonly referred to as the
- A. collarbone.
- B. thigh.
- C. hamstring.
- D. shin.

_____ 11. The scapula and acromion are parts of the
- A. pelvis.
- B. shoulder.
- C. ankle.
- D. wrist.

_____ **12.** Inferiorly, the knee connects with the
    A. radius and fibula.   **C.** tibia and fibula.
    B. femur and tibia.   **D.** ulna and tibia.

_____ **13.** The body contains how many different types of muscle?
    A. two   **C.** four
    B. three   **D.** five

_____ **14.** The structure that carries air downward from the larynx to the lungs is the
    A. bronchus.   **C.** epiglottis.
    B. pharynx.   **D.** trachea.

_____ **15.** The chamber that pumps oxygen-rich blood out of the heart for distribution to the rest of the body is the
    A. right atrium.   **C.** left atrium.
    B. right ventricle.   **D.** left ventricle.

_____ **16.** The major artery leading from the heart is the
    A. aorta.   **C.** carotid.
    B. pulmonary.   **D.** femoral.

_____ **17.** The pulse that is located in the foot is the
    A. carotid.   **C.** brachial.
    B. femoral.   **D.** dorsalis pedis.

_____ **18.** The blood vessels where gases, nutrients, and waste products are exchanged between the body's cells and the bloodstream are the
    A. arteries.   **C.** capillaries.
    B. venules.   **D.** arterioles.

_____ **19.** The elements of the blood that are part of the body's immune system and help to defend against infection are
    A. plasma.   **C.** white blood cells.
    B. red blood cells.   **D.** platelets.

_____ **20.** The pressure created in the arteries when blood is forced out of the heart is referred to as
    A. radial.   **C.** femoral.
    B. systolic.   **D.** diastolic.

_____ **21.** The adequate supply of oxygen and nutrients to the organs and tissues of the body, with the removal of waste products, is called
    A. automaticity.   **C.** perfusion.
    B. conduction.   **D.** autonomicity.

_____ **22.** The central nervous system is made up of the brain and the
    A. sensory nerves.   **C.** motor nerves.
    B. spinal cord.   **D.** endocrines.

_____ **23.** The skin layer rich with blood vessels, nerves, and specialized structures such as sweat glands and sebaceous glands is the
    A. epidermis.   **C.** subcutaneous layer.
    B. dermis.   **D.** arrector pili.

_____24. The endocrine system produces chemicals called
      A. hormones.   **C.** dioxins.
      B. carotenes.   **D.** biles.

_____25. Body functions such as digestion, heart rate, and the activities of involuntary muscles are controlled by the _____ nervous system.
      A. central   **C.** autonomic
      B. peripheral   **D.** automatic

IN THE FIELD

Review the following real-life situation. Then answer the questions that follow.

You and your crew are dispatched for a call about a fall at a home. As the ambulance pulls up to a single-family house, you survey the scene. A truck for AAA Roofers is parked in the driveway. There is scaffolding at the east end of the house. At its base, two men are kneeling over a third that is lying supine on the ground. The scene appears to be safe, so you grab your jump kit and approach. As you do, one of the men runs over to you and tells you that the crew had been removing old shingles from the roof when David lost his footing and fell about 18 feet to the ground.

Your patient is not conscious when you begin your initial assessment. After determining that he is breathing adequately, you note a large laceration on the left side of the patient's lower jaw. You also note that an area on the outside of the patient's left arm, just above the elbow, is swollen and deformed. There is a large laceration on the front of the patient's upper left thigh just above the kneecap, which is bleeding profusely.

1. Which of the body's major systems do you suspect may have been injured as a result of this accident?

2. Describe the location of the injury on the patient's head.

3. Describe the location of the injury to the patient's arm.

4. Describe the location of the injury to the patient's lower extremity.

CHAPTER 4 REVIEW

Write the word or words that best complete each sentence in the space provided.

1. Use of the _____ _____ position ensures that health care providers will employ the same point of reference when terms of direction and location are used.

2. A(n) _____ _____ is the kind of flat surface that would be formed if you sliced straight through an imaginary human body.

3. The _____ line is one that is drawn vertically from the middle of the armpit to the ankle.

4. The elbow is _____ to the shoulder because the elbow is farther away from the torso than the shoulder.

5. Anatomically speaking, the nose is _____ to the mouth.

6. When a patient is lying on his back with legs elevated higher than the head and body on an inclined plane, he is in the _____ position.

7. Bones are connected to bones by _____, while muscles are connected to bones by _____.

8. The top, back, and sides of the skull plus the forehead make up the _____.

9. The spinal column is made up of blocks of bone called _____.

10. The _____ is composed of the ribs, the sternum, and a portion of the spine.

11. The _____ _____ consists of the acetabulum and the ball at the head of the femur.

12. The elbow is an example of a(n) _____ joint.

13. The property that allows the heart to generate and conduct electrical impulses on its own is _____.

14. During respiration, gas exchange with the bloodstream takes place in the small sacs called _____.

15. The section of the respiratory cycle in which the intercostal muscles and diaphragm relax is known as _____.

©2008 by Pearson Education, Inc.
Prehospital Emergency Care, 8th ed.

16. The respiratory anatomy of infants and children differs from that of adults in that the

_____ is narrower, softer, and more flexible.

17. Because the chest walls of infants and children are softer, they rely more on the

_____ for breathing.

18. The upper chambers of the heart are the _____, while the lower chambers

are the _____.

19. The _____ _____ carry oxygenated blood from

the lungs to the heart.

20. The elements of the blood that are essential to the formation of blood clots are

_____.

21. When the left ventricle of the heart is relaxing and refilling, the pressure remaining in the arteries is

the _____ blood pressure.

22. _____ and _____ are two names for the condition

that results when adequate supplies of oxygen are not delivered to and waste products are not

removed from all the body's tissues.

23. The peripheral nervous system is made up of nerves located outside of the

_____ and the _____

_____.

24. The layers of the skin are the _____, the _____,

and the _____ _____.

25. The _____ _____ produces chemicals called

hormones that help to regulate many body activities and functions.

REINFORCEMENT

ANATOMY AND PHYSIOLOGY: TRUE OR FALSE

Indicate if the following statements are true or false by writing T or F in the space provided.

_____ **1.** Anatomy refers to the body's structures and functions.

_____ **2.** The directions "left" and "right" always refer to the EMT's left and right.

_____ **3.** The imaginary midline divides the body into upper and lower halves.

_____ **4.** The term "lateral" refers to a position farther away from the midline.

_____ **5.** Anatomically speaking, the elbow is distal to the hand.

_____ **6.** There is one midclavicular line centered between the two clavicles.

_____ **7.** In the Fowler's position, a patient is lying with the upper body elevated.

_____ **8.** The first 12 vertebrae form the sacral spine.

_____ **9.** The ulna is the inner and larger bone of the lower leg.

_____ **10.** The heart muscle receives its blood supply through the coronary artery system.

_____ **11.** The cricoid cartilage forms the lower portion of the trachea.

_____ **12.** The left ventricle pumps blood to the aorta.

_____ **13.** The cardiac conduction system delivers waste gases to the lungs where they can be expelled from the body.

_____ **14.** The femoral artery is the main source of blood supply to the upper arm.

_____ **15.** The primary function of the red blood cells is to carry oxygen to the body cells and carbon dioxide away from the cells.

_____ **16.** In a blood pressure reading of 120/80, the 120 refers to the diastolic pressure while the 80 refers to the systolic pressure.

_____ **17.** A pulse can be felt at the point where a vein passes over a bone near the skin surface.

_____ **18.** The skin plays an important part in regulating the body's temperature.

_____ **19.** The epidermis contains the hair follicles and sweat glands.

_____ **20.** The thyroid gland makes insulin for the metabolism of calcium.

Student's Name _____

THE CIRCULATORY SYSTEM

Demonstrate your knowledge of the body's circulatory system by correctly labeling its major arteries and veins on the diagram below.

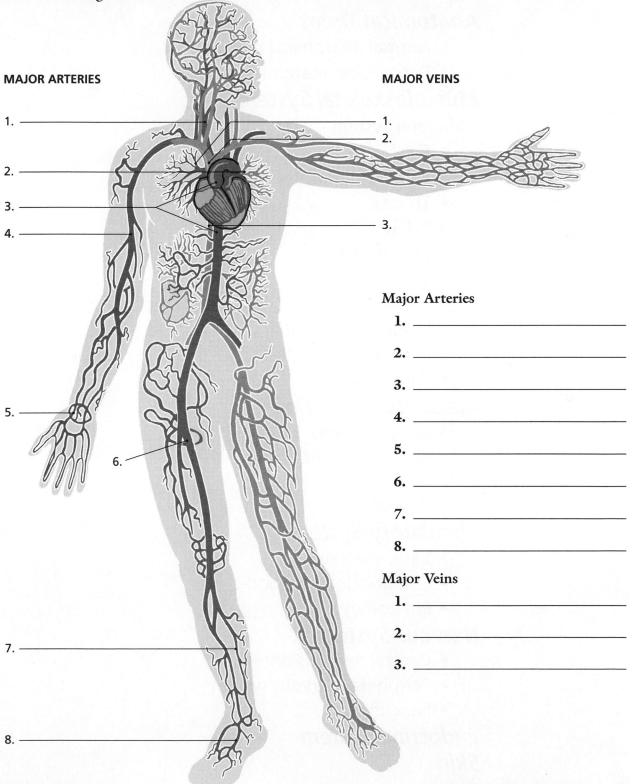

MAJOR ARTERIES

1. _____
2. _____
3. _____
4. _____
5. _____
6. _____
7. _____
8. _____

MAJOR VEINS

1. _____
2. _____
3. _____

Major Arteries

1. _____
2. _____
3. _____
4. _____
5. _____
6. _____
7. _____
8. _____

Major Veins

1. _____
2. _____
3. _____

The Human Body

Anatomical Terms
- Normal anatomical position
- Descriptive anatomical terms

Musculoskeletal System
Skeletal System
- Skull
- Spinal column
- Thorax
- Pelvis
- Extremities
- Joints

Muscular System
- Voluntary muscle
- Involuntary muscle
- Cardiac muscle

Respiratory System
- Basic anatomy
- Anatomy in infants and children
- Physiology

Circulatory System
- Basic anatomy
- Composition of blood
- Physiology

Nervous System
- Central nervous system
- Peripheral nervous system
- Functions

Endocrine System
Skin

HANDOUT 4-2: Chapter 4 Quiz

1. A	8. B	14. D	20. B
2. B	9. B	15. D	21. C
3. A	10. A	16. A	22. B
4. C	11. B	17. D	23. B
5. A	12. C	18. C	24. A
6. A	13. B	19. C	25. C
7. C			

HANDOUT 4-3: In the Field

1. There is a good possibility of injuries to the patient's skin, nervous, cardiovascular, respiratory, and musculoskeletal systems.
2. The injury is on the left mandible.
3. The wound is on the lateral surface of the patient's left arm, superior to the elbow. It could also be noted as an injury to the distal humeral area.
4. The upper thigh wound is on the anterior surface of the left lower extremity superior to the patella.

HANDOUT 4-4: Chapter 4 Review

1. normal anatomical
2. anatomical plane
3. midaxillary
4. distal
5. superior
6. Trendelenburg
7. ligaments, tendons
8. cranium
9. vertebrae
10. thorax
11. hip joint
12. hinge
13. automaticity
14. alveoli
15. exhalation
16. trachea
17. diaphragm
18. atria, ventricles
19. pulmonary veins
20. platelets
21. diastolic
22. Hypoperfusion, shock
23. brain, spinal cord
24. epidermis, dermis, subcutaneous layers
25. endocrine system

HANDOUT 4-5: Anatomy and Physiology: True or False

1. F	6. F	11. F	16. F
2. F	7. T	12. T	17. F
3. F	8. F	13. F	18. T
4. T	9. F	14. F	19. F
5. F	10. T	15. T	20. F

HANDOUT 4-6: The Circulatory System

Major Arteries
1. carotid
2. pulmonary
3. aorta
4. brachial
5. radial
6. femoral
7. posterior tibial
8. dorsal pedis

Major Veins
1. pulmonary
2. superior vena cava
3. inferior vena cava

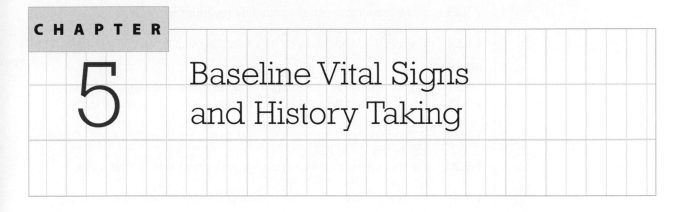

This chapter covers Lesson 1-5 and portions of Lesson 1-7 of the U.S. Department of Transportation's EMT-Basic National Standard Curriculum.

OBJECTIVES

Numbered objectives are from the U.S. Department of Transportation EMT-Basic National Standard Curriculum. Asterisked objectives, if any, pertain to material that is supplemental to the DOT curriculum. Page numbers in parentheses refer to pages in the textbook.

Cognitive

1-5.1   Identify the components of vital signs. (p. 103)
1-5.2   Describe the methods to obtain a breathing rate. (pp. 104–105)
1-5.3   Identify the attributes that should be obtained when assessing breathing. (pp. 104–105)
1-5.4   Differentiate between shallow, labored, and noisy breathing. (p. 105)
1-5.5   Describe the methods to obtain a pulse rate. (pp. 106–107)
1-5.6   Identify the information obtained when assessing a patient's pulse. (pp. 106–108)
1-5.7   Differentiate between a strong, weak, regular, and irregular pulse. (p. 107)
1-5.8   Describe the methods to assess skin color, temperature, and condition (capillary refill in infants and children). (pp. 108–109)
1-5.9   Identify normal and abnormal skin colors. (p. 108)
1-5.10 Differentiate between pale, blue, red, and yellow skin color. (p. 108)
1-5.11 Identify normal and abnormal skin temperature. (p. 108)
1-5.12 Differentiate between hot, cool, and cold skin temperature. (p. 108)
1-5.13 Identify normal and abnormal skin conditions. (p. 109)
1-5.14 Identify normal and abnormal capillary refill in infants and children. (p. 109)
1-5.15 Describe the methods to assess the pupils. (p. 110)
1-5.16 Identify normal and abnormal pupil size. (p. 110)
1-5.17 Differentiate between dilated (big) and constricted (small) pupil size. (p. 110)
1-5.18 Differentiate between reactive and nonreactive pupils and equal and unequal pupils. (pp. 110)
1-5.19 Describe the methods to assess blood pressure. (pp. 112–115)
1-5.20 Define systolic pressure. (p. 111)
1-5.21 Define diastolic pressure. (p. 111)
1-5.22 Explain the difference between auscultation and palpation for obtaining a blood pressure. (pp. 112–113)
1-5.23 Identify the components of the SAMPLE history. (p. 119)
1-5.24 Differentiate between a sign and a symptom. (p. 119)

Total Teaching Time
150 minutes

Resources Needed
- Scored Chapter 4 Quizzes
- Enough blood pressure cuffs, stethoscopes, and penlights for at least one out of every three students
- Inexpensive prizes, such as penlights

Additional Resources
Larmon/Davis, *Basic Life Support Skills*

Elling, *EMT Achieve: Basic Test Preparation*

Limmer/Mistovich/ O'Keefe, *Audio Lecture & Study Guide: EMT*

Mistovich/Kuvlesky, *SUCCESS! for the EMT, Second Edition*

1-5.25 State the importance of accurately reporting and recording the baseline vital signs. (p. 103)

1-5.26 Discuss the need to search for additional medical identification. (p. 119)

Affective

1-5.27 Explain the value of performing the baseline vital signs. (pp. 103–104)

1-5.28 Recognize and respond to the feelings patients experience during assessment. (p. 103)

1-5.29 Defend the need for obtaining and recording an accurate set of vital signs. (pp. 103–104)

1-5.30 Explain the rationale for recording additional sets of vital signs. (pp. 103, 199)

1-5.31 Explain the importance of obtaining a SAMPLE history. (pp. 103, 119–102)

Psychomotor

1-5.32 Demonstrate the skills involved in assessment of breathing.

1-5.33 Demonstrate the skills associated with obtaining a pulse.

1-5.34 Demonstrate the skills associated with assessing skin color, temperature, condition, and capillary refill in infants and children.

1-5.35 Demonstrate the skills associated with assessing the pupils.

1-5.36 Demonstrate the skills associated with obtaining blood pressure.

1-5.37 Demonstrate the skills that should be used to obtain information from the patient, family, or bystanders at the scene.

REVIEW

The last lesson, "The Human Body," described the anatomy and physiology of the human body. Students learned how to identify, locate, and use medical terminology to label structures (anatomy) such as the heart, arteries, veins, and capillaries. They also learned how such structures function (physiology) and work together to form intricate and efficient systems in healthy individuals. Stress to students that this knowledge of the human body will enable them to perform high-quality patient assessment and care and to communicate necessary patient information to other health professionals accurately and concisely. Remind them to go over the content of the last chapter to be sure they are able to use the proper terminology to communicate patient information as well as recognize when a body is functioning normally and when there are life-threatening deviations. Distribute the scored quizzes from the last class. Go over each question on the quiz and handle any concerns students may have about the answers.

INTRODUCTION TO CHAPTER 5

Chapter 5, "Baseline Vital Signs and History Taking," is the fifth lesson in Module 1. This lesson describes the two basic elements of patient assessment: vital signs and the patient SAMPLE history. Tell students that vital signs are measurable items like respirations, pulse, and blood pressure. Explain that accurate measurement and recording of vital signs over a period of time may reveal a trend in the patient's condition, which is valuable information in the continuum of care. Point out that the first set of measurements, or baseline vital signs, provide a "base" to which subsequent measurements can be compared. Stress that the patient SAMPLE history, which addresses signs and symptoms, allergies, medications, and so on, is

©2008 by Pearson Education, Inc.
Prehospital Emergency Care, 8th ed.

just as important as vital signs. This patient history can guide the EMT's pace, shine light on underlying problems, and in the event that the patient loses consciousness, it can provide the only source of information about the patient available to hospital personnel. The EMT uses each detail revealed by the assessment—vital signs and SAMPLE history—to help build a picture of the patient's condition and to inform decisions on emergency care.

Distribute the Chapter 5 Objectives Checklist and give students a few minutes to look it over. Then briefly paraphrase the objectives for this lesson in your own words.

LECTURE

The following suggested lecture outline is based on the Department of Transportation's EMT-Basic National Standard Curriculum. In some places, the DOT curriculum has been rearranged or expanded upon so that it is more complete or easier for the student to understand. The page numbers in parentheses refer to pages in the textbook. The parenthetical references in dark, heavy type are to figures, tables, and scans in the textbook.

BASELINE VITAL SIGNS AND HISTORY TAKING

I. Gathering patient information (p. 103)
   A. Patient assessment (p. 103)
   B. Observe environment (p. 103)
   C. Reassure patient (p. 103)
   D. Treat with respect and dignity (p. 103)
II. Baseline vital signs (pp. 103–104)
   A. Vital signs (pp. 103–104)
     1. Breathing
     2. Pulse
     3. Skin
     4. Pupils
     5. Blood pressure
     6. Pulse oximetry
     7. Trending
     8. Equipment
       a. Sphygmomanometer (blood pressure cuff) in adult and pediatric sizes
       b. Stethoscope
       c. Wristwatch that counts seconds
       d. Penlight to examine pupils
       e. EMT shears
       f. Pen and pocket notebook
      g. Personal protective equipment
III. Breathing (pp. 104–105)**(Fig. 5-1, p. 104)**
   A. Assessed by observing the patient's chest rise and fall (p. 104)
   B. Rate (pp. 104–105)
     1. Determined by counting the number of breaths in a 30-second period and multiplying by 2
     2. Care should be taken not to inform the patient, to avoid influencing the rate **(Table 5-1, p. 104)**
     3. Adult
       a. 12–20 breaths per minute
     4. Child
       a. 15–30 breaths per minute
     5. Infant

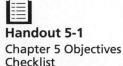

Handout 5-1
Chapter 5 Objectives Checklist

● ➤
Lecture Master
You may wish to display Lecture Master 5 when presenting the lecture to the class.

Teaching Tip
Tell students that to count respirations, they can place a hand on the patient's wrist, as if taking a pulse, and hold the patient's arm close to his or her abdomen while counting breaths. Then they can obtain a pulse rate.

On the Net
Covers equipment needed to basic interpretations.
http://www.medinfo.ufl.edu/year1/bcs/clist/vitals.html

Slides/Videos
Brady Skill Series: EMT-B, "Vital Signs"

                    a. 25–50 breaths per minute
                C. Quality (p. 105)
                    1. Determined while assessing the rate
                    2. Quality can be placed in one of four categories
                        a. Normal
                            (1) Average chest wall motion, not using accessory muscles
                        b. Shallow
                            (1) Slight chest or abdominal wall motion
                        c. Labored
                            (1) An increase in the effort of breathing
                            (2) Grunting and stridor
                            (3) Use of accessory muscles
                            (4) Nasal flaring, supraclavicular and intercostal retractions in infants and children
                            (5) Sometimes gasping
                        d. Noisy
                            (1) Increase in the audible sound of breathing may include snoring, wheezing, gurgling, crowing **(Table 5-2, p. 105)**
                D. Rhythm (p. 105)
                    1. Regular
                    2. Irregular
  IV. **Pulse** (pp. 105–108)**(Fig. 5-2, p. 106)**
                A. Locations (pp. 105–106)
                    1. Carotid
                    2. Femoral
                    3. Radial
                    4. Brachial
                    5. Posterior tibial
                    6. Dorsalis pedis
                B. Initially a radial pulse should be assessed in all patients 1 year or older (p. 106)
                C. In patients younger than 1 year, a brachial pulse should be assessed (p. 106) **(Fig. 5-3, p. 106)**
                D. Rate (pp. 107–108)
                    1. Rate is the number of beats felt in 30 seconds multiplied by 2 **(Table 5-3, p. 107)**
                    2. Pulsus paradoxus
                E. Quality (pp. 107–108) **(Table 5-4, p. 107)**
                    1. Strong
                    2. Weak
                    3. Regular
                    4. Irregular
                F. If peripheral pulse is not palpable, assess carotid pulse (p. 106) **(Fig. 5-4, pp. 106–107)**
                    1. Avoid excess pressure on geriatric patients
                    2. Never attempt to assess carotid pulse on both sides at the same time
  V. **Skin** (pp. 108–109)**(Table 5-5, p. 108)**
                A. The patient's color should be assessed in the nail beds, oral mucosa, and conjunctiva (p. 108)
                    1. In infants and children, palms of hands and soles of feet should be assessed
                B. Color (p. 108)
                    1. Normal skin

✓
Teaching Tip
Consider using moulage
and makeup on a
volunteer to demonstrate
pallor, cyanosis, or
jaundice.

©2008 by Pearson Education, Inc.
Prehospital Emergency Care, 8th ed.

        a. Pink
    2. Abnormal skin colors
        a. Pale
            (1) Indicating poor perfusion (impaired blood flow)
        b. Cyanotic (blue-gray)
            (1) Indicating inadequate oxygenation or poor perfusion
        c. Flushed (red)
            (1) Indicating exposure to heat or carbon monoxide poisoning
        d. Jaundice (yellow)
            (1) Indicating liver abnormalities
        e. Mottled
            (1) Similar to cyanosis, but in a blotchy pattern
C. Temperature (pp. 108–109)
    1. Place the back of your hand on the patient's skin (**Fig. 5-5, p. 109**)
    2. Normal
        a. Warm
    3. Abnormal skin temperatures
        a. Hot
            (1) Indicating fever or an exposure to heat
        b. Cool
            (1) Indicating poor perfusion or exposure to cold
        c. Cold
            (1) Indicating extreme exposure to cold
D. Condition (p. 109)
    1. Normal
        a. Dry
    2. Abnormal
        a. Wet or moist
            (1) Shock (hypoperfusion)
            (2) Poisoning
            (3) Heat-related problem
            (4) Cardiac problem
            (5) Diabetic problem
        b. Dry
            (1) Spinal injury
            (2) Severe dehydration
            (3) Heat-related problem
E. Capillary refill (p. 109) (**Fig. 5-6, p. 109**)
    1. Most reliable in infants and children under 6 years of age
    2. Affected by cold, circulatory problems, and certain medications
    3. Normal
        a. In infants, children, and adult males
            (1) 2 seconds
        b. Adult females
            (1) 3 seconds
        c. Elderly persons
            (1) 4 seconds
    4. Abnormal
        a. May indicate shock (hypoperfusion)
VI. Pupils (p. 110)
    A. Briefly shine a light into the patient's eyes and determine size and reactivity (p. 110) (**Fig. 5-7, p. 110; Table 5-6, p. 110**)

Point to Emphasize

Capillary refill time will vary depending on age, disease status, and environmental temperature.

Point of Interest

In some people, unequal pupils are normal.

On the Net

For information about equipment such as BP cuffs and stethoscopes, go to: http://www. alliedhpi.com

On the Net

Basic information and links about hypertension. http://sln.fi.edu/biosci/healthy/pressure.html

On the Net

Detailed information about blood pressure. http://www.medformation.com/mf/mm_qdis.nsf/qd/nd2500g.htm

    B. Size (p. 110)
        1. Dilated (big)
        2. Normal
        3. Constricted (small)
    C. Equality (p. 110)
        1. Equal
        2. Unequal
    D. Reactivity (p. 110)
        1. Whether or not the pupils change in response to light
            a. Reactive
            b. Change when exposed to light
            c. Nonreactive
            d. Do not change when exposed to light
        2. Equally, unequally, or fixed reactivity

VII. Blood pressure (pp. 111–115)
    A. Assess systolic and diastolic pressures (p. 111) **(Table 5-7, p. 111)**
        1. Systolic blood pressure
            a. First distinct sound (Korothoff sounds) of blood flowing through the artery as the pressure in the blood pressure cuff is released
            b. This is a measurement of the pressure exerted against the walls of the arteries during contraction of the heart
            c. Normal adult is less the 140 mmHg
        2. Diastolic blood pressure
            a. Point during deflation of the blood pressure cuff in which sounds of the pulse beat disappear
            b. It represents the pressure exerted against the walls of the arteries while the left ventricle is at rest
            c. Normal adult is less than 85
    B. Normal blood pressure (pp. 111–112)
        1. Adult male
            a. Systolic equals 100 mmHg + patient age
            b. Systolic greater than 140 mmHg is considered hypertension
            c. Diastolic normally 60–90 mmHg
            d. Diastolic greater than 90 mmHg is considered diastolic hypertension
        2. Adult female
            a. Systolic equals 90 mmHg + patient age
            b. Diastolic normally 60–90 mmHg
            c. Diastolic greater than 90 mmHg is considered diastolic hypertension
        3. Child 1–10 years old
            a. (Child's age × 2) + 80 mmHg
            b. Lower limit of systolic
               (1) (Child's age × 2) + 70 mmHg
        4. Child or adolescent greater than 10 years
            a. Minimum systolic of 90 mmHg
            b. Less than minimum indicates possible hypoperfusion
    C. Pulse pressure (p. 112)
        1. Difference between systolic and diastolic pressures
        2. Less than 25 percent of systolic
            a. Narrow pulse pressure
         3. Greater than 50 percent of systolic
            a. Widened pulse pressure

4. Pulsus paradoxus

    a. Sudden drop in blood pressure of greater than 10 mmHg

D. There are two methods of obtaining blood pressure (pp. 112–115) **(Fig. 5-10, p. 115):**

    1. Auscultation

        a. Listen for the systolic and diastolic sounds using a stethoscope **(Fig. 5-8, p. 114)**

    2. Palpation

        a. Systolic blood pressure may be measured by feeling for return of pulse with deflation of the cuff **(Fig. 5-9, p. 115)**

VIII. Orthostatic vital signs (pp. 115–116) **(Fig. 5-11, p. 116)**

A. Do not attempt orthostatic vital signs in patients with possible spinal injury (p. 115)

B. Technique (pp. 115–116)

    1. Take pulse and blood pressure with patient supine

    2. Stand patient up and wait 2 minutes

        a. Can use sitting position if unable to stand

    3. Retake pulse and blood pressure

C. Positive orthostatic (tilt) test (pp. 115–116)

    1. Increase in heart rate greater than 10–20 bpm

    2. Decrease in blood pressure of 10–20 mmHg

IX. Pulse oximetry (pp. 116–119) **(Fig. 5-12, p. 117)**

A. Method of measuring the oxygen saturation levels in the blood (pp. 116–117)

B. Readings (pp. 116–117)

    1. 97–100 percent SpO_2 normal

    2. <95 percent SpO_2 indicates hypoxia and compromise

C. Treat the patient, not the pulse oximetry reading (p. 118)

D. Indications for pulse oximetry (p. 118)

    1. Any situation where the patient's oxygen status is a concern

    2. The "sixth vital sign"

E. Limitations of the pulse oximeter (pp. 118–119)

    1. Shock (hypoperfusion) may produce abnormally high readings

    2. Hypothermia or cold injury to the extremities will reduce peripheral perfusion

    3. Excessive movement of the patient may produce inaccurate readings

    4. During some types of seizures, the excessive movement will lead to inaccurate readings

    5. If the finger probe is used, nail polish will produce an inaccurate reading. Carbon monoxide will give an abnormally high reading.

    6. Cigarette smokers may have falsely high readings

    7. Anemia may produce abnormally high readings

X. Vital sign reassessment (p. 119)

A. Vital signs should be reassessed and recorded every 15 minutes at a minimum in a stable patient (p. 119)

B. Vital signs should be reassessed and recorded every 5 minutes in the unstable patient (p. 119)

C. Vital signs should be reassessed following all medical interventions (p. 119)

XI. The SAMPLE history (pp. 119–120)

A. Signs/symptoms (p. 119)

    1. Sign

        a. Any condition observed by the EMT

Point to Emphasize
Remind students that signs are things they can see, hear, or touch, while symptoms are what the patient tells them.

        2. Symptom
            a. Any condition described by the patient
    B. Allergies (p. 119)
        1. Types
            a. Medications
            b. Food
            c. Environmental
        2. Consider medical identification tag
    C. Medications (p. 119)
        1. Prescription
            a. Current
            b. Recent
            c. Birth control pills
        2. Nonprescription
            a. Current
            b. Recent
        3. Herbal preparations
        4. Consider medical identification tag
    D. Pertinent past history (p. 119)
        1. Medical
        2. Surgical
        3. Trauma
        4. Consider medical identification tag
    E. Last oral intake (p. 119)
        1. Solid or liquid
        2. Time
        3. Quantity
    F. Events leading to the injury or illness (p. 119)
        1. What was the patient doing?
        2. What happened?

CASE STUDY

Ask a student volunteer to read the Case Study that begins on page 103 of the textbook. You may wish to use the following questions to engage students in a discussion of the Case Study Follow-up that begins on page 120 of the textbook. Provide missing information and clarify ideas as needed.

Q1. What were Mr. Li's baseline vitals?

A1. *Respirations—18 and normal; pulse—78 and regular; skin—pink, warm, and dry; pupils—normal, equal, and reactive; and blood pressure—168/82.*

Q2. What was Mr. Li's SAMPLE history?

A2. *Signs/symptoms—patient lying supine on kitchen floor, unable to get up; complaint of pain in his left hip. Mr. Li says he fell about an hour earlier.*

Allergies—penicillin

Medications—insulin daily to help control blood sugar

Pertinent past history—history of diabetes and both hip joints replaced in 1989

Last oral intake—dinner last night. Ms. Kennedy added that while they were waiting for the ambulance, she gave her father a glass of water.

Slides/Videos

Medic Alert Slides. Medic Alert Foundation, P.O. Box 381009, Turlock, CA 95381-9009.

Point to Emphasize

Stress the importance of asking patients if they have taken their medications at the same time the patients are asked if they have any prescribed medications.

©2008 by Pearson Education, Inc.
Prehospital Emergency Care, 8th ed.

Events leading to injury—Mr. Li slipped and fell from the chair at about 9:00 A.M.

Q3. Why did you take Mr. Li's vital signs every 15 minutes instead of more frequently?

A3. *Because his vital signs are good and his condition is considered stable.*

IN REVIEW

Assess students' ability to apply what they have just learned by discussing the Review Questions on page 122 in the textbook.

Q1. Identify the components of vital signs, and state how often they should be taken.

A1. *The components of vital signs are breathing, pulse, skin, pupils, and blood pressure. In a stable patient, vital signs should be taken every 15 minutes and as often as necessary to ensure proper care. In an unstable patient, vital signs should be taken every 5 minutes. Vital signs should also be taken after every medical intervention. (pp. 103–104, 119)*

Q2. Explain how to assess a patient's breathing rate and quality of breathing. Also state the normal ranges of respirations per minute for the adult, child, and infant.

A2. *Breathing is assessed by observing the patient's chest rise and fall. Breathing rate is determined by counting the number of breaths in a 30-second period and multiplying by 2. Quality of breathing can be determined while rate is being assessed. Normal respirations are 12–20/minute for adults, 15–30/minute for children, and 25–50/minute for infants. (pp. 104–105)*

Q3. Describe what you would observe when a patient is breathing normally and when a patient is breathing abnormally.

A3. *In normal breathing, the chest expands out at least one inch, accessory muscles of the abdomen are not used to breathe, rate is normal, and inhalations and exhalations are about the same length. In shallow breathing, there is only slight chest or abdominal wall motion. In labored breathing, there may be grunting and stridor, use of accessory muscles, nasal flaring, and gasping. In infants and children, there may also be retraction of the skin around the collarbone and between the ribs. In noisy breathing, snoring, wheezing, gurgling, or crowing may be heard. (p. 105)*

Q4. State the general circumstances under which you would choose to take a radial pulse, a brachial pulse, or a carotid pulse.

A4. *Take a radial pulse in all patients 1 year or older. Take a brachial pulse in patients younger than 1 year. When a peripheral pulse cannot be obtained, take the pulse at the carotid artery. (p. 106)*

Q5. Explain how to take a pulse. Also identify normal resting pulse rates in an adult, adolescent, school-age child, preschool child, and infant.

A5. *To take a pulse, use the tips of two or three fingers—not the thumb—to palpate the artery and count the number of beats in a 30-second period, then multiply by 2. Normal resting rates are 60–80 beats/minute for an adult, 60–105 beats/minute for an adolescent, 60–120* *beats/minute for a school-age child, 80–150 beats/minute for a preschooler, and 120–150 beats/minute for an infant. (pp. 106–107)*

Q6. Define the terms that you would use to describe pulse quality.

A6. *The quality of the pulse can be characterized as strong, weak, regular, or irregular. A strong pulse usually refers to a normal pulse that is both full and strong. A "bounding" pulse is one that is abnormally strong. A weak pulse is usually quite rapid, in which case it would be called "thready." A regular pulse is usually a normal pulse that occurs at regular intervals with a smooth rhythm. An irregular pulse is one that occurs at irregular intervals between beats. (p. 107)*

Q7. List the places on the body to check for skin color. Also identify normal and abnormal skin colors.

A7. *Check for skin color in the nail beds, oral mucosa, and conjunctiva. In infants and children and in dark-skinned people, check the palms and soles. Normally, skin color in these areas is pink. Abnormal colors include pale, blue-gray, red, yellow, and black-and-blue mottling. (p. 108)*

Q8. Explain how to assess a patient's pupils, and describe normal and abnormal findings.

A8. *Briefly shine a light into the patient's eyes to assess pupil size, equality, and reactivity. Normally, both pupils are the same size and constrict equally in response to light. Abnormal pupils may be dilated or constricted, or unequal in size, and neither or only one pupil may react to light. (p. 110)*

Q9. Explain how to take blood pressure by palpation and by auscultation. Also identify the normal ranges of systolic and diastolic blood pressure for an adult male and an adult female.

A9. *To take blood pressure by palpation, feel for the return of the pulse as the cuff is deflated. By auscultation, listen for the systolic and diastolic sounds through a stethoscope. (p. 113–115) (For normal blood pressure rates, see Table 5-7, p. 111 of the textbook.)*

Q10. Name the categories of information you need to obtain through a SAMPLE history.

A10. *The SAMPLE history includes signs and symptoms, allergies, medication, pertinent past history, last oral intake, and events leading to the injury or illness. (pp. 119–120)*

CRITICAL THINKING

Assess students' ability to respond to real-life emergency situations by discussing the Critical Thinking questions on page 122 in the textbook.

Q1. What is the significance of the gurgling sound?

A1. *The gurgling sound indicates that the patient has some type of fluid (blood, vomit, etc.) in his airway.*

Q2. How would you document the pulse rate?

A2. *Documentation of this patient's pulse rate should include the beat-per-minute count (45 bpm), whether it is strong or weak, and the location* *of the pulse being assessed. It could be documented as "radial pulse is 45 bpm and strong" or "radial pulse is bradycardic at 45 bpm but strong." The location is important to note because it provides an indication of perfusion. If a radial pulse is found, it typically implies better perfusion than if only a carotid or femoral pulse was able to be palpated. Also, keep in mind that a heart rate less than 60 bpm in the adult is termed bradycardia and a heart rate greater than 100 bpm in the adult is known as tachycardia.*

Q3. What does the pulse oximeter reading indicate?

A3. *The pulse oximeter reading (SpO2) of 76% on room air indicates that the patient is severely hypoxic and requires immediate assisted ventilation with supplemental oxygen connected to the ventilation device. A respiratory rate of 45 per minute in an adult is beyond the upper range of normal in an adult patient and will not allow for adequate breathing. High respiratory rates will decrease the time for adequate lung filling and will lead to poor tidal volumes and inadequate breathing.*

Q4. What do the skin signs indicate?

A4. *The cyanosis would indicate a poor oxygenation status, most likely due to the high respiratory rate and poor tidal volume. The warm and dry skin would indicate an adequate blood pressure is present.*

Q5. What other vitals signs would be important to assess in this patient?

A5. *Responding EMTs should also assess this patient's pupils for size, equality, and reactivity to light.*

Q6. When would you attempt to gather a SAMPLE history?

A6. *Since the patient is unresponsive and transport time is a critical factor in trauma situations, the SAMPLE history should be gathered while en route to the hospital.*

Q7. How would you gather the SAMPLE history?

A7. *Since the patient is unresponsive, his spouse would be the best source for a SAMPLE history.*

SKILLS DEMONSTRATION AND PRACTICE

Using a student as a patient, demonstrate the following:

1. Assess breathing.
2. Take radial pulse.
3. Take carotid pulse.
4. Assess skin color, temperature, and condition (including capillary refill for infants and children).
5. Assess pupils.
6. Measure blood pressure by auscultation.
7. Measure blood pressure by palpation.

Help students form groups of three. If the number of students does not divide equally by threes, it is acceptable to have groups of two or four. Provide blood pressure cuffs, stethoscopes, and penlights for each group, and direct the students to take turns being the patient, the EMT, and an observer. Visit each group several times to monitor progress and skill accuracy. Provide assistance, if necessary.

WRITE SAMPLE HISTORIES

Have students break into pairs. Tell them that the members of each pair should take turns playing the roles of patient and EMT. Then direct students to perform a SAMPLE history on each other as quickly and accurately as possible. Encourage them to be creative but realistic. When they are done, have them sign the back of each other's SAMPLE histories. However, advise students not to sign the back of their partner's paper if the SAMPLE history was collected inaccurately. After the pairs have completed their first two SAMPLE histories, have them form new pairs with other students. Challenge them to perform as many accurate SAMPLE histories (and collect as many signatures) as possible within 10 minutes. The person with the most signatures wins.

Rotate among the pairs. Listen to the SAMPLE histories being taken. Correct performance as needed. Referee any disputes. Stop when the allotted time has passed. Determine which students have the most signatures. Provide each winning student with a prize, such as a penlight.

ASSIGNMENTS

Assign students to read Chapter 6, "Lifting and Moving Patients," before the next class. Also ask them to complete Chapter 5 of the Workbook.

EVALUATION

Chapter Quiz Distribute copies of the Chapter Quiz provided in Handout 5-2 to evaluate student understanding of this chapter. Remind students not to refer to their textbooks or notes while taking the quiz.

Test Manager You may wish to create a custom-tailored test using Prentice Hall *TestGen for Prehospital Emergency Care, Eighth Edition* to evaluate student understanding of this chapter.

Online Test Preparation (for students and instructors) Additional test preparation is available through *EMT Achieve: Basic Test Preparation* at http://www.prenhall.com/EMTAchieve. Instructors can also monitor student mastery online.

REINFORCEMENT

Handouts If classroom discussions or performance on the quiz indicates that some students have not fully mastered the chapter content, you may wish to assign some or all of the Reinforcement Handouts for this chapter.

Reading/Reference
Textbook, pp. 123–149

Workbook
Chapter 5 Activities

Chapter Quiz
Handout 5-2

TestGen
Chapter 5 Test

Online Test Preparation
Send your students to http://www.prenhall.com/EMTAchieve

Handouts 5-3 to 5-5
Reinforcement Activities

TECH EXTRAS

Brady Skills Series EMT-B Videos/CD Have your students watch the skills come to life on either VHS or CD-ROM.

PowerPoint Presentation(for instructors) The PowerPoint material developed for this chapter offers useful reinforcement of chapter content.

Student CD A wide variety of material on this CD-ROM will reinforce and also expand student knowledge and skills.

Companion Website(for students) Additional review quizzes and links to EMS resources will contribute to further reinforcement of this chapter. Please visit http://www.prenhall.com/mistovich.

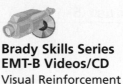

Brady Skills Series EMT-B Videos/CD
Visual Reinforcement

PowerPoint Presentation
Chapter 5

Student CD
Chapter 5

Companion Website
http://www.prenhall.com/mistovich

OBJECTIVES CHECKLIST

Cognitive		Date Mastered
1-5.1	Identify the components of vital signs.	
1-5.2	Describe the methods to obtain a breathing rate.	
1-5.3	Identify the attributes that should be obtained when assessing breathing.	
1-5.4	Differentiate between shallow, labored, and noisy breathing.	
1-5.5	Describe the methods to obtain a pulse rate.	
1-5.6	Identify the information obtained when assessing a patient's pulse.	
1-5.7	Differentiate between a strong, weak, regular, and irregular pulse.	
1-5.8	Describe the methods to assess skin color, temperature, and condition (capillary refill in infants and children).	
1-5.9	Identify normal and abnormal skin colors.	
1-5.10	Differentiate between pale, blue, red, and yellow skin color.	
1-5.11	Identify normal and abnormal skin temperature.	
1-5.12	Differentiate between hot, cool, and cold skin temperature.	
1-5.13	Identify normal and abnormal skin conditions.	
1-5.14	Identify normal and abnormal capillary refill in infants and children.	
1-5.15	Describe the methods to assess the pupils.	
1-5.16	Identify normal and abnormal pupil size.	
1-5.17	Differentiate between dilated (big) and constricted (small) pupil size.	
1-5.18	Differentiate between reactive and nonreactive pupils and equal and unequal pupils.	
1-5.19	Describe the methods to assess blood pressure.	
1-5.20	Define systolic pressure.	
1-5.21	Define diastolic pressure.	
1-5.22	Explain the difference between auscultation and palpation for obtaining a blood pressure.	
1-5.23	Identify the components of the SAMPLE history.	
1-5.24	Differentiate between a sign and a symptom.	
1-5.25	State the importance of accurately reporting and recording the baseline vital signs.	
1-5.26	Discuss the need to search for additional medical identification.	

©2008 by Pearson Education, Inc.
Prehospital Emergency Care, 8th ed.

Affective	Date Mastered
1-5.27 Explain the value of performing the baseline vital signs.	
1-5.28 Recognize and respond to the feelings patients experience during assessment.	
1-5.29 Defend the need for obtaining and recording an accurate set of vital signs.	
1-5.30 Explain the rationale for recording additional sets of vital signs.	
1-5.31 Explain the importance of obtaining a SAMPLE history.	

Psychomotor	Date Mastered
1-5.32 Demonstrate the skills involved in assessment of breathing.	
1-5.33 Demonstrate the skills associated with obtaining a pulse.	
1-5.34 Demonstrate the skills associated with assessing the skin color, temperature, condition, and capillary refill in infants and children.	
1-5.35 Demonstrate the skills associated with assessing the pupils.	
1-5.36 Demonstrate the skills associated with obtaining blood pressure.	
1-5.37 Demonstrate the skills that should be used to obtain information from the patient, family, or bystanders at the scene.	

CHAPTER 5 QUIZ

Write the letter of the best answer in the space provided.

_____ 1. Which of the following is *not* a vital sign?
    A. pulse   **C.** respiration
    B. mental status   **D.** blood pressure

_____ 2. An EMT's first set of patient measurements is called the _____ vital signs.
    A. initial   **C.** palpated
    B. baseline   **D.** preliminary

_____ 3. The vital sign that is more reliable in infants and children than in adults is called
    A. skin color.   **C.** pupillary reaction.
    B. capillary refill.   **D.** blood pressure.

_____ 4. The term used to describe a weak, rapid pulse is
    A. mottled.   **C.** thready.
    B. reedy.   **D.** bounding.

_____ 5. In cases of shock or early stages of blood loss, an EMT would expect the pulse to be
    A. rapid, regular, and full.   **C.** slow.
    B. rapid, regular, and thready. **D.** absent.

_____ 6. The first pulse taken by an EMT on patients 1 year and older is the _____ pulse.
    A. carotid   **C.** femoral
    B. radial   **D.** dorsalis pedis

_____ 7. A heart rate greater than 100 beats per minute in an adult patient is called
    A. tachycardia.   **C.** pulse pressure.
    B. bradycardia.   **D.** rapid pulse point.

_____ 8. The act of breathing out is called
    A. inhalation.   **C.** respiration.
    B. exhalation.   **D.** inspiration.

_____ 9. All of the following are signs of labored breathing *except*
    A. nasal flaring.   **C.** grunting.
    B. retractions.   **D.** jaundice.

_____ 10. The skin color that indicates anemia or emotional distress is
    A. pale.   **C.** flushed.
    B. blue-gray.   **D.** jaundiced.

_____ 11. The skin color that indicates inadequate breathing or heart attack is
    A. flushed.   **C.** jaundiced.
    B. blue-gray.   **D.** yellow.

_____ 12. The skin condition that may indicate a spinal injury is
    A. hot.   **C.** damp.
    B. cool and dry.   **D.** abnormally dry.

_____ **13.** When checking pupils, an EMT should look for all of the following *except*
   A. size.
   B. equality.
   C. reactivity.
   D. color.

_____ **14.** In cases of stroke or head injury, the pupils are likely to be
   A. dilated.
   B. constricted.
   C. unequal.
   D. equal.

_____ **15.** A normal systolic blood pressure for a 40-year-old female would be
   A. 90.
   B. 100.
   C. 130.
   D. 150.

_____ **16.** When deflating the cuff of a sphygmomanometer, the systolic blood pressure is the
   A. first beats.
   B. last sound.
   C. dullest sound.
   D. loudest beats.

_____ **17.** What is the difference between the systolic and diastolic blood pressure readings called?
   A. tachycardia
   B. bradycardia
   C. pressure point
   D. pulse pressure

_____ **18.** For unstable patients, an EMT should take vital signs every _____ minutes.
   A. 20
   B. 15
   C. 10
   D. 5

_____ **19.** In distinguishing signs from symptoms, an example of a symptom would be
   A. chest pain.
   B. slow pulse.
   C. retractions.
   D. cyanosis.

_____ **20.** The "L" in SAMPLE stands for
   A. length of illness.
   B. last doctor's visit.
   C. length of chief complaint.
   D. last oral intake.

IN THE FIELD

Read the following real-life situation. Then answer the questions that follow.

You're looking out the window of the fire station watching the snow fall. The blare of the speaker breaks the peace: "Engine 3 respond to an elderly woman complaining of shortness of breath, 18 Warren Street. Time out 0600."

"Just around the corner," you say to your partner. As expected, you arrive on the scene in just a few minutes. You survey a quiet neighborhood, known for housing many retirees. Nothing in the immediate environment of the house indicates possible danger. The crew dons gloves as it walks up to the door. After you knock at the door, a woman's voice invites you to enter.

Upon entering, you find an elderly woman sitting upright on an overstuffed chair in the living room. She is awake and responsive to your questions. Her chief complaint is that she "can't breathe." Your general impression is that she is in some degree of breathing distress. The woman has an open airway, but her breathing is labored and noisy. One crew member starts to administer high-concentration oxygen by nonrebreather mask.

While oxygen is administered, you continue with patient assessment. The woman's pulse is rapid, faster than 100 beats per minute. You advise the lieutenant that the patient is "high priority." The lieutenant, in turn, advises the incoming ambulance of the patient's condition and priority. The ambulance reports that weather conditions will delay their arrival by several minutes.

One crew member proceeds to obtain vital signs as you begin the patient interview. You ask the patient to describe her symptoms. You ask, "Have you had any coughing or bloody sputum?" She responds to your questions with choppy answers, a sign of difficulty breathing. You ask if the patient has any allergies. You also find out if she is taking any medications. Finally, you inquire whether she has had similar episodes like this one.

The crew member taking the vital signs interrupts briefly to relate his findings. He reports that the patient's heart rate is 110 beats per minute, strong and slightly irregular. He also indicates a blood pressure of 160/110 and a respiratory rate of 28, with labored breathing and a pulse ox of 82 percent on high-flow O_2.

The woman offers, "Had a nagging cough for several days. Last night I had so much trouble breathing that I got up to sit in the easy chair. I've been sleeping on and off all night." She denies any allergies but did suffer a heart attack several years ago and a subsequent "heart failure." She is on Digoxin, Lasix, and potassium supplements.

You ask the patient when she last had anything to eat or drink. Her answer completes your history. As you write down the information, the ambulance pulls up.

1. What are the patient's baseline vital signs?

2. How long should the crew member spend in taking the patient's pulse? Why?

3. Which parts of the passage describe the patient's symptoms?

4. What priority would you assign this patient?

CHAPTER 5 REVIEW

Write the word or words that best complete each sentence in the space provided.

1. The outward signs of what is going on inside a patient's body are the

    _____ _____.

2. The first set of vital signs an EMT obtains is called _____ vital signs.

3. The rhythmic beat generated by the contraction of the left ventricle is called the

    _____.

4. In patients younger than 1 year, an EMT should first attempt to assess a(n)

    _____ pulse.

5. In an adolescent, a normal resting pulse rate would be _____ to

    _____ beats per minute.

6. If the pulse rate, rhythm, or character is not normal, an EMT should continue taking the count for

    _____ seconds.

7. For determination of vital signs, an EMT is concerned with two respiratory factors:

    _____ and _____.

8. An adult patient is breathing outside of normal rates when respirations are above

    _____ breaths per minute or below _____ breaths

    per minute.

9. Snoring, wheezing, gurgling, and crowing are examples of _____

    breathing.

10. The harsh, high-pitched sound that indicates labored breathing is _____.

11. In addition to checking nail beds, oral mucosa, and conjunctiva, assess the skin color of infants,

    children, and dark-skinned patients on the _____ and

    _____.

12. Pupils that are _____ are too large.

13. The proper term for a blood pressure cuff is _____.

14. The force of blood against the walls of the blood vessels is known as the

    _____ _____.

©2008 by Pearson Education, Inc.
Prehospital Emergency Care, 8th ed.

15. The bladder of a blood pressure cuff should be centered over the _____

    artery.

16. Taking blood pressure by use of the fingertips is known as _____.

17. A patient's _____ are conditions that an EMT cannot observe but can only

    learn about when the patient describes them.

18. On way to get an accurate patient _____ is to use the acronym SAMPLE.

19. The "A" in SAMPLE stands for _____.

20. When gathering information from your patient, try as much as possible to ask

    _____ _____ questions.

REINFORCEMENT

BASELINE VITAL SIGNS AND HISTORY TAKING

Write the letter of the term in the space provided next to the appropriate description.

_____ **1.** Pressure created when the heart contracts

_____ **2.** Pulse felt in the major artery in the neck

_____ **3.** Harsh, high-pitched sound of labored breathing

_____ **4.** Force of blood against the walls of blood vessels

_____ **5.** Objective physical evidence of a patient's condition

_____ **6.** Pulse felt in the major artery of the upper arm

_____ **7.** To get smaller, as in the pupils of the eyes

_____ **8.** Feeling, as for the return of a pulse when taking blood pressure

_____ **9.** Act of breathing in and out

_____ **10.** Patient conditions that cannot be observed

_____ **11.** Measurements, or outward indications of what is going on inside the body

_____ **12.** Black center of the eye

_____ **13.** Listening, as in use of a stethoscope for characteristic sounds

_____ **14.** To get larger, as in the pupils of the eyes

_____ **15.** Pulse felt at the wrist

A. auscultation

B. blood pressure

C. brachial

D. carotid

E. constrict

F. dilate

G. palpation

H. pupil

I. radial

J. respiration

K. signs

L. stridor

M. symptoms

N. systolic

O. vital signs

Baseline Vital Signs and History Taking

Vital Signs
Breathing
- Rate
- Quality
- Rhythm

Pulse
- Rate
- Quality and Rhythm

Skin Signs
- Color
- Temperature
- Condition
- Capillary Refill

Pupils

Blood Pressure
- Auscultation
- Palpation

Reassessment

SAMPLE History
Signs/symptoms

Allergies

Medications

Pertinent past history

Last oral intake

Events leading to illness/injury

HANDOUT 5-2: Chapter 5 Quiz

1.	B	**6.**	B	**11.**	B	**16.**	A
2.	B	**7.**	A	**12.**	D	**17.**	D
3.	B	**8.**	B	**13.**	D	**18.**	D
4.	C	**9.**	D	**14.**	C	**19.**	A
5.	B	**10.**	A	**15.**	C	**20.**	D

HANDOUT 5-3: In the Field

1. First complete set of vital signs: heart rate 110 beats per minute, blood pressure 160/110, respiration rate of 28 and labored.

2. Because the pulse is irregular, the crew member should take it for 60 seconds.

3. Symptoms include conditions described by the patient, such as her nagging cough for several days, the lack of sleep the prior night, the fact that she needs to sit upright.

4. The patient is high priority because she has breathing difficulty. She also has a sustained rapid pulse. Tell students that the decision for high-priority transport is made early by EMTs, especially in the absence of advanced life support.

HANDOUT 5-4: Chapter 5 Review

1. vital signs
2. baseline
3. pulse
4. brachial
5. 60, 105
6. 60
7. rate, quality
8. 20, 12
9. noisy
10. stridor

11. palms, soles
12. dilated
13. sphygmomanometer
14. blood pressure
15. brachial
16. palpation
17. symptoms
18. history
19. allergies
20. open-ended

HANDOUT 5-5: Baseline Vital Signs and History Taking

1.	N	**5.**	K	**9.**	J	**13.**	A
2.	D	**6.**	C	**10.**	M	**14.**	F
3.	L	**7.**	E	**11.**	O	**15.**	I
4.	B	**8.**	G	**12.**	H		

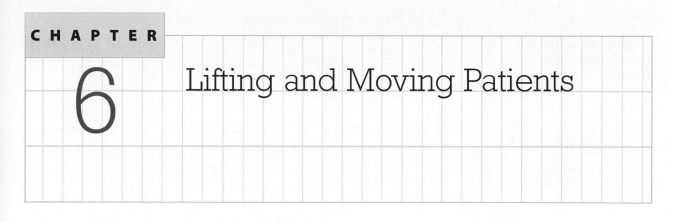

CHAPTER 6

Lifting and Moving Patients

This chapter covers Lesson 1-6 of the U.S. Department of Transportation's EMT-Basic National Standard Curriculum.

OBJECTIVES

Numbered objectives are from the U.S. Department of Transportation EMT-Basic National Standard Curriculum. Asterisked objectives, if any, pertain to material that is supplemental to the DOT curriculum. Page numbers in parentheses refer to pages in the textbook.

Cognitive

1-6.1   Define body mechanics. (p. 125)
1-6.2   Discuss the guidelines and safety precautions that need to be followed when lifting a patient. (pp. 124–127)
1-6.3   Describe the safe lifting of cots and stretchers. (p. 130)
1-6.4   Describe the guidelines and safety precautions for carrying patients and/or equipment. (pp. 127–130)
1-6.5   Discuss one-handed carrying techniques. (p. 129)
1-6.6   Describe correct and safe carrying procedures on stairs. (pp. 139–141)
1-6.7   State the guidelines for reaching and their application. (p. 129)
1-6.8   Describe correct reaching for log rolls. (p. 129)
1-6.9   State the guidelines for pushing and pulling. (pp. 129–130)
1-6.10 Discuss the general considerations of moving patients. (p. 130)
1-6.11 State three situations that may require the use of an emergency move. (p. 130–131)
1-6.12 Identify the following patient carrying devices (pp. 136–145):
— Wheeled ambulance stretcher
— Portable ambulance stretcher
— Stair chair
— Scoop stretcher
— Long spine board
— Basket stretcher
— Flexible stretcher

Affective

1-6.13 Explain the rationale for properly lifting and moving patients. (p. 123)

Psychomotor

1-6.14 Working with a partner, prepare each of the following devices for use, transfer a patient to the device, properly position the patient on the device, move the device to the ambulance, and load the patient into the ambulance:

Total Teaching Time
415 minutes

Resources Needed
- Scored Chapter 5 Quizzes
- Wheeled ambulance stretcher
- Moderately heavy equipment (for one-handed lifting)
- Stair chair
- Long spine board
- Moderately heavy equipment (for pushing and pulling)
- Seven people to serve as patients
- Seven EMTs to serve as teaching assistants
- Ambulance
- Station 1: A shirt (not a T-shirt) and blanket
- Station 2: Long board
- Station 3: Two stretchers or other patient carrying devices
- Station 4: Wheeled ambulance stretcher and portable ambulance stretcher
- Station 5: Stair chair and scoop stretcher
- Station 6: Long spine board, basket stretcher, and flexible stretcher
- Station 7: Ambulance stretcher and hospital stretcher

Additional Resources

Larmon/Davis, Basic Life Support Skills

Elling, EMT Achieve: Basic Test Preparation

Limmer/Mistovich/ O'Keefe, Audio Lecture & Study Guide: EMT

Mistovich/Kuvlesky, SUCCESS! for the EMT, Second Edition

Handout 6-1

Chapter 6 Objectives Checklist

•➤

Lecture Master

You may wish to display Lecture Master 6 when presenting the lecture to the class.

Slides/Videos

"EMT-Free." Ferno-Washington, Inc., 70 Weil Way, Wilmington, OH 45177. Lifting and moving techniques with EMT-Basic back care in mind.

— Wheeled ambulance stretcher
— Portable ambulance stretcher
— Stair chair
— Scoop stretcher
— Long spine board
— Basket stretcher
— Flexible stretcher

1-6.15   Working with a partner, the EMT-Basic will demonstrate techniques for the transfer of a patient from an ambulance stretcher to a hospital stretcher.

REVIEW

The last lesson, "Baseline Vital Signs and History Taking," described two essential elements of patient assessment: vital signs and a patient history. Students learned how to obtain a patient's vital signs—respiration; pulse; skin color, temperature, and condition; pupils; and blood pressure. They learned that vital signs reflect the patient's condition and that several sets reflect changes—improvement or deterioration. Students learned how to gather a SAMPLE history and how that information can affect the treatment given to the patient.

Distribute the scored quizzes from the last class. Go over each question on the quiz and handle any concerns students may have about the answers.

INTRODUCTION TO CHAPTER 6

Chapter 6, "Lifting and Moving Patients," is the sixth and last lesson in Module 1. The knowledge about the use of proper body mechanics students gain in this chapter will form a solid foundation for their health, longevity, and effectiveness as an EMT. Stress the fact that many EMTs are injured every year because they attempt to lift patients or equipment improperly. Encourage students to practice good body mechanics in all aspects of their lives.

Distribute the Chapter 6 Objectives Checklist and give students a few minutes to look it over. Then briefly paraphrase the objectives for this lesson in your own words.

LECTURE

The following suggested lecture outline is based on the Department of Transportation's EMT-Basic National Standard Curriculum. In some places, the DOT curriculum has been rearranged or expanded upon so that it is more complete or easier for the student to understand. The page numbers in parentheses refer to pages in the textbook. The parenthetical references in dark, heavy type are to figures, tables, and scans in the textbook.

LIFTING AND MOVING PATIENTS

   I. Body mechanics (pp. 124–127)
     A. Basic principles (p. 125)
       1. Use leg, hip, buttock, and contracted abdominal muscles, not back muscles, to lift
       2. Keep weight as close to body as possible (**Fig. 6-1, p. 125**)
       3. Visualize shoulders as stacked on top of the hips and feet and move all three as a unit

4. Reduce the height or distance through which a weight must be moved **(Fig. 6-2, p. 126)**
  B. Use proper posture and stay in shape (p. 125) **(Figs. 6-3, 6-4, p. 126; 6-5, p. 127)**
   1. Lordosis (swayback)
   2. Kyphosis (slouch)
  C. Develop communication and teamwork skills (pp. 125–127)
   1. Size up the scene immediately and accurately
   2. Consider the weight of the patient and recognize the need for additional help
   3. Be aware of the physical abilities and limitations of each team member
   4. Select the most appropriate equipment for the job
 II. General guidelines for lifting and moving (pp. 127–130)
  A. Guidelines for lifting (p. 127)
   1. Consider weight of patient and need for additional help
   2. Know physical ability and limitations
   3. Lift without twisting
   4. Have feet positioned properly
   5. Communicate clearly and frequently with partner
  B. Safe lifting of cots and stretchers (pp. 127–129)
   1. Know or find out the weight to be lifted
   2. Use at least two people
   3. Ensure enough help is available. Use an even number of people to lift so that balance is maintained.
    a. Know or find out the weight limitations of equipment being used
    b. Know what to do with patients who exceed weight limitations of equipment
   4. Lift while keeping back in locked-in position
   5. When lowering cot or stretcher, reverse steps
   6. Avoid bending at the waist
   7. Use the proper techniques
    a. Power lift **(Fig. 6-6, p. 128)**
     (1) Offers best defense against injury
     (2) Useful for rescuers with weak knees or thighs
    b. Power grip **(Fig. 6-7, p. 129)**
     (1) Use with power lift technique
     (2) Gets maximum force from hands
    c. Squat lift **(Fig. 6-8, p. 129)**
     (1) Alternative to power lift
     (2) Useful for rescuers with one weak knee or ankle
    d. One-handed technique for carrying some equipment **(Fig. 6-9, p. 129)**
     (1) Use proper body mechanics
     (2) Avoid leaning too much to either side
    e. Stair-chair technique
     (1) Use to move patients up or down stairs
     (2) Include a "spotter" while performing
  C. Carrying (p. 129)
   1. Keep weight as close to body as possible
   2. Keep back in locked-in position
    a. Do not hyperextend back, or lean back from waist
   3. Never lift and twist simultaneously; first lift, then turn as a unit
    a. Refrain from twisting

Teaching Tip

Stress to students that unless they take care of their backs, their careers in EMS will be short.

Point of Interest

Some ambulance services require that job applicants undergo back X-rays as part of the hiring process.

On the Net

For more on acute lower back problems, go to: text.nlm.nih.gov/ahcpr/lbp/www/lbpctxt.html

On the Net

For a NIOSH lumbar torque study, go to: www.paja.occuphealth.fi/~tles/torque.html

On the Net

Valuable information on how to lift and transport patients safely. http://www.blinncol.edu/twe/emt/emtb/b9-5.PDF

Slides/Videos

Brady Skill Series: EMT-B, "Lifting and Moving Patients"

      b. Use even number of rescuers to maintain balance

    4. Two-rescuer teams should carry loads for 1 minute or less

    5. Use wheeled stretchers or other rolling devices to carry patients and equipment, whenever possible

  D. Reaching (p. 129)

    1. Guidelines for reaching

      a. Keep back in locked-in position

      b. When reaching overhead, avoid hyperextended position

      c. Avoid twisting the back while reaching

      d. Application of reaching techniques

      e. Avoid reaching more than 15–20 inches in front of the body

      f. Avoid situations where prolonged (more than a minute) strenuous effort is needed in order to avoid injury

    2. Correct reaching for log rolls

      a. Keep back straight while leaning over patient

      b. Lean from the hips

      c. Use shoulder muscles to help with roll

  E. Pushing and pulling guidelines (pp. 129–130) **(Fig. 6-10, p. 130)**

    1. Push, rather than pull, whenever possible

    2. Keep back locked-in

    3. Keep line of pull through center of body by bending knees

      a. Keep weight close to the body

      b. Push from the area between the waist and shoulder

      c. If weight is below waist level, use kneeling position

    4. Avoid pushing or pulling from an overhead position, if possible

      a. Keep elbows bent with arms close to the sides

III. Lifting and moving patients (pp. 130–135)

  A. Body mechanics (p. 130)

  B. Emergency moves (pp. 130–132)

    1. Immediate danger to the patient or rescuer

    2. Conditions warranting consideration of an emergency move

      a. Immediate environmental danger to the patient or rescuer

      b. Inability to gain access to other patients who need life-saving care

      c. Inability to provide life-saving care because of patient's location or position

      d. Types of emergency moves

      e. Armpit-forearm drag **(Fig. 6-11, p. 131)**

      f. Shirt drag **(Fig. 6-12, p. 131)**

      g. Blanket drag **(Fig. 6-13, p. 132)**

  C. Urgent moves (p. 132)

    1. Patient is suffering an immediate threat to life and must be moved

      a. Rapid extrication

    2. Designed primarily for removing a patient quickly from a motor vehicle

    3. Must be performed quickly but without compromising patient's spine

    4. Operating within vehicle places rescuer's back in vulnerable position

      a. Procedure

      b. First rescuer brings patient's head into neutral in-line position and provides manual stabilization

Teaching Tip

Have another trained EMT on hand to help you demonstrate these techniques.

Reading/Reference

O'Neill, E. "Unconventional Patient Moves," Emergency Medical Services, May 2002.

On the Net

Moving patients; suggestions to reduce risks. http://www.nursingworld.org/AJN/2000/sep/Health.htm

    c. Second rescuer applies a cervical-spine immobilization device

    d. Third rescuer places a long backboard by vehicle door and then moves to passenger seat

    e. Second rescuer supports patient's thorax as the third frees the patient's legs

    f. At direction of second rescuer, second and third rescuers rotate until patient's back in open doorway and his feet are on the seat

    g. Since the first rescuer usually cannot support the patient's head any longer, another rescuer should support the head until the first rescuer exits the vehicle and takes support of the head from the door opening

    h. The end of the long backboard is placed on the seat next to the patient's buttocks; assistants support the other end of the board as the first and second rescuers lower the patient onto it

    i. The second and third rescuers slide the patient into the proper position on the board in short, coordinated moves, as the first rescuer continues manual stabilization

D. Nonurgent moves (p. 132)

  1. No immediate threat to life

  2. General guidelines

  3. Take time to select best equipment and method of moving patient safely

  4. Move the easiest way that will not cause injury or pain

  5. Move patient as a unit

  6. Keep patient's head and neck in neutral position

  7. Take all necessary spinal precautions

  8. Work as a coordinated team

  9. Assign one rescuer to give commands (usually one applying in-line stabilization)

E. Direct ground lift (no suspected spine injury) (pp. 133–134) (Fig. 6-14, p. 133)

  1. Lift is not recommended for the heavier patient

  2. Rescuer's back is vulnerable; rescuers should take the following precautions:

    a. Keep back straight

    b. Bend at hips, not waist

    c. Lift with legs and gluteal muscles, not with back muscles

F. Extremity lift (no suspected extremity injuries) (p. 134) (Fig. 6-15, p. 134)

  1. Use to lift patient from ground to a patient carrying device

  2. Do not use for patients with suspected spinal or extremity injuries

  3. Rescuer's back is vulnerable; rescuers should take the following precautions:

    a. Maintain a straight back and contract abdominal muscles while lifting

    b. Keep head in line with back (don't extend head forward or backward)

    c. Lift with legs and gluteal muscles, not back muscles

G. Direct carry (transferring a supine patient from bed to wheeled stretcher or from any carrying device to another) (pp. 134–135) (Fig. 6-16, p. 135)

H. Draw sheet method (transferring supine patient from bed to wheeled stretcher or from any carrying device to another) (p. 135) **(Fig. 6-17, p. 136)**

IV. Packaging for transportation (pp. 135–147)

    A. Packaging (pp. 135–136)

        1. Readying the patient for transport

    B. General considerations (pp. 135–136)

        1. Make sure that carrying device is locked in open position before positioning patient

        2. Use appropriate lifting, moving, or carrying technique to place patient on device

        3. Generally place a sheet or blanket on device, and when patient is positioned, cover patient with a sheet or blanket

        4. Secure patient with straps, securing all so that they will not cause rescuer to trip or fall

        5. Secure both patient and carrying device securely in ambulance before ambulance moves

        6. Take all necessary spinal precautions before, during, and after packaging

    C. Equipment (pp. 136–145) **(Table 6-2, pp. 137–138)**

        1. Wheeled stretcher (ambulance gurney) **(Figs. 6-18, 6-19, p. 138)**

            a. Safest, most comfortable means of transferring a patient

            b. Most can accommodate weights to 400 pounds

            c. Weighs about 70 pounds and is constructed of aluminum alloy

            d. Can be adapted to almost any patient position

            e. Allows two rescuers to carry in narrow spaces

            f. Comes in two basic types **(Fig. 6-20, p. 139)**

                (1) Lift-in

                (2) Roll-in

             g. Loading and unloading

                (1) Lift-in type—requires two attendants, one on each side **(Fig. 6-21, p. 140–141)**

                (2) Roll-in type—uses special wheels **(Fig. 6-22, p. 141)**

            h. Bariatric stretchers and devices **(Fig. 6-23, p. 142)**

        2. Portable stretcher **(Fig. 6-24, p. 142)**

            a. Is standard equipment

            b. Is made of a continuous tubular metal frame with canvas or coated fabric bottom and straps

            c. Is particularly useful when patient must be removed from a narrow space

            d. Is often used as an auxiliary to the wheeled stretcher

            e. Is easily loaded into ambulance and off-loaded when in ambulance

            f. Comes in three styles

                (1) Basic

                (2) Basic with folding wheels and posts

                (3) Breakaway

            g. Is variation of pole stretcher (canvas litter) **(Fig. 6-24b, p. 142)**

        3. Stair chair **(Figs. 6-25, p. 142; 6-26 and 6-27, p. 143)**

            a. Useful in narrow corridors and doorways, small elevators, stairways

            b. Should not be used when patient has

        (1) Altered mental status
        (2) Suspected spinal injury
        (3) Injuries to lower extremities

    4. Backboards (**Fig. 6-28 and 6-29, p. 144**)
      a. Standard equipment, lightweight plastic with molded handholds
      b. Protect patient from rocky ground and act as spinal immobilizer
      c. Two basic types
        (1) Long backboard
        (2) Short backboard
          (a) Used to immobilize noncritical sitting patients before moving them to long backboard
          (b) May be vest-type or corset-type

    5. Scoop (orthopedic) stretcher (**Fig. 6-30, p. 145**)
      a. Designed for patients weighing up to 300 pounds
      b. Made to be assembled and disassembled around patient
      c. Can be used in confined areas where conventional stretchers will not fit
      d. Is all metal so picks up temperature of environment
      e. Is not recommended for patients with suspected spinal injury
      f. Requires two rescuers and access to patient from all sides (**Fig. 6-31, p. 145–146**)

    6. Basket stretcher (Stokes basket) (**Fig. 6-32, p. 146**)
      a. Two styles
        (1) Welded metal frame fitted with a contoured chicken-wire web
        (2) Tubular aluminum frame riveted to a molded polyethylene shell
      b. Will fit onto wheeled stretchers
      c. Allows EMT to completely immobilize patient who is already on a backboard
      d. Can be moved over any terrain
      e. Can accommodate wheeled stretcher mattress to increase patient comfort and insulate from cold

    7. Flexible (Reeves) stretcher (**Fig. 6-33, p. 147**)

D. Patient positioning (pp. 145–147)
    1. Unresponsive patient without suspected spine injury
      a. Once in ambulance, place in left lateral recumbent position facing rescuer
    2. Patient with chest pain, discomfort, or breathing difficulties
      a. Place in position of comfort, usually sitting up if hypotension is not present
      b. Patient with suspected spine injury
      c. Immobilize on long backboard
      d. Patient in shock (hypoperfusion)
      e. Place supine; may elevate end of backboard or legs 8–12 inches, depending on local protocol
      f. Pregnant patient in third trimester
      g. Position on left side
      h. Alert patient who is nauseated or vomiting
      i. Place in sitting or recovery position
      j. Special needs patients

Point of Interest

Some of the best resources for information about patient lifting and moving equipment are the various EMS journals. Fill out the reader information cards in them and send them back. Manufacturers will send plenty of information that will be useful for reference.

    k. Pregnant women
        (1) Generally position on left side and follow local protocol
    l. Infants and toddlers
        (1) Can usually be carried in an infant car seat
    m. Elderly patients
        (1) Because of osteoporosis, take care to avoid bone fractures
    n. Handicapped patients
        (1) Use common sense, and communicate with patient on position of comfort

ENRICHMENT (OPTIONAL)

The following sections contain information that is valuable as background for the EMT, but that goes substantially beyond the U.S. Department of Transportation's EMT-Basic National Standard Curriculum.

  V. Packaging patients for air transport (pp. 147–148)
    A. Basic guidelines (pp. 147–148)
      1. Decontaminate any patient contaminated with hazardous materials
      2. If possible, have patient's airway managed with endotracheal tube before arrival at aircraft
      3. Leave chest accessible if patient is intubated
      4. If patient is to be transported by helicopter and is immobilized on long backboard, make sure to use a backboard that will fit in the helicopter
      5. Be sure patient is well secured to backboard
      6. Secure all equipment, blankets, sheets, and so on with tape, and secure all loose equipment at the scene against rotor wash
      7. Tell patient what to expect in the way of noise and rotor wash
      8. Cover the patient's eyes, ears, and exposed wounds to protect them from noise and rotor wash
      9. Consider having the engine company wet the landing zone to prevent blowing dust and debris
     10. Make sure that you and all other rescuers remove any loose clothing and hats to avoid their being blown into the rotor or engine
     11. Do not approach the aircraft with the patient until instructed to do so by the pilot or crew
     12. Lay an IV bag on the patient's chest rather than holding it up
     13. Minimize the number of people under a helicopter rotor at all times

CASE STUDY FOLLOW-UP

Ask a student volunteer to read the Case Study that begins on page 124 of the textbook. You may wish to use the following questions to engage the students in a discussion of the Case Study Follow-up that begins on page 148 of the textbook. Provide missing information and clarify ideas as needed.

Q1. During your scene size-up, what do you do to make this routine transfer safer?

A1. *Shovel the short walk to the front of the house and apply salt to melt the ice.*

Q2. What device do you use to safely transport Mrs. Sanchez from the upstairs bedroom to the ambulance?

A2. *A stair chair.*

Q3. At the top of the stairway, before moving Mrs. Sanchez down the stairs, what do you and your partners do?

A3. *Review the upcoming moves at the direction of the training officer and check the straps on the stair chair.*

Q4. What procedure do you use to lift the stair chair and descend the stairs?

A4. *One EMT gets behind the chair at the head while the taller one stands at the foot facing the patient. The training officer gets in position to spot behind the EMT at the foot and rests a hand on his or her back. As the EMT at the head tilts the chair back, the one at the foot grasps it by its legs. The training officer calls out how many steps there are ahead. Both EMTs lift simultaneously and start the descent. The spotter counts out steps as they descend.*

IN REVIEW

Assess students' ability to apply what they have just learned by discussing the Review Questions on page 149 in the textbook.

Q1. List the four basic principles of body mechanics.

A1. *The four basic principles of body mechanics are: Keep the weight of the object as close to the body as possible; use the leg, hip, and gluteal muscles plus contracted abdominal muscles (not the back) to move an object; "stack" the shoulders, hips, and feet and move them as a unit; reduce the height or distance through which the object must be moved. (p. 125)*

Q2. Explain how to perform the power grip, and when you should use it.

A2. *To perform the power grip, palm and fingers should come in complete contact with the object and fingers should be bent at the same angle. A power grip should always be used for getting the maximum force from your hands when lifting or moving an object. (p. 127, 129)*

Q3. Explain how to perform the power lift, and when you should use it.

A3. *To perform the power lift, place feet shoulder width apart and turn them out slightly; bend knees and tighten the muscles of the abdomen; keep the back straight, with head facing forward in a neutral position; straddle the object, keeping feet flat with weight evenly distributed and just forward of the heels; place hands about 10 inches apart, and use a power grip to lift. The back should remain locked in as the force is driven through the heels and arches of your feet. Your upper body should come up before the hips. A power-lift technique helps prevent injury while lifting and protects the patient with a safe and stable move. Use it whenever possible. It is also the lift of choice for rescuers with weak knees or thighs. (pp. 127–128)*

Q4. Name the three categories of patient moves, and explain when each should be used.

A4. *The three categories for moving patients are emergency moves—when there is immediate danger to the patient or rescuer; urgent moves— there must be an immediate threat to the patient's life; and nonurgent moves—in which no immediate threat to life exists. (pp. 130–132)*

Q5. List some of the guidelines and safety precautions for carrying.

A5. *Guidelines and safety precautions for carrying include: Keep the weight as close to your body as possible; keep your back in a locked-in position; do not hyperextend your back; keep shoulders, hips, and feet (base) in alignment; refrain from twisting; strenuous effort should be sustained for no longer than 1 minute; whenever possible, carry patients and equipment on devices that can be rolled. (p. 129)*

Q6. Explain, briefly, how to perform (a) a direct ground lift, (b) an extremity lift, (c) a direct carry, and (d) the draw sheet method.

A6. *(a) Direct ground lift—Two or three rescuers kneel beside a patient who is on the floor or ground, place arms under the patient, roll the patient to their chests, stand, and place the patient on the stretcher. (b) Extremity lift—One rescuer reaches under the patient's armpits and grasps the patient's wrists. The second rescuer grasps the patient under the knees. They lift the patient together. (c) Direct carry—Two rescuers place a stretcher perpendicular to the patient's bed. They place their arms under the patient, lift and curl the patient to their chests, rotate, and place the patient on the stretcher. (d) Draw sheet method— Two rescuers place a stretcher next to the patient's bed. They reach across the stretcher, grasp the loosened bottom bed sheet, and pull the patient onto the stretcher. (pp. 133–135)*

Q7. Name the device that is recommended for carrying a patient up and down stairs, whenever possible, and explain the function of the spotter.

A7. *The stair chair is recommended for carrying a patient up or down stairs. The spotter directs the move, for example, warning the rescuers of the number of stairs ahead. (pp. 139, 143)*

Q8. Name types of patient carrying devices you would consider using if the spaces you need to traverse are too narrow or too confined for a wheeled stretcher.

A8. *In a narrow or confined space, a portable stretcher, a stair chair, a backboard, a scoop stretcher, or a flexible stretcher may be used. (pp. 139–143)*

Q9. Explain the proper body mechanics for reaching while doing a log roll.

A9. *When performing a log roll, correct reaching consists of leaning from the hips, not the waist; keeping the back straight; and using the stronger shoulder muscles to assist whenever possible. (p. 129)*

Q10. Explain the safety guidelines for pushing and pulling.

A10. *Whenever possible, push rather than pull. If the object must be pulled, keep the weight close to your body and bend your knees slightly. When pushing, push from the areas between your waist and shoulders. If the weight is below waist level, use the kneeling position to avoid bending. Keep elbows bent, with arms close to the sides of the body. Avoid pushing or pulling from an overhead position, if possible. (pp. 129–130)*

CRITICAL THINKING

Assess students' ability to respond to real-life emergency situations by discussing the Critical Thinking questions on page 149 in the textbook.

Q1. What is the significance of the gurgling sound?

A1. *The gurgling sound indicates that the patient has some type of fluid (blood, vomit, etc.) in his airway.*

Q2. How would you document the pulse rate?

A2. *Documentation of this patient's pulse rate should include the beat-per-minute count (45 bpm), whether it is strong or weak, and the location of the pulse being assessed. It could be documented as "radial pulse is 45 bpm and strong" or "radial pulse is bradycardic at 45 bpm but strong." The location is important to note because it provides an indication of perfusion. If a radial pulse is found, it typically implies better perfusion than if only a carotid or femoral pulse was able to be palpated. Also, keep in mind that a heart rate less than 60 bpm in the adult is termed bradycardia and a heart rate greater than 100 bpm in the adult is known as tachycardia.*

Q3. What does the pulse oximeter reading indicate?

A3. *The pulse oximeter reading (SpO_2) of 76% on room air indicates that the patient is severely hypoxic and requires immediate assisted ventilation with supplemental oxygen connected to the ventilation device. A respiratory rate of 45 per minute in an adult is beyond the upper range of normal in an adult patient and will not allow for adequate breathing. High respiratory rates will decrease the time for adequate lung filling and will lead to poor tidal volumes and inadequate breathing.*

Q4. What do the skin signs indicate?

A4. *The cyanosis would indicate a poor oxygenation status, most likely due to the high respiratory rate and poor tidal volume. The warm and dry skin would indicate an adequate blood pressure is present.*

Q5. What other vitals signs would be important to assess in this patient?

A5. *Responding EMTs should also assess this patient's pupils for size, equality, and reactivity to light.*

Q6. When would you attempt to gather a SAMPLE history?

A6. *Since the patient is unresponsive and transport time is a critical factor in trauma situations, the SAMPLE history should be gathered while en route to the hospital.*

Q7. How would you gather the SAMPLE history?

A7. *Since the patient is unresponsive, his spouse would be the best source for a SAMPLE history.*

SKILLS DEMONSTRATION AND PRACTICE

ACTIVITY 1: Working with an EMT partner, explain and demonstrate for the class how to perform each of the following lifts or moves:

- power lift
- squat lift
- one-handed carrying technique

- stair-chair technique
- reaching
- pushing and pulling

Set up the following five practice stations and write the station names and their locations on a chalkboard, flip chart, or overhead transparency:

1. power lift/squat lift
2. one-handed carrying technique
3. stair-chair technique
4. reaching
5. pushing and pulling

Divide the class into teams of two. If there is an odd number of students, it is acceptable to have a team of three, provided that each student practices each skill. Direct each team to visit the five practice stations listed. At each station, arrange for there to be a "patient" and an EMT who will help the teams practice the skill.

Visit each station to monitor progress of practice. Provide assistance to the EMTs, if necessary. Make sure that each team visits each practice station. When each team has completed each station, make sure that students return to the main classroom.

ACTIVITY 2: Write the following on a blackboard, a flipchart, or an overhead transparency to display to students:

1. Emergency moves
2. Urgent moves
3. Nonurgent moves
4. Wheeled ambulance stretcher and portable ambulance stretcher
5. Stair chair and scoop stretcher
6. Long spine board, basket stretcher, and flexible stretcher
7. Ambulance stretcher to hospital stretcher

Divide students into teams of two. If there are an odd number of students, it is acceptable to have a team of three provided that each student practices each skill.

Explain that each team is to visit the seven listed practice stations. Tell students that at each station there will be a "patient" and a teaching assistant who will demonstrate and help students practice each skill. At stations 4–6, students must prepare each moving device for use, transfer the patient to the device, properly position the patient on the device, move the device to the ambulance, and load the patient into the ambulance. At station 7, students must transfer the patient from an ambulance stretcher to a hospital stretcher.

Direct each team to its first practice station. Visit each station to monitor progress of practice. Provide help to the teaching assistants, if necessary. Make sure that each team visits each practice station.

When each team has completed each station, make sure that students return to the main classroom.

Reading/Reference
Textbook, pp. 150–213

Workbook
Chapter 6 Activities

ASSIGNMENTS

Assign students to read Chapter 7, "Airway Management, Ventilation, and Oxygen Therapy," before the next class. Also ask them to complete Chapter 6 of the Workbook.

EVALUATION

Chapter Quiz Distribute copies of the Chapter Quiz provided in Handout 6-2 to evaluate student understanding of this chapter. Remind students not to refer to their textbooks or notes while taking the quiz.

Test Manager You may wish to create a custom-tailored test using Prentice Hall *TestGen for Prehospital Emergency Care,* Eighth Edition to evaluate student understanding of this chapter.

Online Test Preparation (for students and instructors) Additional test preparation is available through *EMT Achieve: Basic Test Preparation* at http://www.prenhall.com/EMTAchieve. Instructors can also monitor student mastery online.

REINFORCEMENT

Handouts If classroom discussions or performance on the quiz indicates that some students have not fully mastered the chapter content, you may wish to assign some or all of the Reinforcement Handouts for this chapter.

TECH EXTRAS

Brady Skills Series EMT-B Videos/CD Have your students watch the skills come to life on either VHS or CD-ROM.

PowerPoint Presentation (for instructors) The PowerPoint material developed for this chapter offers useful reinforcement of chapter content.

Student CD A wide variety of material on this CD-ROM will reinforce and also expand student knowledge and skills.

Companion Website (for students) Additional review quizzes and links to EMS resources will contribute to further reinforcement of this chapter. Please visit http://www.prenhall.com/mistovich.

Chapter Quiz
Handout 6-2

TestGen
Chapter 6 Test

Online Test Preparation
Send your students to
http://www.prenhall.com/
EMTAchieve

Handouts 6-3 to 6-6
Reinforcement Activities

**Brady Skills Series
EMT-B Videos/CD**
Visual Reinforcement

**PowerPoint
Presentation**
Chapter 6

Student CD
Chapter 6

Companion Website
http://www.prenhall.com/
mistovich

OBJECTIVES

OBJECTIVES CHECKLIST

Cognitive	Date Mastered
1-6.1 Define body mechanics.	
1-6.2 Discuss the guidelines and safety precautions that need to be followed when lifting a patient.	
1-6.3 Describe the safe lifting of cots and stretchers.	
1-6.4 Describe the guidelines and safety precautions for carrying patients and/or equipment.	
1-6.5 Discuss one-handed carrying techniques.	
1-6.6 Describe correct and safe carrying procedures on stairs.	
1-6.7 State the guidelines for reaching and their application.	
1-6.8 Describe correct reaching for log rolls.	
1-6.9 State the guidelines for pushing and pulling.	
1-6.10 Discuss the general considerations of moving patients.	
1-6.11 State three situations that may require the use of an emergency move.	
1-6.12 Identify the following patient carrying devices: Wheeled ambulance stretcher Portable ambulance stretcher Stair chair Scoop stretcher Long spine board Basket stretcher Flexible stretcher	

Affective	Date Mastered
1-6.13 Explain the rationale for properly lifting and moving patients.	

Psychomotor	Date Mastered
1-6.14 Working with a partner, prepare each of the following devices for use, transfer a patient to the device, properly position the patient on the device, move the device to the ambulance, and load the patient into the ambulance: —Wheeled ambulance stretcher —Portable ambulance stretcher —Stair chair —Scoop stretcher —Long spine board —Basket stretcher —Flexible stretcher	
1-6.15 Working with a partner, the EMT will demonstrate techniques for the transfer of a patient from an ambulance stretcher to a hospital stretcher.	

CHAPTER 6 QUIZ

Write the letter of the best answer in the space provided.

_____ 1. When you are lifting a heavy object, avoid using the muscles of your
   A. back.   **C.** shoulders.
   B. arms.   **D.** legs.

_____ 2. One technique that can greatly reduce risk of back injuries when lifting and moving patients is
   A. not allowing the weight to get close to your body.
   B. keeping the lifted weight in close to your body.
   C. keeping your feet together.
   D. locking out your knees.

_____ 3. When reaching for a patient or a piece of equipment, an EMT should reach in front of her body no more than _____ inches.
   A. 8 to 12   **C.** 15 to 20
   B. 20 to 24   **D.** 30 to 36

_____ 4. The lifting technique that should be used by an EMT with one weak leg or one weak ankle is the
   A. power lift.   **C.** power grip.
   B. back lift.   **D.** squat lift.

_____ 5. When performing a log roll, an EMT should
   A. bend over the patient.   **C.** twist and pull simultaneously.
   B. lean from the hips.   **D.** lean from the waist.

_____ 6. The preferred device for carrying a conscious medical patient down a flight of stairs is the
   A. stair chair.   **C.** ambulance stretcher.
   B. Reeves device.   **D.** backboard.

_____ 7. Which one of the conditions below is not one that permits the use of an emergency move?
   A. The scene is hazardous.
   B. Care of life-threatening injuries requires repositioning.
   C. The patient's position is hampering a police investigation.
   D. You must reach other patients.

_____ 8. When your assessment of a patient trapped in wreckage reveals that the patient is suffering from an immediate threat to life, you would order a(n) _____ move.
   A. emergency   **C.** immediate
   B. urgent   **D.** rapid

_____ 9. The technique used when quickly removing a patient from a vehicle is called
   A. log rolling.   **C.** rapid extrication.
   B. the long axis drag.   **D.** the Stokes move.

_____ 10. Unresponsive patients with no suspected spinal injuries should be placed in the
   A. position of comfort.   **C.** left lateral recumbent position.
   B. Fowler's position.   **D.** Trendelenburg position.

©2008 by Pearson Education, Inc.
Prehospital Emergency Care, 8th ed.

IN THE FIELD

Read the following real-life situation. Then answer the question that follows.

Bob said, "Clay overreacted," and Andy replied, "Yeah, he endangered the patient. Suppose the guy had a broken neck or something! He's just lucky the guy was all right." Overhearing this conversation, you are naturally curious and ask, "What happened?"

The two other EMTs tell you that there was a motor-vehicle collision, a high-speed crash, where the cars were found T-boned and the passengers seriously injured. When Clay's ambulance arrived, it was assigned by EMS command to the patients in car B.

After approaching the cars, Clay did a quick scene size-up, including assessing for scene safety. The position in which the cars came to rest after impact made access on the driver's side impossible, so Clay looked into the passenger-side window of car B. He could see that the driver, who appeared unresponsive, had a large cut over his left eyebrow that was bleeding profusely. An initial assessment of the passenger revealed no obvious injuries.

It was at this point that Clay called EMS command and asked for more manpower as well as the heavy rescue team. He then immediately extricated the passenger in order to gain access to the driver. Despite the fact that Clay now had access to the driver and could start patient care, he was unable to extricate the driver without the assistance of heavy rescue. Eventually, the heavy rescue team disentangled the driver from the dash. He was then transported to the trauma center.

1. What did Clay decide to do that Andy and Bob had such a problem with? Did he do the right thing?

2. Which patient moving technique should have been used?

3. If the driver had not appeared to be seriously injured, what should have happened differently?

REINFORCEMENT

CHAPTER 6 REVIEW

Write the word or words that best complete each sentence in the space provided.

1. The proper use of your body to facilitate lifting and moving a patient is called

   _____ _____.

2. A major cause of lower back injuries is lifting and _____ simultaneously.

3. When lifting a patient carrying device, it is best to use a(n) _____ number

   of people.

4. Never reach more than _____ inches away from your body for equipment.

5. To get the best hold possible on a piece of equipment, use the _____

   _____.

6. When faced with a choice of pushing or pulling an object, whenever possible, try to

   _____.

7. Always keep the weight of an object to be lifted or moved as _____ to the

   body as possible.

8. To move a heavy object, use the _____, _____,

   and _____ muscles plus contracted abdominal muscles.

9. When moving patients up or down stairs, always try to use a(n) _____

   _____.

10. To help prevent injury when lifting or moving patients or objects, maintain a normal

    _____ curve of the _____

    _____.

11. A(n) _____ move is used when no immediate threat to life exists and the

    patient can be moved when ready for transport.

12. The greatest danger to the patient in any emergency move is the possibility of aggravating a(n)

    _____ _____.

13. The _____ _____ is the safest and most

    comfortable means of transferring a patient.

14. The _____ _____ is a way of transferring a supine

    patient from a bed to a wheeled stretcher or from any patient carrying device to another.

©2008 by Pearson Education, Inc.
Prehospital Emergency Care, 8th ed.

15. _____ is a term that means readying the patient for transport.

16. A patient with chest pain or difficulty breathing should be placed in a(n)

_____ _____ _____.

17. During a(n) _____ _____, the patient is stabilized

manually before being removed from a vehicle onto a long spine board.

18. A patient with suspected spinal injury should be immobilized on a(n)

_____ _____.

19. To slide a patient from an ambulance stretcher to a hospital bed, the EMT would use the

_____ _____ method.

20. A pregnant patient in the third trimester should be transported on her

_____ _____.

LIFTING AND MOVING: LISTING

1. List four basic principles of body mechanics.

2. List three basic techniques used in lifting and moving patients and equipment.

3. List at least three ways of ensuring good teamwork and performance when teams of rescuers are carrying out lifts and moves.

MOVING PATIENTS: MATCHING

Part I. Write the letter of the patient carrying device in the space provided next to the situation it is appropriate for.

_____ **1.** A conscious patient is found seated in the front seat of a car after a collision.

A. Long backboard

_____ **2.** An elderly woman has fallen between the toilet and the bathtub.

B. Scoop stretcher

_____ **3.** A hunter has twisted her knee in the woods.

C. Basket stretcher

_____ **4.** A child has fallen out of a tree fort.

D. Stair chair

_____ **5.** A middle-age male has chest pain in his two-story brownstone house.

E. Short backboard

Part II. Write the letter of the type of move in the space provided beside the patient move it describes.

_____ **1.** Blanket drag

A. Emergency move

_____ **2.** Draw sheet method

B. Urgent move

_____ **3.** Rapid extrication

C. Nonurgent move

_____ **4.** Armpit-forearm drag

_____ **5.** Direct carry

Lifting and Moving Patients

Body Mechanics
Basic Principles

Posture and Fitness

Communication and Teamwork

General Guidelines for Lifting and Moving
Power Lift

Power Grip

Squat Lift

One-Handed Carrying

Stair-Chair Technique

Reaching

Pushing and Pulling

Lifting and Moving Patients
Emergency Moves

- Armpit-forearm drag
- Shirt drag
- Blanket drag

Urgent Moves

- Rapid extrication

Nonurgent Moves

- Direct ground lift
- Extremity lift
- Direct carry method
- Draw sheet method

Packaging for Transportation

Patient Carrying Devices

- Wheeled stretcher
- Portable stretcher
- Stair chair
- Backboard
- Scoop stretcher
- Basket stretcher
- Flexible stretcher

Patient Positioning

Packaging Patients for Air Transportation

HANDOUT 6-2: Chapter 6 Quiz

1. A	**5.** B	**8.** B
2. B	**6.** A	**9.** C
3. C	**7.** C	**10.** C
4. D		

HANDOUT 6-3: In the Field

1. Clay decided to perform an urgent move of the stable patient based on urgent need to gain access to the unstable patient. Emergency medical practice allows this deviation from the rule that potentially injured trauma patients need spinal immobilization before movement if such delays in packaging the patient would compromise other patients.

2. Clay would have used the rapid extrication technique, explained in detail in Chapter 34, "Injuries to the Spine." This technique is used to move patients when an initial assessment has determined an urgent move is needed to save that patient's life or the life of another to whom access is blocked by the first patient.

3. Based on the mechanism of injury, both patients should have received spinal immobilization via short board or vest-like extrication device, then been transferred to a long backboard.

HANDOUT 6-4: Chapter 6 Review

1. body mechanics
2. twisting
3. even
4. 20
5. power grip
6. push
7. close
8. leg, hip, gluteal (buttocks)
9. stair chair
10. inward, lower back

11. nonurgent
12. spinal injury
13. wheeled stretcher
14. direct carry
15. Packaging
16. position of comfort
17. rapid extrication
18. long backboard
19. draw sheet
20. left side

HANDOUT 6-5: Lifting and Moving: Listing

1. Keep the weight of the object as close to the body as possible; to move a heavy object, use the leg, hip, and gluteal (buttocks) muscles plus contracted abdominal muscles; visualize the shoulders as stacked on top of the hips and the hips on top of the feet and move them as a unit; reduce the height or distance through which the object must be moved.

2. Power lift; squat lift; power grip. Students may also cite one-handed carrying techniques and stair-chair technique.

3. Any three of the following: All members should be properly trained in proper techniques; partners should be closely matched in size and strength; team members should use commands that are easy to understand; they should communicate often; even numbers of rescuers should be used when lifting and moving.

HANDOUT 6-6: Moving Patients: Matching

Part I	Part II
1. E	**1.** A
2. B	**2.** C
3. C	**3.** B
4. A	**4.** A
5. D	**5.** C

7 Airway Management, Ventilation, and Oxygen Therapy

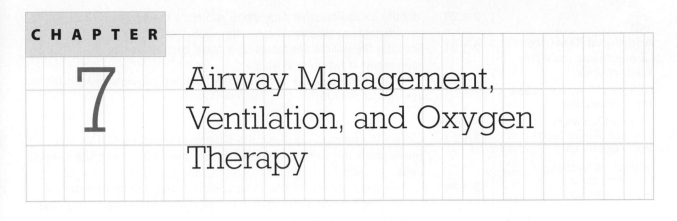

This chapter covers Lessons 2-1 and 2-2 of the U.S. Department of Transportation's EMT-Basic National Standard Curriculum.

OBJECTIVES

Numbered objectives are from the U.S. Department of Transportation's EMT-Basic National Standard Curriculum. Asterisked objectives, if any, pertain to material that is supplemental to the DOT curriculum. Page numbers refer to pages in the textbook.

Cognitive

2-1.1 Name and label the major structures of the respiratory system on a diagram. (pp. 154–157)

2-1.2 List the signs of adequate breathing. (p. 178)

2-1.3 List the signs of inadequate breathing. (pp. 178–180)

2-1.4 Describe the steps in performing the head-tilt, chin-lift. (pp. 164–165)

2-1.5 Relate the mechanism of injury to opening the airway. (p. 165)

2-1.6 Describe the steps in performing the jaw thrust. (p. 166)

2-1.7 State the importance of having a suction unit ready for immediate use when providing emergency care. (p. 167)

2-1.8 Describe the techniques of suctioning. (p. 169)

2-1.9 Describe how to artificially ventilate a patient with a pocket mask. (pp. 188–190)

2-1.10 Describe the steps in performing the skill of artificially ventilating a patient with a bag-valve mask while using the jaw thrust. (pp. 193–195)

2-1.11 List the parts of a bag-valve-mask system. (p. 191)

2-1.12 Describe the steps in performing the skill of artificially ventilating a patient with a bag-valve mask for one and two rescuers. (p. 192)

2-1.13 Describe the signs of adequate artificial ventilation, using the bag-valve mask. (p. 192)

2-1.14 Describe the signs of inadequate artificial ventilation, using the bag-valve mask. (pp. 192–193)

2-1.15 Describe the steps in artificially ventilating a patient with a flow-restricted, oxygen-powered ventilation device. (p. 195)

2-1.16 List the steps in performing the actions taken when providing mouth-to-mouth and mouth-to-stoma artificial ventilation. (pp. 186, 200)

2-1.17 Describe how to measure and insert an oropharyngeal (oral) airway. (p. 171)

2-1.18 Describe how to measure and insert a nasopharyngeal (nasal) airway. (pp. 172–173)

2-1.19 Define the components of an oxygen delivery system. (pp. 201–209)

Total Teaching Time
290 minutes

Resources Needed

- Scored Chapter 6 Quizzes Numbers required will vary based on number of practice stations:
- EMTs to serve as teaching assistants
- CPR mannequins
- Pocket masks, one per student
- Other barrier shields used in your area
- BVM unit with full oxygen cylinder
- Flow-restricted, oxygen-powered ventilation device with full oxygen cylinder
- Tracheostomy mannequin
- Portable suction unit with soft and rigid catheters
- Oropharyngeal airways, assorted sizes for adults, infants, and children
- Nasopharyngeal airways, assorted sizes for adults, infants, and children
- Water-based lubricant
- Several sizes of oxygen cylinders
- Several types of regulators/flowmeters
- Nonrebreather face masks—adult, infant, and child sizes
- Nasal cannula
- Infant and child CPR mannequins

Additional Resources

Larmon/Davis, *Basic Life Support Skills*

Elling, *EMT Achieve: Basic Test Preparation*

Limmer/Mistovich/ O'Keefe, *Audio Lecture & Study Guide: EMT*

Mistovich/Kuvlesky, *SUCCESS! for the EMT, Second Edition*

2-1.20   Identify a nonrebreather face mask and state the oxygen flow requirements needed for its use. (pp. 205, 207–208)

2-1.21   Describe the indications for using a nasal cannula versus a nonrebreather face mask. (p. 208)

2-1.22   Identify a nasal cannula and state the flow requirements needed for its use. (pp. 208–209)

Affective

2-1.23   Explain the rationale for basic life support artificial ventilation and airway protective skills taking priority over most other basic life support skills. (p. 152)

2-1.24   Explain the rationale for providing adequate oxygenation through high-inspired oxygen concentrations to patients who, in the past, may have received low concentrations. (p. 204)

Psychomotor

2-1.25   Demonstrate the steps in performing the head-tilt, chin-lift.

2-1.26   Demonstrate the techniques in performing the jaw thrust.

2-1.27   Demonstrate the techniques of suctioning.

2-1.28   Demonstrate the steps in providing mouth-to-mouth artificial ventilation with body substance isolation (barrier shields).

2-1.29   Demonstrate how to use a pocket mask to artificially ventilate a patient.

2-1.30   Demonstrate the assembly of a bag-valve-mask unit.

2-1.31   Demonstrate the steps in performing the skill of artificially ventilating a patient with a bag-valve mask for one and two rescuers.

2-1.32   Demonstrate the steps in performing the skill of artificially ventilating a patient with a bag-valve mask while using the jaw thrust.

2-1.33   Demonstrate artificial ventilation of a patient with a flow-restricted, oxygen-powered ventilation device.

2-1.34   Demonstrate how to artificially ventilate a patient with a stoma.

2-1.35   Demonstrate how to insert an oropharyngeal (oral) airway.

2-1.36   Demonstrate how to insert a nasopharyngeal (nasal) airway.

2-1.37   Demonstrate the correct operation of oxygen tanks and regulators.

2-1.38   Demonstrate the use of a nonrebreather face mask and state the oxygen-flow requirements needed for its use.

2-1.39   Demonstrate the use of a nasal cannula and state the flow requirements needed for its use.

2-1.40   Demonstrate how to artificially ventilate the infant and child patient.

2-1.41   Demonstrate oxygen administration for the infant and child patient.

REVIEW

In the last chapter, "Lifting and Moving Patients," students learned how to safely lift patients or equipment, using proper body mechanics. Remind them that their knowledge and use of proper body mechanics will provide a necessary foundation for their health, longevity, and effectiveness as EMTs. Distribute the scored quizzes from the last class. Go over each question on the quiz and handle any concerns students may have about the answers.

Tell students that they have now completed Module 1, Preparatory. Invite several students to summarize in a sentence or phrase the key concepts of each chapter they have studied so far. Students' summaries might include the basics of the emergency medical services system and the role of an EMT; how to protect themselves from injury and illness; basic medical, legal, and ethical issues that affect the EMT; the structures and functions of the human body; how to measure vital signs and obtain a patient's medical history; and how to prepare to lift and move patients.

INTRODUCTION TO MODULE 2/CHAPTER 7

Point out to students that Module 2, Airway, is a single chapter devoted to "Airway Management, Ventilation, and Oxygen Therapy." Emphasize that establishing and maintaining an airway, ensuring effective ventilation, and providing oxygen to the patient are part of the initial assessment conducted on every patient regardless of injuries or illness. Without an airway, the patient will rapidly deteriorate and die; all other care is futile if an adequate airway cannot be cleared and maintained.

Distribute the Chapter 7 Objectives Checklist and give students a few minutes to look it over. Then briefly paraphrase the objectives for this lesson in your own words.

LECTURE

The following suggested lecture outline is based on the Department of Transportation's EMT-Basic National Standard Curriculum. In some places, the DOT curriculum has been rearranged or expanded upon so that it is more complete or easier for the student to understand. The page numbers in parentheses refer to pages in the textbook. The parenthetical references in dark, heavy type are to figures, tables, and scans in the textbook.

AIRWAY MANAGEMENT, VENTILATION, AND OXYGEN THERAPY

I. Respiratory system review (pp. 154–162)
  A. Anatomy of the respiratory system (pp. 154–157)
    1. The upper airway (**Fig. 7-1, p. 155**)
      a. Nose and mouth
      b. Pharynx
        (1) Oropharynx
        (2) Nasopharynx
      c. Epiglottis
        (1) A leaf-shaped structure that prevents food and liquid from entering the trachea during swallowing
      d. Larynx (**Fig. 7-2, p. 156**)
    2. The lower airway (**Fig. 7-3, p. 152**)
      a. Trachea (windpipe)
      b. Cricoid cartilage
        (1) Firm cartilage ring forming the lower portion of the larynx
      c. Bronchi and bronchioles
        (1) Two major branches of the trachea to the lungs. Bronchus subdivides into smaller air passages, or bronchioles, which end at the alveoli.
        (2) Carina
      d. Lungs
        (1) Surrounded by pleura
          (a) Visceral

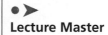

Handout 7-1
Chapter 7 Objectives Checklist

Lecture Master
You may wish to display Lecture Master 7 when presenting the lecture to the class.

Teaching Tip
Use an anatomical model to help show respiratory anatomy.

Slides/Videos
"Airway," *Pulse,* Apr. 2000.

Teaching Tip
Obtain a set of beef lungs from your local butcher. The anatomy is very similar to that of humans.

     (b) Parietal
   (2) Between pleura is pleural space, which contains serous fluid
  e. The diaphragm
 B. Mechanics of breathing (pp. 157–158)
  1. Inhalation (active)
   a. Diaphragm and intercostal muscles contract, increasing the size of the thoracic cavity
    (1) Diaphragm moves slightly downward, flares lower portion of rib cage
    (2) Ribs move upward/outward
   b. Air flows into the lungs
  2. Exhalation
   a. Diaphragm and intercostal muscles relax, decreasing the size of the thoracic cavity
    (1) Diaphragm moves upward
    (2) Ribs move downward/inward
   b. Air flows out of the lungs
  3. Control of respiration
   a. Chemoreceptors
   b. Located in the carotid arteries, aorta, and medulla oblongata
   c. Measure
    (1) Level of oxygen
    (2) Level of carbon dioxide
    (3) pH
   d. Stimulus
    (1) Hypercarbia
     (a) Elevated level of carbon dioxide
   e. Hypoxia
    (1) Condition when elevated level CO_2 is normal (COPD) and patient switches to decreased oxygen as primary stimulus to breath
 C. Respiratory physiology (pp. 158–160)
  1. Oxygenation
   a. Normally occurs as a result of respiration
   b. May occur as a result of artificial ventilation
  2. Hypoxia
   a. Inadequate amount of oxygen being delivered to cells
   b. Signs of mild/moderate hypoxia
    (1) Tachypnea
    (2) Dyspnea
    (3) Pale, cool, clammy skin (early)
    (4) Tachycardia
    (5) Restlessness and agitation
    (6) Disorientation and confusion
    (7) Headache
   c. Signs of severe hypoxia
    (1) Tachypnea
    (2) Dyspnea
    (3) Cyanosis (**Fig. 7-4, p. 160**)
    (4) Tachycardia that leads to dysrhythmias
    (5) Confusion
    (6) Loss of coordination
    (7) Sleepy appearance
    (8) Head bobbing, with droopy eyelids

         (9) Slow reaction time

         (10) Altered mental status

      d. In newborns and infants, bradycardia may be an early sign of hypoxia

   3. Alveolar/capillary exchange **(Fig. 7-5, pp. 161)**

      a. Oxygen-rich air enters the alveoli during each inspiration

      b. Oxygen enters the capillaries as carbon dioxide enters the alveoli

      c. Carbon dioxide is exhaled from the alveoli and out of the lungs

   4. Capillary/cellular exchange

      a. Cells give up carbon dioxide to the capillaries

      b. Capillaries give up oxygen to the cells

 D. Airway anatomy in infants and children (pp. 160–162) **(Fig. 7-6, p. 161; Fig. 7-7, p. 162)**

   1. Mouth and nose

      a. In general, all structures are smaller and more easily obstructed than in adults

   2. Pharynx

      a. Infants' and children's tongues take up proportionally more space in the mouth than adults

   3. Trachea and lower airway

      a. Infants and children have narrower tracheas that are obstructed more easily by swelling

      b. The trachea is softer and more flexible in infants and children

   4. Cricoid cartilage

      a. Like other cartilage in the infant and child, the cricoid cartilage is less developed and less rigid

   5. Chest wall and diaphragm

      a. Chest wall is softer

      b. Infants and children tend to depend more heavily on the diaphragm for breathing

   6. Oxygen reserves

II. Airway Assessment (pp. 162–167)

 A. Airway Functions and Considerations (pp. 162–163) **(Fig. 7-8, p. 163)**

   1. The airway and respiratory tract is the conduit that allows air to move from the atmosphere and into the alveoli for gas exchange

   2. No matter what the patient condition, the airway must remain patent at all times

   3. Any obstruction (food, blood, swelling, vomit) of the airway will lead to some degree of poor gas exchange and potential hypoxia

   4. The size of the obstruction will affect the amount of air available for gas exchange; the tongue may create only a partial airway obstruction, whereas a piece of food may completely stop air flow into the trachea and lungs

 B. Abnormal upper airway sounds (pp. 163–164)

   1. Snoring (sonorous sounds)

      a. Upper airway is partially obstructed by the tongue or by relaxed tissues in the pharynx

   2. Crowing

a. Sound like a crow cawing that occurs when the muscles around the larynx spasm and narrow the opening into the trachea

   3. Gurgling (pp. 000–000)

      a. Sound like gargling, usually indicates the presence of blood, vomitus, secretions, or other liquid in the airway

   4. Stridor (pp. 000–000)

      a. Harsh, high-pitched sound heard during inspiration

      b. It is characteristic of a significant upper airway obstruction from swelling in the larynx

      c. Stridor may also be heard if a mechanical obstruction by food or other objects is present

 C. Opening the mouth (p. 164)

   1. Crossed-finger technique to open mouth (**Fig. 7-9, p. 164**)

 D. Opening the airway (pp. 164–176)

   1. Head-tilt, chin-lift, maneuver when no neck injury suspected—review technique learned in BLS course (**Figs. 7-10, pp. 165**)

   2. Head-tilt, chin-lift in infants and children (**Fig. 7-11, p. 166**)

   3. Jaw-thrust maneuver when EMT-Basic suspects spinal injury—review technique learned in BLS course (**Fig. 7-12, p. 166**)

   4. Jaw thrust in infants and children (**Fig. 7-13, p. 167**)

   5. Positioning the patient for Airway Control (**Fig. 7-14, p. 167**)

III. Suction equipment and technique (pp. 167–170)

 A. Standard precautions during suctioning (pp. 167–168)

 B. Suction Equipment (pp. 168–169)

   1. Mounted suction devices (**Fig. 7-15, p. 168**)

   2. Portable suction devices (**Fig. 7-16, p. 168**)

      a. Electrical

      b. Oxygen-powered

      c. Hand-powered (**Fig. 7-17, p. 168**)

   3. Suction catheters

      a. Hard or rigid ("tonsil sucker," "tonsil tip")

         (1) Used to suction the mouth and oropharynx of an unresponsive patient

         (2) Should be inserted only as far as you can see

         (3) Use rigid catheter for infants and children, but take caution not to touch back of airway

      b. Soft (French)

         (1) Useful for suctioning the nasopharynx and in other situations where a rigid catheter cannot be used

         (2) Should be measured so that it is inserted only as far as the base of the tongue

 C. Techniques of suctioning (p. 169) (**Fig. 7-18, p. 170**)

   1. Suction device should be inspected on a regular basis before it is needed. A properly functioning unit with a gauge should generate a 300 mmHg vacuum. A battery-operated unit should have a charged battery.

   2. Turn on the suction unit

   3. Attach a catheter

   4. Use a rigid catheter when suctioning mouth or oropharynx

5. Often will need to suction nasal passages; should use a bulb syringe or French catheter with low to medium suction
6. Insert the catheter into the oral cavity without suction, if possible; insert only to the base of the tongue
7. Apply suction; move the catheter tip side to side
8. Suction for no more than 15 seconds at a time
9. In infants and children, suction for approximately 5 seconds

D. Special considerations when suctioning (p. 169)
1. If the patient has secretions or emesis that cannot be removed quickly and easily by suctioning, the patient should be log rolled and the oropharynx should be cleared
2. If patient produces frothy secretions as rapidly as suctioning can remove, suction for 15 seconds, artificially ventilate for 2 minutes, then suction for 15 seconds, and continue in that manner; consult medical direction for this situation
3. Monitor heart rate during suctioning
4. For a patient who is being artificially ventilated, before and after suctioning hyperoxygenate for 5 minutes
5. If necessary, rinse the catheter and tubing with water to prevent obstruction of the tubing from dried material

IV. **Airway adjuncts** (pp. 170–173)
A. Special considerations (pp. 170–171)
1. Be sure the adjunct is clean and clear of obstructions
2. Use the proper size airway adjunct
3. Airway adjuncts do not protect the airway from aspiration of secretions, blood, vomitus, or other foreign substances into the lungs
4. The mental status of the patient will determine whether or not an adjunct can be used
5. If the patient becomes more responsive or gags, remove the airway adjunct
6. A head-tilt, chin-lift or jaw-thrust maneuver must still be maintained, even when an airway adjunct is in place and properly positioned

B. Oropharyngeal (oral) airways (pp. 171) **(Figs. 7–19, p. 171)**
1. Oropharyngeal airways may be used to assist in maintaining an open airway on unresponsive patients without a gag reflex; patients with a gag reflex will vomit
2. Inserting the oropharyngeal airway **(Fig. 7-20, p. 172)**
   a. Select the proper size; it should extend from level of front teeth to angle of jaw
   b. Open the patient's mouth
   c. In adults, to avoid obstructing the airway with the tongue, insert the airway upside down, with the tip facing toward the roof of the patient's mouth
   d. Advance the airway gently until resistance is encountered; turn the airway 180 degrees so that it comes to rest with the flange on the patient's teeth **(Fig. 7-21, p. 173)**
   e. Another method of inserting an oral airway is to insert it right side up, using a tongue depressor to press the tongue down and forward to avoid obstructing the airway; this is the preferred method for airway insertion in an infant or child **(Fig. 7–22, p. 173)**

Teaching Tip
Throughout the lecture, keep a variety of airway adjuncts on hand. Perform mini-demonstrations of appropriate techniques as you lecture.

Point to Emphasize
Remind students that the techniques they practice on mannequins will feel much different when performed on live patients.

Reading/Reference
Slovis, et al., "10
Commandments of
Airway Management,"
JEMS, Jul. 2005.

    C. Nasopharyngeal (nasal) airways (pp. 171–173) **(Figs. 7–23, p. 173)**

        1. Nasopharyngeal airways are less likely to stimulate vomiting and may be used on patients who are responsive but need assistance keeping the tongue from obstructing the airway; even though the tube is lubricated, this is a painful stimulus

        2. Inserting the nasopharyngeal airway **(Fig. 7-24, p. 174 and Fig. 7-25, p. 175)**

            a. Select the proper size; measure from the tip of the nose to the tip of the patient's ear; also consider the diameter of the airway in the nostril

            b. Lubricate the airway (outside of the tube) with a water-soluble lubricant

            c. Insert the airway posteriorly; the bevel should be toward the base of the nostril or toward the septum

            d. If the airway cannot be inserted into one nostril, try the other nostril

V. Assessment of breathing (pp. 173–177)

    A. Relationship of tidal volume and respiratory rate in assessment of breathing (pp. 173–177)

        1. Tidal volume

        2. Minute volume

            a. Minute volume (MV) = Respiratory rate (f) tidal volume (V_T)

        3. Alveolar ventilation

            a. The amount of air breathed in that reaches the alveoli

            b. Dead air space

VI. Assessing for adequate breathing (pp. 177–180)

    A. Look (p. 177)

    B. Listen (p. 177)

    C. Feel (p. 177)

    D. Auscultate (p. 177–178) **(Fig. 7–26, p. 177)**

    E. Adequate breathing (p. 178)

        1. Rate

            a. Adult

               (1) 10–24 breaths per minute

            b. Child

               (1) 15–30 breaths per minute

            c. Infant

               (1) 25–50 breaths per minute

        2. Rhythm

            a. Regular

        3. Quality

            a. Breath sounds

               (1) Present and equal

            b. Chest expansion

               (1) Adequate and equal

            c. Minimum effort of breathing (use of abdominal muscles normal in infants and children)

            d. Depth (tidal volume)

               (1) Adequate

    F. Inadequate breathing (pp. 178–180) **(Fig. 7-27, p. 179)**

        1. Respiratory failure

        2. Respiratory arrest

        3. Signs of inadequate breathing

            a. Rate

Slides/Videos
"Airway Emergencies,"
*Case Studies in Prehospital
Care.* St. Louis, MO:
American Safety Video
Publishers.

        (1) Outside of normal ranges
        (2) Tachypnea
        (3) Bradypnea
    b. Rhythm
        (1) Irregular
    c. Quality
        (1) Breath sounds, diminished or absent
        (2) Chest expansion, unequal or inadequate
        (3) Increased effort to breathe (in infants and children, use of accessory muscles)
    d. Depth (tidal volume)
        (1) Shallow and inadequate
        (2) Minimal chest wall movement
        (3) Inadequate chest rise with inhalation
    e. Skin that is pale or cyanotic, cool and clammy
    f. Retractions above clavicles, between the ribs and below rib cage, especially in children
    g. Nasal flaring, especially in children
    h. Seesaw breathing in infants, where abdomen and chest move in opposite directions
    i. Agonal respirations (occasional gasping breaths) seen just before death

VII. Making the decision to ventilate or not (pp. 180–183) **(Fig. 7-28, pp. 181–182) (Table 7-1, p. 183)**
    A. Adequate respiratory rate and an adequate tidal volume with each breath = Adequate breathing (pp. 180–181)
    B. Inadequate respiratory rate and an adequate tidal volume = Inadequate breathing (p. 182)
    C. Adequate respiratory rate and an inadequate tidal volume = Inadequate breathing (pp. 182–183)

VIII. Techniques of artificial ventilation (pp. 183–198)
    A. Basic considerations (pp 183–186)
      1. Preferred ventilation methods, in order, are **(Fig. 7–29, p. 183)**:
        a. Mouth-to-mask
        b. Two-person bag-valve mask
        c. Flow-restricted, oxygen-powered ventilation device
        d. One-person bag-valve mask
      2. Standard precautions
        a. Disposable gloves and protective eyewear are required
        b. If large amounts of blood or other body fluids are present, use a face mask
        c. If TB is suspected, wear a HEPA respirator
      3. Adequate ventilation **(Fig. 7-30a, p. 185)**
        a. Indications of adequate ventilation
        b. Rate is sufficient
        c. Tidal volume is consistent and sufficient to cause chest to rise with each ventilation
        d. Heart rate returns to normal
        e. Color improves
      4. Inadequate ventilation **(Fig. 7-30b, p. 185)**
        a. Rate is too slow or too fast
        b. Chest does not rise and fall with each ventilation
        c. Heart rate does not return to normal
        d. Color does not improve
      5. Cricoid pressure, or Sellick's maneuver **(Fig. 7-30c, p. 186)**

   a. Reduces complications associated with artificial ventilation via mouth-to-mask, BVM, or other device

   b. Protects airway from regurgitation

   c. Prevents aspiration

   d. Protects against gastric inflation

   e. Used only on unresponsive adult

   f. Requires a rescuer whose only function is to apply pressure to the cricoid cartilage

B. Mouth-to-mask ventilation (p. 186)

C. Mouth-to-mask and bag-valve ventilation: General considerations (pp. 186–188)

 1. Ventilation volumes and duration of ventilation

  a. Ventilation rates for the patient with a pulse (Table 7-2, p. 187)

   (1) Adult

    (a) Adolescent and older

    (b) 10–12 ventilations per minute

    (c) One every 5–6 seconds

   (2) Child

    (a) 1 year to adolescent

    (b) 12–20 ventilations per minute

    (c) One every 3–5 seconds

   (3) Infant

    (a) Up to 1 year

    (b) 12–20 ventilations per minute

    (c) One every 3–5 seconds

   (4) Newborn

    (a) Birth to 30 days

    (b) 40–60 ventilations per minute

    (c) One every 1–1.5 seconds

  b. Ventilation rates for the patient without a pulse

   (1) Adult

    (a) Adolescent and older

    (b) One person

     (i) 30 compressions to 2 ventilations

    (c) Two person

     (i) 30 compressions to 2 ventilations

   (2) Child

    (a) 1 year to adolescent

    (b) One person

     (i) 30 compressions to 2 ventilations

    (c) Two person

     (i) 15 compressions to 2 ventilations

   (3) Infant

    (a) Up to 1 year

    (b) One person

     (i) 30 compressions to 2 ventilations

    (c) Two person

     (i) 15 compressions to 2 ventilations

   (4) Newborn

    (a) Birth to 30 days

    (b) One person

     (i) 3 compressions to 1 ventilations

    (c) Two person

     (i) 3 compressions to 1 ventilations

    c. Ventilation rates for the patient without a pulse with an advanced airway in place
      (1) Adult
        (a) Adolescent and older
        (b) 100 compressions per minute with no pause for ventilation
        (c) 8–10 ventilations per minute
        (d) 1 ventilation every 6–7.5 seconds
      (2) Child
        (a) 1 year to adolescent
        (b) 100 compressions per minute with no pause for ventilation
        (c) 8–10 ventilations per minute
        (d) 1 ventilation every 6–7.5 seconds
      (3) Infant
        (a) Up to 1 year
        (b) 100 compressions per minute with no pause for ventilation
        (c) 8–10 ventilations per minute
        (d) 1 ventilation every 6–7.5 seconds
      (4) Newborn
        (a) Birth to 30 days
        (b) 3 compressions per 1 ventilation
        (c) 30 ventilations per minute
        (d) 1 ventilation every third compression
  2. Gastric inflation
D. Mouth-to-mask ventilation (pp. 188–190) **(Fig. 7-32, p. 188)**
  1. General considerations
  2. Mouth-to-mask technique—no suspected spine injury **(Fig. 7-33, p. 189)**
    a. Connect one-way valve to port
    b. Connect oxygen tubing to oxygen inlet, and set oxygen flow to 15 liters per minute
    c. Open the airway with head-tilt, chin-lift
    d. Get in position
      (1) Cephalic technique, or at patient's head, if you are working with a partner
      (2) Lateral technique, or at patient's side, if you are working alone
    e. Place mask on patient's face, holding it with a "C-E" technique:
      (1) Thumbs and index fingers form a "C" around the mask chimney
      (2) Middle, ring, and little fingers grasp the mandible just in front of the earlobes to form "E"
      (3) Using the "E" fingers, lift mandible upward and lift chin
    f. Place mouth around one-way valve and ventilate
      (1) Blow steadily for 1 second until chest rises (tidal volume of approx. 6–7 mL/kg)
      (2) When chest rises adequately, stop ventilation to allow for exhalation
    g. If chest does not rise adequately, reposition patient's head and try again; if that fails, assume foreign body airway obstruction and follow guidelines for removing it

3. Mouth-to-mask technique (suspected spine injury)
  a. Connect a one-way valve to the ventilation port of the mask and connect tubing that is attached to an oxygen supply to the oxygen inlet; set the oxygen flow for 15 lpm
  b. Position yourself, if possible, at the top of the patient's head or at the side
  c. Open the airway with the jaw-thrust maneuver
  d. Place the mask on the patient's face
  e. Deliver the ventilation as you would in the non-spine injured patient
4. Ineffective ventilations
  a. Reposition head and neck to ensure open airway
  b. Change from head-tilt, chin-lift to a jaw-thrust maneuver
  c. Readjust face mask and ensure a seal
  d. Administer a greater tidal volume
  e. Insert an oral or nasal airway
E. Bag-valve-mask technique (pp. 190–195)
  1. Consists of self-inflating bag, one-way valve, face mask, and oxygen reservoir, and needs to be connected to oxygen
  2. General considerations
    a. Has volume of approximately 1,600 mL
    b. Provides less volume than mouth-to-mask
    c. Difficult for single rescuer to maintain airtight seal
    d. Two rescuers can work the device more effectively
    e. Adjunct airways (oral or nasal) may be necessary
  3. BVM should have: **(Fig. 7-34, p. 191)**
    a. Self-refilling bag that is easily cleaned and sterilized
    b. Non-jam valve that allows maximum oxygen flow of 30 liters per minute
      (1) No pop-off valve or disabled pop-off valve
    c. Standard 15/22 fittings
    d. Oxygen inlet and reservoir that allow for high concentrations of oxygen
    e. True nonrebreather valve
    f. Adaptability to all environmental conditions and temperature extremes
    g. Available in a variety of infant, child, and adult sizes
    h. Transparent masks to detect vomitus, blood, secretions during ventilation
  4. Bag-valve-mask technique—No suspected spine injury
  5. Two-person BVM ventilation **(Fig. 7-35, p. 192)**
    a. Position self at top of patient's head for optimal performance
    b. After opening airway, select correct mask size **(Fig. 7-36, p. 192)**
    c. Place apex of mask over bridge of nose; then lower mask over mouth and into cleft above chin
    d. Position thumbs over top half of mask, index and middle fingers over bottom half, ring and little fingers to bring jaw up to mask
    e. Hold mask, using a "C-E" technique
    f. Have another rescuer connect the bag valve to the mask, if not done already

On the Net
Skills and techniques for using a BVM effectively.
http://www.enw.org/MaskVentilation.htm

g. Have other rescuer squeeze the bag with two hands while watching for adequate chest rise and fall

h. Deliver ventilation at the proper rate and volume

    (1) Adult

        (a) 1 ventilation every 5-6 seconds (10-12 ventilations/minute)

    (2) Children & Infants

        (a) 1 ventilation every 3-5 seconds (12-20 ventilations/minute)

6. One-person BVM ventilation **(Fig. 7-37, p. 193)**

  a. Apply mask to patients' face with one hand

  b. Position thumb over part of mask covering bridge of nose; position index finger over part covering cleft above chin

  c. Seal mask firmly by pushing down with thumb and index finger while pulling up on mandible with other fingers to maintain a head-tilt, chin-lift

  d. Hold mask in place with "E-C" technique using only one hand

  e. Squeeze bag with your other hand, while observing chest rise

  f. Bag may be alternatively compressed against your body or forearm to deliver greater tidal volume

7. Bag-valve-mask problems

  a. Reposition airway and repeat ventilation attempt

  b. Reposition fingers and mask to attain a tight seal

  c. If still not able to ventilate, consider a foreign body airway obstruction; follow guidelines for removing it

  d. Make sure BVM system is properly connected and operational

  e. If still not able to ventilate, use an alternative method (e.g., pocket mask or FROPVD)

  f. If unable to maintain an open airway, insert oral or nasal airway

  g. If patient's abdomen is rising with each ventilation or abdomen appears to be distended:

    (1) Excessive air may be entering esophagus and stomach; reposition head and neck and resume ventilation

    (2) Ventilations may be too fast or too great tidal volume. Squeeze bag slowly to deliver volume over a 1-second period and allow for adequate exhalation after each one. Lower tidal volume can be used once oxygen is connected to BVM at 15 liters per minute.

8. Bag-valve-mask technique—patient with suspected spinal injury **(Fig. 7-38, p. 194)**

  a. While providing manual in-line stabilization of head and neck, open airway using jaw-thrust maneuver

  b. Select correct mask size

    (1) Do so while another rescuer maintains in-line stabilization

On the Net

Airway management
of the trauma victim.
http://www.trauma.org/
anaesthesia/airway.html

    (2) If alone, kneel at patient's head and hold it between your thighs and knees to prevent movement

  c. Position your thumbs over top half of mask, and index and middle fingers over bottom half

  d. Place top of mask over bridge of nose, and lower mask over mouth until bottom half fits snugly in cleft above chin

  e. Place middle, ring, and little fingers under mandible and bring jaw up to mask, without tilting head back or moving neck

  f. Have another rescuer connect the BVM to mask, if not already done

  g. Maintain mask seal

    (1) Place thumbs at bridge of nose and index fingers over bottom half of mask

    (2) Use thumbside edges of palms to hold mask down on face

    (3) Use middle, ring, and little fingers to maintain jaw thrust

  h. Ventilate

    (1) have another rescuer squeeze the bag with two hands to deliver volume over 1–2 seconds

  i. Deliver ventilation at the proper rate and volume **(Table 7-2, p. 187)**

    (1) Adult

      (a) 1 ventilation every 5–6 seconds (10–12 ventilations/minute)

    (2) Children & Infants

      (a) 1 ventilation every 3–5 seconds (12–20 ventilations/minute)

  j. If BVM is not already connected to oxygen, ventilate for 1 minute at a higher tidal volume over 1–2 seconds; then have another rescuer make the connection, setting the flow at 15 liters per minute, attach reservoir, and resume ventilation at a lower tidal volume (6–7 mL/kg)

  k. Maintain manual in-line stabilization until patient is completely immobilized on a long backboard

  l. Once patient is immobilized, follow two-person BVM technique, using jaw thrust to maintain a patent airway

F. Flow-restricted, oxygen-powered ventilation device (FROPVD) (pp. 195–196) **(Fig. 7-39, p. 196)**

  1. Use only with adult patients

  2. FROPVDs should provide:

    a. Peak flow rate of 100 percent oxygen at up to 40 liters per minute

    b. Inspiratory pressure relief valve that opens at approx. 60 cm of water and vents remaining volume to atmosphere or ceases gas flow

    c. Audible alarm that sounds when relief valve pressure is exceeded

    d. Satisfactory operation under a variety of environmental conditions and extremes of temperature

    e. Trigger or on/off button positioned so that both hands of rescuer can remain on mask to hold seal

  f. Standard 15/22 fittings

  g. Rugged, compact, easy to hold, and operate design

 3. FROPVD technique

  a. Ensure proper function of device, and check oxygen source to ensure an adequate supply

  b. Open airway, and then insert an oral or nasal airway

  c. Apply mask to patient's face in same manner as for BVM

  d. Connect the FROPVD to mask, if not already done

  e. Activate valve by depressing trigger or button on valve

  f. When chest begins to rise, deactivate valve by releasing trigger or button

  g. Deliver ventilation at the proper rate and volume **(Table 7-2, p. 187)**

   (1) Adult

    (a) 1 ventilation every 5–6 seconds (10–12 ventilations/minute)

   (2) Children & Infants

    (a) 1 ventilation every 3–5 seconds (12–20 ventilations/minute)

 4. FROPVD problems

  a. Reposition head and chin

  b. Recreate mask seal

  c. If still not effective, consider an airway obstruction and follow procedure for removing it

  d. If oxygen source that powers device runs out or user cannot effectively use the device, use an alternative means to ventilate patient (e.g., pocket mask or BVM device)

G. Automatic transport ventilator (ATV) (pp. 196–197) **(Fig. 7-40, p. 196)**

 1. General Considerations

 2. ATV recommended features

  a. Time or volume-cycled (not pressure cycled)

  b. Standard 15/22 connector

  c. Lightweight (less than or equal to 4 kg)

  d. Satisfactory operation in extremes of temperature

  e. Default peak inspiratory pressure limit of 60 cm H_2O that is adjustable from 20 to 80 cm H_2O and easily accessible

  f. Audible alarm that alerts operator when lung compliance is low or airway pressure is high

  g. Ability to deliver 50–100 percent oxygen

  h. Inspiratory time of 2 seconds for adults and 1 second for children

  i. Adjustable inspiratory flow of 30 L/minute for adult and 15 L/minute for child

  j. Rate of 10 breaths per minute for adults and 20 breaths per minute for children

 3. ATV technique

  a. Consult medical direction for ventilator settings, and follow manufacturer's recommendations

  b. Check ATV to ensure proper functioning

  c. Attach ATV to mask, and seal mask on face by using same technique as BVM

  d. Select tidal volume and rate to be delivered

    e. Turn unit on

    f. Observe for adequate chest rise and fall; adjust tidal volume, if needed

    g. Continuously monitor device for proper functioning and patient's chest rise and fall

    h. If failure of device is detected or suspected, immediately discontinue and begin ventilation with a pocket mask or BVM device

H. Ventilation of the patient who is breathing spontaneously (pp. 197–198)

    1. The patient has a reduced minute volume due to either an inadequate respiratory rate or inadequate tidal volume (hypoventilation)

    2. The patient with an adequate respiratory rate but an inadequate tidal volume/shallow breathing (hypopnea)

    3. The patient has an adequate tidal volume but has a respiratory rate that is too slow (bradypnea)

        a. You must deliver ventilation at a rate of 10 to 12 per minute in the adult and 12–20 per minute in the child and infant.

    4. The patient has a respiratory rate that is too fast (tachypnea) that leads to an inadequate tidal volume (hypopnea)

        a. You must deliver ventilation at a rate of 10–12 per minute in the adult and 12–20 per minute in the child and infant.

I. Hazards of overventilation of patients (p. 198)

    1. Cardiac arrest patient

    2. Hyperventilation/prolonged ventilation decrease volume of ejected blood

    3. Decrease perfusion of coronary and cerebral vessels

    4. Excessive rate and volume trap air in alveoli causing thoracic pressure to remain higher than it should

    5. Alveoli compress capillaries in the lungs and obstruct blood flow to the left atrium

    6. More ventilation is not good for the patient

    7. What is good for the patient is establishing and maintaining a patent airway, providing good ventilations at the right rate and tidal volume, and providing supplemental oxygen with ventilations

IX. Special considerations in airway management and ventilation (pp. 198–201)

    A. A patient with a stoma or tracheostomy tube (pp 199–200) **(Figs 7-41, p. 199; Fig. 7-42, p. 200)**

        1. Bag-valve-mask-to-tracheostomy tube ventilation

        2. Bag-valve mask-to-stoma ventilation

            a. Remove all coverings (e.g., scarves and ties) from the area of the stoma

            b. Clear the stoma of any foreign matter; you will not need to perform a head-tilt, chin-lift or jaw-thrust maneuver on a patient with a stoma

            c. You will not need to perform a head-tilt, chin-lift or jaw-thrust maneuver on a patient with astoma.

            d. Select a mask, most often a child or infant mask, that fits securely over the stoma and can be sealed against the neck

    e. If the chest does not rise, seal the nose and mouth with one hand so that air will not leak out of the mouth and nose

  3. Mouth-to-stoma ventilation

    a. Not recommended due to possible contamination with infectious disease

    b. Use a bag-valve mask device with an infant- or child-sized mask

B. Infant and child patients (pp. 200–201)

  1. Place in correct neutral position for an infant and extend a little past neutral for a child

  2. Avoid excessive ventilation volumes and pressure; use only enough to make chest rise

  3. Ventilate with bag-valve mask until adequate chest rise occurs. Do not use pop-off valve; must be disabled (placed in closed position) in order to adequately ventilate child or infant

  4. Ventilation rate for infants and children is 12–20 per minute or one ventilation every 32.5 seconds.

C. Patients with facial injuries (p. 201)

  1. Buinttrauma can cause excessive swelling

  2. Bleeding into the pharynx may be severe.

D. Foreign body airway obstructions (p. 201)

  1. Use foreign body airway obstruction (FBAO) procedures learned in BLS training

  2. When foreign-body airway obstruction persists, EMTs should perform three cycles of the FBAO procedure, then transport, continuing the FBAO procedure en route

E. Dental appliances (p. 201)

X. Oxygen delivery (pp. 201–209)

A. Oxygen cylinders (p. 202) (**Fig. 7-43, p. 201**)

  1. When full, all cylinders are at same pressure (about 2,000 psi)

  2. Sizes available for emergency care

    a. D cylinder—350 liters

    b. E cylinder—625 liters

    c. M cylinder—3,000 liters

    d. G cylinder—5,300 liters

    e. H cylinder—6,900 liters

  3. Duration of flow (**Table 7-3, p. 202**):

    a. Tank pressure measured by gauge in psi

    b. Minus safe residual pressure, always set at 200 psi

    c. Multiplied by constant

      (1) D = 016

      (2) E = 028

      (3) M = 156

      (4) G = 241

      (5) H = 314

      (6) K = 314

    d. Divided by flow rate expected to be delivered or being delivered to the patient in liters per minute

    e. Equals duration of flow in minutes

B. Safety precautions (pp. 202–203)

  1. No combustible materials touching cylinder, regulator, fittings, valves, or hoses

  2. No smoking in area

      3. Store below 125° F

      4. Never use cylinder without a safe, properly fitting regulator valve

      5. Never use regulator valve that has been modified from another gas

      6. Keep all valves closed when cylinder is not in use, even when empty

      7. Keep cylinders secured to prevent toppling

      8. Never place any part of body over cylinder valve

C. Pressure regulators (p. 203)

      1. High-pressure regulators

      2. Therapy regulators

D. Oxygen humidifiers (pp. 203–204) **(Fig. 7-44, p. 203)**

E. Indications for oxygen use (pp 204)

      1. Cardiac or respiratory arrest

      2. Hypoxia in a patient with adequate respiratory rate and adequate tidal volume

      3. Medical conditions that can cause hypoxia

      4. Altered mental status, including unresponsiveness

      5. Injuries to any body cavity or central nervous system, including head, spine, chest, abdomen, and pelvis

      6. Multiple fractures and multiple soft tissue injuries

      7. Severe bleeding, either internal or external

      8. Any evidence of hypoperfusion (shock)

      9. When either respiratory rate or tidal volume is inadequate, begin positive pressure ventilation with oxygen connected at 15 liters per minute

F. Hazards of oxygen administration (pp. 204–205)

      1. Oxygen is stored in tanks at a pressure of 2,000 psi

      2. Oxygen is an accelerant to combustion

      3. Oxygen and oil do not mix while under pressure

      4. Oxygen toxicity is a very rare event in the prehospital environment

      5. Damage to the retina of the eye through scar tissue formation may occur in premature newborns with excessive oxygen administration

      6. Respiratory depression or respiratory arrest in patients with chronic obstructive pulmonary disease, abbreviated as COPD (emphysema and chronic bronchitis) may occur from administration of high-flow oxygen

G. Oxygen administration procedures(p. 205) **(Fig. 7-45, pp. 206–207)**

      1. Remove protective seal

      2. Quickly open, then shut the valve

      3. Attach regulator-flowmeter to tank

      4. Attach oxygen device to flowmeter

      5. Open flowmeter to desired setting

      6. Apply oxygen device to patient

      7. When complete, remove device from patient; then turn off valve and remove all pressure from the regulator

H. Terminating oxygen therapy (p. 205)

I. Transferring the oxygen source: portable to on-board (p. 205)

J. Oxygen delivery equipment (pp. 205–209)

      1. Nonrebreather **(Fig. 7-46, p. 208)**

a. Preferred method of giving oxygen to prehospital patients
   b. Up to 90 percent oxygen can be delivered
   c. Nonrebreather bag must be full before mask is placed on patient
   d. Flow rate should be adjusted so that when patient inhales, bag does not collapse (15 liters per minute)
   e. Patients who are cyanotic, cool, clammy, or short of breath need oxygen; patients with chronic obstructive pulmonary disease and infants and children who require it should receive high-concentration oxygen
   f. Masks come in different sizes for adults, children, and infants; be sure to select the correct size mask
2. Nasal cannula (**Fig. 7-47, pp. 208–209**)
   a. Rarely the best method of delivering adequate oxygen to the prehospital patient
   b. Should be used only when patients will not tolerate a nonrebreather mask, despite coaching from the EMT
   c. Other delivery devices *not* recommended for use by EMTs in prehospital setting
3. Other oxygen delivery devices
   a. Simple face mask
   b. Partial rebreather
   c. Venturi mask (**Figs. 7-37, p. 193 and 7-38, p. 194**)

CASE STUDY FOLLOW-UP

Ask a student volunteer to read the Case Study that begins on page 154 of the textbook. You may wish to use the following questions to engage students in a discussion of the Case Study Follow-up that begins on page 210 of the textbook. Provide missing information and clarify ideas as needed.

Q1. Why are you cautious as you approach the scene?

A1. *Because the bar has been the site of frequent fights, stabbings, and shootings.*

Q2. Why do you instruct your partner to take in-line stabilization?

A2. *Because the mechanism of injury/nature of illness is unclear.*

Q3. After log rolling the patient onto a backboard, how do you secure his airway?

A3. *By immediately suctioning the vomitus out of the mouth, then performing a jaw-thrust maneuver. As the patient is not responsive, even to a painful pinch, and has no gag reflex, an oropharyngeal airway is inserted.*

Q4. How do you ventilate the patient?

A4. *With positive pressure ventilation via a bag-valve mask and supplemental oxygen. One EMT holds in-line stabilization with knees and thighs, maintains the jaw thrust and seals the mask to the patient's face with one hand, and squeezes the bag against his side with the other.*

Q5. What do you do when that patient vomits in the ambulance?

A5. *Begin suctioning immediately while the immobilized patient is tilted on the board to help drain the vomitus from his mouth. Once the vomitus is cleared, ventilation is continued.*

IN REVIEW

Assess students' ability to apply what they have just learned by discussing the Review Questions on page 213 in the textbook.

Q1. Describe the two manual methods used to open an airway and explain the circumstances in which each should be used.

A1. *The two manual methods used to open an airway are the head-tilt, chin-lift and the jaw-thrust maneuver. In the head-tilt, chin-lift, the head is extended backward as the chin is lifted; it is used in nontrauma situations. In the jaw-thrust, only the mandible (jaw) is moved up and forward without extending the head or moving the neck; it is used when spinal injury is suspected. (pp. 164–167)*

Q2. Name the two airway adjuncts that can be inserted to assist in establishing and maintaining an open airway and explain the circumstances in which each should be used.

A2. *The two airway adjuncts are the oropharyngeal and the nasopharyngeal airway. Both are used to prevent the tongue from blocking the airway. The oropharyngeal airway cannot be used when the patient has a gag reflex; the nasopharyngeal airway can often be tolerated by a patient with reduced responsiveness (who needs assistance in maintaining a patent airway) but who still has a gag reflex. (pp. 171–173)*

Q3. Outline the assessment techniques you would use to determine if the patient's breathing is adequate or inadequate.

A3. *The assessment techniques to determine if the patient's breathing is adequate or inadequate are the following: Look—at general appearance, respiratory rate, chest rise and fall, retractions; Listen— patient speech, air movement in and out of nose and mouth; Feel—air escaping from the nose and mouth; Auscultate—breath sounds equal and present bilaterally. (pp. 177–180)*

Q4. Name the signs of adequate breathing.

A4. *The signs of adequate breathing are the following: Rate—within normal limits; Rhythm—regular; Quality—equal, full, and present breath sounds bilaterally, good expansion of the chest, no retractions or excessive muscle use; Depth (tidal volume)—feel adequate volume of air, see good chest rise on inspiration. (p. 178)*

Q5. Name the signs of inadequate breathing.

A5. *The signs of inadequate breathing are the following: Rate—bradypnea (too slow) or tachypnea (too fast); Rhythm—irregular pattern; Quality— diminished or absent breath sounds, poor rise and fall of the chest, poor air movement; Depth—shallow and inadequate. (pp. 178–180)*

Q6. Name the recommended methods that the EMT can use to artificially ventilate the patient.

A6. *The recommended methods that the EMT can use to artificially ventilate the patient, in order of preference, are mouth-to-mask;*

©2008 by Pearson Education, Inc.
Prehospital Emergency Care, 8th ed.

two-person bag-valve mask; flow-restricted, oxygen-powered ventilation device; one-person bag-valve mask. (p. 183)

Q7. Explain the difference in the technique for ventilation of a patient with and without a suspected spinal injury.

A7. *The difference in the technique for ventilation of a patient with and without a suspected spinal injury is as follows: In-line stabilization must be established and maintained while ventilating the patient with a suspected spinal injury until the patient is completely immobilized to the backboard. The nontrauma patient with no suspected spinal injury does not require in-line stabilization during ventilation. (p. 193)*

Q8. List the indications that the patient is being ventilated adequately.

A8. *Indications that the patient is being ventilated adequately are the following: Rate is sufficient, tidal volume is consistent and causes the chest to rise adequately, adequate exhalation occurs without any air being trapped, the heart rate returns to normal, and color improves. (p. 184)*

Q9. Describe the appropriate procedure for initiating oxygen administration.

A9. *The appropriate procedure for initiating oxygen administration is as follows: (1) Check the cylinder to be sure it contains oxygen and remove the protective seal on the tank valve. (2) Quickly open, then shut, the cylinder valve for 1 second to remove any dust or debris from the valve assembly. (3) Place the yoke of the regulator over the valve and align the pins, being sure the regulator washer is present and in the proper place; hand tighten the T-screw on the regulator. (4) Slowly open the main cylinder valve about one-half turn to charge the regulator and check the pressure gauge to be sure an adequate amount of oxygen is available. (5) Attach the oxygen mask or nasal cannula tubing to the nipple of the regulator. (6) Open the regulator flowmeter control and set the oxygen flow at the desired liters per minute. (7) With the oxygen flowing, apply the oxygen mask or nasal cannula to the patient. (pp. 205–207)*

Q10. Describe the appropriate procedure for terminating oxygen administration.

A10. *The appropriate procedure for terminating oxygen administration is as follows: (1) Remove the oxygen mask or nasal cannula from the patient. (2) Turn off the oxygen regulator flowmeter control, and then turn off the cylinder valve. (3) Open the regulator valve to allow the oxygen trapped in the regulator to escape until the pressure gauge reads zero, then turn off completely the regulator flowmeter control. (p. 205)*

CRITICAL THINKING

Assess students' ability to respond to real-life emergency situations by discussing the Critical Thinking questions on page 213 in the textbook.

Q1. What is the status of the patient's airway?

A1. *The snoring sounds during respiration indicate that the patient's airway is partially blocked—presumably by either his tongue or relaxed tissue in the pharynx.*

Q2. How would you manage the airway in this particular patient?

A2. *Remove any pillows from under the patient's head. Immediately perform a head-tilt, chin-lift maneuver to open the airway. If snoring sounds are still heard, reposition the airway. If the sounds are still present, insert an airway adjunct. This patient would likely accept either a nasopharyngeal or oropharyngeal airway. If he will not accept an oropharyngeal airway, proceed with insertion of a nasopharyngeal airway.*

Q3. What is the status of his ventilation?

A3. *The rate of 5–6 breaths per minute coupled with the minimal chest movements and pulse oximeter reading of 79 percent indicates that the patient's ventilations are inadequate for proper oxygenation. He has both an inadequate respiratory rate and an inadequate tidal volume, creating an inadequate ventilatory status.*

Q4. What emergency care would you provide to manage the ventilation?

A4. *The patient requires immediate ventilatory assistance with a bag-valve-mask or other ventilation device. He should be ventilated at a rate of 10–12 times per minute. Supplemental oxygen must be attached to and delivered via the ventilation device.*

Q5. What is the oxygenation status of the patient?

A5. *Even though his skin signs aren't yet indicating it, this patient's slow, shallow respirations and poor pulse oximeter reading indicate that his oxygenation status is poor and he is hypoxic.*

Q6. What intervention would you provide to manage the oxygenation status?

A6. *The positive pressure ventilation and supplemental oxygen delivery through the ventilation device will improve the oxygenation status.*

SKILLS DEMONSTRATION AND PRACTICE

Set up the 10 practice stations described below. Have an EMT at each station to demonstrate the skills and equipment needed for it and to help students practice the skill. If 10 EMTs or 10 stations are not practical for your setting, reduce the number of stations by combining demonstration and practice stations. Group the listed skills in meaningful clusters and be sure all the listed skills are demonstrated and practiced.

Write the station names on a chalkboard, flip chart, or overhead transparency. (Items in parentheses following station names are the equipment needed at each station. You do not have to include this information on the written list.)

1. Ventilating using head-tilt, chin-lift and jaw-thrust (CPR mannequin)

2. Suctioning (portable suctioning device, rigid and soft suction catheters, CPR mannequin)

3. Ventilating using barrier shields and pocket masks (pocket masks for each student, other barrier shields used in your area, CPR mannequin)

4. Bag-valve mask to assemble and use on neck-injured and non-neck-injured patients (BVM unit including full oxygen cylinder, CPR mannequin)

©2008 by Pearson Education, Inc.
Prehospital Emergency Care, 8th ed.

5. Flow-restricted, oxygen-powered ventilation (FROPVD with full oxygen cylinder, CPR mannequin)

6. Stomas (tracheostomy mannequin, portable suction unit with soft suction catheter, FROPVD with full oxygen cylinder, BVM unit)

7. Oropharyngeal and nasopharyngeal airways (several sizes of oropharyngeal and nasopharyngeal airways, water-based lubricant, CPR mannequin)

8. Oxygen tanks and regulators (several sizes of oxygen cylinders and several types of regulators/flowmeters)

9. Nonrebreather face masks and nasal cannulae (nonrebreather face mask, nasal cannula, full oxygen cylinder with regulator)

10. Infants and children (infant and child CPR mannequins, portable suction unit with a rigid suction catheter, FROPVD, BVM unit with full oxygen cylinder, several sizes of infant and child masks and oral and nasal airways)

Divide the class into 10 groups. You can do this by having students count off "1, 2, 3, . . . 10" until each student has been numbered. All like-numbered students will constitute a group. Have each team rotate through each of the 10 practice stations listed, being sure to give the location of each demonstration and practice station.

Direct teams to their initial stations. Group 1 can begin with Station 1, Group 2 can begin Station 2, etc. Visit each station to monitor progress of practice. Provide help to the teaching assistants, if necessary. Make sure that each team visits each practice station. When each team has completed each station, make sure that students return to the main classroom.

ASSIGNMENTS

Assign students to read Chapter 8, "Scene Size-Up," before the next class. Also ask them to complete Chapter 7 of the Workbook.

EVALUATION

Chapter Quiz Distribute copies of the Chapter Quiz provided in Handout 7-2 to evaluate student understanding of this chapter. Remind students not to refer to their textbooks or notes while taking the quiz.

Test Manager You may wish to create a custom-tailored test using Prentice Hall *TestGen for Prehospital Emergency Care, Eighth Edition* to evaluate student understanding of this chapter.

Online Test Preparation (for students and instructors) Additional test preparation is available through *EMT Achieve: Basic Test Preparation* at http://www.prenhall.com/EMTAchieve. Instructors can also monitor student mastery online.

REINFORCEMENT

Handouts If classroom discussions or performance on the quiz indicates that some students have not fully mastered the chapter content, you may wish to assign some or all of the Reinforcement Handouts for this chapter.

Reading/Reference
Textbook, pp. 218–238

Workbook
Chapter 7 Activities

Chapter Quiz
Handout 7-2

TestGen
Chapter 7 Test

Online Test Preparation
Send your students to
http://prenhall.com/
EMT Achieve

Handouts 7-3 to 7-7
Reinforcement Activities

**Brady Skills Series
EMT-B Videos/CD**
Visual Reinforcement

**PowerPoint
Presentation**
Chapter 7

Student CD
Chapter 7

Companion Website
http://www.prenhall.com/
mistovich

TECH EXTRAS

Brady Skills Series EMT-B Videos/CD Have your students watch the skills come to life on either VHS or CD-ROM.

PowerPoint Presentation (for instructors) The PowerPoint material developed for this chapter offers useful reinforcement of chapter content.

Student CD A wide variety of material on this CD-ROM will reinforce and also expand student knowledge and skills.

Companion Website (for students) Additional review quizzes and links to EMS resources will contribute to further reinforcement of this chapter. Please visit http://www.prenhall.com/mistovich.

OBJECTIVES CHECKLIST

Cognitive		Date Mastered
2-1.1	Name and label the major structures of the respiratory system on a diagram.	
2-1.2	List the signs of adequate breathing.	
2-1.3	List the signs of inadequate breathing.	
2-1.4	Describe the steps in performing the head-tilt, chin-lift.	
2-1.5	Relate mechanism of injury to opening the airway.	
2-1.6	Describe the steps in performing the jaw thrust.	
2-1.7	State the importance of having a suction unit ready for immediate use when providing emergency care.	
2-1.8	Describe the techniques of suctioning.	
2-1.9	Describe how to artificially ventilate a patient with a pocket mask.	
2-1.10	Describe the steps in performing the skill of artificially ventilating a patient with a bag-valve mask while using the jaw thrust.	
2-1.11	List the parts of a bag-valve-mask system.	
2-1.12	Describe the steps in performing the skill of artificially ventilating a patient with a bag-valve mask for one and two rescuers.	
2-1.13	Describe the signs of adequate artificial ventilation, using the bag-valve mask.	
2-1.14	Describe the signs of inadequate artificial ventilation, using the bag-valve mask.	
2-1.15	Describe the steps in artificially ventilating a patient with a flow-restricted, oxygen-powered ventilation device.	
2-1.16	List the steps in performing the actions taken when providing mouth-to-mouth and mouth-to-stoma artificial ventilation.	
2-1.17	Describe how to measure and insert an oropharyngeal (oral) airway.	
2-1.18	Describe how to measure and insert a nasopharyngeal (nasal) airway.	
2-1.19	Define the components of an oxygen delivery system.	
2-1.20	Identify a nonrebreather face mask and state the oxygen flow requirements needed for its use.	
2-1.21	Describe the indications for using a nasal cannula versus a nonrebreather face mask.	
2-1.22	Identify a nasal cannula and state the flow requirements needed for its use.	

OBJECTIVES

Affective	Date Mastered
2-1.23 Explain the rationale for basic life support artificial ventilation and airway protective skills taking priority over most other basic life support skills.	
2-1.24 Explain the rationale for providing adequate oxygenation through high-inspired oxygen concentrations to patients who, in the past, may have received low concentrations.	

Psychomotor	Date Mastered
2-1.25 Demonstrate the steps in performing the head-tilt, chin-lift.	
2-1.26 Demonstrate the techniques in performing the jaw thrust.	
2-1.27 Demonstrate the techniques of suctioning.	
2-1.28 Demonstrate the steps in providing mouth-to-mouth artificial ventilation with body substance isolation (barrier shields).	
2-1.29 Demonstrate how to use a pocket mask to artificially ventilate a patient.	
2-1.30 Demonstrate the assembly of a bag-valve-mask unit.	
2-1.31 Demonstrate the steps in performing the skill of artificially ventilating a patient with a bag-valve mask for one and two rescuers.	
2-1.32 Demonstrate the steps in performing the skill of artificially ventilating a patient with a bag-valve mask while using the jaw thrust.	
2-1.33 Demonstrate artificial ventilation of a patient with a flow-restricted, oxygen-powered ventilation device.	
2-1.34 Demonstrate how to artificially ventilate a patient with a stoma.	
2-1.35 Demonstrate how to insert an oropharyngeal (oral) airway.	
2-1.36 Demonstrate how to insert a nasopharyngeal (nasal) airway.	
2-1.37 Demonstrate the correct operation of oxygen tanks and regulators.	
2-1.38 Demonstrate the use of a nonrebreather face mask and state the oxygen flow requirements needed for its use.	
2-1.39 Demonstrate the use of a nasal cannula and state the flow requirements for its use.	
2-1.40 Demonstrate how to artificially ventilate the infant and child patient.	
2-1.41 Demonstrate oxygen administration for the infant and child patient.	

CHAPTER 7 QUIZ

Write the letter of the best answer in the space provided.

_____ 1. The first step of emergency care in the patient with inadequate breathing is
   A. checking for the patient's pulse.
   B. manually stabilizing the cervical spine.
   C. opening and maintaining the patient's airway.
   D. looking for and controlling severe bleeding.

_____ 2. Inadequate breathing or inadequate blood circulation can cause
   A. kyphosis.
   B. hyperglycemia.
   C. lordosis.
   D. hypoxia.

_____ 3. Signs of inadequate breathing include all of the following *except*
   A. retractions above the clavicles, between ribs, and below rib cage.
   B. cyanosis of the lips, ear lobes, or nail beds.
   C. bradypnea.
   D. pink skin and respiratory rate between 10 and 24 per minute.

_____ 4. Stimulation of the back of a patient's throat when suctioning may cause
   A. convulsions.
   B. a slowed heart rate.
   C. unequal pupils.
   D. cyanosis.

_____ 5. A 24-year-old female patient has fallen from the roof of her house and is unconscious. The best method of opening her airway is the _____ maneuver.
   A. head-tilt, chin-lift
   B. jaw-thrust
   C. head-tilt, neck-lift
   D. tongue-jaw lift

_____ 6. Methods of artificial ventilation, in order of preference, are
   1. one-person bag-valve mask.
   2. mouth-to-mask.
   3. flow-restricted, oxygen-powered ventilation device.
   4. two-person bag-valve mask.

   A. 2, 4, 3, and 1
   B. 2, 4, 1, and 3
   C. 1, 4, 3, and 2
   D. 4, 3, 1, and 2

_____ 7. Signs of inadequate artificial ventilation of an adult patient include
   A. a heart rate that returns to normal.
   B. failure of the patient's skin color to improve.
   C. the patient's chest rising and falling with each ventilation.
   D. a ventilation rate of 10–12 per minute.

_____ 8. When high-concentration oxygen is attached to a bag-valve mask, the concentration of oxygen delivered to the patient is approximately
   A. 16%.
   B. 24%.
   C. 100%.
   D. 90%.

_____ 9. All the following are important features of bag-valve-mask systems *except* a
    A. non-jam valve system.
    B. 15/22mm respiratory fitting.
    C. nonrebreathing valve.
    D. pop-off valve.

_____ 10. The most difficult part of delivering BVM artificial ventilations for a single rescuer is
    A. obtaining an adequate mask seal.
    B. squeezing the bag completely.
    C. maintaining an open airway.
    D. preventing the patient from vomiting.

_____ 11. Oropharyngeal airways can be used on unconscious patients, *except* those who
    A. are in cardiac arrest.
    B. have a gag reflex.
    C. are younger than 8 years.
    D. have a contagious respiratory disease.

_____ 12. Because the oropharyngeal airway is likely to stimulate the patient's gag reflex, the rescuer should
    A. use only nasal airways.   **C.** be prepared to suction.
    B. use the next smaller size.   **D.** not use one.

_____ 13. The nasopharyngeal airway is often utilized because it
    A. comes in more sizes than the oropharyngeal airway.
    B. often does not stimulate the patient's gag reflex.
    C. can be used even if clear (CSF) fluid is seen in the nose or ears.
    D. is made of rigid, clear plastic, which is less likely to cause bleeding.

_____ 14. Which of the following is *true* regarding suctioning a patient's airway?
    A. Never suction the airway for longer than 15 seconds.
    B. Suction only as you insert the catheter into the mouth.
    C. BSI precautions are not important if there is no visible blood.
    D. You may hyperventilate a patient before and after suctioning.

_____ 15. One advantage of a "tonsil tip" catheter over a "French" catheter is that it
    A. is flexible and can be inserted deeper into the pharynx.
    B. is more effective for particulate matter.
    C. can suction the nose.
    D. can be inserted well beyond the base of the tongue.

_____ 16. Before suctioning, a patient who is artificially ventilated should be
    A. placed in a position of comfort.
    B. hypoventilated.
    C. hyperventilated.
    D. fully immobilized.

_____ 17. A nasal cannula should be used to deliver oxygen to a patient who
    A. has a chronic lung disease.
    B. requires a high concentration of oxygen.
    C. will not tolerate a nonrebreather mask.
    D. uses a cannula with a home oxygen system.

_____ **18.** Administer oxygen to any patient who needs supplemental oxygen *unless*
    A. the patient is an infant.
    B. the patient has COPD.
    C. medical direction instructs otherwise.
    D. the patient has TB.

_____ **19.** Oxygen cylinder sizes vary, but all are considered "full" when pressure is equal to _____ psi.
    A. 1,000   **C.** 2,000
    B. 1,500   **D.** 2,500

_____ **20.** An insufficiency in the supply of oxygen to the body's tissues is called
    A. hypoxia.   **C.** respiratory compromise.
    B. hyperventilation.   **D.** bronchoconstriction.

_____ **21.** The use of which of the following methods is contraindicated with children?
    A. mouth-to-mask
    B. flow-restricted, oxygen-powered ventilation device
    C. two-person bag-valve mask
    D. one-person bag-valve mask

_____ **22.** To ease insertion, nasopharyngeal airways must be lubricated with
    A. lubricant with petroleum jelly.
    B. any petroleum-based lubricant, such as WD-40.
    C. any silicone-based lubricant.
    D. any water-soluble lubricant.

_____ **23.** When a patient who has a full set of dentures needs ventilations
    A. leave the dentures in place if they are secure and then ventilate.
    B. remove the dentures in all circumstances before ventilating.
    C. an endotracheal intubation must be performed.
    D. an ATV should be used.

_____ **24.** A suction device, whether portable or mounted, must generate a vacuum of _____ mmHg.
    A. 100   **C.** 300
    B. 200   **D.** 400

_____ **25.** When a nasal cannula is used, the flow rate should be no more than _____ liters per minute.
    A. 1 to 6   **C.** 10 to 12
    B. 6 to 10   **D.** 12 to 14

REINFORCEMENT

IN THE FIELD

Review the following real-life situation. Then answer the questions that follow.

You and your EMT partner, Cindy, are assigned to a suburban station on a cold February morning. At 0613, you are dispatched to an apartment building for a breathing problem. You arrive at the building about 7 minutes later and are met by the patient's wife, who is quite anxious. You put on your personal protective equipment, get the ambulance cot and your equipment, and follow the woman to the sixth floor of the building. On the way up in the elevator, the patient's wife tells you her husband, Mike, is having a very hard time breathing, and he looks a little blue.

You arrive at the apartment and find your patient, a 23-year-old male, seated in a chair, leaning forward on his legs. His skin is pale, his lips are cyanotic, and you hear wheezing as he breathes. You introduce yourself and Cindy to the patient as you begin assessing his condition. It is obvious he is quite anxious, so you attempt to calm him as you explain what you are doing. Mike cannot speak in full sentences but tells you that he has had asthma for about 15 years. He usually uses an inhaler but ran out of the medicine about 5 days ago. His breathing got worse 2 days ago, when the elevator was not working and he had to climb up the five flights to his apartment. You obtain a pulse ox reading and place the patient on oxygen, using a nonrebreather mask at 15 liters per minute. Cindy begins taking Mike's vital signs. His blood pressure is 96/74; his pulse is 110; and his respirations are 28 per minute. You decide that Mike needs immediate transport to the hospital, about 25 minutes away. As you get Mike placed on your cot, sitting up for comfort, you use your portable radio to request an ALS rendezvous.

1. As you begin patient contact, describe your initial impression, and explain why you feel this way.

2. Is this patient considered a high priority for immediate transport? Explain your rationale.

3. What signs and symptoms indicated to you that the patient was having severe respiratory difficulty?

4. Why was an ALS rendezvous requested for this patient?

REINFORCEMENT

CHAPTER 7 REVIEW

Write the word or words that best complete each sentence in the space provided.

1. The most basic components of emergency medical care are to establish and maintain a(n) _____, ensure effective ventilation, and provide oxygen to the patient.

2. The EMT's chief responsibilities are finding and correcting immediately all _____ - _____ problems.

3. Respiratory _____ occurs when respiratory rate and/or tidal volume is insufficient.

4. When breathing stops completely, the patient is in _____ _____.

5. Minimal or uneven chest movements, diminished breath sounds, and noisy breathing are signs of _____ _____.

6. A blue or gray color to the patient's skin or nail beds is called _____, which is a sign of breathing difficulty.

7. The procedure commonly used for opening the airway of a patient when no trauma is suspected is the _____ - _____, - _____ - _____ maneuver.

8. The two passageways found at the lower end of the pharynx are the _____ and _____.

9. The trachea is protected by a small flap of tissue called the _____.

10. When one rescuer is using a bag-valve-mask device, the most difficult part of delivering artificial ventilations is maintaining an _____ _____.

11. When delivering artificial ventilations to a nonbreathing patient, give one ventilation every _____ seconds to an adult and one every _____ seconds to a child.

12. _____ is the process by which the blood and cells become saturated with oxygen.

13. The most common cause of an obstructed airway in the unresponsive patient is the _____.

14. Use an oropharyngeal airway for all unresponsive patients who do not exhibit a(n)

_____ _____.

15. A properly sized oropharyngeal airway should extend the distance from the level of the patient's

_____ _____ to the angle of the patient's

_____.

16. Lubricate the outside of a nasopharyngeal airway with a sterile _____ - soluble lubricant.

17. _____ is an excessive rapid breathing rate and may indicate inadequate

oxygenation and breathing.

18. It is possible to add moisture to oxygen by adding a(n) _____ to the

regulator.

19. A nonrebreather mask is the EMT's best way to deliver high concentrations of oxygen to a

breathing patient because it can provide concentrations of oxygen ranging from

_____ to _____ %.

20. A surgical opening into the neck and trachea, also known as a tracheostomy, is a(n)

_____.

AIRWAY: LISTING

1. List four factors of breathing that must be assessed when determining whether a patient's breathing is adequate.

2. List and describe four sounds that may indicate airway obstruction.

3. List eight signs of inadequate breathing.

4. List, in order of preference, four methods of providing positive pressure ventilations to patients.

AIRWAY: TRUE OR FALSE

Indicate if the following statements are true or false by writing T or F in the space provided.

_____ **1.** The trachea is the passageway through which food travels into the stomach.

_____ **2.** The nose, mouth, pharynx, and trachea are all parts of the respiratory system.

_____ **3.** During mouth-to-mask ventilations of infant and child patients, each breath should be delivered over 2 to 2.5 seconds.

_____ **4.** A pinkish skin coloration is one sign of adequate breathing.

_____ **5.** Excessive use of neck and intercostal muscles is a sign of inadequate breathing in an adult.

_____ **6.** Cyanosis is the term used to describe a bluish skin color.

_____ **7.** A nonrebreather mask is the preferred method for delivering supplemental oxygen to patients in the prehospital setting.

_____ **8.** Head, neck, or spinal injury should be suspected in any unconscious trauma patient.

_____ **9.** The head-tilt, chin-lift maneuver should be used to open the airway of a patient with a suspected neck injury.

_____ **10.** When using the head-tilt, chin-lift maneuver to open a patient's airway, place your fingertips on the bony part of the chin, not the soft tissues under the lower jaw.

_____ **11.** When opening an unconscious patient's airway, you may need to insert your thumb into the patient's mouth.

_____ **12.** When using the jaw-thrust maneuver to open a patient's airway, stabilize the patient's head with your knees.

_____ **13.** Use of a pocket mask with supplemental oxygen to ventilate a patient can deliver a higher tidal volume of air than use of a bag-valve-mask device.

_____ **14.** A pop-off valve is an undesirable feature of some older bag-valve-mask devices.

_____ **15.** BVMs should have a standard 15/22 mm connection to properly fit face masks and endotracheal tubes.

_____ **16.** If a nasopharyngeal airway is too long, it can enter the esophagus and cause massive gastric distension.

_____ **17.** With a BVM device, a mask seal can more easily be maintained when ventilations are performed by two rescuers.

_____ **18.** Nonbreathing adult patients should be ventilated at a rate of 10–12 times per minute.

_____19. If the chest does not rise and fall during BVM ventilation, you should reposition the head to ensure an open airway.

_____20. Using a nasal cannula with supplemental oxygen will deliver nearly 100% oxygen concentration to your patient.

_____21. A pediatric-sized BVM mask can be used to establish a seal around a stoma.

_____22. Flow-restricted, oxygen-powered ventilation devices may have an audible alarm when the relief valve is activated.

_____23. If a patient rejects an oropharyngeal airway at your first attempt, reopen the airway and insert it more aggressively.

_____24. To ease insertion of a nasopharyngeal airway, it should be lubricated with petroleum jelly.

_____25. The EMT should never suction a patient for more than 5 seconds at a time.

REINFORCEMENT

AIRWAY: MATCHING

Write the letter of the term in the space next to the appropriate description below.

_____ **1.** The active process of breathing air into the lungs

A. ATV

_____ **2.** A small flap of tissue that closes over the trachea during swallowing

B. bilaterally

_____ **3.** The portion of the pharynx that extends from the nostrils to the soft palate

C. bradypnea

_____ **4.** On both sides

D. cyanosis

_____ **5.** Inflation of the stomach

E. diaphragm

_____ **6.** A bluish color of the skin and mucous membranes that indicates poor oxygenation of tissue

F. epiglottis

_____ **7.** Innermost covering of the lungs

G. exhalation

_____ **8.** A reduction of oxygen delivery to the tissues

H. gastric distension

_____ **9.** A breathing rate that is faster than the normal rate

I. hypoxia

_____ **10.** A breathing rate that is slower than the normal rate

J. inhalation

_____ **11.** A positive-pressure ventilation device that delivers ventilations automatically

K. intercostal

_____ **12.** A harsh, high-pitched sound heard on inspiration; indicates swelling of the larynx

L. nasopharynx

_____ **13.** The passive process of breathing air out of the lungs

M. tachypnea

_____ **14.** The major muscle of respiration, which separates the chest cavity from the abdominal cavity

N. stridor

_____ **15.** Describing the muscles between the ribs

O. visceral pleura

©2008 by Pearson Education, Inc.
Prehospital Emergency Care, 8th ed.

Airway Management, Ventilation, and Oxygen Therapy

Respiratory System Review
Anatomy

Physiology

Ensuring an Open Airway
Opening the Mouth

Opening the Airway

Suction Equipment and Techniques

Airway Adjuncts

Assessment of Breathing
Adequate Breathing

Inadequate Breathing

Techniques of Artificial Ventilation
Basic Considerations

Basic Techniques

- Mouth-to-mask
- Bag-valve mask
- Flow-restricted, oxygen-powered ventilation device
- Automatic transport ventilator

Oxygen Delivery
Basics, Precautions, and Procedures

Oxygen Delivery Devices

Special Considerations

HANDOUT 7-2: Chapter 7 Quiz

1. C	8. C	14. A	20. A
2. D	9. D	15. B	21. B
3. D	10. A	16. C	22. D
4. B	11. B	17. C	23. A
5. B	12. C	18. C	24. C
6. A	13. B	19. C	25. A
7. B			

HANDOUT 7-3: In the Field

1. Your general impression would be of a 23-year-old male, seated in a tripod position, pale skin, and audibly wheezing. He is having a difficult time breathing and is a priority patient.

2. Any patient with breathing difficulty is considered a high priority.

3. The patient was seated in a tripod position, leaning forward. His skin color was pale, he is cyanotic, and you can hear wheezing. These are all signs of inadequate breathing.

4. An ALS rendezvous was requested due to the real possibility that his condition could worsen, requiring a higher level of treatment. The paramedics could establish an IV line for medications, if needed, intubate if necessary, and administer medication in the form of a breathing treatment while en route.

HANDOUT 7-4: Chapter 7 Review

1. airway
2. life-threatening
3. failure
4. respiratory arrest
5. inadequate breathing
6. cyanosis
7. head-tilt, chin-lift
8. trachea, esophagus
9. epiglottis
10. adequate seal
11. 4 to 5, 3
12. Oxygenation
13. tongue
14. gag reflex
15. front teeth, jaw
16. water
17. Tachypnea
18. humidifier
19. 80, 100
20. stoma

HANDOUT 7-5: Airway: Listing

1. Rate, rhythm, quality, and depth of breathing

2. Snoring—sonorous sounds; crowing—air rushing through a spasming larynx makes a crow-like sound; gurgling—a sound like gargling; stridor—harsh, high-pitched sound heard during inspirations

3. Any eight of the following: chest expansion is absent, minimal, or unequal; use of accessory muscles; no air can be felt or heard at the nose or mouth, or the amount of air exchanged is evaluated to be below normal; respiratory rate is too fast or too slow; rhythm of breathing is irregular; patient's skin is cool and clammy; patient exhibits nasal flaring; patient is unable to speak or cannot speak full sentences; cyanosis visible in skin, lips, tongue, ear lobes, or nail beds; breathing is very shallow, very deep, or appears labored; breath sounds are diminished or absent; noises such as wheezing, crowing, stridor, snoring, gurgling, or gasping are heard; retractions above the clavicles and between and below the ribs, especially in children.

4. Mouth-to-mask; two-person bag-valve mask; flow-restricted, oxygen-powered ventilation device; one-person bag-valve mask

HANDOUT 7-6: Airway: True or False

1. F	8. T	14. T	20. F
2. T	9. F	15. T	21. T
3. F	10. T	16. T	22. T
4. T	11. F	17. T	23. F
5. T	12. F	18. T	24. F
6. T	13. T	19. T	25. F
7. T			

HANDOUT 7-7: Airway: Matching

1. J	5. H	9. M	13. G
2. F	6. D	10. C	14. E
3. L	7. O	11. A	15. K
4. B	8. I	12. N	

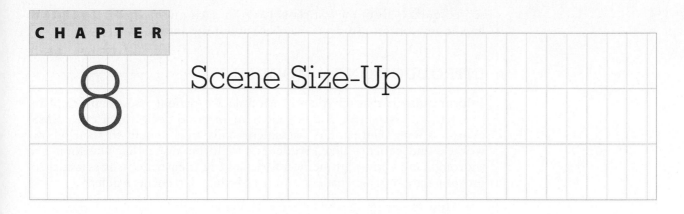

This chapter covers Lesson 3-1 and portions of Lesson 3-9 of the U.S. Department of Transportation's EMT-Basic National Standard Curriculum.

OBJECTIVES

Numbered objectives are from the U.S. Department of Transportation EMT-Basic National Standard Curriculum. Asterisked objectives, if any, pertain to material that is supplemental to the DOT curriculum. Page numbers in parentheses refer to pages in the textbook.

Cognitive

3-1.1   Recognize hazards/potential hazards. (pp. 221–231)

3-1.2   Describe common hazards found at the scene of a trauma and a medical patient. (pp. 220–231)

3-1.3   Determine if the scene is safe to enter. (pp. 221–231)

3-1.4   Discuss common mechanisms of injury/nature of illness. (pp. 231–233)

3-1.5   Discuss the reason for identifying the total number of patients at the scene. (pp. 226, 234)

3.1-6   Explain the reason for identifying the need for additional help or assistance. (pp. 222–229, 234)
— Explain how to gain scene control. (pp. 230–231)
— Explain how to establish rapport with the patient. (pp. 230, 234, 235–236)

Affective

3-1.7   Explain the rationale for crew members to evaluate scene safety prior to entering. (pp. 218, 220)

3-1.8   Serve as a model for others, explaining how patient situations affect your evaluation of mechanism of injury or illness. (pp. 231–234)

Psychomotor

3-1.9   Observe various scenarios and identify potential hazards.

Objectives 3-1.4, 5, 6, and 8 are also addressed in Chapter 9, "Patient Assessment."

REVIEW

Review with students Chapter 7, "Airway Management, Ventilation, and Oxygen Therapy," reminding them that "A" in the ABCs of CPR stands for Airway—the first priority in treating every patient they care for. Point out that without an airway, the patient will not be able to survive. Distribute the

Total Teaching Time
105 minutes

Resources Needed
- Scored Chapter 7 Quizzes
- Trauma kit with BSI equipment and a selection of airways
- Portable suction unit

Additional Resources
Larmon/Davis, *Basic Life Support Skills*

Elling, *EMT Achieve: Basic Test Preparation*

Limmer/Mistovich/O'Keefe, *Audio Lecture & Study Guide: EMT*

Mistovich/Kuvlesky, *SUCCESS! for the EMT, Second Edition*

scored quizzes from the last class. Go over each question on the quiz and handle any concerns students may have about the answers.

INTRODUCTION TO MODULE 3

Inform students that the focus of Module 3 is patient assessment. Explain that patient assessment is a key element in good prehospital care. EMS providers with keen patient assessment skills are a benefit to their fellow workers and patients alike. Students should be aware that developing a thorough and consistent method for assessing their patients is essential to providing good-quality patient care. In Module 3, students will learn

- How to size up a scene before entering it
- How to perform an initial assessment of a patient's condition
- How to perform a more detailed history and physical examination of patients who are sick or injured
- The importance of periodically rechecking a patient's condition
- How to communicate with other health care professionals
- How to document contacts with patients—what the EMT found and did

INTRODUCTION TO CHAPTER 8

Tell students that this chapter, "Scene Size-up," describes the first part of the patient assessment process. Remind them that the prehospital setting is an extremely uncontrolled environment with many subtle hazards confronting EMTs. Explain that good sense developed through experience and study makes it easier to recognize such hazards. But caution them never to let experience lead to complacency and a letting down of their guard. The costs of failing to recognize the hazards of an unstable scene can be high for themselves, their partners, and their patients. On every call, stress that they identify and pay close attention to the scene size-up characteristics, follow basic guidelines before entering the scene, and follow their intuition when things do not seem right.

Distribute the Chapter 8 Objectives Checklist and give students a few minutes to look it over. Then briefly paraphrase the objectives for this lesson in your own words.

LECTURE

The following suggested lecture outline is based on the Department of Transportation's EMT-Basic National Standard Curriculum. In some places, the DOT curriculum has been rearranged or expanded upon so that it is more complete or easier for the student to understand. The page numbers in parentheses refer to pages in the textbook. The parenthetical references in dark, heavy type are to figures, tables, and scans in the textbook.

SCENE SIZE-UP

I. **Body substance isolation review** (pp. 220–221)
    A. Personal protective equipment (PPE) (pp. 220–221)
        1. Eye protection
        2. Gloves
        3. Gown
        4. Mask

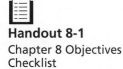

Handout 8-1
Chapter 8 Objectives Checklist

Lecture Master
You may wish to display Lecture Master 8 when presenting the lecture to the class.

Slides/Videos
Brady Skill Series: EMT-B, "Initial Assessment and Scene Size-Up"

Reading/Reference
Smith, M., "Taskmaster: Managing Yourself and Others On Scene," *EMS Magazine,* Dec. 2005.

On the Net
Keeping things safe. http:// www.firefightersforums .com/articles/Scene_Size_ Up.shtml

©2008 by Pearson Education, Inc.
Prehospital Emergency Care, 8th ed.

II. Determining scene safety (pp. 221–231)
  A. Basics (p. 221)
    1. Definition
        a. Assessment to ensure the well-being of the EMT
    2. Personal protection
        a. Is it safe to approach the patient?
  B. Dispatch information (pp. 221–222)
  C. Consider scene characteristics (pp. 222–229) **(Fig. 8-1, p. 222)**
    1. Crash scenes **(Fig. 8-2, p. 224)**
        a. Protecting yourself and others at the crash scene from being struck by traffic
    2. Other rescue scenes **(Fig. 8-3, p. 224)**
    3. Unstable surfaces
        a. Slopes
        b. Ice
        c. Water **(Fig. 8-4, p. 225)**
    4. Toxic substances and low oxygen areas
    5. Crime scenes
        a. Arriving at the scene
        b. Studying the crowd
        c. Approaching the scene **(Figs. 8-5, and 8-6, p. 227; Fig. 8-7, p. 228)**
        d. At the patient's side
    6. Barroom scenes
        a. Potential danger due to alcohol
    7. Car passengers
  D. Protection of the patient (pp. 229–230)
  E. Protection of bystanders (p. 230)
  F. Control the scene (pp. 230–231)
  G. Maintaining situation awareness (p. 231)
III. Determining the nature of the problem (pp. 231–234)
  A. Trauma (pp. 231–233)
    1. Mechanism of injury
        a. Determine the mechanism of injury from the patient, family, or bystanders and inspection of the scene.
    2. Falls
    3. Automobile crashes **(Fig. 8-8, p. 232)**
    4. Motorcycle crashes
    5. Recreational vehicle crashes
    6. Contact sports involving intentional or unintentional collision
    7. Recreational sports (e.g., skiing, diving, basketball)
    8. Pedestrian collision with a car, bus, truck, bike, or other force
    9. Blast injuries from an explosion
    10. Stabbings **(Fig. 8-9, p. 233)**
    11. Shootings
    12. Burns
  B. Medical (pp. 233–234)
    1. Nature of illness
        a. Determine from the patient, family, or bystanders why EMS was activated.
IV. Determining the total number of patients (p. 234)
  A. Obtain additional help prior to contact with patients: law enforcement, fire, rescue, ALS, utilities. EMT is less likely to call for help if involved in patient care. (p. 234)

Teaching Tip
Consider inviting your local utility company's safety representative to deliver a short lesson on electrical or natural gas hazards at emergency scenes.

Point to Emphasize
As observers of the scene, EMTs are in a key position to spot clues that might alert doctors and nurses of the receiving hospital to potential dangers. Encourage them to photograph the scene, if possible.

Reading/Reference
Limmer, D., "Crime Scene Interaction," *JEMS,* Mar. 2002.

    B. If there are more patients than the responding unit can effectively handle. (p. 234)

        1. Initiate a multiple-casualty plan.

        2. Begin triage.

    C. If the responding crew can manage the situation, consider spinal precautions and continue care. (p. 234)

V. Gaining scene control and establishing rapport (pp. 234–236)

    A. Achieve smooth transition of care.

    B. Reduce the patient's anxiety.

        1. Bring order to the environment

        2. Introduce yourself

        3. Gain patient consent

        4. Position yourself

        5. Use communication skills

        6. Be courteous

        7. Use touch when appropriate

    C. Maintain control (p. 236)

CASE STUDY FOLLOW-UP

Ask a student volunteer to read the Case Study that begins on page 219 of the textbook. You may wish to use the following questions to engage students in a discussion of the Case Study Follow-up that begins on page 236 of the textbook. Provide missing information and clarify ideas as needed.

Q1. As you approach the street, why do you shut off the siren and the emergency lights?

A1. *To draw less attention to the scene and to avoid attracting a crowd.*

Q2. Because the house is completely dark and there appears to be no activity in or around it, what additional information do you obtain from dispatch?

A2. *As much additional information as the dispatcher can provide. In this case, the dispatcher called back to the party who phoned in the call and determined that a person had come from the darkened house, which had no phone, and requested that an emergency call be made. The call thus seems legitimate.*

Q3. How do you approach the darkened house?

A3. *With extreme caution. First, dispatch is informed of the plan to approach the scene and a radio check-up is arranged to ensure EMT safety. All the scene lights on the ambulance are turned on and its floodlight is focused on the front door. One EMT walks in front, carrying the flashlight, while the other follows about 8 feet behind with the jump kit. As the lead EMT walks up the front steps to the door, the other stays at the bottom of the steps, watching the rest of the house. The lead EMT stands to the knob side of the door when knocking.*

Q4. Once inside the house, what do you discover about the scene?

A4. *There is an elderly woman lying on the couch. Her husband says, "My wife isn't feeling well," and sits in an armchair. The fuses have blown and the only light in the room is from a small, battery-powered television set. There is a bottle of the medication Diabenase, used in treating diabetes, on a table next to the couch. The woman, Mrs. Ziegler, says, "My legs are swollen. They've been like this all week." The scene seems secure. There is no apparent mechanism of injury, and the patient appears to be suffering from a medical condition. There are no other patients to worry about at the scene.*

IN REVIEW

Assess students' ability to apply what they have just learned by discussing the Review Questions on page 238 in the textbook.

Q1. Define scene size-up.

A1. *Scene size-up is the EMT's initial evaluation of a scene to which he or she has been called. (p. 220)*

Q2. List three goals of the scene size-up.

A2. *Three goals of scene size-up are to ensure scene safety, to determine whether a patient is suffering from trauma or a medical problem, and to determine the total number of patients so that additional resources can be called if needed. (p. 220)*

Q3. List basic guidelines an EMT should follow at potentially dangerous or unstable scenes.

A3. *The basic guidelines an EMT should follow at potentially dangerous or unstable scenes include: Do not enter unstable scenes; take extra precautions at such scenes; call for assistance if a scene is outside the EMT's area of training or expertise; retreat if the scene turns hazardous. (p. 222)*

Q4. List guidelines to follow to protect the EMT from moving traffic at a crash scene or while managing patients on a highway or roadway.

A4. *Limit your time on-scene to reduce your exposure to traffic; shut down traffic on the roadway, if necessary, to ensure your safety; place flares or cones far enough from the crash scene to give oncoming traffic plenty of warning of the crash scene; place apparatus and vehicles strategically so that they protect the scene; wear bright safety reflective clothing or a vest at the crash scene to make you highly visible both day and night; do as much work as possible away from and out of the traffic flow; don't turn your back to moving traffic; don't jump highway dividers to provide emergency care while leaving yourself exposed to moving traffic; reduce any unnecessary scene lighting that may distract or may impair visibility of oncoming traffic; turn the wheels of the parked emergency vehicles so that they are pointed away from the scene; avoid stopping and standing between vehicles. (p. 223–224)*

Q5. Explain the special problems an EMT is likely to encounter in confined areas like a cave, well, or sewer.

A5. *Confined areas are likely to pose a threat because of the concentration of toxic gases or because they are low-oxygen areas. (p. 226)*

Q6. Explain how EMTs should approach a house that they feel may be the scene of a crime.

A6. *In approaching the possible scene of a crime, approach on the grass, not the sidewalk; walk single file, with the person in front holding the flashlight, if used, to the side of his body, rearmost person carrying equipment; look for possible places of concealment or cover while approaching the house; change position while taking time to survey the* *building; stand to the knob side of the door when knocking; reassess the situation before entering; leave doors open when entering. (pp. 226–228)*

Q7. Explain the chief determination about the nature of the patient's problem an EMT should make during scene size-up.

A7. *The chief determination about the nature of the patient's problem during scene size-up is whether it is a trauma or a medical problem. (p. 231)*

Q8. Define mechanism of injury.

A8. *Mechanism of injury is how the patient was injured—the strength, direction, and nature of the forces applied to her body. (p. 231)*

Q9. List clues to mechanism of injury that the EMT should be alert to at an automobile crash.

A9. *Clues to mechanism of injury that the EMT should be alert to at an automobile crash include the following: (1) Outside the vehicle— deformity greater than 20 inches, intrusion into the passenger compartment, axle displacement, rollover. (2) Inside the vehicle— impact marks on the windshield, missing rearview mirror, collapsed steering wheel, broken seat, side-door damage, deformed dashboard, deformed pedals. (p. 232)*

Q10. List clues at a scene that might indicate the nature of a patient's illness.

A10. *Clues to the nature of a patient's illness may include prescription and nonprescription medications, drugs, drug paraphernalia, alcohol, oxygen equipment, and environmental conditions. (p. 233–234)*

Q11. Explain why the EMT must determine the total number of patients at a call during the scene size-up.

A11. *The total number of patients must be determined so that additional personnel or resources can be promptly summoned if the number of patients is beyond the capacity of the initial EMS team to handle. (pp. 234)*

CRITICAL THINKING

Assess students' ability to respond to real-life emergency situations by discussing the Critical Thinking questions on page 238 in the textbook.

Q1. What body substance isolation precautions do you anticipate?

A1. *At the very least, the responding EMTs should use exam gloves and consider eye protection.*

Q2. What indicators will you look for to determine if the scene is safe to enter?

A2. *The first step would be to consult with law enforcement to ensure that the scene is safe to enter. The EMTs would then stay alert for the presence of weapons and any other signs of potential continued violence.*

Q3. What criteria will you use to categorize the patient as trauma or medical?

A3. *If the patient received a physical injury caused by a blunt or penetrating force, which she obviously did, she would be considered a trauma patient.*

©2008 by Pearson Education, Inc.
Prehospital Emergency Care, 8th ed.

Q4. How will you determine if more than one patient is present on the scene?

A4. *In order to determine if there are more patients or victims at this scene, the responding EMTs should question law enforcement, the patient, and any bystanders. They should also visually observe the scene and look for blood or other signs of violence that don't appear to be related to their patient.*

Q5. What other resources may be needed at the scene?

A5. *Based on the information provided, the other resources that may be needed at this scene include law enforcement and ALS (advanced life support) personnel.*

Q6. When will you call for additional resources, if needed?

A6. *In this situation law enforcement should be requested prior to the arrival of EMS and any additional medical resources required should be called for immediately—prior to beginning any patient care.*

ROLE PLAY

Ask two volunteers willing to play the role of EMTs responding to a 9-1-1 call to step outside the classroom. Provide them with a trauma jump kit containing BSI equipment and a selection of airways. A portable suction unit should also be provided. Tell them to review their notes on scene size-up while waiting for the "dispatch call." Return to the classroom and ask for four more volunteers. Describe this situation to them:

It is 0200 at an all-night fast-food restaurant. A young man comes in and gives his order to an employee behind the register. When the employee opens the cash register to make change, the young man pulls out a gun, shoots the employee, then grabs all of the bills in the register and flees. The employee is bleeding, unconscious, and has shallow, gurgling respirations. A customer—a witness to the shooting—becomes hysterical. The manager rushes out of his office, sees the wounded employee, and calls 9-1-1 for an ambulance. A police officer First Responder arrives before the ambulance, secures the area, and begins administering first aid to the employee. When the EMTs arrive, the manager rushes out of the restaurant to call them in.

Determine which volunteers will play the roles of the wounded employee, the customer, the manager, and the police officer. Use moulage to simulate a gunshot wound to the left chest of the employee. When the volunteers at the "restaurant" are ready, "dispatch" the EMT team. Dispatch information should include the following facts: the time, the location of the restaurant, and the report of a shooting there. Also inform them that the nearest hospital is 20 minutes away and that police have been notified.

The role play should start from the moment the EMTs arrive. Allow the role play to progress naturally. Intervene only if the players seem to be at a loss for what to do. End the play when the patient's airway has been secured. (The EMTs should not be asked to treat the patient any further since they have not yet reached this point in training.) Hold a debriefing with the entire class when the role play is over. Discuss the following points:

- What did the EMTs do correctly to size up the scene and treat the patient?
- What, if anything, should have been done differently?

Reading/Reference
Textbook, pp. 239–328

Workbook
Chapter 8 Activities

Chapter Quiz
Handout 8-2

TestGen
Chapter 8 Test

Online Test Preparation
Send your students to
http://www.prenhall.com/
EMTAchieve

Handouts 8-3 to 8-5
Reinforcement Activities

**Brady Skills Series
EMT-B Videos/CD**
Visual Reinforcement

**PowerPoint
Presentation**
Chapter 8

- What clues to the mechanism of injury might be present at this scene?
- What resources might have to be activated on a call such as this one?
- How important is BSI in this case?

Stress the importance of verifying that the police have secured a scene like this one before entering it. Point out that if the team failed to do so, they too might become shooting victims or hostages.

ASSIGNMENTS

Assign students to read Parts 1 and 2 of Chapter 9, "Patient Assessment," before the next class. Also ask them to complete Chapter 8 of the Workbook.

EVALUATION

Chapter Quiz Distribute copies of the Chapter Quiz provided in Handout 8-2 to evaluate student understanding of this chapter. Remind students not to refer to their textbooks or notes while taking the quiz.

Test Manager You may wish to create a custom-tailored test using Prentice Hall *TestGen for Prehospital Emergency Care, Eighth Edition* to evaluate student understanding of this chapter.

Online Test Preparation (for students and instructors) Additional test preparation is available through *EMT Achieve: Basic Test Preparation* at http://www.prenhall.com/EMTAchieve. Instructors can also monitor student mastery online.

REINFORCEMENT

Handouts If classroom discussions or performance on the quiz indicates that some students have not fully mastered the chapter content, you may wish to assign some or all of the Reinforcement Handouts for this chapter.

TECH EXTRAS

Brady Skills Series EMT-B Videos/CD Have your students watch the skills come to life on either VHS or CD-ROM.

PowerPoint Presentation (for instructors) The PowerPoint material developed for this chapter offers useful reinforcement of chapter content.

Student CD A wide variety of material on this CD-ROM will reinforce and also expand student knowledge and skills.

Companion Website (for students) Additional review quizzes and links to EMS resources will contribute to further reinforcement of this chapter. Please visit http://www.prenhall.com/mistovich.

Student CD
Chapter 8

Companion Website
http://www.prenhall.com/
mistovich

OBJECTIVES

OBJECTIVES CHECKLIST

Cognitive	Date Mastered
3-1.1 Recognize hazards/potential hazards.	
3-1.2 Describe common hazards found at the scene of a trauma and a medical patient.	
3-1.3 Determine if the scene is safe to enter.	
3-1.4 Discuss common mechanisms of injury/nature of illness.	
3-1.5 Discuss the reason for identifying the total number of patients at the scene.	
3-1.6 Explain the reason for identifying the need for additional help or assistance. — Explain how to gain scene control. — Explain how to establish rapport with the patient.	

Affective	Date Mastered
3-1.7 Explain the rationale for crew members to evaluate scene safety prior to entering.	
3-1.8 Serve as a model for others, explaining how patient situations affect your evaluation of mechanism of injury or illness.	

Psychomotor	Date Mastered
3-1.9 Observe various scenarios and identify potential hazards.	

CHAPTER 8 QUIZ

Write the letter of the best answer in the space provided.

_____ 1. Which of the following is *not* a part of the scene size-up?
   A. determining the mechanism of injury
   B. determining the number of patients
   C. establishing an airway
   D. taking body substance isolation precautions

_____ 2. Body substance isolation (BSI) precautions may include
   A. gloves, eyewear, and mask. **C.** a PFD.
   B. turnout gear. **D.** a rescue helmet.

_____ 3. The scene size-up should take place
   A. only at the beginning of a call.
   B. at the beginning and throughout the entire call.
   C. at the beginning and at the end of the call.
   D. after life-threatening conditions have been corrected.

_____ 4. EMTs should *not* enter a known crime scene
   A. at any time.
   B. unless a patient has a life-threatening condition.
   C. until it has been secured by police.
   D. without approval of medical direction.

_____ 5. The EMT should suspect the presence of toxic substances
   A. in a confined space.
   B. at a home where multiple family members have the same complaint.
   C. at a fire.
   D. in all of the situations above.

_____ 6. When responding to a known crime scene, you should initially
   A. stabilize the patient.
   B. turn on all lights and sirens.
   C. contact medical control.
   D. turn off the siren and emergency lights several blocks before arrival.

_____ 7. In assessing potential injuries from a fall during scene size-up, determine
   A. if the patient requires any emergency care.
   B. the surface that the patient landed on.
   C. the patient's pertinent past history.
   D. signs and symptoms.

_____ 8. When controlling the scene, the EMT should
   A. eliminate light sources.
   B. leave all furniture in place.
   C. be compassionate in providing care.
   D. always treat the patient where found.

_____ 9. During scene size-up at a multiple-vehicle crash, it is important to determine the number of patients because
   A. on-scene resources may be inadequate for them all.
   B. run reports are required for each patient.
   C. ALS must be called if there are more than two patients.
   D. the media must be given accurate information.

_____ 10. Which of the following may be useful in determining nature of illness/mechanism of injury?
   A. the patient
   B. bystanders
   C. family members
   D. all of the above

IN THE FIELD

Review the following real-life situation. Then answer the questions that follow.

Your unit is dispatched to a motor-vehicle collision on a well-traveled road. You are the EMT in charge. The dispatch time is 0130 hours. It is raining with a wind out of the north at 5 miles per hour, and a temperature of 32°F (0°C). The caller has stated that there is only a single car involved.

1. What scene size-up considerations should you have in mind as you approach the scene?

You are the first emergency unit to reach the scene. You observe that a mid-size passenger car has struck a power pole head on. You see a victim in the car moving around. Power lines are down, and there is a strong smell of gasoline in the air.

2. What actions should you take, based on scene size-up?

3. List any additional resources that you would call for this scene.

CHAPTER 8 QUIZ

REINFORCEMENT

Write the word or words that best complete each sentence in the space provided.

1. Determining scene safety means looking for possible threats to the safety of

_____, _____, and

_____.

2. Before approaching patients at a crash scene, EMTs must assess the _____.

3. The forces that may have caused injury to a patient are called the _____.

4. A key element of _____ precautions is always to wear the appropriate

personal protective gear on-scene.

5. The _____ is an anticipation that certain types of mechanisms will produce

specific types of injuries.

6. Suspect hazardous materials or an oxygen-depleted environment in calls involving

_____, _____, or _____.

7. With a medical patient, finding out what is or may be wrong with the patient is called identifying

the _____.

8. Important sources of information for determining what is wrong with a medical patient include the

patient, _____, _____, and

_____ at the scene.

9. At crime scenes in which guns might be involved, EMTs should position the emergency vehicle

outside the _____.

10. If your scene size-up indicates that you do not have sufficient resources to handle the call, you

should request _____.

REINFORCEMENT

SCENE SIZE-UP: LISTING

1. List the three basic goals of the scene size-up.

2. List three categories of people with which the EMT must be concerned in ensuring scene safety.

3. List four significant external signs of vehicle impact to look for and document during the scene size-up.

4. List three potential sources of information about the nature of a patient's illness.

5. List seven ways you can reduce a patient's anxiety at the emergency scene.

Scene Size-up

Determine Scene Safety
Dispatch Information
Take BSI Precautions
Scene Characteristics
- Crash scenes
- Other rescue scenes
- Crime scenes
- Barrooms

Protect Patient
Protect Bystanders
Control the Scene
Maintain Situation Awareness
Determine the Nature of the Problem
Mechanism of Injury
- Falls
- Auto crashes
- Motorcycle crashes
- Recreational vehicle crashes
- Penetrating trauma
- Blast injuries

Nature of the Illness

Determine the Number of Patients
Gain Scene Control and Establish Rapport
Achieve Smooth Transition of Care
Reduce Patient Anxiety
Maintain Control

HANDOUT 8-2: Chapter 8 Quiz

1. C	**4.** C	**7.** B	**9.** A
2. A	**5.** D	**8.** C	**10.** D
3. B	**6.** D		

HANDOUT 8-3: In the Field

1. Because it is late, dark, and stormy, you should be especially alert for the possibility of victims or bystanders in the roadway as you approach. Watch for unusual traffic patterns. See if you can spot arcing from downed power lines or a glow that might indicate fire. Consider the possibility of a crime scene.

2. You should look for clues to escaped hazardous materials, keep looking for collision victims or bystanders, and look for smoke. Because the power lines are down and there is a smell of spilled fuel, you would park your unit away from the wreck, upwind if possible. Be sure the unit is at least one full span of wires from power poles to which broken wires are attached. Mark the danger zone not with flares, but with reflective triangles. Because the weather is wet and the temperature is so cold, you should be alert to the possibility of icing and consider expanding the danger zone. Do not enter the scene until it is safe to do so.

3. Request fire department and power company backup. Be sure to call for a law enforcement unit to handle traffic control and consider having the road salted or sanded.

HANDOUT 8-4: Chapter 8 Review

1. crew, patient, bystanders
2. total scene
3. mechanism of injury
4. body substance isolation
5. index of suspicion
6. spills, leaks, confined spaces
7. nature of illness
8. relatives, bystanders, evidence
9. killing zone
10. additional resources

HANDOUT 8-5: Scene Size-up: Listing

1. Identify hazards and ensure scene safety; identify the nature of the problem—mechanism of injury and/or nature of illness; determine whether factors such as the number of patients or unusual scene characteristics require additional resources.

2. Self and other team members, patients, bystanders

3. Deformity to the vehicle greater than 20 inches, intrusion into the passenger compartment, displacement of a vehicle axle, rollover

4. The patient, family members or bystanders, physical evidence at the scene

5. Bring order to the environment, introduce yourself, gain patient consent, position yourself properly, use communication skills, be courteous, use touch when appropriate.

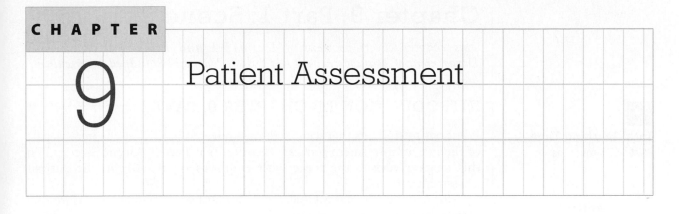

REVIEW

Have several volunteers highlight what they learned about scene size-up during the last lesson. Point out that scene size-up is the first and most important aspect of patient assessment. It begins as the EMT approaches the scene. The EMT surveys the scene to determine if there are any threats to the EMT him- or herself, to the patient, or to others. Remind students that the scene size-up also includes determining the nature of the call and obtaining additional help, if necessary. Distribute the scored quizzes from the last class. Go over each question on the quiz and handle any concerns students may have about the answers.

INTRODUCTION TO CHAPTER 9

Tell students that this chapter is structured differently from others in the book because its subject—patient assessment—is so important. Patient assessment is the cornerstone of good prehospital care, and the best EMS providers are renowned for their patient assessment abilities. Students should know that if they can develop a consistent, thorough method for assessing their patients, they will be well on the way to providing the best patient care possible. Provide an overview of the steps of the patient assessment process. You may wish to direct students to look at Figure 9-1 on page 244 of their textbook as you explain the steps.

COMPONENTS OF PATIENT ASSESSMENT

1. Scene size-up
2. Initial assessment
3. Focused history and physical exam
4. Detailed physical exam
5. Ongoing assessment
6. Communication and documentation

Explain that, due to the amount of the material contained in this chapter, it has been divided into six separate lessons—one for each component of patient assessment. (You may wish to cover Parts 1 and 2 during a single class period. You may also wish to cover Parts 5 and 6 during a single class period. There are two quizzes for this chapter. Quiz A covers material from Parts 1, 2, and 3 and can be given at the end of Part 3. Quiz B covers material from Parts 4, 5, and 6 and can be given at the end of Part 6. Or you may choose to give both quizzes at the end of Part 6.)

Additional Resources

Larmon/Davis, *Basic Life Support Skills*

Elling, *EMT Achieve: Basic Test Preparation*

Limmer/Mistovich/O'Keefe, *Audio Lecture & Study Guide: EMT*

Mistovich/Kuvlesky, *SUCCESS! for the EMT, Second Edition*

Chapter 9, Part 1: Scene Size-up

This chapter covers portions of Lesson 3-1 and Lesson 3-9 of the U.S. Department of Transportation's EMT-Basic National Standard Curriculum.

Total Teaching Time
Part 1: 75 minutes

Resources Needed
- Scored Chapter 8 Quizzes
- Jump kit with BSI equipment
- Paper cut-out of a gun

Lecture Master
You may wish to display Lecture Master 9-1 when presenting the lecture.

✓ Teaching Tip
Consider inviting a local police or fire department representative to deliver a short lesson on personal safety at emergency scenes.

✓ Teaching Tip
Caution students that dispatcher information must be verified and updated during scene size-up.

INTRODUCTION TO CHAPTER 9, PART 1

Point out to students that scene size-up—covered in the last chapter—is part of the patient assessment process. Mention that Part 1, "Scene Size-up," in this chapter revisits the topic with emphasis on its role in the patient assessment process.

Review the Chapter 8 Objectives Checklist with students to ensure that they have grasped its key points.

LECTURE

Instead of a standard lecture for this part of the chapter, read the key phases of the scene size-up listed below and ask students to explain each phase more fully.

PART 1: SCENE SIZE-UP

I. Phases of the scene size-up (p. 241)
  A. Take necessary body substance isolation precautions. (pp. 241)
  B. Evaluate scene hazards and ensure safety. (p. 241)
    1. Personal protection
    2. Protection of the patient
    3. Protection of bystanders
  C. Determine the mechanism of injury or the nature of the illness. (p. 241)
    1. Trauma patient
    2. Medical patient
  D. Establish the number of patients. (p. 241)
  E. Ascertain the need for additional resources to manage the scene or patients. (p. 241)

CASE STUDY

Note: The case studies will not be reviewed until the last lesson of this chapter.

IN REVIEW

Note: The In Review Questions will not be covered until the last lesson of this chapter.

ROLE PLAY

Ask two volunteers willing to play the role of EMTs who are responding to a 9-1-1 call to step outside the classroom. Provide them with a jump kit and describe the following situation to them:

You are dispatched to a mobile home in a rural area. According to the dispatcher, the patient is an adult female who is "acting crazy." The emphasis of the scene is on scene size-up. However, you should also utilize the other information and skills you have learned to date. Do not worry about administering patient care.

Return to the room and ask for two more volunteers. Describe the following situation to them:

You are a married couple, Rose and Phil, but your relationship is not good. Phil is currently unemployed and frequently drinks too much. Rose works at a minimum-wage job all day. She also has to take care of all the housekeeping responsibilities because her husband considers them "women's work." Very depressed about this situation, Rose has just started counseling—against her husband's wishes. One night when she gets home from work, she finds her husband sitting at the kitchen table, obviously drunk, cleaning his hunting rifle. The first words out of his mouth are, "You're late. Where's my dinner?" An argument begins and grows more heated. Weeping uncontrollably, Rose curls into a ball on the floor and keeps saying, "I can't take it anymore." Phil continues yelling at her and orders her to "get a hold of yourself." This only makes matters worse. Finally, Phil calls 9-1-1.

Determine which of the two volunteers will act as the husband and which as the wife. Place the paper gun on a table in obvious view.

When the volunteers "at home" are ready, dispatch the EMT team. The role play should start from the moment the EMTs arrive. Allow the role play to progress naturally. End the play when the scene has been sized up and brought under control. (The EMTs should not be asked to treat the patient any further, since they have not yet reached this point in training.)

When the role play has ended, discuss the following questions with the class:

- What did the EMTs do correctly to size up the scene and gain control of the situation?
- What, if anything, should have been done differently?

ASSIGNMENT

If you are treating Part 2 as a separate lesson, direct students to review Chapter 9, Part 2, "Initial Assessment," before the next class; otherwise begin the lesson for Part 2 now.

EVALUATION

Note: The quiz will not be given until the end of Part 3 or Part 6 of this chapter.

REINFORCEMENT

You may wish to have students review the Reinforcement Handouts that accompanied Chapter 8. In addition, or as an alternative, you could have students review the "In the Field" handouts for subsequent parts of this chapter and discuss what scene size-up concerns each scenario raises.

Reading/Reference
Textbook, pp. 241–261

Steps for Scene Safety

Take Necessary BSI Precautions

Evaluate Scene Hazards and Ensure Scene Safety

   Personal protection

   Protection of the patient

   Protection of bystanders

Determine the Mechanism of Injury or the Nature of the Illness

   Trauma patient

   Medical patient

Establish the Number of Patients

Ascertain the Need for Additional Resources to Manage the Scene or the Patient(s).

Chapter 9, Part 2: Initial Assessment

Covers Lesson 3-2 and portions of Lesson 3-9 of the U.S. Department of Transportation's EMT-Basic National Standard Curriculum

OBJECTIVES

Numbered objectives are from the U.S. Department of Transportation EMT-Basic National Standard Curriculum. Asterisked objectives, if any, pertain to material that is supplemental to the DOT curriculum. Page numbers in parentheses refer to pages in the textbook.

Cognitive

3-2.1 Summarize the reasons for forming a general impression of the patient. (pp. 243–247)

3-2.2 Discuss methods of assessing altered mental status. (pp. 247–250)

3-2.3 Differentiate between assessing the altered mental status in the adult, child, and infant patient. (p. 248)

3-2.4 Discuss methods of assessing the airway in the adult, child, and infant patient. (pp. 250–252)

3-2.5 State reasons for management of the cervical spine once the patient has been determined to be a trauma patient. (p. 246–247)

3-2.6 Describe methods used for assessing if a patient is breathing. (pp. 252–254)

3-2.7 State what care should be provided to the adult, child, and infant patient with adequate breathing. (p. 254)

3-2.8 State what care should be provided to the adult, child, and infant patient without adequate breathing. (p. 254)

3-2.9 Differentiate between a patient with adequate and inadequate breathing. (p. 254)

3-2.10 Distinguish between methods of assessing breathing in the adult, child, and infant patient. (pp. 252–254)

3-2.11 Compare the methods of providing airway care to the adult, child, and infant patient. (pp. 251)

3-2.12 Describe the methods used to obtain a pulse. (pp. 255–256)

3-2.13 Differentiate between obtaining a pulse in an adult, a child, and an infant patient. (p. 255)

3-2.14 Discuss the need for assessing the patient for external bleeding. (p. 256)

3-2.15 Describe normal and abnormal findings when assessing skin color. (pp. 257–258)

3-2.16 Describe normal and abnormal findings when assessing skin temperature. (p. 258)

3-2.17 Describe normal and abnormal findings when assessing skin condition. (p. 258)

3-2.18 Describe normal and abnormal findings when assessing skin capillary refill in the infant and child patient. (p. 258)

3-2.19 Explain the reason for prioritizing a patient for care and transport. (pp. 258–261)

Affective

3-2.20 Explain the importance of forming a general impression of the patient. (pp. 243–247)

Total Teaching Time
Part 2: 180 minutes

Resources Needed

- 4 nonstudent volunteers to serve as patients
- 4 EMTs to serve as teaching assistants
- 4 complete jump kits containing BSI equipment, assorted cervical collars, stethoscopes, BP cuffs, and penlights
- 4 portable oxygen cylinders
- 4 portable suction units
- Wristwatches with second hands

3-2.21 Explain the value of performing an initial assessment. (p. 242)

Psychomotor

3-2.22 Demonstrate the techniques for assessing mental status.
3-2.23 Demonstrate the techniques for assessing the airway.
3-2.24 Demonstrate the techniques for assessing if the patient is breathing.
3-2.25 Demonstrate the techniques for assessing if the patient has a pulse.
3-2.26 Demonstrate the techniques for assessing the patient for external bleeding.
3-2.27 Demonstrate the techniques for assessing the patient's skin color, temperature, condition, and capillary refill (infants and children only).
3-2.28 Demonstrate the ability to prioritize patients.

REVIEW

Point out that during the last lesson students learned about scene size-up—the first and most important aspect of patient assessment. Emphasize that this step begins as the EMT approaches the scene. The EMT surveys the scene to determine if there are any threats to him- or herself, to the patient, or to others. The scene size-up also allows the EMT to determine the nature of the call, gain control of the situation, and obtain additional help, if needed.

INTRODUCTION TO CHAPTER 9, PART 2

Once the EMT completes scene size-up, an initial assessment is performed on the patient or patients who have been identified. The purpose of an initial assessment is to find and correct immediately life-threatening problems and determine what else to assess and how much time to spend doing that. Tell students that in this lesson they will be learning how to perform an initial assessment.

Distribute the Chapter 9, Part 2, Objectives Checklist and give students a few minutes to look it over. Then briefly paraphrase the objectives for this lesson in your own words.

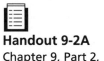

Handout 9-2A
Chapter 9, Part 2,
Objectives Checklist

●➤

Lecture Master
You may wish to display
Lecture Master 9-2 when
presenting the lecture to
the class.

LECTURE

The following lecture outline is based on the Department of Transportation's EMT-Basic National Standard Curriculum. In some places, the DOT curriculum has been rearranged and expanded upon so that it is more complete or easier for students to understand. This outline is offered for your convenience as you present your lecture. The page numbers in parentheses refer to pages in the textbook. References in dark, heavy type are to figures and tables in the textbook. Point out the flowchart in Figure 9-1 on page 244, which shows the sequence of events in the initial assessment. Direct students to follow along during the lecture.

II. Form a general impression of the patient (pp. 243–247) **(Fig. 9-1, p. 244)**
- **A.** Estimate patient's age (pp. 243)
- **B.** Determine if the patient is injured or ill (pp. 243, 245) **(Figs. 9-2, 9-3, p. 245; Table 9-1, p. 245)**
- **C.** Obtain the chief complaint (pp. 245–246) **(Fig. 9-4, p. 246)**
- **D.** Identify immediate life threats (p. 246) **(Table 9-2, p. 247)**
- **E.** Establish manual in-line stabilization (pp. 246–247) **(Fig. 9-5, p. 247)**
- **F.** Position the patient for assessment (p. 247) **(Fig. 9-6, p. 248)**

III. Assess mental status (pp. 247–250)
- **A.** Assess the level of mental status (pp. 247–250) **(Fig. 9-7, p. 249; Table 9-3, p. 249)**
  - **1.** Alertness and orientation
  - **2.** Responds to verbal stimulus
  - **3.** Responds to painful stimulus
    - **a.** Trapezius pinch
    - **b.** Supraorbital pressure
    - **c.** Sternal rub
    - **d.** Armpit pinch
    - **e.** Nail bed pressure
    - **f.** Pinch thumb–index finger web
    - **g.** Pinch finger, toe, hand, or foot
    - **h.** Problems with some types of painful stimuli **(Fig. 9-8, p. 250)**
  - **4.** Unresponsive
    - **a.** No gag or cough
  - **5.** Document the level of responsiveness

IV. Assess the airway (pp. 250–252)
- **A.** Responsive patient (p. 251)
  - **1.** Is the patient talking or crying?
  - **2.** If yes, assess for adequacy of breathing.
  - **3.** If no, open airway.
- **B.** Unresponsive or severely altered mental status patient (p. 251)
  - **1.** Is the airway open? **(Fig. 9-9, p. 250; Table 9-4, p. 251)**
  - **2.** Open the airway.
  - **3.** For medical patients
    - **a.** Perform the head-tilt, chin-lift.
      - **(1)** Clear
      - **(2)** Not clear
        - **(a)** Clear the airway
  - **4.** For trauma patients
    - **a.** Perform the jaw thrust.
      - **(1)** Stabilize a sitting patient's head from the rear and a supine patient's head from the top
    - **b.** Clear
    - **c.** Not clear
      - **(1)** Clear the airway
- **C.** Indications of partial airway occlusion (pp. 251–252)
  - **1.** Snoring
  - **2.** Gurgling
  - **3.** Crowing
  - **4.** Stridor

V. Assess breathing (pp. 252–255)

Point to Emphasize

The general impression is extremely valuable. EMTs will hone this "sixth sense" as they assess more and more patients.

Point to Emphasize

Don't be too quick to base your general impression strictly on dispatch information. Avoid "tunnel vision."

Teaching Tip

Remind students what they learned about medical/legal issues in Chapter 3. Review the importance of obtaining consent.

Slides/Videos

Brady Skill Series: EMT-B

"Introduction to Patient Assessment"

"Trauma Patient with No Significant Mechanism of Injury"

"Trauma Patient with a Significant Mechanism of Injury"

"Detailed Physical Exam"

"Medical Patient—Responsive"

"Medical Patient—Unresponsive"

"Ongoing Assessment"

A. Assess the rate and quality of the patient's breathing (pp. 252–254) (**Fig. 9-10, p. 252; Table 9-5, p. 252**)
  1. Look
  2. Inadequate tidal volume
  3. Abnormal respiratory rate
      a. Bradypnea
      b. Tachypnea
  4. Retractions
  5. Use of the neck muscles
  6. Nasal flaring
  7. Excessive abdominal muscle use
  8. Tracheal tugging
  9. Cyanosis
  10. Asymmetrical movement of the chest wall
  11. Listen
  12. Feel
B. Absent or inadequate breathing (p. 254)
  1. Absence of breathing (apnea)
  2. Inadequate breathing
      a. Insufficient or ineffective respiratory rate
      b. Signs of inadequate oxygenation; signs of serious respiratory distress
C. Adequate breathing (p. 154)
D. Adequate oxygenation (pp. 254–255)

VI. Assess circulation (pp. 255–258)(**Table 9-6, p. 255**)
  A. Assess the patient's pulse (pp. 255–256) (**Figs. 9-11, p. 255; 9-12, p. 256**)
    1. Radial pulse.
    2. In a patient 1 year old or younger, palpate a brachial pulse.
    3. If no radial pulse is felt, palpate carotid pulse.
    4. If pulseless, medical patient is 1 year of age or older, start CPR and apply automated external defibrillator (AED).
    5. If medical patient is younger than 1 year of age, start CPR.
    6. If trauma patient, start CPR.
  B. Identify major bleeding (p. 256)
    1. If bleeding is present, control it. (**Fig. 9-13, p. 256**)
  C. Assess perfusion (pp. 257–258)
    1. Skin color (**Fig. 9-14, p. 257**)
        a. Normal
            (1) Pink
        b. Abnormal
            (1) Pale or mottled
            (2) Cyanotic or blue-gray
            (3) Flushed or red
            (4) Jaundiced or yellow
    2. Skin temperature
        a. Normal
            (1) Warm
        b. Abnormal
        c. Hot
            (1) Cool
            (2) Cold
            (3) Clammy (cool and moist)
    3. Skin condition
        a. Normal
            (1) Dry

On the Net
For more on AED availability and usage, go to: www.mei.com

Point to Emphasize
Most bleeding stops with direct pressure. The use of a tourniquet is rarely indicated.

Point to Emphasize
Stress the importance of skin signs in determining the circulatory status of a patient.

Point to Emphasize
Remind students that capillary refill is an *unreliable* indicator of peripheral perfusion in adults.

☑

Teaching Tip
Point out that it's better to err on the side of caution and provide transport when determining priority patients.

©2008 by Pearson Education, Inc.
Prehospital Emergency Care, 8th ed.

                    b. Abnormal
                        (1) Moist
                    4. Capillary refill **(Fig. 9-15, p. 259)**
                    5. Shock (Hypoperfusion)
VII. **Establish patient priority** (pp. 258–261)**(Table 9-7, p. 260; Table 9-8, p. 261)**
        A. General impression (pp. 260–261)
        B. Mental status (pp. 260–261)
        C. Airway (pp. 260–261)
        D. Breathing (pp. 260–261)
        E. Circulation (pp. 260–261)

CASE STUDY FOLLOW-UP

Note: The case studies will not be reviewed until the last lesson of this chapter.

IN REVIEW

Note: The In Review will not be covered until the last lesson of this chapter.

SKILLS DEMONSTRATION AND PRACTICE

Arrange to have four people serve as patients and four EMTs to serve as teaching assistants at the stations listed below. Assign roles to each patient based on the stations. You may use moulage to simulate trauma patients if desired. (The equipment needed is in parentheses, followed by suggested scenarios.)

List of Practice Stations

- Station A—Responsive trauma patient (a wristwatch with a second hand, BSI equipment, towel, sterile dressings, gauze bandages, and several sizes of cervical collars): An adult who has accidentally cut his finger at home with a kitchen knife. When the EMTs arrive, the cut is bleeding profusely.

- Station B—Unresponsive trauma patient (a wristwatch with a second hand, BSI equipment, sterile dressings, gauze bandages, several sizes of cervical collars, oxygen equipment, oxygen mask, and an assortment of airways): A teenager who was shot at school by a rival gang member. When the EMTs arrive, the teenager is lying in a pool of blood and is unable to speak.

- Station C—Responsive medical patient (BSI equipment, a wristwatch with a second hand): An adult with severe chest pain that radiates to the left arm. The patient has a history of unstable angina and takes nitroglycerin. She has taken three nitroglycerin pills, each 15 minutes apart, without relief. When the EMTs arrive, she is alert and anxious, sweating profusely.

- Station D—Unresponsive medical patient (BSI equipment, a wristwatch with a second hand, oxygen equipment, oxygen mask, and an assortment of airways): An adult with diabetes who about mid-morning began acting confused and "drunk." A coworker called 9-1-1. When the EMTs arrive, the patient is unconscious.

Divide the students into groups of two. Have half the students count off "1, 2, 3," until they have all been numbered. Then have remaining students count off "1, 2, 3," until all students have been numbered. Pair like-numbered students. If there is an odd number of students, it is acceptable to have teams of three. Direct each team to rotate through each of the four stations. At each station, have the teaching assistant demonstrate initial assessment skills for the type of patient featured there. The teaching assistant should then help students practice the assessment. Give the location of each station.

Call four pairs at random and direct each pair to its first station. Visit each station to monitor progress of practice. Provide help to the teaching assistants as needed. Advise students when it is time to rotate to the next station. When each pair has completed all four stations, make sure that students return to the main classroom.

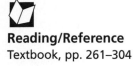

Reading/Reference
Textbook, pp. 261–304

ASSIGNMENT

Direct students to review Chapter 9, Part 3, "Focused History and Physical Exam," before the next class.

EVALUATION

Note: The quiz will not be given until the end of Part 3 of this chapter.

REINFORCEMENT

Handouts 9-2B to 9-2D
Reinforcement Activities

Reinforcement Handouts are provided for students whose participation in class discussions or performance on the quiz indicates they have not fully mastered the content of Part 2. You may wish to assign some or all of these handouts to those students.

OBJECTIVES CHECKLIST

Cognitive		Date Mastered
3-2.1	Summarize the reasons for forming a general impression of the patient.	
3-2.2	Discuss methods of assessing altered mental status.	
3-2.3	Differentiate between assessing the altered mental status in the adult, child, and infant patient.	
3-2.4	Discuss the methods of assessing the airway in the adult, child, and infant patient.	
3-2.5	State reasons for management of the cervical spine once the patient has been determined to be a trauma patient.	
3-2.6	Describe methods used for assessing if a patient is breathing.	
3-2.7	State what care should be provided to the adult, child, and infant patient with adequate breathing.	
3-2.8	State what care should be provided to the adult, child, and infant patient without adequate breathing.	
3-2.9	Differentiate between a patient with adequate and inadequate breathing.	
3-2.10	Distinguish between methods of assessing breathing in the adult, child, and infant patient.	
3-2.11	Compare the methods of providing airway care to the adult, child, and infant patient.	
3-2.12	Describe the methods used to obtain a pulse.	
3-2.13	Differentiate between obtaining a pulse in an adult, a child, and an infant patient.	
3-2.14	Discuss the need for assessing the patient for external bleeding.	
3-2.15	Describe normal and abnormal findings when assessing skin color.	
3-2.16	Describe normal and abnormal findings when assessing skin temperature.	
3-2.17	Describe normal and abnormal findings when assessing skin condition.	
3-2.18	Describe normal and abnormal findings when assessing skin capillary refill in the infant and child patient.	
3-2.19	Explain the reason for prioritizing a patient for care and transport.	

Affective		Date Mastered
3-2.20	Explain the importance of forming a general impression of the patient.	
3-2.21	Explain the value of performing an initial assessment.	

Psychomotor		Date Mastered
3-2.22	Demonstrate the techniques for assessing mental status.	
3-2.23	Demonstrate the techniques for assessing the airway.	
3-2.24	Demonstrate the techniques for assessing if the patient is breathing.	
3-2.25	Demonstrate the techniques for assessing if the patient has a pulse.	
3-2.26	Demonstrate the techniques for assessing the patient for external bleeding.	
3-2.27	Demonstrate the techniques for assessing the patient's skin color, temperature, condition, and capillary refill (infants and children only).	
3-2.28	Demonstrate the ability to prioritize patients.	

©2008 by Pearson Education, Inc.
Prehospital Emergency Care, 8th ed.

IN THE FIELD

Read the following real-life situation. Then answer the questions that follow.

One morning, you and your partner are dispatched to "an elderly man who is having trouble breathing." Upon arrival at the scene, the man's wife meets you at the door and says, "I'm worried about my husband. He's been feeling sick lately—tired, coughing, fever. I think it's the flu."

The woman leads you into the bedroom. Here you see a man in his 80s, supine on the bed with his head propped up on three pillows. From where you stand in the doorway, he appears pale and sweaty. Many boxes of tissues surround the bed. Upon seeing you, the patient gasps, "I can't breathe."

You now begin your initial assessment. The patient is awake, but he speaks in short, choppy sentences, only one or two words per breath. He answers your questions, but is confused about his surroundings and the time of day. As you start taking vital signs, he becomes resistive, and you try to calm his fears. You note that his breathing is rapid and shallow. He has a rapid, weak radial pulse, and his skin is cool and clammy.

1. Based on the first two paragraphs, what is your general impression of the man's condition?

2. Based on your initial assessment, what treatments are needed? (List the steps in order.)

3. Should the patient be rapidly transported? Why or why not?

INITIAL ASSESSMENT: LISTING

1. List the six steps of initial assessment.

2. List and describe the four levels of responsiveness on the AVPU scale.

3. List at least six criteria for rapid transport of a patient.

©2008 by Pearson Education, Inc.
Prehospital Emergency Care, 8th ed.

INITIAL ASSESSMENT: TRUE OR FALSE

Indicate if the following statements are true or false by writing T or F in the space provided.

_____ **1.** Once a patient's ABCs have been assessed during the initial assessment, the EMT can determine the patient's priority for treatment and transport.

_____ **2.** Immediately treat life-threatening problems with circulation, breathing, and airway in that order before continuing with the initial assessment.

_____ **3.** The patient's race is a key factor in forming a general impression.

_____ **4.** If you suspect possible spinal injury, ask the patient to nod her head slightly and report if she feels any pain when doing so.

_____ **5.** During the initial assessment, the AVPU scale is used to help determine a patient's mental status.

_____ **6.** If a responsive patient cannot speak or cry, assume that his airway is not open.

_____ **7.** Provide positive pressure ventilation with supplemental oxygen to all responsive patients who are breathing adequately.

_____ **8.** Immediately begin CPR and use an AED on any pulseless patient.

_____ **9.** At room temperature, a capillary refill time of up to 4 seconds in an infant indicates normal perfusion.

_____ **10.** A responsive patient who is not obeying commands should be considered a priority for rapid transport.

The Initial Assessment

General Impression
Age and Sex
Medical or Trauma
Chief Complaint
Life Threats

Mental Status
A—Alert
P—Painful
V—Verbal
U—Unresponsive

Airway
Open or Closed

Breathing
Adequate or Inadequate

Circulation
Pulse
- Rate
- Quality

Bleeding
Skin Signs

Chapter 9, Part 3: Focused History and Physical Exam

Covers Lessons 3-3, 3-4, and portions of Lesson 3-9 of the U.S. Department of Transportation's EMT-Basic National Standard Curriculum.

OBJECTIVES

Numbered objectives are from the U.S. Department of Transportation EMT-Basic National Standard Curriculum. Asterisked objectives, if any, pertain to material that is supplemental to the DOT curriculum. Page numbers in parentheses refer to pages in the textbook.

Focused History and Physical Exam—Trauma Patient

Cognitive

3-3.1 Discuss the reasons for reconsideration concerning the mechanism of injury. (pp. 264–265)

3-3.2 State the reasons for performing a rapid trauma assessment. (pp. 263–264)

3-3.3 Recite examples and explain why patients should receive a rapid trauma assessment. (p. 263)

3-3.4 Describe the areas included in the rapid trauma assessment and discuss what should be evaluated. (pp. 268–283)

3-3.5 Differentiate when the rapid assessment may be altered in order to provide patient care. (p. 270)

3-3.6 Discuss the reason for performing a focused history and physical exam. (pp. 261–262)

Affective

3-3.7 Recognize and respect the feelings that patients might experience during assessment. (pp. 216, 270)

Psychomotor

3-3.8 Demonstrate the rapid trauma assessment that should be used to assess a patient based on mechanism of injury.

Focused History and Physical Exam—Medical Patient

Cognitive

3-4.1 Describe the unique needs for assessing an individual with a specific chief complaint with no known prior history. (pp. 291–304)

3-4.2 Differentiate between the history and physical exam that are performed for responsive patients with no known prior history and responsive patients with a known prior history. (pp. 302–304)

3-4.3 Describe the needs for assessing an individual who is unresponsive. (pp. 292–302)

3-4.4 Differentiate between the assessment that is performed for a patient who is unresponsive or has an altered mental status and other medical patients requiring assessment. (pp. 292–304)

Affective

3-4.5 Attend to the feelings that these patients might be experiencing. (p. 216)

Psychomotor

3-4.6 Demonstrate the patient assessment skills that should be used to assist a patient who is responsive with no known history.

Total Teaching Time
Part 3: 270 minutes (plus optional 10 minutes for Quiz A)

Resources Needed

- 4 nonstudent volunteers to serve as patients

- 4 EMTs to serve as teaching assistants.

- 4 complete jump kits containing BSI equipment, assorted cervical collars, stethoscopes, BP cuffs, and penlights

- 4 portable oxygen cylinders

- 4 portable suction units

3-4.7 Demonstrate the patient assessment skills that should be used to assist a patient who is unresponsive or has an altered mental status.

REVIEW

Point out that during the last lesson, "Initial Assessment," students learned that upon arrival at a scene, they may encounter a patient with a problem or problems that are immediately life threatening. Such a patient may die within minutes unless he or she receives immediate treatment and transport to a hospital. For this patient, there is not enough time to go through all the steps of a thorough assessment. Therefore, every assessment begins with a process called the initial assessment, designed to identify and treat immediately life-threatening conditions and to set priorities for further assessment and treatment or immediate transport.

INTRODUCTION TO CHAPTER 9, PART 3

Students have learned two steps in the patient assessment process: scene size-up and initial assessment. Tell them that Part 3, "Focused History and Physical Exam," the third lesson of Chapter 9, describes the focused history and physical exam. Explain that adequate time must be spent at the scene to assess the patient correctly and to give proper emergency care. Stress, however, that with seriously ill and injured patients, time must not be wasted at the scene. These patients need to get to a hospital as quickly as possible. Point out to students that the key to striking the right balance between care and speed is focus. Instead of performing a time-consuming, comprehensive assessment on every patient, the EMT hones in on what is important for this particular patient. The process is known as the focused history and physical exam.

Tell students that the focused history and physical exam are somewhat different for patients with trauma and medical problems, so each will be discussed separately.

Distribute the Chapter 9, Part 3, Objectives Checklist and give students a few minutes to look it over. Then briefly paraphrase the objectives for this lesson in your own words.

Handout 9-3A
Chapter 9, Part 3,
Objectives Checklist

Lecture Master
You may wish to display
Lecture Master 9-3A when
presenting the first part of
the lecture to the class.

LECTURE

The following lecture outline is based on the Department of Transportation's EMT-Basic National Standard Curriculum. In some places, the DOT curriculum has been rearranged or expanded upon so that it is more complete or easier for students to understand. This outline is offered for your convenience as you present your lecture. The page numbers in parentheses refer to pages in the textbook. References in dark, heavy type are to figures in the textbook.

Point out the flowchart in Figure 9-16 on page 264, which shows the sequence of events in the focused history and physical exam for the trauma patient, and direct students to follow along during the lecture.

VIII. Reevaluate the mechanism of injury (pp. 264–265)
  A. Significant mechanism of injury (p. 265)
    1. Ejection from vehicle
    2. Death in same passenger compartment
    3. Falls
        a. More than 15 feet or three times patient's height
    4. Rollover of vehicle
    5. High-speed vehicle collision
    6. Vehicle–pedestrian collision
    7. Motorcycle crash
    8. Unresponsiveness or altered mental status
    9. Penetrations of the head, neck, chest, or abdomen
        (Fig. 9-17, p. 265)
    10. Explosion (blast) injuries
    11. Hidden injuries
    12. Seatbelts
        a. If buckled, may have produced injuries.
        b. If patients had seatbelts on, it does not mean they do
            not have injuries.
    13. Airbags
        a. May not be effective without seatbelt.
        b. Patient can hit wheel after deflation.
        c. Lift the deployed airbag and look at the steering wheel
            for deformation.
            (1) "Lift and look" under the bag after the patient has
                been removed.
            (2) Any visible deformation of the steering wheel
                should be regarded as an indicator of potentially
                serious internal injury, and appropriate action
                should be taken.
    14. Collision resulting in prolonged extrication
    15. Special considerations for infants and children
        a. Falls more than 10 feet
        b. Bicycle collision
        c. Vehicle in medium-speed collision
        d. Any vehicle collision where the infant or child was
            unrestrained

**IX. Trauma patient with significant mechanism of injury, altered
mental status, suspected multiple injuries, or critical finding in
the initial assessment** (pp. 265–288) **(Fig. 9-19, pp. 271–273)**
  A. Continue spinal stabilization. (p. 266)
  B. Consider ALS request. (p. 266)
  C. Reconsider transport decision. (p. 266)
  D. Reassess mental status. (pp. 266–268) **(Table 9-9, p. 267 and
      Table 9-10, p. 268)**
  E. Perform a rapid trauma assessment. (pp. 268–283) **(Fig. 9-18,
      pp. 269–270; Fig. 9-19, pp. 271–273)**
    1. DCAP-BTLS
        a. Deformities
        b. Contusions
        c. Abrasions
        d. Punctures/penetrations
        e. Burns
        f. Tenderness

Teaching Tip
You might wish to start the class by demonstrating a complete trauma assessment to give students an idea of how the sequence of steps is carried out in real time.

On the Net
Patient assessment and treatment scenarios.
http://www.trauma.org/res us/moulage/moulage.html

Point to Emphasize
Stress that patients must be treated based on mechanism of injury as well as assessment findings.

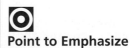

Reading/Reference
Bledsoe B., et al., "25 Physical Examination Perals" *JEMS*, Mar. 2005.

Point to Emphasize
The rapid trauma assessment is helpful in finding life-threatening injuries.

Teaching Tip
At first, don't allow students to use the short form "DCAP-BTLS." Having them say what each letter stands for helps to ingrain the terms in the students' memory.

    g. Lacerations
    h. Swelling
2. Techniques
    a. Inspect (look)
    b. Palpate (feel)
    c. Auscultate (listen)
3. Assess the head
    a. Techniques
        (1) Inspect (look)
        (2) Palpate (feel)
    b. Scalp and skull **(Fig. 9-19a, p. 271)**
        (1) DCAP-BTLS
            (a) Deformities
            (b) Contusions
            (c) Abrasions
            (d) Punctures/penetrations
            (e) Burns
            (f) Tenderness
            (g) Lacerations
            (h) Swelling
        (2) Crepitation
    c. Face **(Fig. 9-19b, p. 271)**
        (1) DCAP-BTLS
            (a) Deformities
            (b) Contusions
            (c) Abrasions
            (d) Punctures/penetrations
            (e) Burns
            (f) Tenderness
            (g) Lacerations
            (h) Swelling
    d. Ears
        (1) Cerebrospinal fluid (CSF) **(Fig. 9-20, p. 275)**
    e. Pupils **(Fig. 9-21, p. 276)**
    f. Nose
    g. Mouth
4. Assess the neck **(Figs. 9-19c, 9-19b, p. 271)**
    a. Techniques
        (1) Inspect (look)
        (2) Palpate (feel)
    b. DCAP-BTLS
        (1) Deformities
        (2) Contusions
        (3) Abrasions
        (4) Punctures/penetrations
        (5) Burns
        (6) Tenderness
        (7) Lacerations
        (8) Swelling
    c. Jugular vein distention (JVD) **(Fig. 9-22, p. 277)**
    d. Crepitation
    e. Apply cervical spinal immobilization collar (CSIC) **(Fig. 9-19e, p. 272)**
5. Assess the chest **(Fig. 9-19f, p. 272; Fig. 9-23, p. 278)**
    a. Techniques

Slides/Videos

"Issues in Spinal Care." Laerdal Medical Corp., One Labriola Ct., Armonk, NY 10504

      (1) Inspect (look)
      (2) Palpate (feel)
      (3) Auscultate (listen)
    b. DCAP-BTLS
      (1) Deformities
      (2) Contusions
      (3) Abrasions
      (4) Punctures/penetrations
      (5) Burns
      (6) Tenderness
      (7) Lacerations
      (8) Swelling
    c. Paradoxical motion
    d. Crepitation
    e. Breath sounds
      (1) Locations (**Fig. 9-19g, p. 272**)
        (a) Apices
        (b) Midclavicular line, bilaterally
        (c) Midaxillary line, bilaterally
      (2) Present
      (3) Diminished
      (4) Absent
      (5) Equal
6. Assess the abdomen (**Fig. 9-19h, p. 272; 9-24, p. 281**)
    a. Techniques
      (1) Inspect (look)
      (2) Palpate (feel)
    b. DCAP-BTLS
      (1) Deformities
      (2) Contusions
      (3) Abrasions
      (4) Punctures/penetrations
      (5) Burns
      (6) Tenderness
      (7) Lacerations
      (8) Swelling
    c. Firm
    d. Soft
    e. Distended
7. Assess the pelvis (**Fig. 9-19i, p. 273**)
    a. Techniques
      (1) Inspect (look)
      (2) Palpate (feel)
    b. DCAP-BTLS
      (1) Deformities
      (2) Contusions
      (3) Abrasions
      (4) Punctures/penetrations
      (5) Burns
      (6) Tenderness
      (7) Lacerations
      (8) Swelling
    c. If no pain is noted, gently compress the pelvis to determine tenderness or motion.
8. Assess all four extremities (**Figs. 9-19j through 9-19n, p. 273**)

✓

Teaching Tip
Have students listen to each other's lung sounds frequently.

◎

Point to Emphasize
Late assessment of blunt abdominal trauma is one of the leading factors in the deaths of patients with abdominal injuries.

◎

Point to Emphasize
Do not let students rock the pelvis to check stability.

      a. Techniques
        (1) Inspect (look)
        (2) Palpate (feel)
      b. DCAP-BTLS
        (1) Deformities
        (2) Contusions
        (3) Abrasions
        (4) Punctures/penetrations
        (5) Burns
        (6) Tenderness
        (7) Lacerations
        (8) Swelling
      c. Distal pulse
      d. Motor function
      e. Sensation
  9. Assess the posterior body
      a. Roll patient with spinal precautions and assess posterior body
      b. Techniques
        (1) Inspect (look)
        (2) Palpate (feel)
      c. DCAP-BTLS
        (1) Deformities
        (2) Contusions
        (3) Abrasions
        (4) Punctures/penetrations
        (5) Burns
        (6) Tenderness
        (7) Lacerations
        (8) Swelling
F. Assess baseline vital signs. (pp. 283–286)
  1. Breathing
  2. Pulse
  3. Skin
  4. Pupils
  5. Blood pressure
  6. Pulse oximeter **(Fig. 9-25, p. 285)**
G. Blood glucose test (pp. 285–286) **(Fig. 9-26, p. 286)**
H. Obtain SAMPLE history. (pp. 286–287)
  1. Signs and symptoms
  2. Allergies
  3. Medications
  4. Pertinent past medical history
  5. Last oral intake
  6. Events leading to the injury
I. Prepare patient for transport. (p. 287) **(Fig. 9-27, p. 287)**
J. Provide emergency care (pp. 287–288)
K. Trauma score (p. 288) **(Table 9-11, p. 289)**
  1. Respiratory rate
  2. Systolic blood pressure
  3. Glasgow Coma Score (GCS)
X. Trauma for patient with no significant mechanism of injury or critical finding (pp. 288–290)
  A. Perform focused trauma assessment (pp. 288–290)
    1. The focused assessment is performed on the specific injury site.

B. Assess baseline vital signs. (p. 290)
    1. Breathing
    2. Pulse
    3. Skin
    4. Pupils
    5. Blood pressure
    6. Pulse oximeter **(Fig. 9-25, p. 285)**
C. Blood glucose (p. 290) **(Fig. 9-26, p. 286)**
D. Obtain SAMPLE history. (p. 290)
    1. Signs and symptoms
    2. Allergies
    3. Medications
    4. Pertinent past medical history
    5. Last oral intake
    6. Events leading to the injury
E. Provide emergency care (p. 290)
F. Prepare patient for transport. (p. 290) **(Fig. 9-27, p. 287)**
G. Sometimes perform rapid trauma assessment. (p. 290)

The next section of the lecture for Chapter 9, Part 3 deals with medical patients. Point out the flowchart in Figure 9-28 on page 292, which shows the sequence of events in the focused history and physical exam for these patients and direct students to follow along during the lecture.

PART 3: FOCUSED HISTORY AND PHYSICAL EXAM—MEDICAL PATIENT

XI. Unresponsive medical patients (pp. 292–302)
  A. Perform rapid medical assessment. (pp. 293–299) **(Fig. 9-29, pp. 294–295)**
    1. Assess the head.
    2. Assess the neck.
    3. Assess the chest.
    4. Assess the abdomen. **(Fig. 9-30, p. 297; Fig. 9-31, p. 298)**
    5. Assess the pelvic region
    6. Assess the extremities.
    7. Assess the posterior body.
  B. Assess baseline vital signs. (p. 299)
    1. Breathing
    2. Pulse
    3. Skin
    4. Pupils
    5. Blood pressure
    6. Pulse oximeter
  C. Blood glucose test. (p. 299)
  D. Position the patient. (p. 300) **(Fig. 9-32, p. 301)**
  E. Obtain SAMPLE history. (pp. 300–302) **(Figs. 9-33, 9-34, p. 301)**
    1. Signs and symptoms
    2. Allergies
    3. Medications
    4. Pertinent past medical history
    5. Last oral intake
    6. Events leading to the illness
  F. Provide emergency care (p. 302)
  G. Make transport decision. (p. 302)

Teaching Tip

Remind students to talk to the patient, explaining what is going on as the exam is carried out. Doing so will make the exam easier for both the patient and the EMT.

Lecture Master

You may wish to display Lecture Master 9-3B when presenting the concluding part of the lecture to the class.

Teaching Tip

You might wish to start the presentation by demonstrating a complete medical assessment to give students an idea of how the sequence of steps is carried out in real time.

Teaching Tip

Point out that when EMTs work as a team the baseline vital signs can often be gathered simultaneously with the patient history.

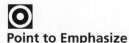

Point to Emphasize

The same person should gather both the SAMPLE and OPQRST histories.

XII. Responsive medical patient (pp. 302–304)
  A. Assess history of present illness including complaints and signs or symptoms. (p. 302)
  B. OPQRST questions (pp. 302–303)
    1. Onset
    2. Provocation/palliation
    3. Quality
    4. Radiation
    5. Severity
    6. Time
  C. Obtain SAMPLE history. (p. 303)
    1. Signs and symptoms
    2. Allergies
    3. Medications
    4. Pertinent past medical history
    5. Last oral intake
    6. Events leading to the illness
  D. Perform focused medical assessment. (p. 303)
  E. Assess baseline vital signs. (p. 303)
    1. Breathing
    2. Pulse
    3. Skin
    4. Pupils
    5. Blood pressure
    6. Pulse oximeter
  F. Provide emergency care. (p. 303)
  G. Make transport decision. (pp. 303–304)

CASE STUDY FOLLOW-UP

Note: The case studies will not be reviewed until the last lesson of this chapter.

IN REVIEW

Note: The In Review will not be covered until the last lesson of this chapter.

PRACTICE SCENARIOS

Arrange for four vacant classrooms or other private areas to serve as practice scenario stations. Before class, set up the following scenarios and brief each nonstudent volunteer on his or her role based on the patient descriptions below. Use moulage to simulate trauma patients if desired.

- Station A—Responsive trauma patient: an adult patient who has fallen from a ladder while painting the outside of his house. His right leg and left wrist are broken.

- Station B—Unresponsive trauma patient: a teenager who has been thrown from a car in a crash. Her neck is broken and she is unconscious.

- Station C—Responsive medical patient: a pregnant woman who is in labor. She thinks the baby is going to come very soon.

- Station D—Unresponsive medical patient: a college student who has tried to commit suicide by taking an overdose of sleeping pills. His roommate came home, found him, and called 9-1-1. When the EMTs arrive, the student is unconscious.

At the beginning of the class, tell students they are going to practice the focused history and physical exam skills they have just learned. Divide the class into teams of two. If there is an odd number of students, it is acceptable to have teams of three. Tell students that you have set up the following four practice scenarios: (1) responsive trauma patient, (2) unresponsive trauma patient, (3) responsive medical patient, and (4) unresponsive medical patient. Instruct the teams to visit all the practice stations and to respond to the on-scene conditions they find. Remind students that the emphasis of the scene is the focused history and physical exam, but encourage them to utilize the information and skills they have learned to date about patient assessment and treatment. Also advise them that there will be a teaching assistant at each station to observe their performance and provide feedback.

Call pairs of students at random and direct them to each scenario. Periodically visit each station to monitor progress. Provide help to the teaching assistants, if necessary. Make sure that each team visits all stations. Assist students waiting to visit the stations with their patient assessment skills. When each pair has completed all the stations, make sure that they return to the main classroom.

ASSIGNMENT

Direct students to review Chapter 9, Part 4, "Detailed Physical Exam," before the next class.

EVALUATION

If you choose to give a quiz now, distribute Handout 9-3B. If not, distribute it at the end of Part 6.

REINFORCEMENT

Reinforcement Handouts are provided for students whose participation in class discussions or performance on the quiz indicates they have not fully mastered the content of Part 3. You may wish to assign some or all of these handouts to those students.

Reading/Reference
Textbook, pp. 304–318

Handout 9-3B
Chapter 9 Quiz A

Handouts 9-3C to 9-3H
Reinforcement Activities

OBJECTIVES

OBJECTIVES CHECKLIST

TRAUMA PATIENT

Cognitive		Date Mastered
3-3.1	Discuss the reasons for reconsideration concerning the mechanism of injury.	
3-3.2	State the reasons for performing a rapid trauma assessment.	
3-3.3	Recite examples and explain why patients should receive a rapid trauma assessment.	
3-3.4	Describe the areas included in the rapid trauma assessment and discuss what should be evaluated.	
3-3.5	Differentiate when the rapid assessment may be altered in order to provide patient care.	
3-3.6	Discuss the reason for performing a focused history and physical exam.	

Affective		Date Mastered
3-3.7	Recognize and respect the feelings that patients might experience during assessment.	

Psychomotor		Date Mastered
3-3.8	Demonstrate the rapid trauma assessment that should be used to treat a patient based on mechanism of injury.	

MEDICAL PATIENT

Cognitive		Date Mastered
3-4.1	Describe the unique needs for assessing an individual with a specific chief complaint with no known prior history.	
3-4.2	Differentiate between the history and physical exam that are performed for responsive patients with no known prior history and responsive patients with a known prior history.	
3-4.3	Describe the needs for assessing an individual who is unresponsive.	
3-4.4	Differentiate between the assessment that is performed for a patient who is unresponsive or has an altered mental status and other medical patients requiring assessment.	

Affective		Date Mastered
3-4.5	Attend to the feelings that these patients might be experiencing.	

Psychomotor		Date Mastered
3-4.6	Demonstrate the patient assessment skills that should be used to assist a patient who is responsive with no known history.	
3-4.7	Demonstrate the patient assessment skills that should be used to assist a patient who is unresponsive or has an altered mental status.	

EVALUATION

CHAPTER 9 QUIZ A: PARTS 1–3

Write the letter of the best answer in the space provided.

_____ 1. Establishing the number of patients is an important part of the
         A. initial assessment.   **C.** detailed assessment.
         B. scene size-up.   **D.** general impression.

_____ 2. The main purpose of the initial assessment is to
         A. obtain the chief complaint.
         B. establish scene safety.
         C. discover and treat immediately life-threatening conditions.
         D. obtain a full set of vital signs and a SAMPLE history.

_____ 3. The patient's age, sex, and chief complaint are part of the:
         A. general impression.   **C.** dispatch information.
         B. patient profile.   **D.** scene size-up.

_____ 4. On the AVPU scale, a patient who responds or attempts to respond only when spoken to is rated
         A. A.   **C.** V.
         B. P.   **D.** U.

_____ 5. The sound that is an indication that the tongue and epiglottis are partially blocking the airway is
         A. stridor.   **C.** gurgling.
         B. crowing.   **D.** snoring.

_____ 6. If assessment reveals pale, cool, clammy skin in conjunction with a significant mechanism of injury, an altered mental status, or severe bleeding, assume that the patient is
         A. having a heart attack.   **C.** not a priority.
         B. having a stroke.   **D.** in shock.

_____ 7. Which of the following is an indication that rapid transport of a patient is required?
         A. a temperature of 105°F   **C.** systolic blood pressure of 110
         B. lordosis   **D.** diaphoresis

_____ 8. The three major steps in the focused history and physical exam are conducting a physical exam, taking baseline vital signs, and
         A. providing emergency care.
         B. packaging the patient for transport.
         C. obtaining a SAMPLE history.
         D. stabilizing the cervical spine.

_____ 9. A trauma patient with a significant mechanism of injury should receive a
         A. focused trauma assessment.   **C.** focused medical assessment.
         B. detailed physical exam.   **D.** rapid trauma assessment.

_____ 10. Which of the following is *not* normally considered a significant mechanism of injury in adult patients?
         A. fall of 10 feet   **C.** blast injury from an explosion
         B. seatbelt injury   **D.** rollover of a vehicle

_____11. In the rapid trauma assessment, the "B" of DCAP-BTLS stands for
   A. breaks.   C. burns.
   B. bruises.   D. bleeding.

_____12. When two or more adjacent ribs are fractured in two or more places, the condition is termed
   A. seesaw movement.   C. decorticate motion.
   B. Battle's sign.   D. flail segment.

_____13. During the rapid trauma assessment, check all extremities for
   A. PMS.   C. IRT.
   B. QRS.   D. JVD.

_____14. The rapid trauma assessment should take about _____ minute(s).
   A. $\frac{1}{2}$ C. 5
   B. 2 to $2\frac{1}{2}$ D. 5 to 7

_____15. The respiratory rate, the systolic blood pressure, and the GCS are the major components of the
   A. revised trauma score.   C. radio report.
   B. patient narrative.   D. dispatch information.

_____16. The first element of the focused history and physical exam for a responsive medical patient is
   A. taking baseline vital signs.
   B. performing a focused medical assessment.
   C. performing a rapid medical assessment.
   D. obtaining a SAMPLE history.

_____17. The exam that is based on the responsive patient's chief complaint and symptoms is the
   A. revised medical exam.   C. Glasgow survey.
   B. focused medical assessment.   D. rapid medical assessment.

_____18. When assessing a responsive medical patient's chief complaint, the "T" of OPQRST stands for
   A. tenderness.   C. termination.
   B. tension.   D. time.

_____19. An assessment finding of jugular vein distention may indicate
   A. hypotension.   C. heart failure.
   B. hypoglycemia.   D. kidney failure.

_____20. For transport, the unresponsive medical patient should normally be placed in the _____ position.
   A. Fowler's   C. Trendelenburg
   B. recovery   D. prone

REINFORCEMENT

IN THE FIELD

Review the following real-life situation. Then answer the questions that follow.

"We knew that the patient was sick when we entered the room. He went back and sat in his living room chair and he had that 'sick look' about him. He was awake and responsive, but he was breathing kind of hard. And his skin was pale and pasty looking. We didn't wait for more information. We got the oxygen on him right away.

"We introduced ourselves and told him we were EMTs with the fire department. He told us how he had chest pain that started about 1 hour ago. He was working on his income taxes when it started up all of a sudden. He said that he lives alone and didn't know who else to call. He described the pain as 'kind of crushing, like the last time I had a heart attack.' When he said that, I made sure that the company officer called for a paramedic unit.

"He told us that the pain was pretty bad, an 8 on a scale of 0 to 10, where zero is no pain and 10 is the worst he's had in his life. The oxygen appeared to make him feel better, and he agreed that it did. It had been 5 minutes since we got there and about 20 minutes since the pain started. While we waited for the ambulance and paramedics, I continued with my SAMPLE history while my partner started to get a baseline set of vital signs."

1. Based on the patient's presentation, what other questions could the EMT have asked about the present chief complaint?

2. What would the EMT proceed to do next if the ambulance was not yet on-scene?

3. If this patient had been unconscious when the EMTs arrived, where might they have possibly found more information?

CHAPTER 9 REVIEW A: PARTS 1–3

Write the word or words that best complete each sentence in the space provided.

1. _____ _____ -_____ is the first component of patient assessment.

2. During the initial assessment, any life-threatening condition that is identified must be _____ _____.

3. A patient's age, sex, appearance, and chief complaint are all elements of the _____ _____.

4. The patient's answer to the question "Why did you call EMS?" is called the _____ _____.

5. To determine a patient's level of responsiveness, use the _____ _____.

6. Once the patient's level of responsiveness is determined during the initial assessment, move on to assess the _____.

7. The best method of assessing breathing is by _____, _____, and _____.

8. Assessment of circulation includes checking capillary refill, pulse, skin color, temperature, and condition, as well as checking for possible major _____.

9. The last step in the initial assessment is _____ _____.

10. Once you have conducted a scene size-up and an initial assessment, your next step is to conduct a _____ _____ _____ _____ _____.

11. For the _____ patient, the steps of the focused history and physical exam are performed in this sequence—physical exam, baseline vital signs, history.

12. A trauma patient with no significant mechanism of injury will generally receive a(n) _____ trauma assessment.

13. To assess a patient's level of orientation, ask specific questions about

_____, _____, and

_____.

14. If assessment reveals that a patient has a deteriorating mental status associated with possible head

injury, you should, if possible, hyperventilate at _____ ventilations per

minute via BVM device.

15. If assessment reveals tracheal tugging, you should suspect _____

_____.

16. As part of the rapid trauma assessment, check the extremities for distal

_____, _____, _____,

and _____.

17. An unresponsive medical patient should receive a(n) _____ medical

assessment.

18. Your critical findings are unequal pupils with altered mental status and a facial droop. You should

consider establishing a(n) _____, providing

_____, _____, _____,

and administering _____.

19. When assessing the responsive medical patient's condition, use the _____

and _____ questions.

20. Reassess vital signs during transport every _____ minutes for critical

patients and every _____ minutes for noncritical patients.

REINFORCEMENT

TRAUMA PATIENT ASSESSMENT: ORDERING

Put in order the following steps of the focused history and physical exam for a trauma patient with a significant mechanism of injury. Place 1 before the first step taken, 2 before the second step, and so on.

_____ Assess baseline vital signs.

_____ Transport the patient.

_____ Consider a request for ALS support.

_____ Perform a detailed physical exam.

_____ Obtain a SAMPLE history.

_____ Continue spinal stabilization.

_____ Perform the ongoing assessment.

_____ Reassess mental status.

_____ Perform rapid trauma assessment.

_____ Reconsider the transport decision.

REINFORCEMENT

TRAUMA PATIENT ASSESSMENT: LISTING

1. List six mechanisms of injury that have a high incidence of producing critical trauma in adults.

2. List four significant mechanisms of injury for infants and children.

3. List what the letters of the memory aid DCAP-BTLS stand for.

MEDICAL PATIENT ASSESSMENT: MATCHING

Below are listed the steps of the focused history and physical exam for responsive and unresponsive medical patients. Write the letters of the steps in the order you would perform them for each type of patient.

A. Obtain SAMPLE history.

B. Make transport decision.

C. Assess baseline vital signs.

D. Perform ongoing assessment.

E. Perform focused medical assessment.

F. Position patient.

G. Perform detailed physical exam.

H. Perform rapid medical assessment.

I. Perform components of detailed physical exam.

J. Transport.

K. Assess complaints plus signs and symptoms.

Responsive Medical Patient

1. _____

2. _____

3. _____

4. _____

5. _____

6. _____

7. _____

Unresponsive Medical Patient

1. _____

2. _____

3. _____

4. _____

5. _____

6. _____

7. _____

REINFORCEMENT

FOCUSING ON THE FOCUSED HISTORY

Below are parts of one patient's SAMPLE history. In the space provided, write the elements of the OPQRST and SAMPLE memory aids that each part of the history represents. When you are done, read the history out loud, like a radio report, in the order suggested by the memory aids. Does the report make sense presented this way?

OPQRST	SAMPLE
A. Onset	**G.** Signs, symptoms
B. Provocation	**H.** Allergies
C. Quality	**I.** Medications
D. Radiation	**J.** Pertinent past history
E. Severity	**K.** Last oral intake
F. Time	**L.** Events leading up to illness

_____ **1.** The pain is a 6 on a scale of 0 to 10.

_____ **2.** I was working on my car in the garage.

_____ **3.** I'm sick to my stomach, too.

_____ **4.** I'm not allergic to anything.

_____ **5.** Do you think this has something to do with my high blood pressure?

_____ **6.** I ate lunch at noon.

_____ **7.** The pain started about an hour ago.

_____ **8.** I take one baby aspirin a day.

_____ **9.** The pain is sharp.

_____ **10.** I think I might have lifted something too heavy.

_____ **11.** I've felt fine today until this.

_____ **12.** The pain goes into my left armpit.

Focused History and Physical Exam—Trauma Patients

Reconsider Mechanism of Injury

Significant Mechanisms

Patient with Significant Mechanism of Injury

Continue Spinal Stabilization

Consider ALS Request

Reconsider Transport

Reassess Mental Status

Perform Rapid Trauma Assessment—DCAP-BTLS

- Head
- Neck (apply CSIC)
- Chest
- Abdomen
- Pelvis
- Extremities
- Posterior body

Assess Baseline Vital Signs

Obtain SAMPLE History

Transport

Perform Detailed Physical Exam

Perform Ongoing Assessment

Patient with No Significant Mechanism of Injury

Perform Focused Trauma Assessment

Obtain Baseline Vital Signs

Obtain SAMPLE History

Perform Components of Detailed Physical Exam

Transport

Perform Ongoing Assessment

Assessment of the Medical Patient

Unresponsive Medical Patient

Perform Rapid Medical Assessment

- Head
- Neck
- Chest
- Abdomen
- Pelvis
- Extremities
- Posterior body

Assess Baseline Vital Signs

Position Patient

Obtain SAMPLE History

- Signs/symptoms
- Allergies
- Medications
- Pertinent past history
- Last oral intake
- Events leading to illness

Transport

Perform Detailed Physical Exam

Perform Ongoing Assessment

Responsive Medical Patient

Assess Patient Complaints

- Onset
- Provocation/palliation
- Quality
- Radiation
- Severity
- Time

Obtain SAMPLE History

Perform Focused Medical Assessment

Assess Baseline Vital Signs

Make Transport Decision

Perform Components of Detailed Physical Exam

Perform Ongoing Assessment

Chapter 9, Part 4: Detailed Physical Exam

Covers Lesson 3-5 and portions of Lesson 3-9 of the U.S. Department of Transportation's EMT-Basic National Standard Curriculum.

Total Teaching Time
Part 4: 130 minutes

Resources Needed
- Complete jump kit containing BSI equipment, assorted cervical collars, stethoscopes, BP cuffs, and penlights

OBJECTIVES

Numbered objectives are from the U.S. Department of Transportation EMT-Basic National Standard Curriculum. Asterisked objectives, if any, pertain to material that is supplemental to the DOT curriculum. Page numbers in parentheses refer to pages in the textbook.

Cognitive

3-5.1 Discuss the components of the detailed physical exam. (pp. 305–306)
3-5.2 State the areas of the body that are evaluated during the detailed physical exam. (pp. 305–317)
3-5.3 Explain what additional care should be provided while performing the detailed physical exam. (pp. 305, 318)
3-5.4 Distinguish between the detailed physical exam that is performed on a trauma patient and that of the medical patient. (pp. 305–317)

Affective

3-5.5 Explain the rationale for the feelings that these patients might be experiencing. (pp. 216, 306, 316)

Psychomotor

3-5.6 Demonstrate the skills involved in performing the detailed physical exam.

REVIEW

In the last lesson, "Focused History and Physical Exam," students learned that for seriously ill and injured patients, time must not be wasted at the scene. These patients need to get to a hospital as quickly as possible. On the other hand, enough time must be spent at the scene to assess the patient adequately and to give proper emergency care. EMT-Basics can strike the right balance between care and speed by engaging in a focused history and physical exam.

INTRODUCTION TO CHAPTER 9, PART 4

Part 4, "Detailed Physical Exam," is the fourth lesson of Chapter 9. The initial assessment and the focused history and physical exam are done rapidly because of the necessity of getting the seriously injured or ill patient into the ambulance and to the hospital without delay. However, there are times, either at the scene or en route to the hospital, when an EMT may have time to do a more complete patient assessment, known as the detailed physical exam.

Distribute the Chapter 9, Part 4, Objectives Checklist and give students a few minutes to look it over. Then briefly paraphrase the objectives for this lesson in your own words.

Handout 9–4A
Chapter 9, Part 4, Objectives Checklist

LECTURE

The following lecture outline is based on the Department of Transportation's EMT-Basic National Standard Curriculum. In some places, the DOT curriculum has been rearranged or expanded upon so that it is more complete or easier for students to understand. This outline is offered for your convenience as you present your lecture. The page numbers in parentheses refer to pages in the textbook. References in dark, heavy type are to figures in the textbook.

Point out the flowchart in Figure 9-35 on page 305, which shows the sequence of events in the detailed physical exam and direct students to follow along during the lecture.

PART 4: DETAILED PHYSICAL EXAM

XIII. Detailed Physical Exam (pp. 304–318)**(Fig. 9-35, p. 305)**
   A. Patient and injury specific, for example, cut finger, would not require the detailed physical exam. (p. 305)
   B. Perform only after all life-threatening injuries and conditions have been managed. (p. 305)
   C. Usually done in back of ambulance on way to hospital. (p. 305)
   D. Perform the detailed physical exam (pp. 305–318)
      1. Assess the head **(Figs. 9-36, p. 306)**
         a. Techniques
            (1) Inspect (look)
            (2) Palpate (feel)
         b. DCAP-BTLS
            (1) Deformities
            (2) Contusions
            (3) Abrasions
            (4) Punctures/penetrations
            (5) Burns
            (6) Tenderness
            (7) Lacerations
            (8) Swelling
      2. Assess the ears **(Figs. 9-36b and c, p. 306–307)**
         a. Techniques
            (1) Inspect (look)
            (2) Palpate (feel)
         b. DCAP-BTLS
            (1) Deformities
            (2) Contusions
            (3) Abrasions
            (4) Punctures/penetrations
            (5) Burns
            (6) Tenderness
            (7) Lacerations
            (8) Swelling
         c. Drainage
      3. Assess the face **(Fig. 9-36d, p. 307)**
         a. Techniques
            (1) Inspect (look)
            (2) Palpate (feel)
         b. DCAP-BTLS
            (1) Deformities

©2008 by Pearson Education, Inc.
Prehospital Emergency Care, 8th ed.

Lecture Master
You may wish to display Lecture Master 9-4 when presenting the lecture to the class.

Point of Interest
The detailed physical exam is similar to the old secondary survey.

Teaching Tip
Remind students to talk to the patient, explaining what is going on as the exam is carried out. Doing so will make the exam easier for both patient and EMT.

Point to Emphasize
What is not exposed cannot be evaluated. Students should expose patients appropriately, bearing in mind considerations of privacy and potential heat loss.

Teaching Tip
Remind students that they can easily practice these exams at home on spouses, other family members, or even the family dog or cat.

              (2) Contusions
              (3) Abrasions
              (4) Punctures/penetrations
              (5) Burns
              (6) Tenderness
              (7) Lacerations
              (8) Swelling
   4. Assess the eyes (**Figs. 9-36e–g, p. 307; Fig. 9-37, p. 312**)
      a. Techniques
              (1) Inspect (look)
              (2) Palpate (feel)
      b. DCAP-BTLS
              (1) Deformities
              (2) Contusions
              (3) Abrasions
              (4) Punctures/penetrations
              (5) Burns
              (6) Tenderness
              (7) Lacerations
              (8) Swelling
      c. Discoloration
      d. Unequal pupils
      e. Foreign bodies
      f. Blood in anterior chamber
   5. Assess the nose (**Fig. 9-36h, p. 307**)
      a. Techniques
              (1) Inspect (look)
              (2) Palpate (feel)
      b. DCAP-BTLS
              (1) Deformities
              (2) Contusions
              (3) Abrasions
              (4) Punctures/penetrations
              (5) Burns
              (6) Tenderness
              (7) Lacerations
              (8) Swelling
      c. Drainage
      d. Bleeding
   6. Assess the mouth (**Fig. 9-36i, p. 308**)
      a. Techniques
              (1) Inspect (look)
              (2) Palpate (feel)
      b. Auscultate (listen)
              (1) Deformities
              (2) Contusions
              (3) Abrasions
              (4) Punctures/penetrations
              (5) Burns
              (6) Tenderness
              (7) Lacerations
              (8) Swelling
      c. Teeth
      d. Obstructions
      e. Swollen or lacerated tongue

Point to Emphasize
Stress with students the need to be alert to potential airway obstructions when assessing the nose and mouth.

  f. Odors

  g. Discoloration

 7. Assess the neck (**Fig. 9-36j, p. 308**)

  a. Techniques

   (1) Inspect (look)

   (2) Palpate (feel)

  b. DCAP-BTLS

   (1) Deformities

   (2) Contusions

   (3) Abrasions

   (4) Punctures/penetrations

   (5) Burns

   (6) Tenderness

   (7) Lacerations

   (8) Swelling

  c. Jugular vein distention (JVD)

  d. Crepitation

 8. Assess the chest (**Figs. 9-36k and l, p. 308**)

  a. Techniques

   (1) Inspect (look)

   (2) Palpate (feel)

   (3) Auscultate (listen)

  b. DCAP-BTLS

   (1) Deformities

   (2) Contusions

   (3) Abrasions

   (4) Punctures/penetrations

   (5) Burns

   (6) Tenderness

   (7) Lacerations

   (8) Swelling

  c. Crepitation

  d. Paradoxical motion

  e. Breath sounds

   (1) Locations

    (a) Apices

    (b) Midclavicular line, bilaterally

    (c) Midaxillary line, bilaterally

   (2) Present

   (3) Diminished

   (4) Absent

   (5) Equal

 9. Assess the abdomen (**Fig. 9-36m, p. 308**)

  a. Techniques

   (1) Inspect (look)

   (2) Palpate (feel)

  b. DCAP-BTLS

   (1) Deformities

   (2) Contusions

   (3) Abrasions

   (4) Punctures/penetrations

   (5) Burns

   (6) Tenderness

   (7) Lacerations

   (8) Swelling

       c. Firm

       d. Soft

       e. Distention

  10. Assess the pelvis (**Fig. 9-36n, p. 308**)

       a. Techniques

          (1) Inspect (look)

          (2) Palpate (feel)

       b. DCAP-BTLS

          (1) Deformities

          (2) Contusions

          (3) Abrasions

          (4) Punctures/penetrations

          (5) Burns

          (6) Tenderness

          (7) Lacerations

          (8) Swelling

       c. If the patient does not complain of pain or is unresponsive, gently flex and compress the pelvis to determine stability.

  11. Assess all four extremities (**Figs. 9-36o–u, pp. 309–310**)

       a. Techniques

          (1) Inspect (look)

          (2) Palpate (feel)

       b. DCAP-BTLS

          (1) Deformities

          (2) Contusions

          (3) Abrasions

          (4) Punctures/penetrations

          (5) Burns

          (6) Tenderness

          (7) Lacerations

          (8) Swelling

       c. Distal pulse

       d. Sensation

       e. Motor function

  12. Assess the posterior body.

       a. Techniques

          (1) Inspect (look)

          (2) Palpate (feel)

       b. DCAP-BTLS

          (1) Deformities

          (2) Contusions

          (3) Abrasions

          (4) Punctures/penetrations

          (5) Burns

          (6) Tenderness

          (7) Lacerations

          (8) Swelling

  13. Reassess vital signs. (**Fig. 9-38, p. 317**)

       a. Breathing

       b. Pulse

       c. Skin

       d. Pupils

       e. Blood pressure

       f. Pulse oximeter

E. Continue emergency care. (p. 318)

CASE STUDY FOLLOW-UP

Note: The case studies will not be reviewed until the last lesson of this chapter.

IN REVIEW

Note: The In Review will not be covered until the last lesson of this chapter.

ROLE PLAY AND PRACTICE

Ask two volunteers to play the role of EMTs who are responding to a 9-1-1 call. Take the two EMT players outside of the classroom and provide them with a complete jump kit containing BSI equipment, assorted cervical collars, stethoscopes, BP cuffs, and penlights. Describe the following situation to them:

You are called by the police, who found a man unconscious. You should act appropriately on what you find there. The emphasis of the scene is on the detailed physical exam. However, you should utilize all the skills you have learned to date. We will call you to the scene in just a minute. Invite two more volunteers to act the parts of a police officer and the patient. Have the patient and the police officer come to the front of the classroom. Describe the following situation to them and the class: The patient is a middle-age adult who was mugged late at night while walking home from a local bar. The patient is unconscious on a sidewalk and has a large contusion on the back of the head. The police officer found the patient during a routine foot patrol of the neighborhood. The police officer administered EMR-level aid and requested an ambulance. No witnesses are present to explain what happened to the patient.

Tell the patient and the police officer to take their places and to start acting. Call the EMTs back into the classroom. Allow the role play to progress naturally. Intervene only if the players seem to be at a loss for what to do. If the EMTs fail to put on the proper BSI equipment, remind them to do so. If the EMTs decide to call their on-line medical director (you), direct them to transport the patient.

End the role play when the detailed physical exam has been completed. (The EMTs should not be asked to treat the patient further since they have not yet reached this point in training.)

With the entire class, discuss the following:

- What did the EMTs do well?
- What, if anything, should they have done differently?

Divide students into pairs and direct them to take turns practicing a detailed physical exam on each other.

ASSIGNMENTS

Direct students to review Chapter 9, Part 5, "Ongoing Assessment," and Part 6, "Communication and Documentation," before the next class.

Reading/Reference
Textbook, pp. 318–323

EVALUATION

Note: The quiz will not be given until the end of Part 6 of this chapter.

REINFORCEMENT

Handouts 9-4B to 9-4C
Reinforcement Activities

Reinforcement Handouts are provided for students whose participation in class discussions or performance on the quiz indicates they have not fully mastered the content of Part 4. You may wish to assign some or all of these handouts to those students.

OBJECTIVES CHECKLIST

Cognitive		Date Mastered
3-5.1	Discuss the components of the detailed physical exam.	
3-5.2	State the areas of the body that are evaluated during the detailed physical exam.	
3-5.3	Explain what additional care should be provided while performing the detailed physical exam.	
3-5.4	Distinguish between the detailed physical exam that is performed on a trauma patient and that of a medical patient.	

Affective		Date Mastered
3-5.5	Explain the rationale for the feelings that these patients might be experiencing.	

Psychomotor		Date Mastered
3-5.6	Demonstrate the skills involved in performing the detailed physical exam.	

IN THE FIELD

Read the following real-life situation. Then answer the questions that follow.

You and your partner are dispatched at 0130 and arrive on the scene of a motor-vehicle rollover a few minutes later. The firefighters have put up scene lights. To the right of the road, you spot a set of tire tracks. An automobile rests on all four wheels in a ditch. State police are managing traffic.

After the fire department stabilizes the vehicle and you have taken BSI precautions, you approach. Inside the vehicle, you notice a young woman who appears to be sleeping, judging by her snoring. She seems oblivious to all the commotion. You immediately stabilize her head and then try to awaken her. The patient awakens quickly, but she seems confused and her speech is slightly slurred. Her airway is patent, and her breathing is relaxed and displays no apparent difficulty. Her radial pulse is strong and regular at roughly 100 beats per minute. As you work, you notice a strong smell of beer in the car and on the patient.

Your partner points out the damage on both sides of the car and on the roof. You decide to continue manual stabilization of her cervical spine and extricate her from the vehicle onto a long backboard. While you perform this, you ask one of the EMTs from the fire department to take a set of baseline vital signs. You also request a Paramedic intercept through the EMS coordinator.

At this point, you begin to perform the rapid trauma assessment. The assessment reveals no significant injuries to the patient. The vital signs are also within normal limits. In light of her mental status, you choose to move the patient rapidly out of the ditch via a Stokes basket, up a ladder, and into the waiting ambulance.

1. What scene hazards were present? How were they managed?

2. What is the mechanism of injury? Would you consider it significant?

3. Were the assessments correctly performed? Explain.

4. Would a detailed physical exam be appropriate for this patient? If so, when would it be performed?

THE DETAILED PHYSICAL EXAM: ORDERING

Below are the areas to assess during the detailed physical exam. Arrange the steps in the order in which the exam should be performed by writing 1 next to the area that should be assessed first, 2 next to the area that should be assessed next, and so on.

_____ Assess the eyes.

_____ Assess the pelvis.

_____ Assess the ears.

_____ Assess the neck.

_____ Assess the mouth.

_____ Assess the head.

_____ Assess the posterior body.

_____ Assess the extremities.

_____ Assess the nose.

_____ Assess the chest.

_____ Assess the face.

_____ Assess the abdomen.

LECTURE MASTER 9-4

Detailed Physical Exam

When to Perform a Detailed Physical Exam
How to Perform a Detailed Physical Exam

- Assess the Head
- Assess the Neck
- Assess the Chest
- Assess the Abdomen
- Assess the Pelvis
- Assess the Lower Extremities
- Assess the Upper Extremities
- Assess the Posterior Body

Reassess Vital Signs
Continue Emergency Care

Chapter 9, Part 5: Ongoing Assessment

Covers Lesson 3-6 and portions of Lesson 3-9 of the U.S. Department of Transportation's EMT-Basic National Standard Curriculum.

OBJECTIVES

Numbered objectives are from the U.S. Department of Transportation EMT-Basic National Standard Curriculum. Asterisked objectives, if any, pertain to material that is supplemental to the DOT curriculum. Page numbers in parentheses refer to pages in the textbook.

Cognitive

3-6.1 Discuss the reasons for repeating the initial assessment as part of the ongoing assessment. (p. 321)
3-6.2 Describe the components of the ongoing assessment. (pp. 319–323)
3-6.3 Describe trending of assessment components. (p. 323)

Affective

3-6.4 Explain the value of performing an ongoing assessment. (pp. 319–321)
3-6.5 Recognize and respect the feelings that patients might experience during assessment. (p. 316)
3-6.6 Explain the value of trending assessment components to other health care professionals who assume care of the patient. (p. 323)

Psychomotor

3-6.7 Demonstrate the skills involved in performing the ongoing assessment.

REVIEW

In the last lesson, "Detailed Physical Exam," students were reminded that the initial assessment and the focused history and physical exam are done rapidly because of the necessity of getting the seriously injured or ill patient into the ambulance and to the hospital without delay. However, there are cases when, either at the scene or en route to the hospital, EMTs may have time to do a more complete patient assessment, known as the detailed physical exam.

INTRODUCTION TO CHAPTER 9, PART 5

Part 5, "Ongoing Assessment," is the fifth lesson in Chapter 9. Explain to students that the patient's condition is continually subject to change. There may be a change for the better, for example, an unresponsive patient regains consciousness. Or there may be a change for the worse, for example, a patient who was alert and oriented becomes confused. Therefore, the patient should frequently be reevaluated at the scene and en route to the hospital, using the procedures of the ongoing assessment.

   Distribute the Chapter 9, Part 5, Objectives Checklist and give students a few minutes to look it over. Then briefly paraphrase the objectives for this lesson in your own words.

Total Teaching Time
Part 5: 70 minutes

Resources Needed
• Enough blood pressure cuffs, stethoscopes, and penlights for each team of four students

Handout 9-5A
Chapter 9, Part 5, Objectives Checklist

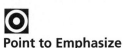

Lecture Master

You may wish to display Lecture Master 9-5 when presenting the lecture to the class.

Point to Emphasize

An ongoing assessment loses some of its value if good baseline vitals were not obtained initially.

Point to Emphasize

Some severely injured patients may need to be monitored every 2 or 3 minutes.

Teaching Tip

Run a practice scenario from start to finish. Don't let students stop when they "load the patient and go." Build into the scenario a transport time long enough to ensure that students perform at least one ongoing assessment.

The following lecture outline is based on the Department of Transportation's EMT-Basic National Standard Curriculum. In some places, the DOT curriculum has been rearranged or expanded upon so that it is more complete or easier for students to understand. This outline is offered for your convenience as you present your lecture. The page numbers in parentheses refer to pages in the textbook.

Point out the flowchart in Figure 9-39 on page 319, which shows the sequence of events in the ongoing assessment, and direct students to follow along.

PART 5: ONGOING ASSESSMENT

   XIV. **Purposes of the ongoing assessment** (pp. 319–321)
      A. Detect any change in condition (p. 321)
      B. Identify missed injuries or conditions (p. 321)
      C. Adjust emergency care (pp. 321)
      D. Stable patient (p. 321)
         1. Repeat and record every 15 minutes
      E. Unstable patient (p. 321)
         1. Repeat and record at a minimum every 5 minutes.
   XV. **Repeat initial assessment.** (pp. 321–322) **(Fig. 9-40a, p. 320)**
      A. Reassess mental status. (p. 321)
      B. Reassess the airway. (pp. 321–322)
      C. Reassess breathing. (p. 322)
      D. Reassess circulation. (p. 322)
         1. Reassess pulse
         2. Reassess bleeding
         3. Reassess the skin
      E. Reestablish patient priorities. (p. 322)
   XVI. **Reassess and record vital signs.** (p. 322) **(Fig. 9-40b, p. 320)**
   XVII. **Repeat focused assessment regarding patient complaint or injuries.** (pp. 322–323) **(Fig. 9-40c, p. 320)**
  XVIII. **Check interventions.** (p. 323) **(Fig. 9-40d, p. 320)**
   XIX. **Note trends in patient condition.** (p. 323) **(Fig. 9-40e, p. 320)**

SKILLS DEMONSTRATION AND PRACTICE

Using four students to act as patients, demonstrate ongoing assessment for the class. Illustrate responsive and unresponsive trauma patients and responsive and unresponsive medical patients. Tell students that they will now apply what they have learned about ongoing assessment to real-life situations.

Help the rest of the class break into groups of three. If the number of students does not divide equally by three, it is acceptable to have groups of two or four. Tell students that each team is to practice the ongoing assessment skills you have just demonstrated. Instruct them to take turns being the patient, the EMT, and an observer. Also, instruct students that the observer may act as a friend or relative of the patient in scenarios in which the patient is unresponsive.

Give students the location of the four classrooms or areas previously set aside for practice. Direct the first four teams to their first stations and tell them they are to rotate through all the stations, using the scenario posted in each. Remind them to change "role" each time they rotate stations. Advise students to practice performing patient assessments as they wait their turn. Provide blood pressure cuff, stethoscope, and penlights for each group.

Visit each group several times to monitor progress and skill accuracy. Provide assistance, if necessary.

CASE STUDY FOLLOW-UP

Note: The case studies will not be reviewed until the last lesson of this chapter.

IN REVIEW

Note: The Review Questions will not be covered until the last lesson of this chapter.

ASSIGNMENT

If you are treating Part 6 as a separate lesson, direct students to review Chapter 9, Part 6, "Communication and Documentation," before the next class; otherwise begin the lesson for Part 6 now.

Reading/Reference
Textbook, pp. 323–324

EVALUATION

Note: The quiz will not be given until the end of Part 6 of this chapter.

REINFORCEMENT

Reinforcement Handouts are provided for students whose participation in class discussions indicates they have not fully mastered the content of Part 5. You may wish to assign some or all of these handouts to those students.

Handouts 9-5B to 9-5C
Reinforcement Activities

OBJECTIVES CHECKLIST

Cognitive	Date Mastered
3-6.1 Discuss the reasons for repeating the initial assessment as part of the ongoing assessment.	
3-6.2 Describe the components of the ongoing assessment.	
3-6.3 Describe trending of assessment components.	

Affective	Date Mastered
3-6.4 Explain the value of performing an ongoing assessment.	
3-6.5 Recognize and respect the feelings that patients might experience during assessment.	
3-6.6 Explain the value of trending assessment components to other health care professionals who assume care of the patient.	

Psychomotor	Date Mastered
3-6.7 Demonstrate the skills involved in performing the ongoing assessment.	

IN THE FIELD

Read the following real-life situation. Then answer the questions that follow.

It is another busy day at the ambulance service. You and your crew have just returned to the station when the tone sounds again. You are dispatched to a home where a 75-year-old female patient was found to be unresponsive.

The site of the call is a quiet suburban street. A man greets you at the curb. He tells you that he had been working in the garden and just came in for lunch. He called his wife, and when he got no answer, looked for her and found her lying on the sofa. He states that she has been "feeling poorly" for the past week.

The patient is still lying on the sofa in the den when you enter the house. She does not respond to your voice, but pulls away from mild painful stimulation. You note snoring and gurgling respirations. The patient's husband informs you that his wife has a history of allergies and shortness of breath. You notice that the patient is breathing at a rate of 40 breaths per minute, with shallow respirations.

While you are performing the initial assessment, your partner is obtaining the patient's vital signs. He informs you that her blood pressure is within normal limits. The patient's heart rate is 104 beats per minute. Skin is warm, pale, and dry; the pulse ox reading is 92 percent.

1. Is this patient breathing adequately?

2. What initial interventions will you perform?

3. List other ways that the EMTs can find out information regarding this patient.

4. How would you check interventions during the ongoing assessment?

ONGOING ASSESSMENT: LISTING

1. List the five steps of the ongoing assessment.

2. The EMT begins the ongoing assessment by repeating the initial assessment to recheck for life-threatening problems. List the steps in this process.

3. List the things that should always be done when checking interventions.

LECTURE MASTER 9-5

Ongoing Assessment

Repeat the Initial Assessment
Mental Status

Airway

Breathing

Circulation

Patient Priority

Reassess and Record Vital Signs

Repeat Focused Assessment

Check Interventions

Note Trends in Patient Condition

Chapter 9, Part 6: Communication and Documentation

Previews Lessons 3-7 and 3-8 of the U.S. Department of Transportation's EMT-Basic National Standard Curriculum.

Total Teaching Time
Part 6: 85 minutes

OBJECTIVES

The objectives for these skills are listed and covered in detail in Chapter 10, "Communication," and Chapter 11, "Documentation."

REVIEW

In the last lesson, Part 5, "Ongoing Assessment," students learned that a patient's condition can change. There may be a change for the better, for example, an unresponsive patient regains consciousness. Or there may be a change for the worse, for example, a patient who was alert and oriented becomes confused. Therefore, frequent patient reevaluation, using the procedures of the ongoing assessment, is essential.

INTRODUCTION AND DISCUSSION OF PART 6

Part 6, "Communication and Documentation," is the last lesson in Chapter 9. Detailed lecture outlines and Lecture Masters for these topics appear in Chapters 10 and 11. You may wish to preview these materials now. After a brief discussion of this topic, discuss the Review Questions and Case Studies for Chapter 9.

Have students recall that the initial information they receive about their patient comes from dispatch. Point out that EMTs communicate at important points, with dispatch and with medical direction as well as with the staff of the medical facility to which they transport their patient. Explain that clear communication with other EMS personnel, the patient, and others at the scene is crucial. A failure of clear communication—both in what others communicate to them and in what they communicate to others—can have a significant adverse effect on the quality of the assessment and care they and others provide to their patient. In addition, stress that a significant portion of the value of patient assessment and care will be lost if what they have learned about the patient's condition and what care they have given the patient are not clearly and adequately documented in their written reports. Tell students that they will learn about communicating clearly in Chapter 10, "Communication," and that in Chapter 11, "Documentation," they will learn how to correctly document their contacts with and care of patients.

CASE STUDY FOLLOW-UP

Ask a student volunteer to read Case Study "Call One—A Trauma Patient," that begins on page 240 of the textbook. You may wish to use the following questions to engage students in a discussion of the Case Study Follow-up that begins on page 325 in the textbook. Provide missing information and clarify ideas as needed.

Q1. During your scene size-up, how did you know when the scene was safe?

A1. *A police officer provided that information.*

Q2. During your initial assessment, how do you address the life-threatening airway and breathing problems?

A2. *By insertion of an oropharyngeal airway and bag-valve-mask ventilation with supplemental oxygen*

Q3. During your focused history and physical exam, how do you protect the patient's spinal column?

A3. *Through application of a cervical spinal immobilization collar while continuing manual in-line stabilization. With assistance from police First Responders, spinal stabilization is maintained as the patient is log-rolled and the posterior thorax and lumbar region and buttocks are exposed. No additional injuries are revealed. While the patient is still on his side, an Emergency Medical Responder slides the backboard next to the patient and the patient is rolled onto it and secured with straps. A head immobilization device is applied.*

Q4. During your detailed physical exam, what additional problems do you identify?

A4. *A small laceration at the left temporal region of the patient's head.*

Q5. During your ongoing assessment, how often did you take this patient's vital signs.

A5. *Every 5 minutes.*

Ask a student volunteer to read Case Study "Call Two—A Medical Patient," that begins on page 240 in the textbook. You may wish to use the following questions to engage students in a discussion of the Case Study Follow-up that begins on page 326 in the textbook. Provide missing information and clarify ideas as needed.

Q1. During your scene size-up, what led you to conclude that this was a medical problem rather than trauma?

A1. *Dispatch had indicated the problem was a woman who could not catch her breath, and there was an oxygen tank in the corner of the woman's room.*

Q2. During your initial assessment, how do you address Mrs. Ortega's respiratory distress?

A2. *Through application of a nonrebreather mask connected to oxygen flowing at 15 liters per minute.*

Q3. During your focused history and physical exam, what do you learn about Mrs. Ortega's past pertinent history?

A3. *Mrs. Ortega has a history of emphysema, a serious lung disease.*

Q4. Why did you not provide positive pressure ventilation for Mrs. Ortega?

A4. *Because, although her breathing was difficult, it was adequate.*

Q5. During your ongoing assessment, how often do you recheck Mrs. Ortega's vital signs?

A5. *Every 15 minutes, because her condition is stable.*

IN REVIEW

Assess students' ability to apply what they learned in Chapter 9 by discussing the In Review on page 328 in the textbook.

Q1. Briefly state the purposes of patient assessment by the EMT.

A1. *The purposes of patient assessment are the following:*
- *To determine whether the patient is injured or has a medical illness*
- *To identify and manage immediately life-threatening injuries or conditions*
- *To determine priorities for further assessment and care on the scene versus immediate transport with assessment and care continuing en route*
- *To examine the patient and gather a patient history*
- *To provide further emergency care based on findings made during the focused history and physical exam and the detailed exam*
- *To monitor the patient's condition, assessing the effectiveness of the care that has been provided and adjusting care as needed*
- *To communicate patient information to the medical facility staff and to document the details of the call (pp. 242–243)*

Q2. List the main components of patient assessment.

A2. *The main components of patient assessment are scene size-up, initial assessment, focused history and physical exam, detailed physical exam, ongoing assessment, and communication and documentation. (p. 241)*

Q3. List the steps of scene size-up.

A3. *The steps of scene size-up are to take BSI precautions, to evaluate scene hazards and ensure scene safety, to determine the MOI or NOI, to establish number of patients, and to ascertain need for additional resources. (p. 241)*

Q4. List the six steps of the initial assessment.

A4. *The six steps of the initial assessment are the following: Form a general impression of the patient. Assess mental status. Assess the airway. Assess breathing. Assess circulation. Establish patient priorities (p. 243).*

Q5. Contrast the order of the three steps of the focused history and physical exam for a responsive medical patient with the order of the steps for an unresponsive medical patient or trauma patient. Explain why the order of the steps differs.

A5. *For a responsive medical patient, the order of the three steps of the focused history and physical exam is (1) history, (2) focused medical assessment, (3) baseline vital signs (p. 000). For an unresponsive medical patient or a trauma patient, the order is (1) rapid trauma or rapid medical assessment, (2) baseline vital signs, (3) history (pp. 000–000). For a responsive medical patient, information about symptoms provided by the patient is usually more important than information from the physical exam, and it is important to get the patient history early in case the patient loses consciousness later. For an unresponsive medical patient or trauma patient, information from the physical exam is more important. (p. 292)*

Q6. Describe the kinds of patients for whom the physical exam should be a rapid head-to-toe assessment (rapid trauma assessment or rapid medical assessment). Describe the kinds of patients for whom the physical exam should be focused on a specific site or area of complaint.

A6. *A rapid head-to-toe assessment should be performed on trauma patients who have a significant mechanism of injury, multiple injuries, altered mental status, or critical findings, and on unresponsive medical patients. A focused exam should be performed on trauma patients who have no significant mechanism of injury, no multiple injuries, alert and oriented mental status, and no critical findings, and on responsive medical patients. (pp. 263–264, 291–292)*

Q7. Name the five categories of measurements that are included in the vital signs.

A7. *The five categories of measurements that are included in the vital signs are respiration, pulse, skin, pupils, and blood pressure. (pp. 283–285)*

Q8. Name the categories of information sought during history taking that the letters in OPQRST and SAMPLE represent.

A8. *OPQRST stands for onset, provocation, quality, radiation, severity, and time. SAMPLE stands for signs and symptoms, allergies, medications, pertinent past history, last oral intake, and events leading to the present problem. (pp. 286–287, 302–303)*

Q9. Under what circumstances should a detailed physical exam not be performed?

A9. *A detailed physical exam should not be performed if it would interfere with necessary ongoing assessment and care for life-threatening conditions in the critical patient. (pp. 305)*

Q10. State how often, at a minimum, during the ongoing assessment, the components of the initial assessment and the vital signs should be reassessed for the following: (a) a critical or an unstable patient, and (b) a stable patient.

A10. *During ongoing assessment, the components of the initial assessment and the vital signs should be reassessed, at a minimum, (a) every 5 minutes for an unstable patient with critical injuries, and (b) every 15 minutes for a stable patient. (p. 321)*

CRITICAL THINKING

Assess students' ability to respond to real-life emergency situations by discussing the Critical Thinking questions on page 328 in the textbook.

SCENARIO 1

Q1. What would be your first immediate action when you arrive at the patient?

A1. *Based on the mechanism of injury, establishing in-line manual spinal stabilization would be the EMT's first action upon arriving at the patient, followed by immediately suctioning the airway.*

Q2. What assessment should you conduct first?

A2. *The first assessment conducted for this patient would be the* initial assessment. *The initial assessment is conducted to identify and manage immediate life threats to the airway, ventilation, oxygenation, and circulation.*

Q3. What are the components of that assessment and in what order would you perform them?

A3. *Since this is a trauma patient, the steps of the initial assessment would be to form a general impression, determine the likelihood of spinal injury, assess mental status, assess the airway, assess breathing, and assess circulation.*

Q4. What life threats are you assessing for and how would you manage them?

A4. *During the general impression, the EMT is looking for any obvious life threats such as blood or vomitus in the airway, open wounds to the chest, flail segment, or major bleeding. The EMT will then assess the airway to determine if it is patent. The tongue, blood, vomitus, bone, teeth, or any other substance would create a potential airway obstruction. Assess the ventilatory status and determine the rate and depth of respiration. Either an inadequate rate or inadequate tidal volume would be a life threat. Assess the pulses and skin temperature, color, and condition. Evidence of poor perfusion is a life threat. Also, assess for any major bleeding.*

Q5. What injuries should you suspect in this patient?

A5. *Based on the mechanism of injury and the patient's presentation, the EMTs should suspect injuries to the patient's head, spine, possibly internal organs, and definitely at least one extremity.*

Q6. What baseline vital signs would you assess?

A6. *An appropriate set of baseline vitals would include pulse rate, respiratory rate, blood pressure, skin signs, pupil condition, and perhaps a pulse oximeter reading.*

Q7. Would you perform a rapid trauma assessment or a focused physical exam?

A7. *Since the mechanism of this patient's injury is significant, he has an altered mental status, and injuries to multiple body systems and regions is probable, a rapid trauma assessment must be performed to identify and manage any other life threats to the patient.*

Q8. What does the change in his mental status indicate?

A8. *The fact that the patient was initially groaning and speaking to bystanders but is now unresponsive indicates that his condition is deteriorating and that his injuries should be considered critical. The hallmark sign of a head (brain) injury is an altered mental status that does not improve or one that deteriorates. It is likely this patient has suffered a head injury.*

Q9. When would you transport?

A9. *This patient would be considered a high priority and should be transported immediately following the rapid trauma assessment, but only after complete spinal immobilization is done.*

Q10. How would you prepare the patient for transport?

A10. The patient should be fitted with a cervical collar and completely immobilized on a long-spine board. (Due to the critical nature of the patient's injuries, it would not be appropriate to take time to splint the angulated arm separately; however, it should be immobilized next to the patient's body using the spine board securing straps.)

Q11. What would you do while en route to the medical facility?

A11. While en route to the medical facility, the EMT caring for the patient should perform ongoing assessments (including performing any critical interventions and repeating vital signs), and, if there is the opportunity, conduct a detailed physical exam and provide proper care for individual injuries (such as splinting the angulated arm). The EMT should also evaluate the trends highlighted by the ongoing assessment process.

SCENARIO 2

Q1. Do you suspect she is a trauma or medical patient?

A1. Since the daughter's description of events and the patient's appearance don't indicate trauma or injury, she would be considered a medical patient. It is still important during your examination to look for any evidence of trauma to be sure that the patient is truly a medical and not a trauma patient.

Q2. What would be your first immediate action when you arrive at the patient?

A2. The first action for this patient would be to determine her mental status through verbal and then painful stimulus, followed immediately by opening her airway with a head-tilt, chin-lift maneuver.

Q3. What assessment should you conduct first?

A3. The first assessment conducted on this patient would be the initial assessment.

Q4. What are the components of that assessment and in what order would you perform them?

A4. Since this is a medical patient, the steps of the initial assessment would be to form a general impression, correct any obvious life threats, assess mental status, assess the airway, assess breathing, and assess circulation.

Q5. What life threats are you assessing for and how would you manage them?

A5. The life threats that the EMT will be assessing for are an occluded airway, inadequate ventilation, inadequate oxygenation, and inadequate circulation.

Q6. Would you collect a SAMPLE history first or do a medical assessment?

A6. The proper procedure is to complete a rapid medical assessment first followed by obtaining baseline vital signs. Finally, the EMT would attempt to collect a SAMPLE history from the relative.

Q7. Would you perform a rapid medical assessment or a focused medical assessment?

A7. *If the patient has an altered mental status, it is important to perform the rapid medical exam.*

Q8. How would you collect a SAMPLE history?

A8. *Since the patient is unresponsive, the daughter would be the best source for obtaining a SAMPLE history.*

Q9. What does the mental status possibly indicate?

A9. *The unresponsiveness of this medical patient could indicate many things including stroke, a diabetic emergency, intoxication, or hypoxia.*

Q10. What would you expect the SpO$_2$ reading to be?

A10. *Pale, cool, clammy skin is an early indication of hypoxia; whereas cyanosis is a late sign. A pulse oximeter reading of less than 95% indicates a hypoxic state; however, based on this patient's skin findings, it is likely the SpO$_2$ reading is well below 95%.*

Q11. When would you transport?

A11. *Since this patient is unresponsive, the EMTs should transport her as soon as they have completed a rapid medical assessment, obtained baseline vital signs, and questioned the daughter to compile a SAMPLE history. If the daughter is riding along to the hospital, it is also an option to gather the SAMPLE history while en route.*

Q12. How would you prepare the patient for transport?

A12. *The patient should be placed in the recovery (also known as coma or lateral recumbent) position on the wheeled stretcher. If the patient requires positive pressure ventilation, she must be placed in a supine position. It is not possible to deliver effective ventilations with the patient in a lateral position.*

Q13. What would you do while en route to the medical facility?

A13. *While en route to the medical facility, the EMT caring for the patient should perform an ongoing assessment (including performing any critical interventions and repeating vital signs), and, if there is the opportunity, conduct a detailed physical exam. The EMT should also evaluate the trends highlighted by the ongoing assessment process.*

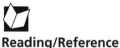

Reading/Reference
Textbook, pp. 329–341

Workbook
Chapter 9 Activities

Handout 9-6A
Chapter 9 Quiz B

TestGen
Chapter 9 Test

ASSIGNMENTS

Assign students to read Chapter 10, "Communication," before the next class. Also ask them to complete Chapter 9 of the Workbook.

EVALUATION

Chapter Quiz Distribute copies of the Chapter Quiz provided in Handout 8-2 to evaluate student understanding of this chapter. Remind students not to refer to their textbooks or notes while taking the quiz.

Test Manager You may wish to create a custom-tailored test using Prentice Hall *TestGen for Prehospital Emergency Care, Eighth Edition* to evaluate student understanding of this chapter.

Online Test Preparation (for students and instructors) Additional test preparation is available through *EMT Achieve: Basic Test Preparation* at http://www.prenhall.com/EMTAchieve. Instructors can also monitor student mastery online.

REINFORCEMENT

Handouts If classroom discussions or performance on the quiz indicates that some students have not fully mastered the chapter content, you may wish to assign some or all of the Reinforcement Handouts for this chapter.

TECH EXTRAS

Brady Skills Series EMT-B Videos/CD Have your students watch the skills come to life on either VHS or CD-ROM.

PowerPoint Presentation (for instructors) The PowerPoint material developed for this chapter offers useful reinforcement of chapter content.

Student CD A wide variety of material on this CD-ROM will reinforce and also expand student knowledge and skills.

Companion Website (for students) Additional review quizzes and links to EMS resources will contribute to further reinforcement of this chapter. Please visit wwwprenhallcom/mistovich.

Online Test Preparation
Send your students to http://www.prenhall.com/ EMTAchieve

Handouts 9-6B to 9-6C
Reinforcement Activities

Brady Skills Series EMT-B Videos/CD
Visual Reinforcement

PowerPoint Presentation
Chapter 9

Student CD
Chapter 9

Companion Website
http://www.prenhall.com/ mistovich

EVALUATION

CHAPTER 9 QUIZ B: PARTS 4–6

Write the letter of the best answer in the space provided.

_____ 1. A detailed physical exam should be performed
  - A. before vital signs are taken.
  - B. before the SAMPLE history.
  - C. only after all life-threatening injuries and conditions have been managed.
  - D. only after approval from medical direction has been received.

_____ 2. The detailed physical exam is most often conducted
  - A. at the scene of the incident.
  - B. in the back of the ambulance en route to the hospital.
  - C. prior to packaging the patient for transport.
  - D. just after packaging the patient for transport.

_____ 3. Which of the following would usually *not* require a detailed physical exam?
  - A. an unresponsive patient
  - B. a patient with multiple injuries
  - C. a patient with a lacerated foot
  - D. a patient with a significant mechanism of injury

_____ 4. When checking for pupillary response during the detailed physical exam, note if both eyes respond equally and simultaneously when a light is shined in one, a response known as
  - A. consensual reflex.
  - B. doll's eyes.
  - C. dysconjugate gaze.
  - D. icterus.

_____ 5. A serious finding during the detailed physical exam is a pulsating mass in the abdomen, which may indicate
  - A. a weakened abdominal aorta.
  - B. progressive appendicitis.
  - C. failure of one or both kidneys.
  - D. liver damage.

_____ 6. For a noncritical patient, the ongoing assessment should be performed every _____ minutes.
  - A. 5
  - B. 10
  - C. 15
  - D. 20

_____ 7. The first step in the ongoing assessment is to
  - A. check interventions.
  - B. reassess and record vital signs.
  - C. repeat the initial assessment.
  - D. repeat the focused assessment.

_____ 8. The chief purposes of the ongoing assessment are to detect any changes in the patient's condition, to identify any missed injuries or conditions, and to
  - A. alert the receiving facility of probable arrival time.
  - B. adjust emergency care as needed.
  - C. fill in any gaps in the SAMPLE history.
  - D. complete packaging of the patient.

_____ **9.** If during the ongoing assessment a patient begins to complain of a symptom not initially identified, the EMT should
    A. inform medical direction and transport immediately.
    B. complete a focused assessment for the area of complaint.
    C. check interventions.
    D. obtain a new set of vital signs.

_____**10.** During the ongoing assessment, the routine in providing emergency care should be
    A. assess, observe, report.
    B. intervene, assess, report.
    C. assess, intervene, reassess.
    D. report, intervene, reassess.

CHAPTER 9 REVIEW B: PARTS 4–6

Write the word or words that best complete each sentence in the space provided.

1. The detailed physical exam is _____ - and _____ - specific.

2. The purpose of the detailed physical exam is to identify all other _____ - _____ _____ and to _____ _____ required for them.

3. The detailed physical exam should be conducted systematically, starting at the _____ .

4. When conducting a detailed physical exam, _____ the injuries as found.

5. Any findings during the detailed physical exam should be _____ and reported to the staff of the receiving facility.

6. To conduct a detailed physical exam, use the techniques of _____ , _____ , and _____ .

7. You can check _____ _____ during the detailed physical exam by asking a patient to say how many fingers you are holding up.

8. The purposes of the ongoing assessment are to determine any _____ in the patient's condition and to _____ the _____ of emergency care.

9. For both the EMT and the hospital staff, it is not only the patient's condition, but also the _____ in the patient's condition that are important.

10. EMTs should perform the ongoing assessment on _____ patients.

PATIENT ASSESSMENT: TRUE OR FALSE

Indicate if the following statements are true or false by writing T or F in the space provided.

_____ **1.** You will perform the initial assessment on every patient after you have finished performing life-saving interventions and, often, after you have done the detailed physical exam.

_____ **2.** Sometimes you may skip the detailed physical exam because you are too busy taking care of life-threatening problems.

_____ **3.** The ongoing assessment must never be skipped except when life-saving interventions prevent doing it.

_____ **4.** In the trauma patient with a significant mechanism of injury, you should obtain a focused history before completing your exam.

_____ **5.** The recording of vital signs should be deferred to the end of the call so that you can focus better on the patient's needs.

_____ **6.** Every responsive medical patient receives a rapid medical assessment.

_____ **7.** When assessing the oxygen delivery system connected to the patient, a good habit to develop is to check the entire path of the oxygen from the tank to the patient.

_____ **8.** The initial assessment is performed only once during patient contact.

_____ **9.** The memory aid, DCAP-BTLS, is used to obtain a patient's past medical history.

_____ **10.** Documenting changes in a patient's condition over time, such as slowing respirations or a rising pulse rate, which may show improvement or deterioration, is known as trending.

HANDOUT 9-2B: In the Field

1. The wife's history of the illness, the patient's chief complaint, age, and physical surroundings would lead an EMT to conclude that an elderly patient has a respiratory problem. Difficulty breathing is a high-priority problem and necessitates a good assessment.

2. The patient's airway is open, but his speech indicates that he is working to breathe. Administer high-concentration oxygen by nonrebreather mask and consider the need to assist him with breathing. Vital signs indicate a high potential for shock, so medical control should be alerted that the patient is ready for immediate transport.

3. The patient needs rapid transport. The patient has difficulty breathing. Although he is responsive, the patient is not following commands. His inability to identify place and time indicates the potential for shock.

HANDOUT 9-2C: Initial Assessment: Listing

1. Form a general impression; assess mental status; assess airway; assess breathing; assess circulation; determine priority.

2. Alert: awake and oriented; Verbal: responds to verbal stimulus; Painful: responds to painful stimuli; Unresponsive: does not respond to any stimulus.

3. Any six of the following: poor general impression; unresponsive; responsive, but not following commands; difficulty breathing; shock; complicated childbirth; chest pain with systolic blood pressure less than 100; uncontrolled bleeding; severe pain anywhere; pulselessness; open chest wound or flail segment; temperature above 104°F; signs of generalized hypothermia; severe allergic reaction; poisoning or overdose of unknown substance.

HANDOUT 9-2D: Initial Assessment: True or False

1. T	4. F	7. F	9. F
2. F	5. T	8. F	10. T
3. F	6. T		

HANDOUT 9-3B: Chapter 9, Quiz A

1. B	6. D	11. C	16. D
2. C	7. A	12. D	17. B
3. A	8. C	13. A	18. D
4. C	9. D	14. B	19. C
5. D	10. A	15. A	20. B

HANDOUT 9-3C: In the Field

1. Was the patient on any medications? Did he take nitroglycerin before EMS arrived? A better understanding of the patient's state when the pain started might have helped.

2. A focused physical exam would be in order using the OPQRST aid (for medical) as well as remembering to check for possible jugular vein distention. Consider a detailed physical exam.

3. Possibly a medical identification device, such as a bracelet or wallet card. They also could have seen if there were any numbers listed near the phone that might help—a doctor's number or that of another family member. Also look for medication bottles to identify potential medical conditions.

HANDOUT 9-3D: Chapter 9, Review A

1. Scene size-up
2. treated immediately
3. general impression
4. chief complaint
5. AVPU scale
6. airway
7. looking, listening, feeling
8. bleeding
9. establishing patient priorities
10. focused history and medical exam
11. trauma
12. focused
13. time, place, person (self)
14. 20–24
15. airway obstruction
16. pulses, motor function, sensation
17. rapid
18. airway, positive pressure ventilation, oxygen
19. SAMPLE, OPQRST
20. 5, 15

HANDOUT 9-3E: Trauma Patient Assessment: Ordering

Order should be reading down: 6, 8, 2, 9, 7, 1, 10, 4, 5, 3

HANDOUT 9-3F: Trauma Patient Assessment: Listing

1. Any six of the following: ejection from vehicle; death in same passenger compartment; falls greater than 15 feet or three times patient's height; rollover of vehicle; high-speed vehicle collision; vehicle–pedestrian collision; motorcycle crash with separation of rider from vehicle; blunt or penetrating trauma resulting in unresponsive or altered mental status; penetrations of the head, neck, chest, or abdomen; blast injuries; seatbelt injuries; impacts causing steering-wheel deformation; prolonged extrication

2. Fall greater than 10 feet, bicycle collision, vehicle collision at medium speed, unrestrained passenger in any vehicle collision

3. Deformities, contusions, abrasions, punctures/penetrations, burns, tenderness, lacerations, swelling

HANDOUT 9-3G: Medical Patient Assessment: Matching

Responsive Medical Patient
Reading down: K, A, E, C, B, I, D
Unresponsive Medical Patient
Reading down: H, C, F, A, J, G, D

HANDOUT 9-3H: Focusing on the Focused History

1.	E	4.	H	7.	F	10.	B
2.	A	5.	J	8.	I	11.	L
3.	G	6.	K	9.	C	12.	D

HANDOUT 9-4B: In the Field

1. Darkness—The fire department lighted the scene. Traffic in road—State police were managing traffic. Uneven slope—The fire department stabilized the vehicle and provided rescue assistance. Possible leaking car fluids—The fire department was available. Body fluids—EMT-Bs have taken body substance isolation precautions.
2. The mechanism of injury is a vehicle rollover, possibly at high speed. This would be significant.
3. After the initial assessment, the EMT correctly decided that this patient was a high-priority patient. The EMT continued manual cervical spine stabilization, requested an ALS intercept, and began a rapid trauma assessment while waiting for the crew to package the patient. The EMT should perform a focused history and physical exam for a trauma patient with a significant mechanism of injury.
4. Given the mechanism of injury, a detailed physical exam would be in order. The rollover could have caused a variety of injuries. Also, the patient is currently stable, which would mean that the EMTs would have the opportunity to perform the assessment during transport.

HANDOUT 9-4C: The Detailed Physical Exam: Ordering

Order should be, reading down: 4, 10, 2, 7, 6, 1, 12, 11, 5, 8, 3, 9

HANDOUT 9-5B: In the Field

1. No. She has gurgling, snoring respirations, a rate much higher than normal, and is breathing shallowly.
2. Complete the initial assessment, ensure that the airway is open and clear, and administer high-flow oxygen.

3. After taking the steps described above, you would complete the other components of patient assessment. If the patient is unable to manage her respirations at any point during the assessment, you would provide positive-pressure ventilations. An airway adjunct such as a nasopharyngeal airway should be inserted. Frequent checks should be made of vital signs during the ongoing assessment.
4. You'd be especially sure to check adequacy of oxygen delivery and ventilations. Check the entire path of oxygen from tank to patient. Check regulator and flowmeter. Look for kinks in tubing. Check that tubing is connected to the mask and that the mask has a good fit. Also continue to monitor pulse oximetry. Good ventilations with oxygen should cause the pulse ox reading to rise.

HANDOUT 9-5C: Ongoing Assessment: Listing

1. Repeat initial assessment; reassess and record vital signs; repeat focused assessment; check interventions; note trends in patient condition.
2. Reassess mental status; reassess airway; reassess breathing; reassess circulation; reestablish patient priorities.
3. Ensure adequacy of oxygen delivery, positive pressure ventilations, bleeding control, CPR or AED, and immobilization.

HANDOUT 9-6A: Chapter 9, Quiz B

1.	C	4.	A	7.	C	9.	B
2.	B	5.	A	8.	B	10.	C
3.	C	6.	C				

HANDOUT 9-6B: Chapter 9, Review B

1. patient, injury
2. life-threatening conditions, provide care
3. head
4. manage (treat)
5. documented
6. inspection, palpation, auscultation
7. visual acuity
8. changes, assess, effectiveness
9. trends (changes)
10. all

HANDOUT 9-6C: Patient Assessment: True or False

1.	F	4.	F	7.	T	9.	F
2.	T	5.	F	8.	F	10.	T
3.	F	6.	F				

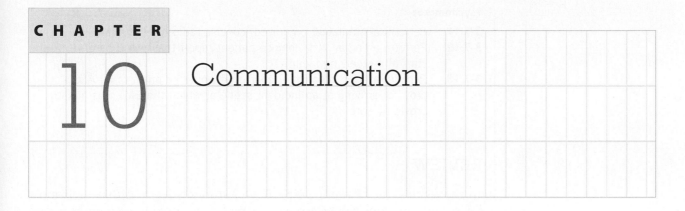

10 Communication

This chapter covers Lesson 3-7 and portions of Lesson 3-9 of the U.S. Department of Transportation's EMT-Basic National Standard Curriculum.

OBJECTIVES

Numbered objectives are from the U.S. Department of Transportation's EMT-Basic National Standard Curriculum. Asterisked objectives, if any, pertain to material that is supplemental to the DOT curriculum. Page numbers refer to pages in the textbook.

Cognitive

3-7.1 List the proper methods of initiating and terminating a radio call. (pp. 333–336)

3-7.2 State the proper sequence for delivery of patient information. (pp. 336–337)

3-7.3 Explain the importance of effective communication of patient information in the verbal report. (pp. 336–337)

3-7.4 Identify the essential components of the verbal report. (p. 337)

3-7.5 Describe the attributes for increasing effectiveness and efficiency of verbal communications. (pp. 336–338)

3-7.6 State legal aspects to consider in verbal communications. (p. 333)

3-7.7 Discuss the communication skills that should be used to interact with the patient. (pp. 337–338)

3-7.8 Discuss the communication skills that should be used to interact with the family, bystanders, and individuals from other agencies while providing patient care and the difference between skills used to interact with the patient and those used to interact with others. (pp. 336–338)

3-7.9 List the correct radio procedures in the following phases of a typical call (pp. 333–337):
— To the scene
— At the scene
— To the facility
— At the facility
— To the station
— At the station

Affective

3-7.10 Explain the rationale for providing efficient and effective radio communications and patient reports. (p. 339)

Total Teaching Time
180 minutes

Resources Needed
- Scored Chapter 10 Quizzes
- Portable two-way radio and a desktop two-way radio or cellular phone and desktop phone with speaker
- Inexpensive items such as pens or penlights for prizes

Additional Resources
Larmon/Davis, *Basic Life Support Skills*

Elling, *EMT Achieve: Basic Test Preparation*

Limmer/Mistovich/O'Keefe, *Audio Lecture & Study Guide: EMT*

Mistovich/Kuvlesky, *SUCCESS! for the EMT, Second Edition*

Psychomotor

3-7.11   Perform a simulated, organized, concise radio transmission.

3-7.12   Perform an organized, concise patient report that would be given to the staff at a receiving facility.

3-7.13   Perform a brief, organized report that would be given to an ALS provider arriving at an incident scene at which the EMT was already providing care.

REVIEW

In the last lesson, "Patient Assessment," students learned that their most important functions will be assessing patients and providing emergency care and transport to a medical facility. Of these functions, performing an accurate and reliable assessment is the most important because all their decisions about care and transport will be based on assessment findings. Emphasize how important it is for them to develop a systematic assessment routine. This will ensure that they assess every patient consistently and appropriately, based on the patient's nature of illness or mechanism of injury.

Distribute the scored quizzes from the last class. Go over each question on the quiz and handle any concerns students may have about the answers.

INTRODUCTION TO CHAPTER 10

Chapter 10, "Communication," is the third chapter in Module 3, "Patient Assessment." Tell students that the job of ambulance crews has evolved from simply transporting patients to hospitals to include administering certain medications and performing procedures such as defibrillation. The responsibilities of ambulance crews are now more complex. Medical knowledge, too, has grown over the years and with it the increasing recognition that time is often a critical factor in aiding patients in emergencies.

Reliable communications systems are an essential part of EMS today. They permit EMTs to reach their patients more quickly and allow hospitals to prepare appropriately for the arrival of those patients. They also link EMTs in the field with doctors, enabling the EMTs to provide more lifesaving services than ever through contact with medical direction. Stress to students the importance of communicating well with their patients and about them to other medical professionals. Good communications skills and the ability to use sophisticated communications equipment are essential for the EMT—and they may be key in saving a life.

Distribute the Chapter 10 Objectives Checklist and give students a few minutes to look it over. Then briefly paraphrase the objectives for this lesson in your own words.

LECTURE

The following suggested lecture outline is based on the Department of Transportation's EMT-Basic National Standard Curriculum. In some places, the DOT curriculum has been rearranged or expanded upon so that it is more complete or easier for the student to understand. The page numbers in

Handout 10-1
Chapter 10 Objectives Checklist

Lecture Master
You may wish to display Lecture Master 10 when presenting the lecture to the class.

parentheses refer to pages in the textbook. The parenthetical references in dark, heavy type are to figures, tables, and scans in the textbook.

COMMUNICATION

I. Components of an emergency communications system (pp. 331–333)
  A. Base station (p. 331)
    1. Radio located at a stationary site **(Fig. 10-1, p. 331)**
  B. Mobile transmitter/receiver (radio) (p. 331) **(Fig. 10-2, p. 331)**
    1. Implies a vehicular mounted device
    2. Usually transmits at lower power than base stations (typically 20–50 watts).
    3. Typical transmission range is 10–15 miles over average terrain.
  C. Portable transmitter/receivers (radio) (pp. 331–332) **(Fig. 10-3, p. 331)**
    1. Implies a handheld device
    2. Typically has power output of 1–5 watts, limiting their range
  D. Repeater (p. 332)
    1. Receives a transmission from a low-power portable or mobile radio on one frequency and retransmits at a higher power on another frequency **(Fig. 10-4, p. 332)**
  E. Digital equipment (p. 332)
    1. Mobile data terminal
  F. Cellular telephones (pp. 332–333) **(Fig. 10-5, p. 333)**
  G. Broadcast regulations (p. 333)
    1. Federal Communications Commission (FCC)
      a. Assigns radio frequencies
      b. Licenses and regulates radio operations
  H. System maintenance (p. 333)
    1. Checked periodically.
    2. Technology changes.
    3. Backup system.
II. Communications within the EMS system (pp. 333–337) **(Fig. 10-6, p. 334)**
  A. Ground rules for radio communication (pp. 333–334)
    1. Turn on the radio and select the correct frequency.
    2. Use EMS frequencies only for EMS communication.
    3. Reduce background noise.
    4. Listen before transmitting.
    5. Push the "press to talk" (PTT) button and wait one second before speaking.
    6. Speak with your lips about 2–3 inches from the microphone. **(Fig. 10-7, p. 334)**
    7. Speak calmly and slowly.
    8. Address the unit being called by its name and number, then identify your unit.
    9. The unit being called will signal for you to begin transmission by saying "go ahead" or whatever is the standard in your system.
    10. If the unit being called responds with "stand by," wait to transmit until further notice.
    11. Keep transmissions brief.

On the Net
For more on portable radio systems, go to: www.wassociates.com

On the Net
For the latest information from the FCC, go to: www.fcc.gov

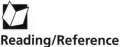

Reading/Reference
"EMS Magazine's Resource Guide: Communications Technologies," *EMS Magazine,* Apr. 2005.

Reading/Reference
Rooker, N., & Jaskoll, S., "Is ICE as Simple as It Sounds?", *EMS Magazine,* Sep. 2005.

Reading/Reference
Careless, J., "The Importance of Rural E9-1-1." *EMS Magazine,* Apr. 2005.

      a. If a transmission should take more than 30 seconds, pause for a few seconds to allow other units the chance to use the frequency for emergency transmissions.

12. Keep your transmission organized and to the point.

13. Use plain English, avoiding slang and meaningless phrases such as "Be advised."

14. Courtesy is assumed, so there is no need to say "Please," "Thank you," or "You're welcome."

15. Also avoid codes and abbreviations unless their use is an accepted part of your system's communications.

16. When transmitting a number that might be confused with another (13 might be heard as 30), say the number ("thirteen"), then the individual digits that make it up ("one-three").

17. Avoid offering a diagnosis. Give only the objective and relevant subjective information that you have gathered in your assessment.

18. When receiving orders or information from dispatch, medical direction, or other medical personnel, use the "echo" method.

      a. Immediately repeat the order word for word.

19. Always write down important information, such as addresses, orders to assist with medication, and so forth that you receive from other parts of the EMS system.

20. The airwaves are public, and scanners can pick up radio and cellular phone messages.

      a. Protect your patient's privacy by not using his name in your transmissions.

      b. Use objective, impartial language in describing the patient's condition.

      c. Do not make personalized or profane comments about the patient or his condition; such statements could be grounds for a slander suit.

21. Use "we" rather than "I" in your transmissions; an EMT rarely acts alone.

22. Use "affirmative" and "negative" rather than "yes" and "no" in transmissions.

23. When you are finished, say "Over." Wait for confirmation that the other unit has received your message and does not need to have anything repeated.

B. Communicating with dispatch (p. 335)

  1. Public Safety Answering Point (PSAP)

  2. Emergency Medical Dispatcher (EMD)

  3. General communication points

      a. Acknowledge the dispatch information

      b. Estimate your time of arrival at the scene while en route and report any special road conditions, unusual delays, etc.

      c. Arrival on the scene

      d. Request any needed additional resources, then help coordinate the response.

      e. In some systems, the unit must also report when they reach the patient after arriving on the scene.

      f. Departure and the destination hospital, number of patients transported (if more than one), and estimated time of arrival at the hospital

g. Arrival at the hospital or another facility

h. Available for another assignment

i. Arrival back at base

C. Communication with medical direction or receiving facility (pp. 335–336)

  1. Basic information

    a. Your unit's identification and its level of service

    b. The patient's age and sex

    c. The patient's chief complaint

    d. A brief, pertinent history of the present illness, including scene assessment and mechanism of injury

    e. Major past illnesses

    f. The patient's mental status

    g. The patient's baseline vital signs

    h. Pertinent findings of your physical examination of the patient

    i. Description of the emergency medical care you (and EMRs) have given the patient

    j. The patient's response to the emergency medical care

    k. Your estimated time of arrival at the facility

  2. Additional guidelines

    a. Be sure that the information you provide to medical direction is accurate and that you report it in a clear, understandable way.

    b. After receiving an order from medical direction to administer a medication or follow a procedure with a patient, repeat the order back word for word. This applies to things that medical direction tells you *not* to do, as well.

    c. If you do not understand an order from medical direction, ask that it be repeated. Then repeat it back to medical direction word for word.

    d. If an order from medical direction appears to be inappropriate, question the order.

      (1) Possibly medical direction misunderstood something in your description of the patient's condition or misspoke in prescribing a course of action.

      (2) Asking questions may prevent the administration of a harmful medication or the application of an inappropriate procedure.

    e. After giving this information, the EMT will continue to assess the patient.

      (1) Additional vital signs may be taken and new information may become available, particularly on long transports.

      (2) In some systems, this information should be relayed to the hospital.

      (3) Information that must be transmitted includes deterioration in the patient's condition.

D. Oral communication (pp. 336–337) **(Fig. 10-8, p. 336)**

  1. After arrival at the hospital, give an oral report to the staff.

    a. Introduce the patient by name (if known).

    b. Summarize the information given over the radio.

      (1) Chief complaint

      (2) History that was not given previously

Point of Interest

Studies have shown a certain degree of inaccuracy in prehospital ETAs. Tell students to think about the trip before giving an estimated time of arrival.

Teaching Tip

Bring a scanner into class. Let students listen to the local EMS frequency and evaluate the various communications they hear.

☑

Teaching Tip

Pass out copies of service run reports (being careful to maintain patient confidentiality). Give the students a few minutes to study them and then give oral reports based on the information provided.

(3) Additional treatment given en route

(4) Additional vital signs taken en route

  c. Give additional information that was collected but not transmitted.

III. Interpersonal communication (pp. 337–338) **(Fig. 10-9, p. 338)**

  A. Communicating with patients (pp. 337–338)

    1. Introduce yourself.

    2. Ask for the patient's name. Also ask what he wishes to be called.

    3. Remember to continue to use the patient's name throughout your contact.

    4. Be sure to say also, "I'm going to help you. Is that all right?"

      a. Don't be surprised if a patient says, "No!" or "I'm okay!" when you ask about providing assistance. Usually he will be responding out of denial because he is simply frightened or confused.

    5. Maintain eye contact when you are speaking with the patient.

      a. In some cultures, direct eye contact is considered rude.

      b. Modify your behavior if you note that a patient is reluctant to make eye contact.

    6. Speak calmly, slowly, and distinctly.

    7. Use language an average person will understand rather than using medical terminology, codes, and abbreviations.

    8. Think about the position you assume in relation to the patient.

      a. If your eye level is above that of the patient, you are in a dominant position, denoting authority and control.

    9. Be courteous.

    10. Explain what you are doing.

    11. Be honest.

    12. Listen when a patient asks you questions and reply as fully as you can, explaining when you cannot answer a question.

      a. Give the patient time to answer a question before you ask another one.

    13. Be sensitive to the power of touch.

  B. Communication with hearing impaired (p. 338)

    1. Lip reading

    2. American Sign Language (ASL)

    3. Write notes

    4. Interpreter

  C. Communication with, non-English-speaking populations (p. 338)

    1. Interpreter

    2. Toll-free interpreter services

  D. Communication with elderly (p. 338)

    1. Take extra time

    2. Potential for visual deficit

    3. Potential for auditory deficit

  E. Communication with children (p. 338)

    1. Parent/caregiver presence

    2. Remain calm and confident

    3. Position at eye level

    4. Explain what you are doing in terms they can understand

ENRICHMENT (OPTIONAL)

The following sections contain information that is valuable as background for the EMT, but that goes substantially beyond the U.S. Department of Transportation's EMT-Basic National Standard Curriculum.

IV. Radio Codes (p. 339)
  A. Some EMS systems use radio codes, such as the Ten-Code system. (p. 339)
  B. Advantages (p. 339)
   1. Shorten radio air time
   2. Provide clear and concise information
   3. Information not understood by the patient, family members, or bystanders
  C. Disadvantages (p. 339)
   1. Useless unless everyone in the system understands them
   2. Medical information is often too complex for codes.
   3. Valuable time may be wasted looking up a code's meaning.

V. Times (p. 339)
  A. Use of military time (p. 339)
   1. 1:00 A.M. to 12 Noon = 0100 to 1200 hours
   2. 1:00 P.M. to Midnight = 1300 to 2400 hours
   3. Aids in keeping of accurate and synchronous clocks by EMTs.

VI. Radio terms (p. 339)
  A. Radio conversations can be shortened by the use of one- or two-word phrases that are universally understood and employed. (p. 339)
  B. Frequently used radio terms (p. 339)
   1. Break
      a. Afford a "pause" so that the hospital can respond or interrupt, if necessary
   2. Clear
      a. End of transmission
   3. Come in
      a. Requesting acknowledgment of transmission
   4. Copy
      a. Message received and understood
   5. ETA
      a. Estimated time of arrival
   6. Go ahead
      a. Proceed with your message
   7. Landline
      a. Refers to telephone communications
   8. Over
      a. End of message, awaiting reply
   9. Repeat/say again
      a. Did not understand message
   10. Spell out
      a. Asking sender to spell out phonetically words that are unclear
   11. Stand by
      a. Please wait
   12. 10-4
      a. Acknowledging that message is received and understood

CASE STUDY FOLLOW-UP

Ask a student volunteer to read the Case Study that begins on page 330 of the textbook. You may wish to use the following questions to engage students in a discussion of the Case Study Follow-up that begins on page 340 of the textbook. Provide missing information and clarify ideas as needed.

Q1. What does your partner say to acknowledge the initial call from dispatch and what additional information does he request?

A1. *"Dispatch, this is Unit 2. We copy and are responding to (the address). Our ETA is 10 minutes. Do you have any more information on the nature of the problem? Over."*

Q2. What does your partner say to dispatch when you arrive at the scene and how does dispatch respond?

A2. *Your partner radios, "Unit 2 to dispatch. We are on the scene at 101 Bate Road." Dispatch responds, "Unit 2 on the scene at 1137 hours."*

Q3. How do you enhance communication with the patient?

A3. *You introduce yourselves to Mr. Behrens.*

Q4. Describe the medical radio report that your partner gave.

A4. *"Columbia Memorial, this is Craryville BLS Unit 2 en route to you with an ETA of 10 minutes. We have a 46-year-old male with a 3-inch laceration of the right hand caused by a Sabre saw. The patient is alert and oriented. The patient says he is allergic to penicillin. His vital signs are blood pressure 146/84, radial pulse 80, respirations 14 and of good quality, skin normal, warm, and moist. We have dressed and bandaged the wound. Bleeding appears to have stopped and patient acknowledges only slight pain from the wound."*

Q5. Describe the oral report your partner gave to the emergency department nurse to whom you transferred the patient.

A5. *"This is Mr. David Behrens. He has a 3-inch laceration to the palm of his right hand from a Sabre saw. Mr. Behrens is allergic to penicillin. We applied a dressing and bandages to the wound, and the bleeding appears to have stopped completely. His vitals are blood pressure 144/82, pulse 80, respirations 14, skin normal."*

IN REVIEW

Assess students' ability to apply what they have just learned by discussing the Review Questions on page 341 in the textbook.

Q1. List the standard components of an EMS communications system.

A1. *The standard components of an EMS communications system are base station, mobile transmitter/receivers, portable transmitter/receivers, repeaters; also cellular phones, encoders, decoders. (pp. 331–333)*

Q2. Explain the function of a repeater.

A2. *The repeater receives transmissions from relatively low-powered elements of a communications system such as mobile or portable transmitters and rebroadcasts them at a higher frequency and power to make coverage of a wide geographical area possible. (p. 332)*

©2008 by Pearson Education, Inc.
Prehospital Emergency Care, 8th ed.

Q3. Explain legal considerations that apply to EMS communications.

A3. *Legal considerations that apply to EMS communications include the following: FCC licenses base station operations, assigns radio call signs, approves equipment, establishes limitations for transmitters, and monitors field operations. FCC also sets regulations to limit interference with emergency radio broadcasts and to bar the use of obscenity and profanity in broadcasts. (pp. 333–334)*

Q4. List the points at which EMTs on a run are expected to communicate with dispatch.

A4. *The points at which EMTs on a run are expected to communicate with dispatch are to acknowledge initial dispatch information, to estimate ETA and any special circumstances affecting it, to announce arrival at the scene and call for additional help if necessary, to announce departure to and ETA at the receiving facility, to announce arrival at the receiving facility, to announce availability for another assignment, and to announce arrival at home base. (p. 335)*

Q5. Explain the procedure that should be followed when medical direction orders an EMT to administer a medication or follow a designated procedure with a patient.

A5. *The procedure that should be followed when medical direction orders an EMT to administer a medication or follow a designated procedure with a patient is as follows: The EMT should follow the "echo" procedure, repeating the order back to medical direction word for word. If the order is not understood, the EMT should ask medical direction to repeat it, then repeat it back to direction word for word. Orders that appear inappropriate should be questioned. (pp. 335–336)*

Q6. List the information that the EMT should provide to the receiving facility while en route with the patient.

A6. *The information that the EMT should provide to the receiving facility while en route with the patient is the EMT's unit identification and level of service, patient's age and sex, chief complaint, pertinent history including scene assessment and mechanism of injury, major past illnesses, patient's mental status, baseline vital signs, pertinent findings of the physical exam, description of emergency care to patient, patient's response to care, and ETA. (p. 336)*

Q7. List the information the EMT is expected to provide in the oral report when turning a patient over to a receiving facility.

A7. *The information the EMT is expected to provide in the oral report when turning a patient over to a receiving facility is the patient's chief complaint, vital signs taken en route, treatment given and response to it, and pertinent history not included in the earlier radio report. (p. 336–337)*

Q8. Explain the importance of eye contact with a patient.

A8. *Eye contact communicates interest and concern and also prepares the way for entry into the patient's "personal space" so that touching of the patient is not perceived as encroachment. An EMT should remain alert to the fact that in some cultures eye contact is considered rude and should be prepared to modify his or her behavior when dealing with people of such cultures. (p. 337)*

Q9. Explain the possible effects on communication with a patient of (a) the EMT's body position and (b) touch.

A9. *(a) The effects of body position may include the following: A position in which the EMT's eye level is above the patient's denotes authority and control; while this may be effective with hostile or aggressive patients, others may find that position intimidating and be more open to communication with the EMT when he or she is at or below their eye level. (b) Touching (taking a hand, patting a shoulder, laying a hand on a forearm) can provide comfort to the patient. (p. 338)*

Q10. Explain what measures an EMT might take when trying to communicate with a patient who is deaf or hearing impaired.

A10. *Measures an EMT might take when trying to communicate with a patient who is deaf or hearing impaired include positioning himself so that his lips are visible to the patient; speaking more loudly, but clearly and distinctly; determining if the patient uses ASL and asking relatives or bystanders to serve as interpreter; considering writing notes on a pad. (p. 338)*

CRITICAL THINKING

Assess students' ability to respond to real-life emergency situations by discussing the Critical Thinking questions on page 341 in the textbook.

Q1. What techniques would you use to communicate with this patient?

A1. *Although many answers would be correct, the three Cs of interpersonal communication (competence, confidence, and compassion) would be the best techniques to keep in mind for communicating with this patient.*

Q2. Are there any special circumstances that you would consider when communicating with this patient?

A2. *This patient does not appear to have any special circumstances which may hinder effective communication.*

Q3. Would you contact medical direction during your management of this patient?

A3. *Based on the deterioration of the patient's mental status and general condition, it would be appropriate to consult with medical direction about the situation. The EMTs may be given specific care instructions or even be diverted to a more appropriate receiving facility.*

Q4. What information is important to relay in the radio report to the receiving medical facility?

A4. *All radio reports to receiving facilities for medical patients should contain the following information: the unit's identification and level of service; the patient's sex, age, and chief complaint; the pertinent history of the present illness; any major past illnesses; the patient's mental status; baseline vital signs; any physical examination findings; any emergency medical care provided (as well as the patient's response to that care); and an accurate estimated time of arrival at the facility.*

Q5. What information would you provide in your oral report to the medical personnel at the receiving medical facility during the transfer of care?

A5. *While physically transferring care of the patient to the receiving facility staff, the EMT should summarize the information provided in the original radio report and include any updates or changes found during the ongoing assessment. Any pertinent history not already provided should also be included in the oral report.*

Q6. What information would you report regarding the change in the patient's condition?

A6. *In this situation, it is critical that the receiving facility be notified of the deterioration of the patient's mental status as well as the changes in each vital sign.*

MEDICAL RADIO REPORT CONTEST

Provide students with the opportunity to apply what they have just learned to a real-life situation. Challenge them to a contest to see who can deliver the best medical radio report. You will need a radio for each student-contestant to take into the hall and a receiver for the classroom—the "base station."

Begin the contest by directing students to review the case history of the two patients discussed in the Chapter 9 Case Studies: the unresponsive trauma patient or the responsive medical patient. (Refer students to page 240 of their textbooks.) Have students reach a consensus on which of these patients they would like to use for the contest. After students have selected the patient, instruct them to compose a medical radio report about the patient. Remind them that they will not have time to write a word-for-word medical radio report in the field. Encourage them to write a few brief notes using key phrases that will help them organize their reports. Set a 5-minute time limit to force students to work quickly.

Before students begin working, pass a box with small strips of paper among students. Direct students to each take a strip, write his or her name on it, and place it in the box as it is passed among them once again. When the 5 minutes are up, take a name from the box and announce the name of the first "contestant" to give his or her report. (Do the same to determine each contestant's turn.) Hand the radio to the first student-contestant. Before the student leaves the classroom, tell him or her that you will be taking the part of the physician or nurse in the emergency department communicating to the EMT en route to the hospital.

As each report is given, have students write the name of the reporter on a sheet of paper. Direct them to take notes that answer these two questions: (1) What were the strengths of this report? (2) How could the report have been improved? Explain that these notes will be used as feedback when all students have given their reports.

When everyone has delivered his or her report, call on the class to provide constructive feedback on a person-to-person basis. Then ask students to write on a small piece of paper the name of the student who delivered the best report. Tally the votes and declare the person with the most votes the winner. If the first vote results in a tie, hold a run-off vote among the individuals who tied.

Provide the winning student with a prize such as a pen or penlight.

Reading/Reference
Textbook, pp. 342–359

Workbook
Chapter 10 Activities

Chapter Quiz
Handout 10-2

TestGen
Chapter 10 Test

Online Test Preparation
Send your students to
http://www.prenhall.com/
EMTAchieve

Handouts 10-3 to 10-7
Reinforcement Activities

**Brady Skills Series
EMT-B Videos/CD**
Visual Reinforcement

**PowerPoint
Presentation**
Chapter 10

Student CD
Chapter 10

Companion Website
http://www.prenhall.com/
mistovich

ASSIGNMENTS

Assign students to read Chapter 11, "Documentation," before the next class. Also ask them to complete Chapter 10 of the Workbook.

EVALUATION

Chapter Quiz Distribute copies of the Chapter Quiz provided in Handout 10-2 to evaluate student understanding of this chapter. Remind students not to refer to their textbooks or notes while taking the quiz.

Test Manager You may wish to create a custom-tailored test using Prentice Hall *TestGen for Prehospital Emergency Care, Eighth Edition* to evaluate student understanding of this chapter.

Online Test Preparation (for students and instructors) Additional test preparation is available through *EMT Achieve: Basic Test Preparation* at http://www.prenhall.com/EMTAchieve. Instructors can also monitor student mastery online.

REINFORCEMENT

Handouts If classroom discussions or performance on the quiz indicates that some students have not fully mastered the chapter content, you may wish to assign some or all of the Reinforcement Handouts for this chapter.

TECH EXTRAS

Brady Skills Series EMT-B Videos/CD Have your students watch the skills come to life on either VHS or CD-ROM.

PowerPoint Presentation (for instructors) The PowerPoint material developed for this chapter offers useful reinforcement of chapter content.

Student CD A wide variety of material on this CD-ROM will reinforce and also expand student knowledge and skills.

Companion Website (for students) Additional review quizzes and links to EMS resources will contribute to further reinforcement of this chapter. Please visit http://www.prenhall.com/mistovich.

OBJECTIVES CHECKLIST

Cognitive		Date Mastered
3-7.1	List the proper methods of initiating and terminating a radio call.	
3-7.2	State the proper sequence for delivery of patient information.	
3-7.3	Explain the importance of effective communication of patient information in the verbal report.	
3-7.4	Identify the essential components of the verbal report.	
3-7.5	Describe the attributes for increasing effectiveness and efficiency of verbal communications.	
3-7.6	State legal aspects to consider in verbal communications.	
3-7.7	Discuss the communication skills that should be used to interact with the patient.	
3-7.8	Discuss the communication skills that should be used to interact with the family, bystanders, and individuals from other agencies while providing patient care and the difference between skills used to interact with the patient and those used to interact with others.	
3-7.9	List the correct radio procedures in the following phases of a typical call: — To the scene — At the scene — To the facility — At the facility — To the station — At the station	

Affective		Date Mastered
3-7.10	Explain the rationale for providing efficient and effective radio communications and patient reports.	

Psychomotor		Date Mastered
3-7.11	Perform a simulated, organized, concise radio transmission.	
3-7.12	Perform an organized, concise patient report that would be given to the staff at a receiving facility.	
3-7.13	Perform a brief, organized report that would be given to an ALS provider arriving at an incident scene at which the EMT was already providing care.	

EVALUATION

CHAPTER 10 QUIZ

Write the letter of the best answer in the space provided.

_____ 1. The initial communication with EMTs about an emergency call is the
   A. hospital radio report.   **C.** dispatch report.
   B. verbal report.   **D.** consult with medical direction.

_____ 2. The two-way radio located at a hospital or dispatch center is a
   A. mobile radio.   **C.** digital radio.
   B. repeater.   **D.** base station.

_____ 3. All of the following patient data should be included in a radio medical report *except*
   A. name and address.   **C.** mental status.
   B. age and sex.   **D.** chief complaint.

_____ 4. The federal agency that assigns and licenses radio frequencies used by EMS units is the
   A. FDA.   **C.** FCC.
   B. HUD.   **D.** DOT.

_____ 5. If an order from medical direction appears to be inappropriate, the EMT should
   A. ignore it.
   B. follow it exactly.
   C. alter the part that appears inappropriate.
   D. question it.

_____ 6. The principles of radio communication encourage transmissions that make use of
   A. codes or slang.   **C.** plain English.
   B. courtesies such as "thank you."   **D.** phrases such as "be advised."

_____ 7. To keep emergency frequencies open, an EMT should pause for several seconds if a transmission takes longer than
   A. 1 minute.   **C.** 2 minutes.
   B. 30 seconds.   **D.** 15 seconds.

_____ 8. To help calm a patient, an EMT should
   A. speak in medical terms.   **C.** use a patient's first name.
   B. explain all procedures.   **D.** downplay expected pain.

_____ 9. In assessing a child, an EMT should
   A. keep the truth from the child.   **C.** ask the parents to leave.
   B. crouch at the child's level.   **D.** stand above the child.

_____ 10. If an on-line physician orders medication, an EMT should
   A. administer it immediately.
   B. repeat back the order word for word.
   C. accept the order without question.
   D. respond "order received."

IN THE FIELD

Review the following real-life situation. Then answer the questions that follow.

The Emergency Medical Dispatcher sends you and your EMT partner to 37 Anne Drive, where a 49-year-old male is complaining of a crushing pain in his chest.

Upon arrival at the house, you and your partner do a quick scene size-up. The man's daughter introduces herself and leads you into the garage. Here you see her father sitting on the floor with his fist clutched to his chest.

Taking BSI precautions, you and your partner put on gloves. After introducing yourself, you crouch down to eye level with the man and ask him his name and age.

"I'm Anthony Cohen," he replies. "I'm 49, but feel like 100. Am I having a heart attack?"

You tell Mr. Cohen that you cannot make a diagnosis but will relay a description of his condition to medical personnel at the hospital. You listen carefully as Mr. Cohen describes his chief complaint, writing down notes as he speaks.

You now begin the initial assessment. You observe that Mr. Cohen is awake and alert and that his airway is open. However, he appears to be splinting his chest wall. His breathing is rapid and shallow. Your partner immediately administers oxygen while you continue the assessment.

As you start to collect vital signs, your partner obtains a history of the present illness as well as a SAMPLE history. She tells Mr. Cohen the purpose of her questions. She also says, "While we talk, my partner will be checking your vital signs—things like your pulse rate."

You record the following vital signs: blood pressure at 160/100, regular and bounding pulse, a pulse rate of 120 beats per minute, breathing at 28 breaths per minute, skin pale and moist, pulse ox of 98 percent.

With Mr. Cohen reporting no prior history of heart problems, you and your partner elect to package him for immediate transport. You request a paramedic intercept en route to the hospital.

1. What aspects of good interpersonal communication are demonstrated in this scenario?

2. What information would you include in a 30-second report to the receiving facility?

CHAPTER 10 REVIEW

Write the word or words that best complete each sentence in the space provided.

1. A(n) _____ _____ is a fixed site that serves as a dispatch and coordination area.

2. A(n) _____ breaks down sound into digital codes while a(n) _____ responds only to those codes.

3. A handheld _____ _____ allows EMTs to be in touch with the members of the EMS while they are away from the ambulance.

4. In the event of power failure or malfunction, EMS systems should have _____ _____ available.

5. The _____ _____ _____ is the agency of the federal government that assigns and licenses radio communications.

6. After receiving an order from medical direction to administer medication, the EMT should _____ _____ _____ word for word.

7. The EMT must communicate with partners and patients plus EMS _____, _____ _____, and medical personnel at the receiving facility.

8. At the conclusion of a call, the EMTs should notify _____ of their return to the station.

9. When caring for a patient with a hearing loss, be sure that your _____ are visible or see if relatives can _____ using American Sign Language.

10. The EMT should never use the patient's _____ in radio transmissions.

COMMUNICATION: MATCHING

Write the letter of the term in the space provided next to the appropriate description.

_____ **1.** A handheld, two-way radio

_____ **2.** Federal agency that assigns and licenses radio frequencies

_____ **3.** A two-way radio mounted on a vehicle

_____ **4.** A unit of measurement for radio output

_____ **5.** A type of portable phone

_____ **6.** A two-way radio at a fixed site, such as a hospital

_____ **7.** A member of the EMS system who receives the initial call for help

_____ **8.** Patient information sent while en route to the hospital

_____ **9.** A device that picks up radio signals from lower-power units

_____ **10.** Patient information given at the hospital

A. base station

B. cellular phone

C. mobile radio

D. portable radio

E. radio report

F. repeater

G. oral report

H. watt

I. FCC

J. EMD

REINFORCEMENT

COMMUNICATION: TRUE OR FALSE

Indicate if the following statements are true or false by writing T or F in the space provided.

_____ **1.** A base station is affixed to an EMS vehicle.

_____ **2.** Wireless communications include radios and cellular telephones.

_____ **3.** The Department of Transportation (DOT) licenses radio frequencies used by EMS agencies.

_____ **4.** The patient's name is included in the radio report.

_____ **5.** The opening statement of every radio report transmits the unit identification.

_____ **6.** Requests for further orders usually come at the end of the radio report.

_____ **7.** An EMT should never question the medications prescribed by an on-line physician.

_____ **8.** Patients from some cultures may consider it impolite to make direct eye contact.

_____ **9.** Standing over a patient enhances the EMT's ability to gather patient information.

_____ **10.** Use of a patient's first name will usually put him or her at ease.

ORGANIZING A RADIO REPORT

Place the following parts of a radio report in correct order of delivery. Write 1 by the first event to be given in the report, 2 by the second event, and so on.

_____ **A.** "The patient has a laceration to the scalp."

_____ **B.** "Our ETA at your location is 5 minutes."

_____ **C.** "Our trauma patient is a 28-year-old male."

_____ **D.** "Respirations are 14, pulse is 100, and BP is 180/90."

_____ **E.** "Medical Center, this is Rescue One."

_____ **F.** "We have administered oxygen and applied a dressing."

_____ **G.** "The patient responds to verbal stimuli."

_____ **H.** "He denies any past medical history."

_____ **I.** "The patient is complaining of a headache."

_____ **J.** "The patient is more responsive after oxygen."

_____ **K.** "The crash was a car versus a pole; estimated speed 45 miles per hour."

LECTURE MASTER 10

Communication

Components
Base Station
Mobile Transmitters/Receivers
Portable Transmitters/Receivers
Repeaters
Digital Equipment
Cellular Phones
Broadcast Regulations
System Maintenance

Communications within the System
Ground Rules
Dispatch
Medical Personnel

Interpersonal Communications
Taking Charge
Communicating with the Patient
Special Considerations

Enrichment
Radio Codes
Times
Radio Terms

HANDOUT 10-2: Chapter 10 Quiz

1. C	**4.** C	**7.** B	**9.** B
2. D	**5.** D	**8.** B	**10.** B
3. A	**6.** C		

HANDOUT 10-3: In the Field

1. The EMT introduces himself and crouches at the patient's level to make eye contact. The EMTs do not guess at a diagnosis, but they do make every effort to provide as much information about procedures as possible.

2. Sample report: This is Community Ambulance to Medic One. We have a 49-year-old male who is complaining of crushing chest pain. He was working in the garage when the pain started. He denies any medical history. At present, the patient is conscious and alert, with shallow respirations at 28, a radial pulse at 120, blood pressure at 160/100, and skin pale and moist. His pupils are dilated, but reactive. Pulse ox of 98 percent. We have administered oxygen, and his chest discomfort has eased. Our ETA is approximately 7 minutes.

HANDOUT 10-4: Chapter 10 Review

1. base station
2. encoder, decoder
3. portable radio (cellular telephone)
4. backup radios (emergency generator)
5. Federal Communications Commission (FCC)
6. repeat the order
7. dispatch, medical direction
8. dispatch
9. lips, sign (translate)
10. name

HANDOUT 10-5: Communication: Matching

1. D	**4.** H	**7.** J	**9.** F
2. I	**5.** B	**8.** E	**10.** G
3. C	**6.** A		

HANDOUT 10-6: Communication: True or False

1. F	**4.** F	**7.** F	**9.** F
2. T	**5.** T	**8.** T	**10.** F
3. F	**6.** T		

HANDOUT 10-7: Organizing a Radio Report

A. 8	**D.** 7	**G.** 6	**J.** 10
B. 11	**E.** 1	**H.** 5	**K.** 4
C. 2	**F.** 9	**I.** 3	

This chapter covers Lesson 3-8 and portions of Lesson 3-9 of the U.S. Department of Transportation's EMT-Basic National Standard Curriculum.

OBJECTIVES

Numbered objectives are from the U.S. Department of Transportation EMT-Basic National Standard Curriculum. Asterisked objectives, if any, pertain to material that is supplemental to the DOT curriculum. Page numbers in parentheses refer to pages in the textbook.

Cognitive

3-8.1   Explain the components of the written report and list the information that should be included in the written report. (pp. 347–349)

3-8.2   Identify the various sections of the written report. (pp. 348–349)

3-8.3   Describe what information is required in each section of the prehospital care report and how it should be entered. (pp. 347–349)

3-8.4   Define the special considerations concerning patient refusal. (p. 350)

3-8.5   Describe the legal implications associated with the written report. (pp. 349–352)

3-8.6   Discuss all state and/or local record and reporting requirements. (p. 352)

Affective

3-8.7   Explain the rationale for patient care documentation. (pp. 343–344)

3-8.8   Explain the rationale for the EMS system gathering data. (pp. 343–344)

3-8.9   Explain the rationale for using medical terminology correctly. (p. 349)

3-8.10 Explain the rationale for using an accurate and synchronous clock so that information can be used in trending. (p. 348)

Psychomotor

3-8.11 Complete a prehospital care report.

REVIEW

In the last lesson, "Communication," students learned that for the EMT, effective communication may be critical in saving a life. As EMTs, they will communicate person-to-person with patients and other members of the EMS system, as well as over the radio or telephone to dispatchers, medical direction, and receiving hospital staff. Their ability to communicate effectively will be crucial to the patient at the scene and en route to the hospital. Remind them that effective communication—clear, concise delivery

Total Teaching Time
170 minutes

Resources Needed
- Scored Chapter 10 Quizzes
- Prehospital care record forms used in your area (two for each student)
- Inexpensive items such as pens or clipboards for prizes

Additional Resources

Larmon/Davis, *Basic Life Support Skills*

Elling, *EMT Achieve: Basic Test Preparation*

Limmer/Mistovich/O'Keefe, *Audio Lecture & Study Guide: EMT*

Mistovich/Kuvlesky, *SUCCESS! for the EMT, Second Edition*

of accurate information—with hospital personnel may make an important difference in the care their patient receives. Distribute the scored quizzes from the last class. Go over each question on the quiz and handle any concerns students may have about the answers.

INTRODUCTION TO CHAPTER 11

Chapter 11, "Documentation," is the fourth and last lesson in Module 3. Tell students that assessing a patient, treating him or her, and transporting him or her to a facility for necessary medical care are the most obvious parts of the job of the EMT. An EMT also prepares documentation for this patient and every patient the EMT comes in contact with. Whether in written form or electronically generated records, documentation is generated and referred to at the scene and en route to the hospital. That same documentation will help ensure that the patient receives the best, most appropriate care at the facility to which he or she is transported. Inform students that the EMT files a prehospital care report (PCR) for each patient and that this "documented" care becomes part of the patient's permanent medical record. In Chapter 12, students will explore various uses of documentation: medical, administrative, legal, educational, and research.

Distribute the Chapter 11 Objectives Checklist and give students a few minutes to look it over. Then briefly paraphrase the objectives for this lesson in your own words.

LECTURE

The following suggested lecture outline is based on the Department of Transportation's EMT-Basic National Standard Curriculum. In some places, the DOT curriculum has been rearranged or expanded upon so that it is more complete or easier for the student to understand. The page numbers in parentheses refer to pages in the textbook. The parenthetical references in dark, heavy type are to figures, tables, and scans in the textbook.

DOCUMENTATION

I. Reasons for documentation (pp. 343–344)
  A. Medical uses (pp. 343–344)
  B. Administrative uses (p. 344)
  C. Legal uses (p. 344)
  D. Educational and research uses (p. 344)
II. Prehospital care report (PCR) (pp. 343–344) **(Fig. 11-1, p. 344)**
  A. Functions (pp. 343–344)
    1. Continuity of care
      a. A form that is not read immediately in the emergency department may be referred to later for important information.
    2. Legal document
      a. A good report has documented
        (1) What emergency medical care was provided
        (2) Status of the patient upon arrival at the scene
        (3) Any changes upon arrival at the receiving facility.
      b. The person who completed the form ordinarily must go to court with the form.
      c. Information should include objective and subjective information and be clear.

Handout 11-1
Chapter 11 Objectives Checklist

Lecture Master
You may wish to display Lecture Master 11 when presenting the lecture to the class.

Point of Interest
Some EMTs keep personal journals of their calls. Point out to students that these journals can be called into court as evidence.

On the Net
How documented information is used in court. http://medical.smis .doi.gov/PDF/casemed.pdf

On the Net
Documentation needed for an approved certificate of course competition. http://www.state.ma.us/ dph/oems/ar323b.pdf

3. Educational

    a. Used to demonstrate proper documentation and how to handle unusual or uncommon cases

4. Administrative

    a. Billing

    b. Service statistics

5. Research

6. Evaluation and continuous quality improvement

B. Format (pp. 344–347)

    1. Types **(Fig. 11-2, pp. 345–346)**

        a. Traditional written form with check boxes and a section for narrative

        b. Computerized version where information is filled in by means of an electronic clipboard or a similar device **(Fig. 11-3 and Fig. 11-4, p. 347)**

    2. Sections

        a. Run data

            (1) Date

            (2) Times

            (3) Service

            (4) Unit

            (5) Names of crew

        b. Patient data

            (1) Patient name

            (2) Address

            (3) Date of birth

            (4) Insurance information

            (5) Sex

            (6) Age

            (7) Nature of call

            (8) Mechanism of injury

            (9) Location of patient

          (10) Treatment administered prior to arrival

          (11) Signs and symptoms

          (12) Care administered

          (13) Baseline vital signs

          (14) SAMPLE history

          (15) Changes in condition

        c. Check boxes

            (1) Be sure to fill in the box completely.

            (2) Avoid stray marks.

        d. Narrative section (if applicable)

            (1) Describe, don't conclude.

            (2) Include pertinent negatives.

            (3) Record important observations about the scene.

            (4) Avoid radio codes.

            (5) Use abbreviations only if they are standard/approved. **(Table 11-1, p. 349)**

            (6) When information of a sensitive nature is documented, note the source of that information.

            (7) State reporting requirements.

            (8) Be sure to spell words correctly, especially medical words.

                (a) If you do not know how to spell a word, find out or use another word.

            (9) For every reassessment, record time and findings.

Teaching Tip

Develop a special form or use a form from a local agency that students can fill out each time they complete a practice scenario in class.

Reading/Reference

Wolfberg, D.M., "Five Good Reasons for Better Documentation," *EMS Magazine,* Nov. 2005

Reading/Reference

Streger, M., "Universal Truths of Patient Care Documentation," *EMS Magazine,* Feb. 2003.

e. Other state or local requirements

  C. Minimum data set (pp. 347–349)

    1. Patient information gathered by the EMT

      a. Chief complaint

      b. Level of consciousness (AVPU)—mental status

      c. Systolic blood pressure for patients older than 3 years

      d. Skin perfusion (capillary refill) for patients younger than 3 years

      e. Skin color and temperature

      f. Pulse rate

      g. Respiratory rate and effort

    2. Administrative information

      a. Time incident reported

      b. Time unit notified

      c. Time of arrival at patient

      d. Time unit left scene

      e. Time of arrival at destination

      f. Time of transfer of care

    3. Accurate and synchronous clocks

III. **Legal concerns** (pp. 349–352)

  A. Confidentiality (pp. 349–350)

    1. The PCR form itself and the information on the form are considered confidential.

    2. HIPAA

  B. Distribution (p. 350)

    1. Local and state protocol and procedures will determine where the different copies of the form should be distributed.

  C. Documentation of patient refusal (p. 350)

    1. Competent adult patients have the right to refuse treatment.

    2. Before the EMT leaves the scene, however, he or she should:

      a. Try again to persuade the patient to go to a hospital.

      b. Ensure the patient is able to make a rational, informed decision (e.g., not under the influence of alcohol or other drugs, or illness/injury effects).

      c. Inform the patient why he should go and what may happen to him if he does not.

      d. Consult medical direction as directed by local protocol.

      e. If the patient still refuses, document any assessment findings and emergency medical care given, then have the patient sign a refusal form. (**Fig. 11-5, p. 351**)

      f. Have a family member, police officer, or bystander sign the form as a witness. If the patient refuses to sign the refusal form, have a family member, police officer, or bystander sign the form verifying that the patient refused to sign.

      g. Complete the prehospital care report.

        (1) Complete patient assessment.

        (2) Care EMT wished to provide for the patient

        (3) Statement that the EMT explained to the patient the possible consequences of failure to accept care, including potential death

        (4) Offer alternative methods of gaining care

        (5) State willingness to return

  D. Falsification issues (pp. 350–351)

    1. When an error of omission or commission occurs, the EMT should not try to cover it up. Instead, document what did or

©2008 by Pearson Education, Inc.
Prehospital Emergency Care, 8th ed.

did not happen and what steps were taken (if any) to correct the situation.

2. Falsification of information on the prehospital care report may lead not only to suspension or revocation of the EMT's certification/license, but also to poor patient care because other health care providers have a false impression of which assessment findings were discovered or what treatment was given.

3. Specific areas of difficulty
   a. Vital signs—document only the vital signs that were actually taken.
   b. Treatment—if a treatment such as oxygen was overlooked, do not chart that the patient was given oxygen.

4. Correction of errors
   a. Errors discovered while the report form is being written
      (1) Draw a single horizontal line through the error, initial it, and write the correct information beside it. (**Fig. 11-6, p. 351**)
      (2) Do not try to obliterate the error—this may be interpreted as an attempt to cover up a mistake.
   b. Errors discovered after the report form is submitted
      (1) Preferably in a different color ink, draw a single line through the error, initial and date it, and add a note with the correct information.
      (2) If information was omitted, add a note with the correct information, the date, and the EMT's initials.

IV. **Special situations/reports/incident reporting** (p. 352)
   A. Multiple-casualty incidents (MCI) (p. 352)
      1. When there is not enough time to complete the form before the next call, the EMT will need to fill out the report later.
      2. The local MCI plan should have some means of recording important medical information temporarily (e.g., triage tag, that can be used later to complete the form).
      3. The standard for completing the form in an MCI is not the same as for a typical call. The local plan should have guidelines.
   B. Special situation reports (p. 352)
      1. Used to document events that should be reported to local authorities or to amplify and supplement primary report
         a. Suspected abuse of a child, spouse, or elderly person
         b. Possible exposure to an infectious disease
         c. Injury to an EMS team member
         d. Other situations that the EMT feels might require special documentation and/or informing of another agency
      2. Should be submitted in a timely manner
      3. Should be accurate and objective
      4. The EMT should keep a copy for his or her own records
      5. The report, and copies if appropriate, should be submitted to the authority described by local protocol
   C. Continuous quality improvement (p. 352)
      1. Information gathered from the prehospital care report can be used to analyze various aspects of the EMS system.

☑

Teaching Tip
Review local and state reporting requirements with students.

2. This information can then be used to improve different components of the system and prevent problems from reoccurring.

ENRICHMENT (OPTIONAL)

The following sections contain information that is valuable as background for the EMT, but that goes substantially beyond the U.S. Department of Transportation's EMT-Basic National Standard Curriculum.

V. Alternative PCR organizations (pp. 352–357)
   A. SOAP (pp. 352–353)
      1. S—subjective
      2. O—objective
      3. A—assessment
      4. P—plan
   B. CHART (p. 353)
      1. C—chief complaint
      2. H—history
      3. A—assessment
      4. R—Rx
      5. T—transport
   C. CHEATED (p. 353)
      1. C—chief complaint
      2. H—history
      3. E—exam
      4. A—assessment
      5. T—treatment
      6. E—evaluation
      7. D—disposition
   D. Medical abbreviations (pp. 353–357) **(Table 11-2, p. 353–357)**
      1. Use only universally accepted/approved abbreviations

CASE STUDY FOLLOW-UP

Ask a student volunteer to read the Case Study that begins on page 343 of the textbook. You may wish to use the following questions to engage students in a discussion of the Case Study Follow-up that begins on page 358 of the textbook. Provide missing information and clarify ideas as needed.

Q1. How do you respond to the patient's initial outburst?

A1. *By remaining calm and politely offering an introduction and saying, "I understand that you've had some problems. We're certainly not here to give you any more trouble. We just want to make sure you're OK. Are you feeling all right? Do you have any pain?"*

Q2. How do you attempt to get Mr. Makynen to allow treatment?

A2. *By speaking to him calmly and not attempting to force treatment on him but trying to help him see that EMT care would be in his best interest because head injuries often display no signs at first but can later develop into potentially life-threatening situations.*

©2008 by Pearson Education, Inc.
Prehospital Emergency Care, 8th ed.

Q3. Since Mr. Makynen continues to refuse treatment, what do you document on the PCR?

A3. *On the PCR, the following should be noted: the mechanism of injury; the bruise to the forehead; and initial findings regarding the patient's alert mental status, open airway, adequate breathing, absence of bleeding, pulse that is rapid but regular and strong, and skin color, temperature, and condition indicating adequate perfusion. Also noted is the patient's denial of pain and loss of consciousness, as well as the witness's report that Mr. Makynen was slumped over the wheel after the collision. The patient's refusal of care, the recommendation that the patient see a doctor, and the explanation of the possible consequences if he does not should be recorded, as well as the patient's final refusal of any further care.*

Q4. What do you do with the PCR after you have written it?

A4. *Show the PCR to Mr. Makynen and allow him to read it and the refusal form and ask him to sign the form.*

Q5. Whom do you ask to witness the refusal form?

A5. *The owner of the van and another bystander.*

IN REVIEW

Assess students' ability to apply what they have just learned by discussing the Review Questions on page 359 in the textbook.

Q1. Explain the various uses of the documentation that the EMT generates after a patient contact.

A1. *Documentation is used to ensure continuity of care, to aid in administrative functions such as insurance and billing, to provide documentation in legal cases, and to provide research and education data. (pp. 343–344)*

Q2. Describe two common formats for the prehospital care report.

A2. *Two common formats for the prehospital care report are a written format with check boxes, write-on lines, and spaces for narrative; and a computerized format. (p. 344)*

Q3. Explain the origin and purpose of the minimum data set.

A3. *The minimum data set is the information that the U.S. Department of Transportation has determined should be on all PCRs in order to help improve and standardize prehospital care. (pp. 347–348)*

Q4. Explain what the phrase "accurate and synchronous clocks" means and why they are important.

A4. *"Accurate and synchronous clocks" means that all parts of an EMS system should use properly set clocks that show the same time and permit the keeping of records that can pinpoint when each step in a patient contact occurred and how long it took. (p. 348)*

Q5. Define pertinent negatives.

A5. *Pertinent negatives are signs and symptoms that a patient might be expected to show in certain circumstances but that the patient denies having. (p. 349)*

Q6. List the steps you should take if a patient refuses treatment.

A6. *Steps to take if a patient refuses treatment include: Make an additional effort to convince the patient; explain the possible consequences of refusal; inform medical direction; document findings in the PCR and have the patient sign a witnessed refusal-of-care form; if the patient won't sign, have the witnesses sign that the patient has refused; suggest alternative methods of getting care; note willingness to return if the patient changes his or her mind. (p. 350)*

Q7. Explain the meaning and importance of the following two documentation rules: "If it wasn't written down, it wasn't done" and "If it wasn't done, don't write it down."

A7. *"If it wasn't written down, it wasn't done" means that no one, including emergency department staff, will know what was done if it wasn't recorded; and you won't be able to prove it was done, for example, in a court of law. "If it wasn't done, don't write it down" means don't falsify information on a report form. (p. 347)*

Q8. Describe how errors on PCRs should be corrected.

A8. *Errors made as a PCR is being filled out should have a single line drawn through them with the EMT's initials and the correct information written alongside or above. Errors discovered after the form is submitted should have a single line drawn through them in different-colored ink; a note should be added with the correct information, the date, and the EMT's initials. (pp. 351–352)*

Q9. Explain how a multiple-casualty incident can affect EMT documentation.

A9. *During a multiple-casualty incident, because of the volume of patients, abbreviated forms, such as triage tags, that contain basic medical information are often attached to patients. PCRs are often completed after the event and may be less detailed than for one-on-one encounters. (p. 352)*

Q10. Describe circumstances in which an EMT might be expected to file special reports with other agencies.

A10. *Circumstances in which an EMT might be expected to file special reports with other agencies include cases of suspected abuse of a child or an elderly person; exposure to infectious diseases; cases of injury to an EMT team member; or any circumstances that EMT deems unusual. (p. 352)*

CRITICAL THINKING

Assess students' ability to respond to real-life emergency situations by discussing the Critical Thinking questions on page 359 in the textbook.

Q1. What can this information be used for?

A1. *The information included in a PCR may be used for the following general reasons: continued patient care, permanent medical records, billing, legal proceedings, education, research, and quality improvement.*

Q2. How will the medical personnel in the medical facility use the information?

A2. *The medical staff at the receiving facility uses the information from the PCR to provide the most appropriate and timely care for the patient. It allows for a better continuity of care of the patient.*

Q3. What will your EMS use the information for?

A3. *EMS systems use the information from PCRs for several reasons, including billing, insurance reporting, educating other EMS personnel, and research studies.*

Q4. What would you document in the patient information section of the minimum data set?

A4. *The patient information section of the minimum data set would include the patient's chief complaint (severe abdominal pain), mental status (alert and oriented deteriorating to verbal), systolic blood pressure (88), skin color and temperature (pale and cold), pulse rate (128), and respiratory rate and effort (24 unlabored with adequate chest rise).*

Q5. What would you document in the administrative section of the PCR?

A5. *The administrative section of a PCR usually includes the EMS unit number; run or call number; crew member names and levels of certification; address of the call; the patient's legal name, age, sex, date of birth, address, social security number, insurance or billing information; the location of the patient; and any care provided prior to EMS arrival.*

Q6. What information would you write in the patient narrative section?

A6. *The patient narrative section of the PCR should include an objective, a relevant and straightforward written "picture" of the entire incident, the patient's chief complaint in his or her own words ("in quotes!"), any pertinent findings at the scene (including a description of any mechanism of injury), the patient's SAMPLE history, and a brief chronological description of the physical exam including any pertinent findings.*

Q7. Should any information not be reported in the PCR?

A7. *Non-pertinent and irrelevant information should never be included in a PCR.*

Q8. If you were to make a mistake while writing the PCR, how would you correct it?

A8. *Any correction to a PCR should be made by drawing a single line through the error, initialing it, and writing the correct information next to it.*

Q9. If the PCR contains a box for a third set of vital signs, what would you document in this patient?

A9. *Since the patient arrived at the receiving facility prior to a third set of vital signs being obtained, the box for the third set would not be used. Depending on local procedures, the completing EMT would most likely leave them blank, draw a single line through them, or write "N/A" (for Not Applicable) in them.*

Q10. How would you collect additional information needed for your PCR?

A10. *Obtaining additional information for a PCR is usually done through personal observation (such as looking around a scene, reading prescription bottles, or examining the patient's identification) and/or through talking with others (such as interviewing the patient, bystanders, or other emergency personnel on scene).*

PREHOSPITAL CARE REPORT CONTEST

Give students the opportunity to apply what they have learned about documentation to a real-life situation. Once again challenge students to a contest—this time to see who can write the best narrative on a prehospital care report. To conduct this contest, you will need enough copies of the PCRs used in your area to give students two copies apiece. Students will use one copy for the contest; the other copy they will keep for professional reference.

As in the last contest, have students prepare by reviewing the case histories of the unconscious trauma patient and the responsive medical patient discussed in the Case Studies for Chapter 9. (Refer students to page 240 of their textbooks.) Once again have students choose by consensus which of these patients they will use to prepare a PCR. Give students 10 minutes to complete their PCRs. Remind them to fill out the entire form—the check boxes as well as the narrative. When students are done, have them take turns reading the narrative portion of the PCR to the rest of the class. Direct the class to take notes, based on the following questions, as each student reads his or her narrative.

- What were the strengths of this narrative?
- How could the narrative have been improved?

After each narrative is read, have students use their notes to give practical feedback.

When all the narratives have been presented, direct students to write on a separate piece of paper the name of the person who they think wrote the best narrative. Tally the votes, and declare the person with the most votes the winner. If the first vote results in a tie, hold a run-off vote among the individuals who tied. Provide the winning student with a prize. Ask students to turn in their PCRs before they leave. Review them and return them along with your comments at the beginning of the next class.

Reading/Reference
Textbook, pp. 360–376

Workbook
Chapter 11 Activities

Chapter Quiz
Handout 11-2

TestGen
Chapter 11 Test

ASSIGNMENTS

Assign students to read Chapter 12, "General Pharmacology," before the next class. Also ask them to complete Chapter 11 of the Workbook.

EVALUATION

Chapter Quiz Distribute copies of the Chapter Quiz provided in Handout 11-2 to evaluate student understanding of this chapter. Remind students not to refer to their textbooks or notes while taking the quiz.

Test Manager You may wish to create a custom-tailored test using Prentice Hall *TestGen for Prehospital Emergency Care, Eighth Edition* to evaluate student understanding of this chapter.

Online Test Preparation (for students and instructors) Additional test preparation is available through *EMT Achieve: Basic Test Preparation* at http://www.prenhall.com/EMTAchieve. Instructors can also monitor student mastery online.

REINFORCEMENT

Handouts If classroom discussions or performance on the quiz indicates that some students have not fully mastered the chapter content, you may wish to assign some or all of the Reinforcement Handouts for this chapter.

TECH EXTRAS

Brady Skills Series EMT-B Videos/CD Have your students watch the skills come to life on either VHS or CD-ROM.

PowerPoint Presentation (for instructors) The PowerPoint material developed for this chapter offers useful reinforcement of chapter content.

Student CD A wide variety of material on this CD-ROM will reinforce and also expand student knowledge and skills.

Companion Website (for students) Additional review quizzes and links to EMS resources will contribute to further reinforcement of this chapter. Please visit http://www.prenhall.com/mistovich.

Online Test Preparation
Send your students to
http://www.prenhall.com/
EMTAchieve

Handouts 11-3 to 11-6
Reinforcement Activities

**Brady Skills Series
EMT-B Videos/CD**
Visual Reinforcement

**PowerPoint
Presentation**
Chapter 11

Student CD
Chapter 11

Companion Website
http://www.prenhall.com/
mistovich

OBJECTIVES CHECKLIST

Cognitive		Date Mastered
3-8.1	Explain the components of the written report and list the information that should be included in the written report.	
3-8.2	Identify the various sections of the written report.	
3-8.3	Describe what information is required in each section of the prehospital care report and how it should be entered.	
3-8.4	Define the special considerations concerning patient refusal.	
3-8.5	Describe the legal implications associated with the written report.	
3-8.6	Discuss all state and/or local record and reporting requirements.	

Affective		Date Mastered
3-8.7	Explain the rationale for patient care documentation.	
3-8.8	Explain the rationale for the EMS system gathering data.	
3-8.9	Explain the rationale for using medical terminology correctly.	
3-8.10	Explain the rationale for using an accurate and synchronous clock so that information can be used in trending.	

Psychomotor		Date Mastered
3-8.11	Complete a prehospital care report.	

OBJECTIVES

CHAPTER 11 QUIZ

Write the letter of the best answer in the space provided.

_____ 1. Documentation of findings helps ensure
    A. that you will not be sued.   **C.** accurate vital signs.
    B. continuity of care.   **D.** payment for the call.

_____ 2. The documentation produced by an EMT is known informally as a
    A. PCR.   **C.** QA.
    B. QI.   **D.** TQM.

_____ 3. A prehospital care report can become all of the following *except*
    A. evidence in a legal case.
    B. part of the hospital's permanent records.
    C. data in a research project.
    D. private property controlled by the patient.

_____ 4. Administrative information on a PCR is often referred to as
    A. PRTs.   **C.** R&D.
    B. run data.   **D.** boilerplate.

_____ 5. The standardized information that should be collected on all PCRs is called the
    A. data element.   **C.** check box.
    B. minimum data set.   **D.** narrative.

_____ 6. The federal agency that has developed a list of minimum elements to be included in all prehospital care reports is the
    A. DOT.   **C.** FCC.
    B. FDA.   **D.** EPA.

_____ 7. An EMT would record the time in which an emergency unit left on a call in the _____ section.
    A. patient data   **C.** CAD
    B. narrative   **D.** administrative information

_____ 8. Unlike a radio report, a prehospital care report will include the patient's
    A. name and address.   **C.** chief complaint.
    B. age and sex.   **D.** vital signs.

_____ 9. All of the following are included in the patient narrative section of a prehospital care report *except*
    A. charges to the patient.   **C.** pertinent negatives.
    B. chief complaint.   **D.** SAMPLE history.

_____ 10. In writing narratives, EMTs usually place quotation marks around
    A. objective observations.   **C.** baseline vital signs.
    B. opposing observations.   **D.** chief complaints.

_____ 11. All of the following can be found in a well-written narrative *except*
    A. pertinent negatives.   **C.** scene information.
    B. radio codes.   **D.** standardized abbreviations.

_____ **12.** The EMT may provide confidential information to all of the following *except*
   A. the patient's family.
   B. the emergency department nurse.
   C. a court under a subpoena.
   D. the police in a criminal investigation.

_____ **13.** If a competent patient refuses care or transport, an EMT should
   A. immediately leave the scene.   **C.** document the refusal.
   B. argue with the patient.   **D.** request police backup.

_____ **14.** Incorrect information in a prehospital care report should be
   A. erased.   **C.** crossed out with a single line.
   B. crossed out completely.   **D.** left unchanged.

_____ **15.** During a multiple-casualty incident (MCI), patient information is usually passed along by
   A. triage tags.   **C.** electronic clipboards.
   B. face-to-face reports.   **D.** cellular phones.

IN THE FIELD

Read the following real-life situation. Then answer the questions that follow.

The emergency medical dispatcher sends you to the scene of a motor-vehicle collision 3 miles west of the convenience store on Fonda Road. The emergency involves a single car that has struck a telephone pole.

When you arrive at the scene, you do a quick scene size-up. The vehicle has only minor damage, and no lines are down. EMRs from the fire department have secured the scene and have initiated CPR on a male patient. You notice no obvious signs of trauma on the patient, except a 1-inch laceration to the forehead.

One of the EMRs reports: "The patient's license indicates that he is in his mid-60s. When we arrived, he was already in cardiac and respiratory arrest. We extricated him from the vehicle and began CPR, while providing manual cervical-spine stabilization."

You write down the EMRs comments in quotes and tell him to continue with CPR. Meanwhile, you insert an oral airway and apply the automated external defibrillator (AED). Readings on the AED advise you to stand clear as it begins to charge. The AED shocks the patient a total of three times in this sequence.

Your EMT partner restarts CPR and continues it for 1 minute. Readings on the AED indicate that the patient has a shockable rhythm. Your partner stands back, and the AED shocks three more times.

The patient now has a weak pulse, but he is still not breathing. You place him on a long spine board and begin transport to the hospital. En route, the patient becomes pulseless. You use the AED again, regaining the pulse on the seventh shock.

You recheck the patient's pulse and find it to be strong—62 beats per minute. Other vital signs show a blood pressure of 112/52 and six spontaneous breaths per minute. You assist his ventilations.

You continue checking vital signs. Upon arrival at the hospital, the patient has a pulse rate of 68, blood pressure of 124/72, and respirations of 16. He has spontaneous eye opening but is not following commands.

Because of the patient's condition, you have been unable to obtain a medical history. You also have no knowledge of prescribed medications or allergies. You did, however, discover some pertinent personal information from the patient's license. Data included: patient name—James Gilligan; date of birth—June 7, 1932; address—73 First Street, Waterford, NY.

You have also recorded these times for your unit, ID# 123 of the Emergency Team. From the AED:

- Call received   0934
- En route   0936
- At scene   0941
- From scene   0955
- At hospital   1013
- In service   1039
- In quarters   1049

- Power on   0943.22
- Shock 1   0943.55
- Shock 2   0944.12
- Shock 3   0944.52
- Shock 4   0946.02
- Shock 5   0946.51
- Shock 6   0947.31
- Shock 7   1007.29

Using the information in this scenario, fill out as many parts of the following prehospital care report as possible. You might substitute the prehospital care report used by an EMS agency in your area.

Prehospital Care Report

M	D	Y																		
DATE OF CALL			RUN NO.																	

4-5057962

AGENCY CODE · VEH. NO.

		MILEAGE		USE MILITARY TIMES
Name	Agency Name	END	CALL REC'D	
Address	Dispatch Information	BEGIN	EN ROUTE	
	Call Location	TOTAL	ARRIVED AT SCENE	
Ph #	CHECK ONE ☐ Residence ☐ Health Facility ☐ Farm ☐ Indus. Facility ☐ Other Work Loc. ☐ Roadway ☐ Recreational ☐ Other	LOCATION CODE	FROM SCENE	

A G E		D O B M	D	Y	S E X ☐ M ☐ F	CALL TYPE AS REC'D. ☐ Emergency ☐ Non-Emergency ☐ Stand-by	COMPLETE FOR TRANSFER ONLY Transferred from ☐☐☐ ☐ No Previous PCR ☐ Unknown if Previous PCR	AT DESTIN IN SERVICE
Physician								
CARE IN PROGRESS ON ARRIVAL ☐ None ☐ Citizen ☐ PD/FD/Other First Responder ☐ Other EMS							Previous PCR Number ☐–☐☐☐☐☐	IN QUARTERS

MECHANISM OF INJURY
☐ MVA (√ seat belt used →) ☐ Fall of ___ feet ☐ GSW ☐ Machinery
☐ Struck by vehicle ☐ Unarmed assault ☐ Knife

☐ Extrication required ___ minutes   Seat belt used? ☐ Yes ☐ No ☐ Unknown

Seat Belt Use Reported By: ☐ Crew ☐ Patient ☐ Police ☐ Other

CHIEF COMPLAINT   **SUBJECTIVE ASSESSMENT**

PRESENTING PROBLEM
If more than one checked, circle primary

☐ Airway Obstruction
☐ Respiratory Arrest
☐ Respiratory Distress
☐ Cardiac Related (Potential)
☐ Cardiac Arrest

☐ Allergic Reaction
☐ Syncope
☐ Stroke/CVA
☐ General Illness/Malaise
☐ Gastro-Intestinal Distress
☐ Diabetic Related (Potential)
☐ Pain

☐ Unconscious/Unresp.
☐ Seizure
☐ Behavior Disorder
☐ Substance Abuse (Potential)
☐ Poisoning (Accidental)

☐ Shock
☐ Head Injury
☐ Spinal Injury
☐ Fracture/Dislocation
☐ Amputation

☐ Major Trauma
☐ Trauma-Blunt
☐ Trauma-Penetrating
☐ Soft Tissue Injury
☐ Bleeding/Hemorrhage

☐ OB/GYN
☐ Burns
Environmental
☐ Heat
☐ Cold
☐ Hazardous Materials
☐ Obvious Death

☐ Other _____

PAST MEDICAL HISTORY		TIME	RESP.	PULSE	B.P.	LEVEL OF CONSCIOUSNESS	GCS	R	PUPILS	L	SKIN	STATUS
☐ None ☐ Allergy to ___ ☐ Hypertension ☐ Stroke ☐ Seizures ☐ Diabetes ☐ COPD ☐ Cardiac ☐ Other (List) ☐ Asthma	V I T A L		Rate: ☐ Regular ☐ Shallow ☐ Labored	Rate: ☐ Regular ☐ Irregular		☐ Alert ☐ Voice ☐ Pain ☐ Unresp.		☐	Normal Dilated Constricted Sluggish No-Reaction	☐	☐ Unremarkable ☐ Cool ☐ Pale ☐ Warm ☐ Cyanotic ☐ Moist ☐ Flushed ☐ Dry ☐ Jaundiced	☐ C ☐ U ☐ P ☐ S
	S I G N S		Rate: ☐ Regular ☐ Shallow ☐ Labored	Rate: ☐ Regular ☐ Irregular		☐ Alert ☐ Voice ☐ Pain ☐ Unresp.		☐	Normal Dilated Constricted Sluggish No-Reaction	☐	☐ Unremarkable ☐ Cool ☐ Pale ☐ Warm ☐ Cyanotic ☐ Moist ☐ Flushed ☐ Dry ☐ Jaundiced	☐ C ☐ U ☐ P ☐ S
Current Medications (List)			Rate: ☐ Regular ☐ Shallow ☐ Labored	Rate: ☐ Regular ☐ Irregular		☐ Alert ☐ Voice ☐ Pain ☐ Unresp.		☐	Normal Dilated Constricted Sluggish No-Reaction	☐	☐ Unremarkable ☐ Cool ☐ Pale ☐ Warm ☐ Cyanotic ☐ Moist ☐ Flushed ☐ Dry ☐ Jaundiced	☐ C ☐ U ☐ P ☐ S

OBJECTIVE PHYSICAL ASSESSMENT

COMMENTS

TREATMENT

☐ Moved to ambulance on stretcher/backboard
☐ Moved to ambulance on stair chair
☐ Walked to ambulance
☐ Airway Cleared
☐ Oral/Nasal Airway
☐ Esophageal Obturator Airway/Esophageal Gastric Tube Airway (EOA/EGTA)
☐ EndoTracheal Tube (E/T)
☐ Oxygen Administered @ ___ L.P.M., Method ___
☐ Suction Used
☐ Artificial Ventilation Method ___
☐ C.P.R. in progress on arrival by: ☐ Citizen ☐ PD/FD/Other First Responder ☐ Other
☐ C.P.R. Started @ Time ▶ ___   Time from Arrest Until C.P.R. ▶ ___ Minutes
☐ EKG Monitored (Attach Tracing) [Rhythm(s) ___]
☐ Defibrillation/Cardioversion No. Times ___   ☐ Manual ☐ Semi-automatic

☐ Medication Administered (Use Continuation Form)
☐ IV Established Fluid ___ Cath. Gauge ___
☐ Mast Inflated @ Time ___
☐ Bleeding/Hemorrhage Controlled (Method Used: ___)
☐ Spinal Immobilization Neck and Back
☐ Limb Immobilized by ☐ Fixation ☐ Traction
☐ (Heat) or (Cold) Applied
☐ Vomiting Induced @ Time ___ Method ___
☐ Restraints Applied, Type ___
☐ Baby Delivered @ Time ___ In Country ___
        ☐ Alive ☐ Stillborn ☐ Male ☐ Female
☐ Transported in Trendelenburg position
☐ Transported in left lateral recumbent position
☐ Transported with head elevated
☐ Other ___

DISPOSITION (See list)   **DISP. CODE**   **CONTINUATION FORM USED** ☐ YES ←

CREW	IN CHARGE	DRIVER'S NAME	NAME	NAME
	☐ EMT ☐ AEMT #	☐ CFR ☐ EMT ☐ AEMT #	☐ CFR ☐ EMT ☐ AEMT #	☐ CFR ☐ EMT ☐ AEMT #

EMS 100A (11/86) provided by NYS-EMS PROGRAM
DOH 3283 (6/94)

AGENCY COPY/WHITE   RESEARCH COPY/YELLOW   HOSPITAL PATIENT RECORD COPY/PINK

NON-HOSPITAL DISPOSITION CODES:

NURSING HOME 001
OTHER MEDICAL FACILITY 002
RESIDENCE 003
TREATED BY THIS UNIT, TRANSPORTED
         BY ANOTHER UNIT 004
REFUSED MEDICAL AID OR
         TRANSPORT 005
CALL CANCELLED 006
STANDBY ONLY (NO PATIENT) 007
NO PATIENT FOUND. 008
OTHER. 010

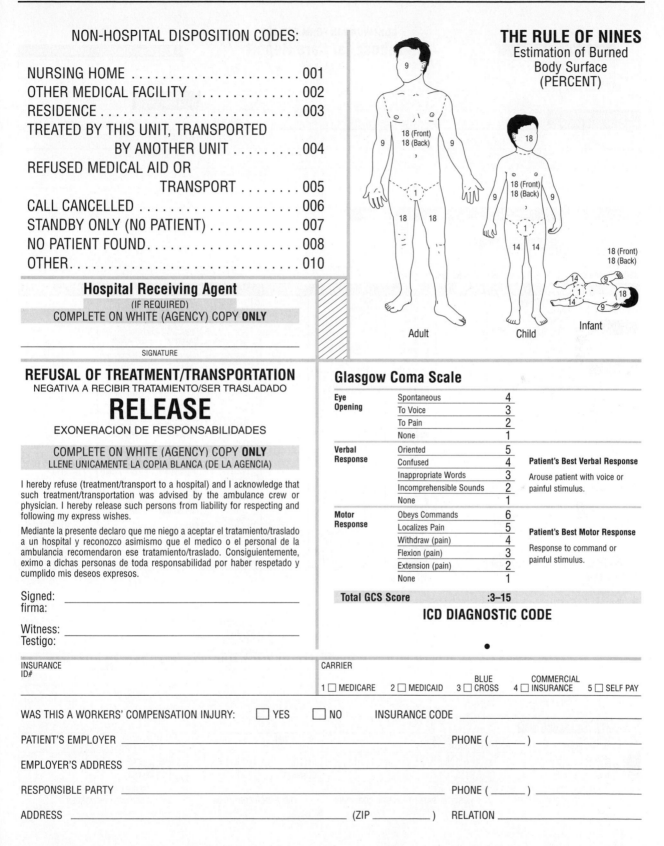

THE RULE OF NINES
Estimation of Burned
Body Surface
(PERCENT)

Adult   Child   Infant

Hospital Receiving Agent
(IF REQUIRED)
COMPLETE ON WHITE (AGENCY) COPY **ONLY**

SIGNATURE

REFUSAL OF TREATMENT/TRANSPORTATION
NEGATIVA A RECIBIR TRATAMIENTO/SER TRASLADADO

RELEASE
EXONERACION DE RESPONSABILIDADES

COMPLETE ON WHITE (AGENCY) COPY **ONLY**
LLENE UNICAMENTE LA COPIA BLANCA (DE LA AGENCIA)

I hereby refuse (treatment/transport to a hospital) and I acknowledge that such treatment/transportation was advised by the ambulance crew or physician. I hereby release such persons from liability for respecting and following my express wishes.

Mediante la presente declaro que me niego a aceptar el tratamiento/traslado a un hospital y reconozco asimismo que el medico o el personal de la ambulancia recomendaron ese tratamiento/traslado. Consiguientemente, eximo a dichas personas de toda responsabilidad por haber respetado y cumplido mis deseos expresos.

Signed: _____
firma:

Witness: _____
Testigo:

Glasgow Coma Scale

Eye Opening	Spontaneous	4	
	To Voice	3	
	To Pain	2	
	None	1	
Verbal Response	Oriented	5	
	Confused	4	**Patient's Best Verbal Response**
	Inappropriate Words	3	Arouse patient with voice or
	Incomprehensible Sounds	2	painful stimulus.
	None	1	
Motor Response	Obeys Commands	6	
	Localizes Pain	5	**Patient's Best Motor Response**
	Withdraw (pain)	4	
	Flexion (pain)	3	Response to command or
	Extension (pain)	2	painful stimulus.
	None	1	

Total GCS Score	:3–15

ICD DIAGNOSTIC CODE
•

INSURANCE ID# _____

CARRIER

1 ☐ MEDICARE 2 ☐ MEDICAID 3 ☐ BLUE CROSS 4 ☐ COMMERCIAL INSURANCE 5 ☐ SELF PAY

WAS THIS A WORKERS' COMPENSATION INJURY: ☐ YES ☐ NO   INSURANCE CODE _____

PATIENT'S EMPLOYER _____ PHONE (_____) _____

EMPLOYER'S ADDRESS _____

RESPONSIBLE PARTY _____ PHONE (_____) _____

ADDRESS _____ (ZIP _____) RELATION _____

CONTINUATION FORM FOR THE
Prehospital Care Report

USE BALL POINT PEN ONLY.

Press Down Firmly. You're Making 4 Copies.

M	D	Y
DATE   RUN NO.

AGENCY CODE   VEH. ID

Name

Agency Name

Enter PCR ID# (Top Center of PCR)

ADDITIONAL HISTORY & PHYSICAL EXAM FINDINGS

Weight in Kilograms

R BREATH SOUNDS L	NECK VEINS	EDEMA	ABDOMEN
Normal	Normal	Pedal	Nomal
Decreased	Distended	Sacral	Tender
Absent	**TRACHEAL SHIFT**	Ascites	Rigid
Rales	R L	Other	Distended
Rhonchi			Other
Wheezes			

SERIAL VITAL SIGNS, EKG, RHYTHMS, MEDICATIONS AND TREATMENT

TIME	RESP.	PULSE	B.P.	LEVEL OF CONSCIOUSNESS	EKG RHYTHMS	DEFIBRILLATION CARDIOVERSION	MEDICATIONS			DOSE	ROUTE
	Rate: □ Regular □ Shallow □ Labored	Rate: □ Regular □ Irregular		□ Alert □ Voice □ Pain □ Unresp.	□ NSR □ Brady □ Asystole □ IVR □ V. Fib. □ V. Tach. □ PVC □ SVT □ Other		□ Epinephrine □ Dopamine □ Naloxone □ Atropine □ Sodium Bicarb. □ Bretylium □ Dextrose □ Isoproterenol □ Nitroglycerin □ Lidocaine □ Lasix □ Other ___				□IV □ET □IM □SL □SQ □PO □Nebulizer
	Rate: □ Regular □ Shallow □ Labored	Rate: □ Regular □ Irregular		□ Alert □ Voice □ Pain □ Unresp.	□ NSR □ Brady □ Asystole □ IVR □ V. Fib. □ V. Tach. □ PVC □ SVT □ Other		□ Epinephrine □ Dopamine □ Naloxone □ Atropine □ Sodium Bicarb. □ Bretylium □ Dextrose □ Isoproterenol □ Nitroglycerin □ Lidocaine □ Lasix □ Other ___				□IV □ET □IM □SL □SQ □PO □Nebulizer
	Rate: □ Regular □ Shallow □ Labored	Rate: □ Regular □ Irregular		□ Alert □ Voice □ Pain □ Unresp.	□ NSR □ Brady □ Asystole □ IVR □ V. Fib. □ V. Tach. □ PVC □ SVT □ Other		□ Epinephrine □ Dopamine □ Naloxone □ Atropine □ Sodium Bicarb. □ Bretylium □ Dextrose □ Isoproterenol □ Nitroglycerin □ Lidocaine □ Lasix □ Other ___				□IV □ET □IM □SL □SQ □PO □Nebulizer
	Rate: □ Regular □ Shallow □ Labored	Rate: □ Regular □ Irregular		□ Alert □ Voice □ Pain □ Unresp.	□ NSR □ Brady □ Asystole □ IVR □ V. Fib. □ V. Tach. □ PVC □ SVT □ Other		□ Epinephrine □ Dopamine □ Naloxone □ Atropine □ Sodium Bicarb. □ Bretylium □ Dextrose □ Isoproterenol □ Nitroglycerin □ Lidocaine □ Lasix □ Other ___				□IV □ET □IM □SL □SQ □PO □Nebulizer
	Rate: □ Regular □ Shallow □ Labored	Rate: □ Regular □ Irregular		□ Alert □ Voice □ Pain □ Unresp.	□ NSR □ Brady □ Asystole □ IVR □ V. Fib. □ V. Tach. □ PVC □ SVT □ Other		□ Epinephrine □ Dopamine □ Naloxone □ Atropine □ Sodium Bicarb. □ Bretylium □ Dextrose □ Isoproterenol □ Nitroglycerin □ Lidocaine □ Lasix □ Other ___				□IV □ET □IM □SL □SQ □PO □Nebulizer
	Rate: □ Regular □ Shallow □ Labored	Rate: □ Regular □ Irregular		□ Alert □ Voice □ Pain □ Unresp.	□ NSR □ Brady □ Asystole □ IVR □ V. Fib. □ V. Tach. □ PVC □ SVT □ Other		□ Epinephrine □ Dopamine □ Naloxone □ Atropine □ Sodium Bicarb. □ Bretylium □ Dextrose □ Isoproterenol □ Nitroglycerin □ Lidocaine □ Lasix □ Other ___				□IV □ET □IM □SL □SQ □PO □Nebulizer
	Rate: □ Regular □ Shallow □ Labored	Rate: □ Regular □ Irregular		□ Alert □ Voice □ Pain □ Unresp.	□ NSR □ Brady □ Asystole □ IVR □ V. Fib. □ V. Tach. □ PVC □ SVT □ Other		□ Epinephrine □ Dopamine □ Naloxone □ Atropine □ Sodium Bicarb. □ Bretylium □ Dextrose □ Isoproterenol □ Nitroglycerin □ Lidocaine □ Lasix □ Other ___				□IV □ET □IM □SL □SQ □PO □Nebulizer

COMMENTS:

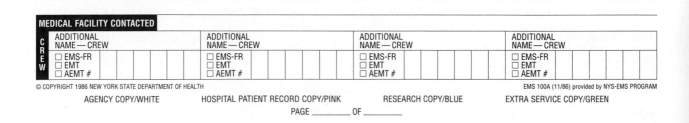

MEDICAL FACILITY CONTACTED

CREW	ADDITIONAL NAME — CREW	ADDITIONAL NAME — CREW	ADDITIONAL NAME — CREW	ADDITIONAL NAME — CREW
	□ EMS-FR □ EMT □ AEMT #	□ EMS-FR □ EMT □ AEMT #	□ EMS-FR □ EMT □ AEMT #	□ EMS-FR □ EMT □ AEMT #

EMS 100A (11/86) provided by NYS-EMS PROGRAM

AGENCY COPY/WHITE   HOSPITAL PATIENT RECORD COPY/PINK   RESEARCH COPY/BLUE   EXTRA SERVICE COPY/GREEN

PAGE ___ OF ___

©2008 by Pearson Education, Inc.
Prehospital Emergency Care, 8th ed.

CHAPTER 11 REVIEW

Write the word or words that best complete each sentence in the space provided.

1. _____ is an important part of the patient care process and serves a variety of functions, including administrative, educational, and research uses.

2. A recent development in prehospital care reports is the _____

   _____, a device that converts handwriting into computerized text.

3. A PCR is a(n) _____ _____ that can sometimes find its way into either criminal or civil court cases.

4. To ensure that runs meet current medical and organizational standards, most EMS agencies have

   a(n) _____ improvement system in place.

5. The U.S. Department of Transportation calls the information it wants on all PCRs the

   _____ _____.

6. The _____ _____ includes unit numbers, date, times, call number, and crew member names.

7. The _____ data includes the patient's name and address, sex, age, and any care rendered before the EMTs arrived.

8. _____ statements can be measured or verified;

   _____ statements reflect an individual's point of view.

9. Because the precise times of events during a call can be both medically and legally important, all EMS systems should use _____ and _____ clocks.

10. When bystander observations and the patient's chief complaint are recorded, they should be placed

    in _____ _____.

11. Documenting _____ _____ lets other medical professionals know that an EMT examined certain areas without making any significant findings.

12. At least _____ complete sets of vital signs should be taken and recorded.

13. If a patient declines emergency treatment or transport, he or she should be asked to sign a(n)

    _____ - _____ - _____

    form.

14. The PCR is considered _____ and must be handled with care and
discretion.

15. In a multiple-casualty incident (MCI), patient information is often passed through the system in the
form of _____ _____.

DOCUMENTATION: LISTING

1. List four basic uses of the prehospital care report (PCR).

2. List the five sections in a typical PCR.

3. List three legal issues that pertain to PCRs and other documents that an EMT may complete.

4. List three things to do to correct an error made while filling out a PCR.

MEDICAL ABBREVIATIONS

Below is a list of symbols and codes that you might encounter when reading a prehospital care report (PCR).

AAO	Awake, alert, and oriented
ACO	Alert, conscious, and oriented
A&O × 3	Alert and oriented to person, place, and time
AAA	Abdominal aortic aneurysm
ABC	Airway, breathing, and circulation
ACLS	Advanced Cardiac Life Support
ALS	Advanced Life Support
ASA	Acetylsalicylic acid (aspirin)
ABD	Abdomen (abdominal)
AMT	Amount
Approx.	Approximately
AMS	Altered mental status
AMA	Against medical advice
AFIB	Atrial fibrillation
BP	Blood pressure
BVM	Bag-valve mask
BS	Breath sounds
BILAT	Bilateral
BSC&=	Breath sounds clear and equal
C-Spine	Cervical spine
CA	Cancer
CVA	Stroke
CHF	Congestive heart failure

REINFORCEMENT

CSF	Cerebrospinal fluid
COPD	Chronic obstructive pulmonary disease
CNS	Central nervous system
CPR	Cardiopulmonary resuscitation
C-Section	Cesarean section
CC	Chief complaint
cc	Cubic centimeter
C/O	Complaining of
CAO × 4	Conscious, alert, and oriented × 4
DOA	Dead on arrival
DT	Delirium tremens
DX	Diagnosis
DKA	Diabetic ketoacidosis
DNR	Do not resuscitate
ETOH	Ethanol (or drinking alcohol)
ET	Endotracheal tube
EGTA	Esophageal gastric tube airway
EKG	Electrocardiogram
EDP	Emotionally disturbed person
FX	Fracture
FB	Foreign body
GSW	Gunshot wound
GYN	Gynecology
HTN	Hypertension (high blood pressure)
HX	History
HEENT	Head, eyes, ears, nose, and throat
IV	Intravenous

ICU	Intensive Care Unit
LOC	Level of consciousness
LUQ	Left upper quadrant
LLQ	Left lower quadrant
L&D	Labor and delivery
LAT	Lateral
LSC=BILAT	Lung sounds clear and equal on both sides
MAST	Military Anti-Shock Trousers
MI	Myocardial infarction (heart attack)
MED	Medicine (medication)
NC	Nasal cannula
NSR	Normal sinus rhythm
NRM	Nonrebreather mask
NKM	No known medications
NKA	No known allergies
N/V	Nausea and vomiting
N/V/D	Nausea, vomiting, and diarrhea
NKDA	No known drug allergies
PMHX	Past medical history
PT	Patient
PE	Pulmonary edema
PVC	Premature ventricular contraction
PEARL	Pupils equal and reactive to light
PALP	Palpation
RX	Medicine
RLQ	Right lower quadrant
RUQ	Right upper quadrant

RXN	Reaction
SOB	Shortness of breath
SX	Symptom
SZ	Seizure
T	Temperature
TIA	Transient ischemic attack (mini-stroke)
TX	Treatment
VS	Vital signs
YO	Years old

LECTURE MASTER 11

Documentation

Reasons
Medical
Administrative
Legal
Education/Research

Prehospital Care Report
Formats
Data

Legal Concerns
Confidentiality
Refusal of Treatment
Falsification
Correcting Errors

Special Considerations
MCIs
Special Reports

HANDOUT 11-2: Chapter 11 Quiz

1. B	**5.** B	**9.** A	**13.** C
2. A	**6.** A	**10.** D	**14.** C
3. D	**7.** D	**11.** B	**15.** A
4. B	**8.** A	**12.** A	

HANDOUT 11-3: In the Field

Work with students as they fill out the prehospital care report. You might invite several EMTs to work with students, thus sharing their knowledge of documentation.

HANDOUT 11-4: Chapter 11 Review

1. Documentation
2. electronic clipboard
3. legal document
4. quality
5. minimum data set
6. administrative information
7. patient
8. Objective, subjective
9. accurate, synchronous
10. quotation marks
11. pertinent negatives
12. two
13. refusal-of-care
14. confidential
15. triage tags

HANDOUT 11-5: Documentation: Listing

1. Becomes part of the patient's permanent hospital record (medical), can serve as a legal document in a civil or criminal case (legal), can be used for administrative purposes such as billing (administrative), supplies data for education research (educational/research)
2. Administrative information, patient data, vital signs, patient narrative, treatment.
3. Confidentiality, patient refusals, falsification
4. Draw a single horizontal line through the error, initial it, and write in the correct information.

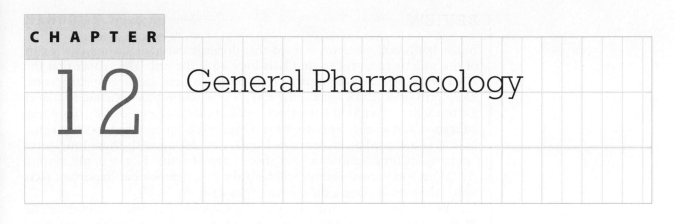

12 General Pharmacology

This chapter covers Lesson 4-1 and portions of Lesson 4-10 of the U.S. Department of Transportation's EMT-Basic National Standard Curriculum.

OBJECTIVES

Numbered objectives are from the U.S. Department of Transportation EMT-Basic National Standard Curriculum. Asterisked objectives, if any, pertain to material that is supplemental to the DOT curriculum. Page numbers in parentheses refer to pages in the textbook.

Cognitive

4-1.1 Identify which medications will be carried on the unit. (pp. 364–365)

4-1.2 State the medications carried on the EMS unit by the generic name. (pp. 364–365)

4-1.3 Identify the medications with which the Emergency Medical Technician/EMT may assist the patient with administering. (pp. 365–366)

4-1.4 State the medications that the Emergency Medical Technician/EMT can assist the patient with by the generic name. (pp. 365–366)

4-1.5 Discuss the forms in which the medications may be found. (pp. 367–368)

* List and explain the various routes of drug administration used by the EMT-Basic. (pp. 366–367)

* List and describe the essential medication information that should be understood by the Emergency Medical Technician/EMT. (pp. 369–370)

* List and describe the key steps in administering medications to a patient. (pp. 370–373)

* Describe the reassessment strategies used following medication administration. (p. 373)

* List sources that can be used to gather medication information. (p. 373)

Affective

4-1.6 Explain the rationale for the administration of medications. (pp. 362, 363–364)

Psychomotor

4-1.7 Demonstrate general steps for assisting the patient with self-administration of medications.

4-1.8 Read the labels and inspect each type of medication.

Total Teaching Time
105 minutes

Resources Needed
- Scored Chapter 11 Quizzes
- PCRs completed by students for Chapter 12
- Several copies each of the *U.S. Pharmacopoeia and Physicians' Desk Reference.*
- Variety of prescription medications—be certain to include different brands of prescribed inhalers, nitroglycerin, and epinephrine auto-injectors among them.

Additional Resources
Larmon/Davis, *Basic Life Support Skills*

Elling, *EMT Achieve: Basic Test Preparation*

Limmer/Mistovich/O'Keefe, *Audio Lecture & Study Guide: EMT*

Mistovich/Kuvlesky, *SUCCESS! for the EMT, Second Edition*

REVIEW

In the last lesson, students learned that documentation is an important part of the patient care process and lasts long after the call. The report that the EMT writes will become a part of the patient's permanent hospital record. As records of an EMS agency, the EMT's reports become valuable resources for research on trends in emergency medical care and a guide for continuing education and quality improvement. Often prehospital care reports written by EMTs are used as evidence in legal cases. Along with these long-term benefits, documentation also has short-term benefits. For example, noting vital signs and patient history will help the EMT remember important facts about the patient during the course of the call.

When you have finished reviewing Chapter 11, return copies of the PCRs students completed as part of the last lesson. Explain that you have made comments on each report.

Generalize about students' performance on the PCRs, noting any strengths you observed. Clarify any items on the PCR with which more than one student had difficulty and provide correct answers as needed. Then distribute the scored quizzes from the last class. Go over each question on the quiz and handle any concerns students may have about the answers.

Take a few minutes to spotlight what students have learned in Module 3. Emphasize students' newfound competencies. Tell them that they have learned the following:

- How to size up a scene before entering it
- How to perform an initial assessment of a patient's condition
- How to perform a more detailed history and physical examination of patients who are sick or injured
- How and why to periodically recheck a patient's condition
- How to communicate with other health care professionals
- How to document what they found and what they did

INTRODUCTION TO MODULE 4

Once the EMT has assessed the patient and taken care of any immediately life-threatening emergencies, it is time to treat the patient's medical emergency or the traumatic injury that prompted the call. Module 4 will help students distinguish between medical emergencies, often caused by a disease or malfunction within the body, and traumatic injuries that are usually caused by an outside force.

Tell students that the focus of Module 4 is medical emergencies. (Module 5 will deal with the treatment of traumatic injuries.) In Module 4, students will learn about some of the medications EMTs can help patients administer to themselves. They will also learn how to handle breathing problems, cardiac emergencies, altered mental status and diabetes-related crises, stroke, seizures and syncope, allergies, poisoning, drug and alcohol emergencies, and acute abdominal pain; environmental and behavioral emergencies; submersion, drowning, and diving emergencies; and, finally, pregnancy problems and how to deliver a baby in an emergency.

INTRODUCTION TO CHAPTER 12

Chapter 12, "General Pharmacology," is the first lesson in Module 4. As EMTs, students will be responsible for either administering or assisting the patient with the administration of some medications. In such cases, the medication will either be prescribed to the patient or will be carried on the EMS unit. Regardless of the source of the medication, medical direction's permission is required, whether as a standing order or as an on-line order, prior to administration.

Emphasize to students how critical it can be that they give their patient the proper medication in an emergency. Once administered, it is not possible to extract the medication or prevent the effects. Therefore, it is not sufficient that students are simply familiar with the medications and proper procedures for their administration; they also must know how to administer them according to local protocols and with the expressed permission of medical direction.

Distribute the Chapter 12 Objectives Checklist and give students a few minutes to look it over. Then briefly paraphrase the objectives for this lesson in your own words.

LECTURE

The following suggested lecture outline is based on the Department of Transportation's EMT-Basic National Standard Curriculum. In some places, the DOT curriculum has been rearranged or expanded upon so that it is more complete or easier for the student to understand. The page numbers in parentheses refer to pages in the textbook. The parenthetical references in dark, heavy type are to figures, tables, and scans in the textbook.

GENERAL PHARMACOLOGY

I. **Administering medications** (pp. 363–364)
   A. Medication (p. 363)
   B. Pharmacology (p. 364)
II. **Medications carried on the EMS unit** (pp. 364–365)
   A. Activated charcoal—will be learned as part of Chapter 19, "Poisoning Emergencies" (p. 364) (**Fig. 12-4, p. 369**)
   B. Oral glucose—will be learned as a part of Chapter 15, "Altered Mental Status—Diabetic Emergencies" (p. 364) (**Fig. 12-3, p. 369**)
   C. Oxygen—learned in Chapter 7, "Airway Management, Ventilation, and Oxygen Therapy" (p. 364) (**Fig. 12-6, p. 369**)
   D. Aspirin—will be learned as part of Chapter 14, "Cardiac Emergencies" (pp. 364–365) (**Fig. 12-1, p. 368**)
III. **Medications prescribed by a physician** (pp. 365–366)
   A. These are prescribed medications the patient has in his or her possession; they are not carried on the EMS unit. EMTs may assist patients in taking these medications, with approval by medical direction. (pp. 365–366)
   B. Prescribed inhaler—will be learned as a part of Chapter 13, "Respiratory Emergencies" (p. 365) (**Fig. 12-5, p. 369**)
   C. Nitroglycerin—will be learned as a part of Chapter 14, "Cardiac Emergencies" (p. 365) (**Fig. 12-1, p. 368**)
   D. Epinephrine—will be learned as a part of Chapter 18, "Allergic Reaction" (pp. 365–366) (**Fig. 12-2, p. 368**)
      1. Some states may permit epinephrine to be carried on the EMS unit
IV. **Medication names** (pp. 366)
   A. Official name (pp. 366)

Handout 12-1
Chapter 12 Objectives Checklist

Lecture Master
You may wish to display Lecture Master 12 when presenting the lecture to the class.

Reading/Reference
Bledsoe, B., D. Clayden, and F. Papa, *Prehospital Emergency Pharmacology.* 5th ed. Brady/Prentice Hall Health, 2001.

Slides/Videos
Brady Skill Series: EMT-B "Administration of Activated Charcoal" "Administration of Glucose" "Metered-Dose Inhaler" "Nitroglycerin" "Epinephrine Auto-Injector" "Nebulizer"

Teaching Tip
Some pharmacies stock inhaler trainers that contain inert gas.

Teaching Tip
Use a package of breath mints to simulate nitroglycerin tablets when students practice assisting in the administration of this medication.

Teaching Tip
Center Laboratories, 35 Channel Dr., Port Washington, NY 11050 has Epi-Pen trainers available.

1. Listed in the *U.S. Pharmacopoeia* (USP), a governmental publication listing all drugs in the United States

    B. Chemical name (p. 366)

      1. Describes the drug's chemical structure

    C. Generic name (p. 366)

      1. Assigned to drug before it becomes officially listed

      2. Simple form of the chemical name

      3. Give examples **(Table 12-1, p. 367)**

    D. Trade (or brand) name (p. 366)

      1. Name a manufacturer uses in marketing the drug.

      2. Give examples **(Table 12-1, p. 367)**

V. Routes of administration (pp. 366–367)

    A. Route by which the medication is administered (p. 366)

    B. Oral (p. 366)

    C. Sublingual (under the tongue) (p. 366)

    D. Inhalation (pp. 366–367)

    E. Injection (p. 367)

VI. Medication form (pp. 367–368)

    A. Medications the EMT carries on the unit or medications that a patient may have a prescription for that the EMT may assist with administration (pp. 367–368)

      1. Compressed powders or tablets—nitroglycerin and aspirin

      2. Liquids for injection—epinephrine

      3. Gels—(oral) glucose

      4. Suspensions—activated charcoal

      5. Fine powder for inhalation—prescribed metered-dose inhaler

      6. Gases—oxygen

      7. Sublingual (under the tongue) spray—nitroglycerin

      8. Liquid/vaporized fixed-dose nebulizers

    B. Each drug is in a specific medication form to allow properly controlled concentrations of the drug to enter into the bloodstream where it has an effect on the target body system. (p. 367)

VII. Essential medication information (pp. 369–370)

    A. Indications (pp. 369–370)

      1. Indication for a drug's use includes the most common uses of the drug in treating a specific illness

    B. Contraindications (p. 370)

      1. Situations in which a drug should not be used because it may cause harm to the patient or offer no effect in improving the patient's condition or illness

    C. Dose (p. 370)

      1. How much of the drug should be given

    D. Actions (p. 370)

      1. Desired effects a drug has on the patient and/or the patient's body systems

    E. Side effects (p. 370)

      1. Any actions of a drug other than those desired; some side effects may be predictable

VIII. Key steps in administration (pp. 370–373)

    A. Obtain an order from medical direction. (pp. 370–371) **(Fig. 12-7, p. 371)**

    B. Select proper medication. (p. 371)

    C. Verify the prescription. (pp. 371–372)

    D. Check expiration date. (p. 372)

    E. Check for discoloration and impurities. (p. 372)

F. Verify form, route, and dose. (p. 372)

G. Medication administration: The five "rights" (p. 372)

    1. Right patient

    2. Right medication

    3. Right route

    4. Right dose

    5. Right date

H. Document administration (p. 373)

IX. Reassessment strategies (p. 373)

  A. Reassess airway, breathing, and circulation (p. 373)

  B. Repeat vital signs. (p. 373)

  C. Must be done as part of the ongoing patient assessment. (p. 373)

  D. Documentation of response to intervention. (p. 373)

X. Sources of medication information (partial listing) (p. 373)

  A. American Hospital Formulary Service—published by the American Society of Hospital Pharmacists (p. 373)

  B. AMA Drug Evaluation—published by the American Medical Association Department of Drugs (p. 373)

  C. *Physicians' Desk Reference (PDR)*—published yearly by the Medical Economics Data Production Company (p. 373)

  D. Package Inserts—information that is packaged with the particular drug (p. 373)

  E. Poison control centers (p. 373)

  F. EMS pocket drug reference guide (p. 373)

  G. ePocrates for the PDA (p. 373)

CASE STUDY FOLLOW-UP

Ask a student volunteer to read the Case Study that begins on page 363 of the textbook. You may wish to use the following questions to engage students in a discussion of the Case Study Follow-up that begins on page 374 of the textbook. Provide missing information and clarify ideas as needed.

Q1. What does your SAMPLE history reveal about the medication that Mr. Brookline takes and the condition for which he takes it?

A1. *Mr. Brookline has a prescription of nitroglycerin related to his past medical history of angina but has not taken the nitroglycerin today.*

Q2. Describe your interaction with medical direction regarding administration of the nitroglycerin.

A2. *Medical direction is contacted by radio for permission to administer the nitroglycerin to Mr. Brookline and report the physical findings, SAMPLE history, and baseline vital signs. Medical direction orders, "Administer one tablet sublingually, recheck the blood pressure within 2 minutes, and reevaluate the intensity of the chest pain. If the chest pain does not subside after 5 minutes and the systolic blood pressure remains greater than 100 mmHg, administer a second tablet and reassess the blood pressure and the chest pain intensity." The order is repeated to medical direction before signing off to ensure that it was received correctly.*

Q3. After you receive permission from medical direction, what do you check before administering the nitroglycerin?

A3. *The medication container is checked to make sure that it is really nitroglycerin, that it is actually prescribed to Jack Brookline, and that the prescription is current and the expiration date has not been passed.*

Q4. What instructions do you give Mr. Brookline regarding the nitroglycerin?

A4. *He is told, "Mr. Brookline, I need you to open your mouth and lift your tongue. I am going to place a nitroglycerin tablet under your tongue. Do not swallow the tablet and be sure to keep your mouth closed until it is completely dissolved. It may burn slightly and you may get a headache."*

Q5. How do you administer the nitroglycerin and what do you do afterward?

A5. *With a gloved hand, a nitroglycerin tablet is placed under the patient's tongue. After the dose is administered, administration, dose, route, and time are recorded.*

IN REVIEW

Assess students' ability to apply what they have just learned by discussing the Review Questions on page 376 in the textbook.

Q1. Name the medications that are carried on the EMS unit.

A1. *Oxygen, oral glucose, activated charcoal, and aspirin (pp. 364–365)*

Q2. Name the medications an EMT may administer or assist in administering if prescribed for the patient.

A2. *Metered-dose inhaler, nitroglycerin, and epinephrine (pp. 365–366)*

Q3. Name four routes by which medications may be administered by the EMT.

A3. *Sublingual, oral, by inhalation, and by injection (pp. 366–367)*

Q4. Name several common forms of medications that may be administered by the EMT.

A4. *Compressed powder or tablet, liquid for injection, gel, suspension, fine powder for inhalation, gas, spray, and liquid for a vaporized fixed-dose nebulizer (pp. 367–368)*

Q5. Define the following six terms related to medications: indications, contraindications, dose, administration, actions, side effects.

A5.
- *Indications—conditions in which a medication should be given*
- *Contraindications—conditions in which a medication should not be given*
- *Dose—the amount of medication to be given*
- *Administration—form and route by which the medication is given*
- *Actions—the therapeutic effects of the medication*
- *Side effects—undesirable effects of the medication (pp. 369–370)*

Q6. Describe the key steps to follow in administering a medication to a patient.

A6. *(1) Obtain an order from medical direction. (2) Select the proper medication. (3) Verify that the medication is prescribed for the patient. (4) Check the expiration date. (5) Check for discoloration or impurities. (6) Verify the proper form, route, and dose. (7) Document the administration of the medication and the patient's response (pp. 370–373)*

Q7. Describe proper reassessment following administration of a medication.

A7. *Repeating vital signs and documenting patient response as part of ongoing assessment (p. 370)*

CRITICAL THINKING

Assess students' ability to respond to real-life emergency situations by discussing the Critical Thinking questions on page 376 in the textbook.

Q1. What medications might you consider administering to this patient?

A1. *Of the medications carried on most BLS ambulances, this patient would be a good candidate for oxygen and aspirin. Nitroglycerin would also be appropriate if carried on the EMS unit and approved by medical direction.*

Q2. What medication would the patient possibly have in his possession?

A2. *Since this patient has no significant medical history and is not currently taking any form of medication, he most likely is not in possession of any.*

Q3. What are the forms of the medications that you would possibly administer to this patient?

A3. *Based on the answer to question #1 above, you would be administering a gas (oxygen) and a compressed powder/tablet (aspirin). Nitroglycerin would be administered in either a tablet or spray form.*

Q4. Why are those forms of medications used?

A4. *Oxygen is only beneficial to individuals in emergency medical situations if it can be inhaled as a gas and aspirin must be administered in tablet form so the patient can chew it into a powder that is absorbable through the highly vascular lining in the mouth. Likewise, nitroglycerin is administered sublingually to allow for fast absorption through the oral mucosal lining.*

Q5. What information must you understand about the medication prior to administering it?

A5. *Prior to administering any medication, the EMT should understand the indications, contraindications, dosing requirements, administration techniques, actions, and potential side effects of it.*

Q6. What are the possible ways to obtain an order for the medication from medical direction?

A6. *As with many aspects of medical direction, there are both on-line and off-line components. Each EMS system has standing orders (off-line medical direction) which specify the medications an EMT can* *administer and in what situations they can be administered. If there is a question or unusual circumstance, EMTs can also contact medical direction via radio or telephone and receive medication orders directly from an on-line physician.*

Q7. What are the five "rights" you would check prior to administering any medication?

A7. *The five "rights" of medication administration are right patient, right medication, right route, right dose, and right date.*

MEDICATIONS EXERCISE

Give students a chance to apply what they have learned about medications an EMT may or may not administer to a real-life situation. Bring into class a variety of medications that patients often take. Medical direction might be a good source for help in selecting these medications. Be sure to include among the medications samples of prescribed inhalers, nitroglycerin, and epinephrine. Also have on hand multiple copies of the *U.S. Pharmacopoeia* and the *Physicians' Desk Reference*.

Then divide the class into teams. Depending on the number of medications available, you can either divide them into batches equal to the number of groups or have all groups work with the same medications. Instruct students to decide, with the help of the textbook and in-class references, which of these medications an EMT is permitted to help patients administer.

To review student choices, take the part of a medical director or invite an actual medical director to visit class. Have each team seek permission to administer each of these drugs in a mock radio report. (If a team has selected three drugs, for example, they should deliver three separate radio reports.) An affirmative answer by either you or the medical director will indicate a correct choice.

Note: This activity also provides a good opportunity to reinforce the communication skills developed in Module 3.

Reading/Reference
Textbook, pp. 377–411

Workbook
Chapter 12 Activities

Chapter Quiz
Handout 12–2

TestGen
Chapter 12 Test

ASSIGNMENTS

Assign students to read Chapter 13, "Respiratory Emergencies," before the next class. Also ask them to complete Chapter 12 of the Workbook.

EVALUATION

Chapter Quiz Distribute copies of the Chapter Quiz provided in Handout 12-2 to evaluate student understanding of this chapter. Remind students not to refer to their textbooks or notes while taking the quiz.

Test Manager You may wish to create a custom-tailored test using Prentice Hall *TestGen for Prehospital Emergency Care, Eighth Edition* to evaluate student understanding of this chapter.

Online Test Preparation (for students and instructors) Additional test preparation is available through *EMT Achieve: Basic Test Preparation* at http://www.prenhall.com/EMTAchieve. Instructors can also monitor student mastery online.

Online Test Preparation
Send your students to
http://www.prenhall.com/
EMTAchieve

REINFORCEMENT

Handouts If classroom discussions or performance on the quiz indicates that some students have not fully mastered the chapter content, you may wish to assign some or all of the Reinforcement Handouts for this chapter.

TECH EXTRAS

Brady Skills Series EMT-B Videos/CD Have your students watch the skills come to life on either VHS or CD-ROM.

PowerPoint Presentation (for instructors) The PowerPoint material developed for this chapter offers useful reinforcement of chapter content.

Student CD A wide variety of material on this CD-ROM will reinforce and also expand student knowledge and skills.

Companion Website (for students) Additional review quizzes and links to EMS resources will contribute to further reinforcement of this chapter. Please visit http://www.prenhall.com/mistovich.

Handouts 12–3 to 12–5
Reinforcement Activities

Brady Skills Series EMT-B Videos/CD
Visual Reinforcement

PowerPoint Presentation
Chapter 12

Student CD
Chapter 12

Companion Website
http://www.prenhall.com/mistovich

OBJECTIVES CHECKLIST

Cognitive		Date Mastered
4–1.1	Identify which medications will be carried on the unit.	
4–1.2	State the medications carried on the EMS unit by the generic name.	
4–1.3	Identify the medications with which the EMT may assist the patient with administering.	
4–1.4	State the medications that the EMT can assist the patient with by the generic name.	
4–1.5	Discuss the forms in which the medications may be found.	
*	List and explain the various routes of drug administration used by the EMT.	
*	List and describe the essential medication information that should be understood by the EMT.	
*	List and describe the key steps in administering medications to a patient.	
*	Describe the reassessment strategies used following medication administration.	
*	List sources that can be used to gather medication information.	

Affective		Date Mastered
4–1.6	Explain the rationale for the administration of medications.	

Psychomotor		Date Mastered
4–1.7	Demonstrate general steps for assisting the patient with self-administration of medications.	
4–1.8	Read the labels and inspect each type of medication.	

CHAPTER 12 QUIZ

Write the letter of the best answer in the space provided.

_____ 1. An EMT is permitted, with medical direction, to administer, or assist the patient in administering, all of the following medications *except*
   A. nitroglycerin.
   B. oxygen.
   C. penicillin.
   D. oral glucose.

_____ 2. A drug or other substance that is used as a remedy for illness is called a(n)
   A. elixir.
   B. treatment.
   C. medication.
   D. prescription.

_____ 3. A chemical substance that is used to treat or prevent a disease or condition is called a
   A. treatment.
   B. prescription.
   C. drug.
   D. preparation.

_____ 4. The study of drugs is referred to as
   A. pharmacology.
   B. pharmacokinetics.
   C. pharmacodynamics.
   D. pharmacytology.

_____ 5. Epinephrine is an example of a drug's _____ name.
   A. chemical
   B. trade
   C. generic
   D. brand

_____ 6. The most common uses of a drug in treating a specific condition are known as
   A. indications.
   B. side effects.
   C. protocols.
   D. contraindications.

_____ 7. A thick slurry of activated charcoal is an example of a
   A. gel.
   B. suspension.
   C. compressed powder.
   D. sublingual spray.

_____ 8. Drugs meeting the requirements of the *U.S. Pharmacopoeia* or *National Formulary* are given a(n) _____ name.
   A. generic
   B. trade
   C. official
   D. chemical

_____ 9. Medications administered sublingually are
   A. swallowed.
   B. inhaled.
   C. dissolved under the tongue.
   D. injected under the skin.

_____ 10. Drug actions that are *not* desired and that occur in addition to the desired therapeutic effects are referred to as
   A. reactions.
   B. contraindications.
   C. indications.
   D. side effects.

REINFORCEMENT

IN THE FIELD

Read the following real-life situation. Then answer the questions that follow.

You receive a call from a 6-year-old girl who states that her "grandma can hardly breathe." When you arrive at the scene, you find a 68-year-old female with labored breathing. She can barely talk as she gasps for air. But after several attempts, the woman indicates that she has just finished mowing the lawn. She thinks the exertion has triggered her respiratory condition.

1. What type of medication do you suspect the patient might take?

You place the patient in a comfortable sitting position and administer high-flow oxygen. You ask your partner to take vital signs while you obtain a medical history. The patient indicates that her physician has prescribed an inhaler for her respiratory condition, but that she has not used it today. The woman tells her granddaughter to bring the medication to you.

2. What are some brand names of the prescribed inhalers that you might expect to see?

3. After examining the patient's medication, you call medical direction for permission to assist the patient in self-administration. In assisting the patient with her medication, what are the key steps that must be followed?

4. What route of administration will be used with this medication?

CHAPTER 12 REVIEW

Write the word or words that best complete each sentence in the space provided.

1. The study of drugs is called _____.

2. Medications have specific _____ effects on the cells, organs, or body systems.

3. _____ _____ is a suspension used to treat a poisoning or an overdose emergency.

4. _____ medications may be administered to patients who are able to swallow.

5. The _____ of a drug are the therapeutic effects that a drug will have.

6. The _____ of a drug is simply how much of the drug should be given to the patient.

7. _____ is a medication that may be administered by the EMT by the intramuscular injection route.

8. The term _____ refers to how a medication is actually given to or taken by a patient.

9. The _____ _____ - _____ may be prescribed for patients with a history of severe allergic reactions.

10. Each drug also has _____, or situations in which the drug should *not* be administered because of the potential harm that could be caused to the patient.

PHARMACOLOGY BASICS: LISTING

1. List the seven medications that an EMT may administer or help a patient to self-administer.

2. List the four types of names by which every drug is known.

3. List the four routes by which the EMT may administer or help a patient to self-administer medications.

4. List eight medication forms.

5. List two common sources from which to gather information about specific medications.

General Pharmacology

Administering Medications
Medications Commonly
Administered by the EMT
   Oxygen
   Oral Glucose
   Activated Charcoal
   Aspirin
   Metered-Dose Inhaler
   Nitroglycerin
   Epinephrine
Medication Names
   Chemical
   Generic
   Trade
   Official
Routes of Administration
   Sublingual
   Oral
   Inhalation
   Injection

Medication Forms

Compressed Powder or Tablet

Liquid for Injection

Gel

Suspension

Fine Powder for Inhalation

Gas

Spray

Liquid/Vaporized Fixed-Dose
Nebulizer

Essential Medication Information

Indications

Contraindications

Dose

Administration

Actions

Side Effects

Administering Medications

Sources of Medication Information

HANDOUT 12-2: Chapter 12 Quiz

1. C	**4.** A	**7.** B	**9.** C
2. C	**5.** C	**8.** C	**10.** D
3. C	**6.** A		

HANDOUT 12-3: In the Field

1. A prescribed inhaler
2. Brand names might include: Alupent®, Ventolin®, Proventil®, Bronkosol®, Serevent®
3. Verify the patient's prescription; check the expiration date; check for discoloration or impurities; verify form, route, and dose; and document the administration drug, dose, route, and time.
4. Inhalation

HANDOUT 12-4: Chapter 12 Review

1. pharmacology
2. physiological
3. Activated charcoal
4. Oral
5. actions
6. dose
7. Epinephrine
8. route
9. epinephrine auto-injector
10. contraindications

HANDOUT 12-5: Pharmacology Basics: Listing

1. Activated charcoal, oral glucose, oxygen, aspirin, metered-dose inhaler, nitroglycerin, epinephrine
2. Generic, chemical, trade (brand), and official
3. Oral, sublingual, inhalation, injection
4. Compressed powder or tablet, liquid for injection, gel, suspension, fine powder for inhalation, gas, spray, and liquid/vaporized fixed-dose nebulizer
5. Any two: American Hospital Formulary Service; AMA Drug Evaluation; *Physicians' Desk Reference* (PDR); package inserts; poison control centers; EMS pocket drug reference guide.

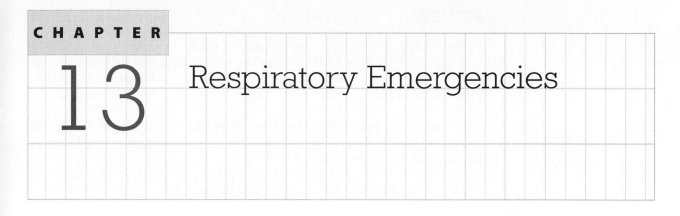

This chapter covers Lesson 4-2 and portions of Lesson 4-10 of the U.S. Department of Transportation's EMT-Basic National Standard Curriculum.

OBJECTIVES

Numbered objectives are from the U.S. Department of Transportation EMT-Basic National Standard Curriculum. Asterisked objectives, if any, pertain to material that is supplemental to the DOT curriculum. Page numbers in parentheses refer to pages in the textbook.

Cognitive

4-2.1   List the structure and function of the respiratory system. (pp. 378–380)

4-2.2   State the signs and symptoms of a patient with breathing difficulty. (pp. 380–387)

4-2.3   Describe the emergency medical care of the patient with breathing difficulty. (pp. 387–393)

4-2.4   Recognize the need for medical direction to assist in the emergency medical care of the patient with breathing difficulty. (pp. 388–389)

4-2.5   Describe the emergency medical care of the patient with breathing distress. (pp. 387–393)

4-2.6   Establish the relationship between airway management and the patient with breathing difficulty. (pp. 379, 381, 387, 395)

4-2.7   List signs of adequate air exchange. (p. 382)

4-2.8   State the generic name, medications forms, dose, administration, action, indications, and contraindications for the prescribed inhaler. (pp. 389–390)

4-2.9   Distinguish between the emergency medical care of the infant, child, and adult patient with breathing difficulty. (pp. 394–395)

4-2.10 Differentiate between upper airway obstruction and lower airway disease in the infant and child patient. (p. 395)

Affective

4-2.11 Defend EMT-Basic treatment regimens for various respiratory emergencies. (pp. 387–393)

4-2.12 Explain the rationale for administering an inhaler. (pp. 388–390)

Psychomotor

4-2.13 Demonstrate the emergency medical care for breathing difficulty.

4-2.14 Perform the steps in facilitating the use of an inhaler.

Total Teaching Time
150 minutes

Resources Needed
- Scored Chapter 12 Quizzes
- Complete jump kit containing BSI equipment
- Oxygen equipment
- Portable suction unit
- Wheeled stretcher
- Practice placebo inhaler

Additional Resources
Larmon/Davis, *Basic Life Support Skills*

Elling, *EMT Achieve: Basic Test Preparation*

Limmer/Mistovich/O'Keefe, *Audio Lecture & Study Guide: EMT*

Mistovich/Kuvlesky, *SUCCESS! for the EMT, Second Edition*

REVIEW

In the last lesson, "General Pharmacology," students learned that, as EMTs, they may carry on their EMS units several medications that they may be able to give under specific conditions. There will be a few other medications that, when prescribed for a patient, they may be permitted—with the approval and advice of medical direction—to assist patients to administer to themselves. The chapter emphasized that the ability of an EMT to administer the proper medication, according to local protocols, in an emergency situation can impact critically on the patient's well-being.

Distribute the scored quizzes from the last class. Go over each question on the quiz and handle any concerns students may have about the answers.

INTRODUCTION TO CHAPTER 13

Chapter 13, "Respiratory Emergencies," is the second lesson in Module 4. Help students understand the seriousness of respiratory emergencies and the high level of anxiety experienced by patients suffering respiratory emergencies. Explain that few things are more frightening to the patient than the inability to breathe easily, and one of the most common symptoms of a respiratory emergency is shortness of breath. Point out that while EMT provide immediate intervention to relieve the patient's physical distress, they must also treat the patient's emotional distress. In Chapter 13, students discover that recognizing the signs and symptoms of respiratory distress, providing immediate intervention, and transport are critical to all patients, but especially to the infant and child. Distribute the Chapter 13 Objectives Checklist and give students a few minutes to look it over. Then briefly paraphrase the objectives for this lesson in your own words.

LECTURE

The following suggested lecture outline is based on the Department of Transportation's EMT-Basic National Standard Curriculum. In some places, the DOT curriculum has been rearranged or expanded upon so that it is more complete or easier for the student to understand. The page numbers in parentheses refer to pages in the textbook. The parenthetical references in dark, heavy type are to figures, tables, and scans in the textbook.

RESPIRATORY EMERGENCIES

I. **Anatomy and physiology review** (p. 378)
  A. Begin the lesson by doing a thorough review of respiratory anatomy and physiology. (Chapters 4 and 7; pp. 69–76, 154–162)
II. **Breathing difficulty** (pp. 378–395)
  A. Terminology (pp. 378–379)
    1. Dyspnea
    2. Apnea
    3. Bronchoconstriction
    4. Bronchospasm
    5. Bonchodilation
  B. Common causes (pp. 379–380)
    1. Mechanical disruption to the airway, lungs, or chest wall
    2. Stimulation of receptors in lungs
    3. Inadequate gas exchange at level of alveoli and capillary
      a. Ventilation disturbance

Handout 13-1
Chapter 13 Objectives Checklist

Lecture Master
You may wish to display Lecture Master 13 when presenting the lecture to the class.

Point of Interest
Inhaled air is warmed and humidified in the nose and oropharynx. By the time air reaches the lungs, it is already close to body temperature.

      b. Perfusion disturbance

      c. Ventilation and perfusion disturbance

   4. Respiratory distress

   5. Respiratory failure

   6. Respiratory arrest

C. Assessment of breathing difficulty (pp. 380–387) (**Fig. 13-9a, p. 396**)

   1. Scene size-up

   2. Initial assessment and management of life threats

      a. General impression

         (1) The patient's position (**Fig. 13-1, p. 380**)

         (2) The patient's face

         (3) The patient's speech

         (4) Altered mental status

         (5) Use of the muscles in the neck and retractions of the muscles between the ribs (intercostal muscles)

         (6) Cyanosis

         (7) Diaphoresis

         (8) Pallor

         (9) Nasal flaring

       (10) Pursed lips

      b. Mental status

      c. Breathing

      d. Circulation

   3. Focused history and physical exam

      a. SAMPLE history (**Tables 13-1, p. 383, 13-2, p. 384**)

      b. Physical exam

         (1) Baseline vital signs, including SpO_2

         (2) Signs and symptoms

            (a) Shortness of breath

            (b) Restlessness, agitation, anxiety

            (c) Increased or irregular heart rate in adults and children; decreased heart rate in infants

            (d) Breathing rates that are faster or slower than normal or irregular

            (e) Cyanosis, pallor, flushing (allergy), moistness

            (f) Audible wheezing

            (g) Diminished ability or inability to speak

            (h) Retractions of accessory muscles in upper chest, between ribs, and muscles of the neck

            (i) Excessive use of diaphragm

            (j) Shallow breathing

            (k) Coughing

            (l) Barrel chest, indicating a chronic respiratory condition (**Fig. 13-3, p. 386**)

           (m) Altered mental status

            (n) Nasal flaring

            (o) Pursed-lip breathing

            (p) Tracheal indrawing

            (q) Indications of chest trauma, such as paradoxical motion

   4. Ongoing assessment of priority patient

D. Emergency care of patient with breathing difficulty (pp. 387–388) (**Fig, 13-9b, p. 397; Fig. 13-10, p. 398**)

   1. Inadequate breathing

Slides/Videos
"Respiratory Emergencies," *Pulse,* Jan. 1999.

a. Establish an open airway.

b. Begin positive pressure ventilation with supplemental oxygen.

c. Transport expeditiously.

2. Adequate breathing

  a. Administer oxygen at 15 liters per minute via nonrebreather mask. **(Fig. 13-2, p. 382)**

  b. Assess baseline vital signs.

  c. Determine if patient has a prescribed metered-dose inhaler. If so, with permission from medical direction, assist patient in self-administration.

  d. Complete focused history and physical exam.

  e. Place patient in position of comfort.

  f. Transport.

E. Metered-dose inhalers (pp. 388–390) **(Fig. 13-4, pp. 389–390; Table 13-3, p. 393; Fig. 13-7, p. 393)**

  1. Medication names

    a. Albuterol (Proventil®, Ventolin®)

    b. Bitolterol mesylate (Tornalate®)

    c. Ipratropium bromide (Atrovent®)

    d. Isoetharine (Bronkosol®)

    e. Metaproterenol (Metaprel®, Alupent®)

    f. Salmeterol xinafoate (Serevent®)

    g. Montelukast (Singulair®)

    h. Levalbuterol (Xoponex®)

    i. Pirbuterol (Maxair®)

  2. Indications

    a. Exhibits signs and symptoms of breathing difficulty

    b. Has physician-prescribed metered-dose inhaler

    c. Has specific authorization by medical direction

  3. Contraindications

    a. Patient not responsive enough to use device

    b. Inhaler is not prescribed for the patient

    c. No permission from medical direction

    d. Patient has already met maximum prescribed dose prior to EMT arrival

  4. Medication form

    a. Handheld metered-dose inhaler

  5. Dosage

    a. Number of inhalations based on medical direction's order

  6. Administration **(Figs. 13-5, pp. 391–392; 13-6, p. 392)**

    a. Ensure right medication, right patient, right route, right dose.

    b. Obtain order from medical direction, either on-line or off-line.

    c. Check the expiration date of the inhaler.

    d. Check to see if the patient has already taken any doses.

    e. Ensure the inhaler is at room temperature or warmer.

    f. Shake the inhaler vigorously for 30 seconds.

    g. Remove nonrebreather mask from patient.

    h. Have the patient exhale deeply.

    i. Have the patient put his lips around the opening of the inhaler.

    j. Have the patient depress the handheld inhaler as he begins to inhale deeply.

Teaching Tip

Have two or three inhalers, some with spacers, available to pass around to students during the lecture.

Point to Emphasize

By the time EMTs arrive on the scene of a respiratory emergency, most patients who had inhalers will have already used them, usually to excess. Students should expect to find rapid heart rates and flushed skin with these patients.

    k. Instruct the patient to hold his breath for 10 seconds or as long as he comfortably can (so medication can be absorbed), and then exhale slowly.

    l. Replace oxygen on patient.

    m. Allow patient to breath a few times and repeat second dose per medical direction.

    n. If patient has a spacer device for use with the inhaler, it should be used. A spacer device is an attachment between inhaler and patient that allows for more effective use of medication.

7. Actions of beta agonist bronchodilators

    a. Dilates bronchioles reducing airway resistance.

8. Side effects

    a. Increased pulse rate

    b. Tremors, shakiness

    c. Nervousness

    d. Dry mouth

    e. Nausea, vomiting

9. Reassessment strategies

    a. Gather vital signs and focused reassessment.

    b. Patient may deteriorate and need positive pressure artificial ventilation.

F. Infant and child considerations (pp. 390–395)

1. Early signs

    a. Increased use of accessory muscles

    b. Retractions during inspiration

    c. Increased breathing rate

    d. Increased heart rate

    e. Nasal flaring

    f. Prolonged exhalation

    g. Frequent coughing

    h. Cyanosis to extremities

    i. Anxiety

2. Late signs

    a. Altered mental status

    b. Slow heart rate

    c. Low blood pressure

    d. Extremely fast, slow, or irregular breathing

    e. Cyanosis to core of body and mucous membranes

    f. Loss of muscle tone (limp appearance)

    g. Diminished or absent breath sounds

    h. Head bobbing with each breath

    i. Grunting during exhalation

    j. See-saw or rocky breathing

    k. Decreased response to pain

    l. Inadequate tidal volume

3. Emergency care

    a. Similar to an adult with difficulty breathing

    b. Allow the child to assume a position of comfort

    c. Apply oxygen by nonrebreather mask on a child who is sitting up in his parent's lap

    d. If at any time the infant or child's breathing becomes inadequate (respiratory failure), remove from the parent, establish an open airway, and begin positive pressure ventilation with supplemental oxygen **(Fig. 13-8, p. 394)**

ENRICHMENT (OPTIONAL)

The following sections contain information that is valuable as background for the EMT, but that goes substantially beyond the U.S. Department of Transportation's EMT-Basic National Standard Curriculum.

III. Assessing breath sounds (pp. 395–397) **(Fig. 13-11, pp. 399–400)**
   A. Wheezing (pp. 397)
   B. Rhonchi (pp. 397)
   C. Crackles or rales (pp. 397)

IV. Conditions that cause breathing difficulty (pp. 397–408)
   A. Obstructive lung disease (pp. 400–401) **(Fig. 13-12, 13-13, p. 401; Fig, 13-14, p. 402)**
   B. Emphysema (pp. 401–402)
      1. Overview of disease process
      2. Assessment
      3. Emergency medical care
   C. Chronic bronchitis (pp. 402–403)
      1. Overview of disease process
      2. Assessment
      3. Emergency medical care
   D. Asthma (pp. 403–404) **(Fig. 13-15, p. 403)**
      1. Overview of disease process
      2. Assessment
      3. Emergency medical care
   E. Pneumonia (pp. 404)
      1. Overview of disease process
      2. Assessment
      3. Emergency medical care
   F. Pulmonary embolism (pp. 404–406) **(Fig. 13-16, p. 405)**
      1. Overview of disease process
      2. Assessment
      3. Emergency medical care
   G. Acute pulmonary edema (pp. 406–407) **(Fig. 13-17, p. 406)**
      1. Overview of disease process
      2. Assessment
      3. Emergency medical care
   H. Spontaneous pneumothorax (pp. 407–408) **(Fig. 13-18, p. 407)**
      1. Overview of disease process
      2. Assessment
      3. Emergency medical care
   I. Hyperventilation syndrome (p. 408)
      1. Overview of disease process
      2. Assessment
      3. Emergency medical care

CASE STUDY FOLLOW-UP

Ask a student volunteer to read the Case Study that begins on page 378 of the textbook. You may wish to use the following questions to engage students in a discussion of the Case Study Follow-up that begins on page 409 of the textbook. Provide missing information and clarify ideas as needed.

Q1. What does your initial assessment reveal about Mrs. Sanders's airway and breathing? What do you do in response?

A1. *The patient gasps for her breath after each word. Her airway is open and her breathing is rapid and labored at a rate of 34 per minute. There are audible wheezes when she exhales. Her radial pulse is about 110 per minute. The skin is moist and slightly pale. This patient is a priority and is immediately given oxygen via a nonrebreather mask at 15 liters per minute.*

Q2. How do you conduct the focused history and physical exam and what do they reveal about Mrs. Sanders's problem?

A2. *The difficulty in breathing is evaluated using the OPQRST mnemonic and asking the patient questions that can be answered with a nod or shake of the head to reduce her need to respond by speaking. Some questions are directed to her husband. Questioning reveals that the breathing difficulty began gradually about 2 hours earlier and got progressively worse. The patient is unable to lie down because this causes her breathing to get much worse. Sitting up is not much better. She has had similar episodes in the past, but none seem to have been this severe. On a scale of 1 to 10, Mrs. Sanders indicates that her difficulty in breathing is about 8 or 9. A SAMPLE history reveals the primary symptom is severe difficulty in breathing. Mrs. Sanders has an allergy to penicillin. The patient has a prescription of Albuterol® in a metered-dose inhaler and took one dose about 15 minutes earlier. She is on no other medication. She has a past medical history of asthma and suffers these attacks maybe once every 4 or 5 months. She has had nothing to eat for about 3 hours but drank a small glass of orange juice about an hour ago. She was cleaning the kitchen when the episode began. A focused physical exam reveals jugular vein distention, significant use of the abdominal muscles when exhaling, breath sounds that are diminished bilaterally, wheezing audible even without a stethoscope, and fingertips slightly cyanotic. The baseline vital signs are blood pressure—134/86; pulse—118 per minute and regular; respirations—32 per minute and labored with audible wheezing; the skin is moist and slightly pale.*

Q3. What do you do before and during administration of the Albuterol®?

A3. *Medical direction is contacted for an order to administer the Albuterol® by MDI. The medication container is checked to ensure it is prescribed to Mrs. Sanders, that it is the correct medication, and that it has not expired. The physical findings and SAMPLE history are reported to medical direction, who orders the administration of one dose. If that dose produces no relief of the symptoms, medical direction is to be recontacted for further orders. Mrs. Sanders is familiar with the MDI and its use, but she is too scared and apprehensive to use it properly and must be verbally coached throughout the procedure.*

Q4. How do you transport Mrs. Sanders to the ambulance?

A4. *Mrs. Sanders is secured in a Fowler's position on a stair chair, and transported down to a stretcher on the first floor, then moved to the stretcher and to the ambulance.*

Assess students' ability to apply what they have just learned by discussing the Review Questions on page 411 in the textbook.

Q1. List the major signs and symptoms of breathing difficulty.

A1. *The major signs and symptoms of breathing difficulty are: shortness of breath; restlessness, agitation, anxiety; increased or irregular heart rate in adults and children; decreased heart rate in infants; breathing rates that are faster or slower than normal or irregular; cyanosis, pallor, flushing, moistness; audible wheezing; diminished ability or inability to speak; retractions of accessory muscles in upper chest, between ribs, and muscles of the neck; excessive use of diaphragm; shallow breathing; coughing; barrel chest; altered mental status; nasal flaring; pursed-lip breathing; tracheal indrawing; indications of chest trauma, such as paradoxical motion. (pp. 380–382)*

Q2. List the signs of adequate breathing.

A2. *The signs of adequate breathing are adequate chest rise and fall, good volume of air being breathed in and out, good breath sounds bilaterally, and adequate breathing rate. (pp. 386–387)*

Q3. List the signs of inadequate breathing.

A3. *The signs of inadequate breathing are poor chest rise and fall, poor volume heard and felt, diminished or absent breath sounds, and inadequate breathing rate. (pp. 386–387, 396)*

Q4. List the steps of emergency care for a patient who is exhibiting signs and symptoms of breathing difficulty but is breathing adequately.

A4. *The steps of emergency care for a patient who is exhibiting signs and symptoms of breathing difficulty but is breathing adequately are: (1) Provide oxygen at 15 liters per minute via a nonrebreather mask. (2) Assess vital signs. (3) If the patient has a prescribed metered-dose inhaler, with permission from medical direction, assist the patient with the administration of the medication. (4) Complete a focused history and physical exam. (5) Place the patient in a position of comfort and transport. (pp. 387, 397–398)*

Q5. List the steps of emergency care for a patient who is in respiratory distress and is breathing inadequately.

A5. *The steps of emergency care for a patient who is in respiratory distress and is breathing inadequately are: (1) Establish an open airway. (2) Begin positive-pressure ventilations with supplemental oxygen. Check for signs of adequate ventilation. (3) Expeditiously transport the patient to the hospital. (pp. 387, 397–398)*

Q6. List the signs of adequate positive-pressure ventilation and the steps to take if ventilation is inadequate.

A6. *The signs of adequate positive-pressure ventilation are: The tidal volume is consistent and sufficient enough to cause the chest to rise with each ventilation; the rate is approximately 10–12/minute for an adult or 20/minute for an infant or a child; heart rate returns to normal; color improves. If ventilation is inadequate, ensure an open airway, ensure a tight seal of the face mask, and adjust the force and rate of ventilations. If still unsuccessful, follow guidelines for removing a foreign body obstruction. (Chapter 7)*

©2008 by Pearson Education, Inc.
Prehospital Emergency Care, 8th ed.

Q7. Explain the steps to administer a medication by MDI.

A7. *The steps to administer a medication by MDI are: (1) Ensure right patient, right medication, right dose, right route, right date. Determine if the patient is alert enough to use the inhaler and if any doses have already been administered prior to your arrival. (2) Obtain an order from medical direction. (3) Ensure that the inhaler is at room temperature or warmer. Shake vigorously for at least 30 seconds. (4) Remove the nonrebreather mask from the patient. Instruct the patient to take the inhaler in his hand and hold it upright. If the patient is unable to hold the device, place your index finger on the top of the metal canister and your thumb on the bottom of the plastic container. (5) Have the patient exhale fully. (6) Have the patient place his lips around the mouthpiece (opening) of the inhaler or open his mouth and place the inhaler 1 to 1.5 inches from the front of the lips (two finger widths). (7) Have the patient begin to slowly and deeply inhale over about 5 seconds as he or you depress the canister. (8) Remove the inhaler and coach the patient to hold his breath for 10 seconds or as long as comfortable. (9) Have the patient exhale slowly through pursed lips. (10) Replace the oxygen mask on the patient. Reassess the breathing status and vital signs. (11) Reassess the patient and consult with medical direction if additional doses are needed. If an additional dose is recommended, wait at least 2 minutes between administrations or longer. If using a spacer, follow the same steps listed above with the following exceptions for (6) and (7): (6) Remove the spacer cap and attach the inhaler to the spacer. (7) Depress the medication canister to fill the spacer with the medication. As soon as the canister is depressed, have the patient place his lips around the mouthpiece and inhale slowly and deeply. (pp. 389–392)*

Q8. List the indications and contraindications for the use of a beta agonist drug.

A8. *Indications for use of a beta agonist drug are: Patient exhibits signs and symptoms of breathing difficulty. The patient has a physician-prescribed metered-dose inhaler. The EMT has received approval from medical direction. The contraindications are: The patient is not responsive enough to use the MDI. The MDI is not prescribed for the patient. Permission has not been granted by medical direction. The patient has already taken the maximum allowed dose prior to your arrival. (p. 389)*

Q9. Describe the early signs of breathing difficulty in the infant or child; list the signs of inadequate breathing and respiratory failure in the infant or child.

A9. *The early signs of breathing difficulty in the infant or child are: increased use of accessory muscles to breathe, retractions during inspiration, tachypnea (increased breathing rate), tachycardia (increased heart rate), nasal flaring, prolonged exhalation, frequent coughing, and cyanosis to the extremities. The signs of inadequate breathing and respiratory failure are: altered mental status (may be completely unresponsive); bradycardia (slow heart rate); hypotension (low blood pressure); extremely fast, slow, or irregular breathing pattern; cyanosis to the core of the body and mucous membranes; loss of muscle tone (limp appearance); diminished or absent breath sounds; head bobbing; grunting; seesaw or rocky breathing; decreased response to pain; inadequate tidal volume. (p. 394)*

Q10. Explain how to distinguish airway obstruction in the infant or child patient caused by disease from airway obstruction from a foreign body; explain how treatment would differ for the two types of airway obstruction.

A10. *Airway obstruction is likely to be caused by a disease if onset is gradual, there are additional signs and symptoms of illness, or if the infant or child has a history of respiratory problems. Airway obstruction is likely to be caused by a foreign body if onset is sudden, there are objects around that the patient could have swallowed or if the choking was witnessed, there are no other signs or symptoms of illness, and there is no history of respiratory problems. Airway obstruction caused by a foreign body may be removed by approved basic life support techniques. Airway obstruction caused by illness should be managed by application of high-flow oxygen by nonrebreather mask or by positive-pressure ventilation with supplemental oxygen, as necessary. (pp. 394–395)*

CRITICAL THINKING

Assess students' ability to respond to real-life emergency situations by discussing the Critical Thinking questions on page 411 in the textbook.

Q1. What would be the immediate emergency care provided during the initial assessment?

A1. *During the initial assessment, the EMT should initiate positive pressure ventilations with supplemental oxygen connected and flowing to the ventilation device.*

Q2. What is the respiratory status of the patient?

A2. *The respiratory rate of 36 per minute and a shallow tidal volume would cause you to categorize this patient as being in respiratory failure. Other signs include the very low SpO_2 reading of 82%; gasping respirations; skin that is pale, cool, and clammy; and the circumoral cyanosis.*

Q3. How would you manage the respiratory status of the patient?

A3. *The EMT should keep the patient in a sitting position, provide positive pressure ventilations with a BVM supplemented with 15 lpm of oxygen and transport without delay.*

Q4. What would you expect to find upon auscultation of the lungs?

A4. *The EMT would most likely notice crackles (rales) and possibly even wheezing on auscultation.*

Q5. What areas of the lungs would be most important to auscultate?

A5. *Auscultating the lower lobes in the posterior thorax will provide the best opportunity to hear any abnormal breath sounds.*

Q6. What would be the most effective method to increase oxygenation in the patient?

A6. *The most effective way to increase this patient's oxygenation would be to provide positive pressure ventilations with a BVM and 15 lpm of oxygen.*

PRACTICE SCENARIO

Give students an opportunity to apply what they have learned by role-playing a real-life situation encountered by an EMS unit responding to a call involving a respiratory complaint. Ask two volunteers to play the role of EMTs and one to be the patient.

Take the two EMT players outside the classroom and provide them with a complete jump kit containing BSI equipment, oxygen equipment, a portable suction unit, and a stretcher. Describe the following scenario to them:

You receive a call from the emergency medical dispatcher for a patient at home having difficulty breathing. The emphasis of the scene is on dealing with respiratory emergencies. However, you should utilize all the skills you have learned to date. You can review basic "run" skills now while you wait for me to call you to the scene.

Return to the classroom and describe this scenario to the student acting the part of the patient.

You are a 30-year-old patient with asthma. You are having a severe attack at home, are struggling to take in enough air, and are very scared. You are standing with your feet wide apart and leaning forward against a table for support. You can hardly speak. You ran out of your prescription inhaler 2 weeks ago and haven't had the money to get a refill, so you bought an over-the-counter medication. (Hand the patient a practice placebo inhaler.) You have taken several doses without relief. Direct the patient to take his or her place and to start acting. Then dispatch the EMTs to the scene. Allow the role play to progress naturally. Intervene only if the players seem to be at a loss for what to do. Bring the play to an end when the EMTs have prepared the patient for transport to the ambulance by placing him or her on the stretcher. Following the role play, discuss the following questions with the class:

- What did the EMTs do well?
- What, if anything, should they have done differently?

You might consider extending practice to the entire class by dividing students into pairs and directing them to take turns administering metered-dose inhalers (using practice placebo inhalers) to each other.

ASSIGNMENTS

Assign students to read Chapter 14, "Cardiac Emergencies," before the next class. Also ask them to complete Chapter 13 of the Workbook.

Reading/Reference
Textbook, pp. 412–463

Workbook
Chapter 13 Activities

Chapter Quiz
Handout 13-2

TestGen
Chapter 13 Test

Online Test Preparation
Send your students to
http://www.prenhall.com/
EMTAchieve

Handouts 13-3 to 13-5
Reinforcement Activities

**Brady Skills Series
EMT-B Videos/CD**
Visual Reinforcement

**PowerPoint
Presentation**
Chapter 13

Student CD
Chapter 13

Companion Website
http://www.prenhall.com/
mistovich

EVALUATION

Chapter Quiz Distribute copies of the Chapter Quiz provided in Handout 13-2 to evaluate student understanding of this chapter. Remind students not to refer to their textbooks or notes while taking the quiz.

Test Manager You may wish to create a custom-tailored test using Prentice Hall *TestGen for Prehospital Emergency Care, Eighth Edition* to evaluate student understanding of this chapter.

Online Test Preparation (for students and instructors) Additional test preparation is available through *EMT Achieve: Basic Test Preparation* at http://www.prenhall.com/EMTAchieve. Instructors can also monitor student mastery online.

REINFORCEMENT

Handouts If classroom discussions or performance on the quiz indicates that some students have not fully mastered the chapter content, you may wish to assign some or all of the Reinforcement Handouts for this chapter.

TECH EXTRAS

Brady Skills Series EMT-B Videos/CD Have your students watch the skills come to life on either VHS or CD-ROM.

PowerPoint Presentation (for instructors) The PowerPoint material developed for this chapter offers useful reinforcement of chapter content.

Student CD A wide variety of material on this CD-ROM will reinforce and also expand student knowledge and skills.

Companion Website (for students) Additional review quizzes and links to EMS resources will contribute to further reinforcement of this chapter. Please visit htttp://www.prenhall.com/mistovich.

OBJECTIVES CHECKLIST

Cognitive		Date Mastered
4-2.1	List the structure and function of the respiratory system.	
4-2.2	State the signs and symptoms of a patient with breathing difficulty.	
4-2.3	Describe the emergency medical care of the patient with breathing difficulty.	
4-2.4	Recognize the need for medical direction to assist in the emergency medical care of the patient with breathing difficulty.	
4-2.5	Describe the emergency medical care of the patient with breathing distress.	
4-2.6	Establish the relationship between airway management and the patient with breathing difficulty.	
4-2.7	List signs of adequate air exchange.	
4-2.8	State the generic name, medications forms, dose, administration, action, indications, and contraindications for the prescribed inhaler.	
4-2.9	Distinguish between the emergency medical care of the infant, child, and adult patient with breathing difficulty.	
4-2.10	Differentiate between upper airway obstruction and lower airway disease in the infant and child patient.	

Affective		Date Mastered
4-2.11	Defend EMT treatment regimens for various respiratory emergencies.	
4-2.12	Explain the rationale for administering an inhaler.	

Psychomotor		Date Mastered
4-2.13	Demonstrate the emergency medical care for breathing difficulty.	
4-2.14	Perform the steps in facilitating the use of an inhaler.	

OBJECTIVES

CHAPTER 13 QUIZ

Write the letter of the best answer in the space provided.

_____ 1. The condition causing breathing difficulty in which the bronchioles of the lower airway are significantly narrowed from constriction of the muscle layer is known as
     A. hypoxia.   **C.** bronchoconstriction.
     B. apnea.   **D.** bronchodilation.

_____ 2. The normal range of breaths per minute for most adults is
     A. 25–50.   **C.** 15–30.
     B. 20–40.   **D.** 12–20.

_____ 3. All of the following are signs of inadequate breathing *except*
     A. present and equal breath sounds.   **C.** cyanotic skin color.
     B. restlessness.   **D.** retractions.

_____ 4. A condition in which the cells in the body are not getting an adequate supply of oxygen is known as
     A. hypoxia.   **C.** hypervolemia.
     B. hypovolemia.   **D.** hypoergia.

_____ 5. A musical whistling sound that is heard in all lung fields upon auscultation of the chest is
     A. rales.   **C.** wheezing.
     B. crackles.   **D.** rhonchi.

_____ 6. In an infant or a child, bradycardia is a sign of
     A. circulatory collapse.   **C.** respiratory failure.
     B. cardiac arrest.   **D.** fatigue.

_____ 7. If a patient is experiencing breathing difficulty but is breathing adequately, he or she should be placed in a
     A. sniffing position.   **C.** prone position.
     B. Trendelenburg position.   **D.** position of comfort.

_____ 8. Which of the following is an example of a commonly encountered obstructive lung disease?
     A. emphysema   **C.** pneumonia
     B. pulmonary edema   **D.** pneumothorax

_____ 9. A medication commonly prescribed for the patient with a history of breathing problems is a(n)
     A. beta blocker.   **C.** bronchodilator.
     B. antiarrhythmic.   **D.** antihistamine.

_____ 10. A condition indicating extreme inspiratory effort in infants and small children in which the chest is drawn inward while the abdomen moves outward is called
     A. nasal flaring.   **C.** retractions.
     B. see-saw breathing.   **D.** grunting.

_____11. All of the following are early signs of breathing difficulty in infants and children *except*
   A. retractions.   C. bradycardia.
   B. nasal flaring.   D. anxiety.

_____12. All of the following are examples of medications delivered via prescribed metered-dose inhalers *except*
   A. Albuterol.   C. Isoetharine.
   B. Epinephrine.   D. Metaproterenol.

_____13. All of the following are medications commonly used for respiratory problems *except*
   A. Tornalate®.   C. Alupent®.
   B. Serevent®.   D. Prozac®.

_____14. A possible side effect from a prescribed inhaler is
   A. tachycardia.   C. cyanosis.
   B. hypotension.   D. altered mental status.

_____15. The total number of MDI doses that an EMT can deliver to a patient with breathing difficulty is
   A. one.   C. three.
   B. two.   D. determined by medical direction.

IN THE FIELD

Read the following real-life situation. Then answer the questions that follow.

Your unit has just received a call from the emergency medical dispatcher. A 68-year-old woman at 181 Shadow Lane reports difficulty breathing. You and your partner head to the scene, arriving 12 minutes after the call.

Upon entry into the house, you find the patient sitting in a chair, leaning forward with her hands on her knees. She appears anxious and has difficulty speaking in full sentences without gasping for breath. She tells you, "I can't seem to get enough air." As she struggles to catch her breath, the patient adds, "My chest is so tight."

You position yourself at eye level with the patient and try to calm her fears. You introduce yourself and explain that you will need to ask several questions before beginning treatment. From your questions, you learn that the patient has a history of emphysema and that she takes Lasix®, theophylline, and Ventolin®. However, she has not taken these medications for several days in an effort to prolong the prescriptions. "Refills are so expensive," she explains.

Upon physical examination, you find the patient alert, but restless. Her pulse rate is 120 beats per minute; her blood pressure is 110/68 mmHg; her respiratory rate is 20 per minute; pulse ox is 88%. Breaths are labored and noisy. Her skin is warm and pale.

1. Is the patient's breathing adequate or inadequate?

2. When you elicited a focused history of the condition, what questions should you have asked the patient?

3. What steps would you take to treat this patient?

4. How would you administer oxygen to the patient?

5. In what position should this patient be transported to the hospital?

CHAPTER 13 REVIEW

Write the word or words that best complete each sentence in the space provided.

1. Respiratory emergencies may range from shortness of breath, or _____, to complete respiratory arrest, or _____.

2. The medication known as a(n) _____ is designed to directly relax and open the bronchioles, resulting in an increase in the effectiveness of breathing.

3. During the _____ _____ - _____, the EMT should seek clues to determine whether the patient's breathing difficulty is due to trauma or to a medical condition.

4. Inadequate oxygenation of the brain causes a(n) _____ _____ _____, which, in turn, can cause the patient to be disoriented or to talk incomprehensibly or mumble.

5. _____ is an ominous and late sign of respiratory distress observable on the patient's skin.

6. Most bronchodilators begin to work almost immediately, and their effects may last up to _____ hours or more.

7. Whenever you have administered a bronchodilator to a patient, you must perform a(n) _____ _____.

8. The term _____ refers to a condition in which the cells of the body are not getting an adequate supply of oxygen.

9. A patient with breathing difficulty who is sitting upright and leaning slightly forward and supporting herself with her arms by holding onto the seat is in the _____ position.

10. Emphysema, chronic bronchitis, and asthma are examples of _____ _____ _____.

11. A device attached to an MDI that holds medication until it is inhaled is a(n) _____.

12. Metered-dose inhalers can only be administered by the EMT with the approval of _____ _____ through on-line or off-line orders.

13. A pulse oximeter reading of less than _____ in a patient with any breathing

difficulty is a sign of hypoxia.

14. If upon assessment you find your patient's breathing rate or tidal volume inadequate, begin

_____ _____ _____.

15. The patient with breathing difficulty is a(n) _____ patient, so consider

advanced life support backup.

©2008 by Pearson Education, Inc.
Prehospital Emergency Care, 8th ed.

PRESCRIBED INHALER

Write in the missing information on the medication flash card below, and save the completed card for future reference.

Prescribed Inhaler

Medication Names

1. Generic: _____

2. Trade: _____

Indications

1. _____

2. _____

3. _____

Contraindications

1. _____

2. _____

3. _____

Medication Form: _____

Dosage: _____

Action: _____

Side Effects

1. _____

2. _____

3. _____

LECTURE MASTER 13

Respiratory Emergencies

Breathing Difficulty
Assessment and Emergency Care

Metered-Dose Inhalers

Breathing Difficulty in the Infant or Child
Assessment and Emergency Care

Assessing Breath Sounds

Conditions that Cause Breathing Difficulty
Obstructive Lung Diseases

Pneumonia

Pulmonary Embolism

Acute Pulmonary Edema

Spontaneous Pneumothorax

Hyperventilation Syndrome

HANDOUT 13-2: Chapter 13 Quiz

1. C	**5.** C	**9.** C	**13.** D
2. D	**6.** C	**10.** B	**14.** A
3. A	**7.** D	**11.** C	**15.** D
4. A	**8.** A	**12.** B	

HANDOUT 13-3: In the Field

1. Adequate, but with the potential to progress to inadequate
2. OPQRST: What were you doing when the breathing difficulty started? Did anything seem to trigger the breathing difficulty? Was the onset gradual or sudden? Was the onset accompanied by chest pain or any other symptoms? Was there a sudden onset of pain? Does lying flat make the breathing difficulty worse? Does sitting up make the breathing difficulty less severe? Is there pain that occurs or increases with breathing? Do you have more trouble breathing in or out? Is the pain sharp (knifelike) or dull? If there is pain associated with breathing difficulty, does it radiate to the back, up the neck, down the arms, or to any other part of the body? How bad is this breathing difficulty on a scale of 1 to 10, with 10 being the worst breathing difficulty you have ever experienced? When did the breathing difficulty start? How long have you had it? If this is a recurring problem, how long does the breathing difficulty usually last? If the breathing difficulty started other than today, could you recall the exact day and time when this started?
3. Perform an initial assessment, administer high-flow oxygen, perform a focused history and physical exam, contact medical direction for permission to assist the patient with her prescribed inhaler, and begin transport to the hospital.
4. Use a nonrebreather mask to administer oxygen at 15 liters per minute.
5. In a position of comfort, most typically Fowler's or semi-Fowler's.

HANDOUT 13-4: Chapter 13 Review

1. dyspnea, apnea
2. bronchodilator
3. scene size-up
4. altered mental status
5. Cyanosis
6. 8
7. ongoing assessment

8. hypoxia
9. tripod
10. obstructive lung diseases
11. spacer
12. medical direction
13. 95 percent
14. positive pressure ventilation
15. priority

HANDOUT 13-5: Prescribed Inhaler

Medication Names:
1. Generic: albuterol, isoetharine, metaproterenol, bitolterol mesylate, salmeterol xinafoate
2. Trade: Proventil®, Ventolin®, Bronkosol®, Bronkometer®, Alupent®, Metaprel®, Tornalate®, Serevent®

Indications:
1. Patient exhibits signs and symptoms of breathing difficulty.
2. Patient has physician-prescribed metered-dose inhaler.
3. Medical direction gives specific authorization, whether on-line or off-line, to administer the medication.

Contraindications:
1. Patient is not responsive enough to use the device.
2. MDI is not prescribed for the patient.
3. Medical direction has not authorized its use.
4. Patient has already taken the maximum allowed dosage prior to EMT's arrival.

Medication Form:
Aerosolized in a metered-dose inhaler

Dosage:
The total number of times the medication can be administered is determined by medical direction.

Action:
Beta agonist that relaxes the bronchiole smooth muscle and dilates the lower airways. This reduces the airway resistance.

Side Effects:
1. Tachycardia
2. Tremors, shakiness
3. Nervousness
4. Dry mouth
5. Nausea, vomiting

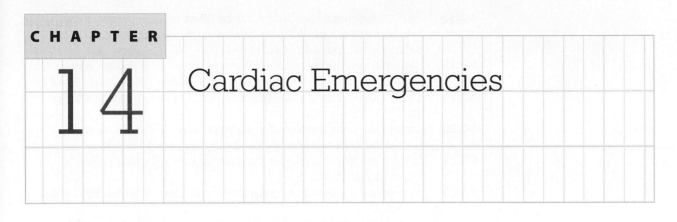

C H A P T E R

14 Cardiac Emergencies

This chapter covers Lesson 4-3 and of Lesson 4-10 of the U.S. Department of Transportation's EMT-Basic National Standard Curriculum.

OBJECTIVES

Numbered objectives are from the U.S. Department of Transportation's EMT-Basic National Standard Curriculum. Asterisked objectives, if any, pertain to material that is supplemental to the DOT curriculum. Page numbers refer to pages in the textbook.

Cognitive

4-3.1 Describe the structure and function of the cardiovascular system. (pp. 414–420)

4-3.2 Describe the emergency medical care of the patient experiencing chest pain/discomfort. (pp. 422–433)

4-3.3 List the indications for automated external defibrillation (AED). (pp. 440–441)

4-3.4 List the contraindications for automated external defibrillation. (pp. 440–441)

4-3.5 Define the role of the EMT-Basic in the emergency cardiac care system. (pp. 426–427)

4-3.6 Explain the impact of age and weight on defibrillation. (pp. 422, 440)

4-3.7 Discuss the position of comfort for patients with various cardiac emergencies. (p. 426)

4-3.8 Establish the relationship between airway management and the patient with cardiovascular compromise. (p. 422)

4-3.9 Predict the relationship between the patient experiencing cardiovascular compromise and basic cardiac life support. (pp. 422, 442)

4-3.10 Discuss the fundamentals of early defibrillation. (p. 435)

4-3.11 Explain the rationale for early defibrillation. (p. 435)

4-3.12 Explain that not all chest pain patients result in cardiac arrest and do not need to be attached to an automated external defibrillator. (pp. 412, 414, 441)

4-3.13 Explain the importance of prehospital ACLS intervention if it is available. (pp. 435, 447)

4-3.14 Explain the importance of urgent transport to a facility with Advanced Cardiac Life Support if it is not available in the prehospital setting. (p. 447)

4-3.15 Discuss the various types of automated external defibrillators. (pp. 437–438)

4-3.16 Differentiate between the fully automated and the semi-automated defibrillator. (p. 437)

Total Teaching Time
320 minutes

Resources Needed
- Scored Chapter 13 Quizzes
- Small breath mints to simulate nitroglycerin and aspirin tablets
- Jump kit
- EMT to serve as teaching assistant
- AED of the type that is most used in your area
- Shockable mannequin
- CPR mannequins

Additional Resources
Larmon/Davis, *Basic Life Support Skills*

Elling, *EMT Achieve: Basic Test Preparation*

Limmer/Mistovich/ O'Keefe, *Audio Lecture & Study Guide: EMT*

Mistovich/Kuvlesky, *SUCCESS! for the EMT, Second Edition*

4-3.17	Discuss the procedures that must be taken into consideration for standard operations of the various types of automated external defibrillators. (pp. 442–446)
4-3.18	State the reasons for ensuring that the patient is pulseless and apneic when using the automated external defibrillator. (pp. 438–440, 441)
4-3.19	Discuss the circumstances that may result in inappropriate shocks. (p. 440)
4-3.20	Explain the considerations for interruption of CPR when using the automated external defibrillator. (pp. 442, 444–445, 446)
4-3.21	Discuss the advantages and disadvantages of automated external defibrillators. (p. 437)
4-3.22	Summarize the speed of operation of automated external defibrillation. (p. 437)
4-3.23	Discuss the use of remote defibrillation through adhesive pads. (p. 437)
4-3.24	Discuss the special considerations for rhythm monitoring. (pp. 438–440)
4-3.25	List the steps in the operation of the automated external defibrillator. (pp. 442–446)
4-3.26	Discuss the standard of care that should be used to provide care to a patient with persistent ventricular fibrillation and no available ACLS. (p. 446–447)
4-3.27	Discuss the standard of care that should be used to provide care to a patient with recurrent ventricular fibrillation and no available ACLS. (p. 446–447)
4-3.28	Differentiate between the single rescuer and multirescuer care with an automated external defibrillator. (p. 445–446)
4-3.29	Explain the reasons for pulses not being checked between shocks with an automated external defibrillator. (p. 444)
4-3.30	Discuss the importance of coordinating ACLS trained providers with personnel using automated external defibrillators. (pp. 435, 447, 451)
4-3.31	Discuss the importance of post-resuscitation care. (pp. 445, 446–447)
4-3.32	List components of post-resuscitation care. (pp. 445, 446–447)
4-3.33	Explain the importance of frequent practice with the automated external defibrillator. (p. 451)
4-3.34	Discuss the need to complete the Automated Defibrillator: Operator's Shift Checklist. (p. 448)
4-3.35	Discuss the role of the American Heart Association in the use of automated external defibrillation. (pp. 433, 435)
4-3.36	Explain the role medical direction plays in the use of automated external defibrillation. (p. 451)
4-3.37	State the reasons why a case review should be completed following the use of the automated external defibrillator. (p. 451)
4-3.38	Discuss the components that should be included in a case review. (p. 451)
4-3.39	Discuss the goal of quality improvement in automated external defibrillation. (p. 451)
4-3.40	Recognize the need for medical direction of protocols to assist in the emergency medical care of the patient with chest pain. (pp. 427, 428, 429, 431)
4-3.41	List the indications for the use of nitroglycerin. (pp. 430–431)
4-3.42	State the contraindications and side effects for the use of nitroglycerin. (pp. 430–431)
4-4.43	Define the function of all controls on an automated external defibrillator, and describe event documentation and battery defibrillator maintenance. (pp. 442–446, 448, 450–451)

©2008 by Pearson Education, Inc.
Prehospital Emergency Care, 8th ed.

Affective

4-3.44   Defend the reasons for obtaining initial training in automated external defibrillation and the importance of continuing education. (pp. 435, 451)

4-3.45   Defend the reason for maintenance of automated external defibrillators. (p. 448, 450–451)

4-3.46   Explain the rationale for administering nitroglycerin to a patient with chest pain or discomfort. (p. 427)

Psychomotor

4-3.47   Demonstrate the assessment and emergency medical care of a patient experiencing chest pain/discomfort.

4-3.48   Demonstrate the application and operation of the automated external defibrillator.

4-3.49   Demonstrate the maintenance of an automated external defibrillator.

4-3.50   Demonstrate the assessment and documentation of patient response to the automated external defibrillator.

4-3.51   Demonstrate the skills necessary to complete the Automated Defibrillator: Operator's Shift Checklist.

4-3.52   Perform the steps in facilitating the use of nitroglycerin for chest pain or discomfort.

4-3.53   Demonstrate the assessment and documentation of patient response to nitroglycerin.

4-3.54   Practice completing the prehospital care report for patients with cardiac emergencies.

REVIEW

In the last lesson, "Respiratory Emergencies," students discovered that few things are more frightening to the patient than the inability to breathe easily. They also learned that shortness of breath is one of the most common symptoms of a respiratory emergency. Have students recall other signs and symptoms that can accompany difficulty in breathing, or respiratory distress, such as agitation, cyanosis, or gurgling. Remind them that patients experiencing respiratory distress need emotional as well as physical care. The EMT's ability to recognize signs and symptoms of respiratory emergencies early and to provide immediate intervention is critical to a patient's well-being, regardless of the patient's age.

Distribute the scored quizzes from the last class. Go over each question on the quiz and handle any concerns students may have about the answers.

INTRODUCTION TO CHAPTER 14

Chapter 14, "Cardiac Emergencies," is the third lesson in Module 4. In this chapter, students will learn that heart disease is America's number one killer. Most often EMTs will be called to assist a responsive patient who has signs and symptoms—particularly chest pain—that may be caused by heart disease. Only occasionally will he or she be called to a patient who is in cardiac arrest or to a patient who goes into cardiac arrest at the scene or en route to the hospital. As EMTs, students must be prepared to treat all patients with signs and symptoms of cardiac compromise as cardiac emergencies. Not every cardiac arrest is preceded by chest pain, nor do all patients with chest pain proceed to cardiac arrest, but for those who do, rapid intervention is vital. Without it, such patients will almost surely die. In cases of cardiac arrest, the actions of properly trained and equipped EMTs can make the difference between life and death.

Distribute the Chapter 14 Objectives Checklist and give students a few minutes to look it over. Then briefly paraphrase the objectives for this lesson in your own words.

Handout 14-1
Chapter 14 Objectives Checklist

LECTURE

The following suggested lecture outline is based on the Department of Transportation's EMT National Standard Curriculum. In some places, the DOT curriculum has been rearranged or expanded upon so that it is more complete or easier for the student to understand. The page numbers in parentheses refer to pages in the textbook. The parenthetical references in dark, heavy type are to figures, tables, and scans in the textbook.

CARDIAC EMERGENCIES

Lecture Master 14
You may wish to display Lecture Master 14 when presenting the lecture to the class.

Teaching Tip
The American Heart Association has excellent charts on cardiac anatomy as well as many other useful teaching materials.

On the Net
For more on cardiac concerns, go to: www.amhrt.org

Teaching Tip
Bring in beef or pork hearts as models when discussing cardiac anatomy and physiology.

Slides/Videos
"Cardiac," *Pulse,* Feb. 2001.

I. **Review of circulatory system anatomy and physiology** (pp. 414–420; also Chapter 4)
   A. Circulatory (cardiovascular) system (pp. 415–417)
      1. The Heart (**Fig. 14-1, p. 415; 14-2, p, 415**)
         a. Structure/function
            (1) Atria
               (a) Right
                  (i) Receives blood from the veins of the body and the heart; pumps oxygen-poor blood to the right ventricle
               (b) Left
                  (i) Receives blood from the pulmonary veins (lungs); pumps oxygen-rich blood to left ventricle
            (2) Ventricles
               (a) Right
                  (i) Pumps blood to the lungs
               (b) Left
                  (i) Pumps blood to the body
            (3) Valves prevent backflow of blood.
         b. Cardiac conductive system (**Fig. 14-6, p. 419**)
            (1) The heart is more than a muscle.
            (2) Specialized contractile and conductive tissue in the heart
            (3) Electrical impulses
      2. The vessels
         a. Arteries
            (1) Function
               (a) Carry blood away from the heart to the rest of the body
            (2) Major Arteries (**Fig. 14-3, p. 418**)
               (a) Coronary arteries
                  (i) Vessels that supply the heart with blood (**Fig. 14-4, p. 419**)
               (b) Aorta
                  (i) Major artery originating from the heart, lying in front of the spine in the thoracic and abdominal cavities

    (ii) Divides at the level of the navel into the iliac arteries

(c) Pulmonary
    (i) Artery originating at the right ventricle
    (ii) Carries oxygen-poor blood to the lungs

(d) Carotid
    (i) Major artery of the neck
    (ii) Supplies the head with blood
    (iii) Pulsations can be palpated on either side of the neck

(e) Femoral
    (i) The major artery of the thigh
    (ii) Supplies the groin and the lower extremities with blood
    (iii) Pulsations can be palpated in the groin area

(f) Radial
    (i) Major artery of the lower hand
    (ii) Pulsations can be palpated at the wrist thumb side

(g) Brachial
    (i) An artery of the upper arm
    (ii) Pulsations can be palpated on the inside of the arm between the elbow and the shoulder
    (iii) Used when determining a blood pressure (BP) using a BP cuff (sphygmomanometer) and a stethoscope

(h) Posterior tibial
    (i) Pulsations can be palpated on the posterior surface of the medial malleolus.

(i) Dorsalis pedis
    (i) An artery in the foot
    (ii) Pulsations can be palpated on the anterior surface of the foot

(3) Arterioles
  (a) Smallest branch of an artery leading to the capillaries

(4) Capillaries
  (a) Found in all parts of the body
  (b) Allow for the exchange of nutrients and waste at the cellular level
  (c) Tiny blood vessels that connect arterioles to venules

(5) Venules
  (a) Smallest branch of the veins leading to the capillaries

(6) Veins (**Fig. 14-3, p. 418**)
  (a) Function
    (i) Vessels that carry blood back to the heart
  (b) Major veins
    (i) Pulmonary vein
      • Carries oxygen-rich blood from the lungs to the left atrium
    (ii) Venae cavae
      • Superior

Point of Interest
A single capillary is 0.0004 inches across and has a wall made up of a single layer of cells.

Teaching Tip
Have students find the various pulses on themselves and/or other students.

- Inferior
- Carries oxygen-poor blood back to the right atrium

   3. The blood **(Fig. 14-5, p. 419)**
      a. Red blood cells
         (1) Give the blood its color
         (2) Carry oxygen to organs
         (3) Carry carbon dioxide away from organs
      b. White blood cells
         (1) Part of the body's defense against infections
      c. Plasma
         (1) Fluid that carries the blood cells and nutrients
      d. Platelets
         (1) Essential for the formation of blood clots

B. The cardiac conduction system (pp. 417–420) **(Fig. 14-6, p. 419)**
   1. Sinoatrial (SA) node
   2. Bachman's bundle
   3. Atrioventricular (AV) node
   4. Bundle of His
   5. Bundle branches
   6. Purkinie fibers

C. Blood pressure (p. 420)
   1. Systolic
      a. Pressure exerted against the walls of the artery when the left ventricle contracts
   2. Diastolic
      a. Pressure exerted against the walls of the artery when the left ventricle is at rest

D. Inadequate circulation (p. 420)
   1. Shock (hypoperfusion)
      a. A state of profound depression of the vital processes of the body
      b. Signs and symptoms
         (1) Pale, cyanotic (blue-gray color), cool, clammy skin
         (2) Rapid, weak pulse
         (3) Rapid and shallow breathing
         (4) Restlessness, anxiety, or mental dullness
         (5) Nausea and vomiting
         (6) Reduction in total blood volume, low or decreasing blood pressure
         (7) Subnormal temperature

II. Cardiac compromise and acute coronary syndromes (pp. 420–422)
   A. Signs and symptoms. May include one or all of the following (pp. 420–424) **(Fig. 14-5, p. 419)**
      1. Squeezing, dull pressure, chest pain commonly radiating down the arms or to the jaw, neck, or back
      2. Sudden onset of sweating (may be a significant finding)
      3. Cool, pale skin
      4. Difficulty breathing (dyspnea)
      5. Anxiety, irritability
      6. Feeling of impending doom
      7. Adnormal pulse rate (may be irregular)
      8. Adnormal blood pressure
      9. Epigastric pain
     10. Nausea/vomiting
     11. Lightheadedness or dizziness

B. Acute coronary syndrome in females (pp. 421–422)
  1. Classical findings
      a. Dull, substernal chest pain or discomfort
      b. Respiratory distress
      c. Nausea, vomiting
      d. Diaphoresis
  2. Nonclassical (atypical) findings
      a. Neck ache
      b. Pressure in the chest
      c. Pains in the back, breast, or upper abdomen
      d. Tingling of the fingers
      e. Unexplained fatigue or weight gain (water weight gain)
      f. Insomnia

III. Assessment and care: cardiac compromise and acute coronary syndromes (pp. 422–427)
  A. Scene size-up and initial assessment (p. 422) **(Table 14-1, p. 423)**
  B. Focused history and physical exam: the SAMPLE history (pp. 422–424)
      1. Onset provocation or palliation
      2. Quality
      3. Radiation
      4. Severity
      5. Time
  C. Fibrinolytic therapy and the EMT's role (pp. 424–425)
      1. Absolute contraindications
      2. Relative contraindications
      3. Immediate transport
          a. History of angina having chest discomfort at rest that lasts longer than 20 minutes
          b. Recent onset of angina that progressively worsens
          c. Nocturnal angina
          d. Angina unrelieved by rest or three nitroglycerin tables over 10 minutes
          e. Chest discomfort that lasts greater than 5–10 minutes after rest
  D. Focused history and physical exam: the physical exam and baseline vital signs (pp. 425–426)
      1. Pupils
      2. Oral cavity
      3. Neck
      4. Chest
      5. Lower and upper extremities
      6. Posterior body
      7. Signs and symptoms **(Fig. 14-7, p. 426)**
          a. Chest discomfort or pain that radiates to chest, neck, jaw, arm, or back
          b. Sudden onset of sweating
          c. Cool, pale skin
          d. Difficulty breathing
  E. Emergency medical care (pp. 426–427)
      1. Oxygen 15 lpm via nonrebreather mask for adequate breathing **(Fig. 14-8, p. 427)**
      2. Provide positive pressure ventilation with supplemental oxygen if breathing is inadequate
      3. Provide calm reassurance
      4. Place in a position of comfort
      5. Assist the patient with prescribed nitroglycerin

6. Administer 160–325 mg of nonenteric aspirin, if local protocol permits
7. Call for ALS backup
8. Initiate early transport
9. Apply pulse oximeter, if available

F. Ongoing assessment (p. 427)
  1. Perform scene size-up and initial assessment.

IV. **Medications** (pp. 426–433)
  A. Aspirin (p. 428) **(Fig. 14-9, p. 428)**
    1. Medication name
      a. Generic
        (1) Aspirin
      b. Trade
        (1) ASA
        (2) Bayer
        (3) Ecotrin
        (4) St. Joseph's
        (5) Bufferin
    2. Indications—must have all of the following criteria
      a. Patient exhibits chest discomfort suggestive of heart attack.
      b. Medical direction has given approval.
    3. Contraindications
      a. Known allergy or hypersensitivity to aspirin
    4. Medication form
      a. Tablet
    5. Dosage
      a. 160 mg to 325 mg as soon as possible after onset of symptoms
    6. Administration
      a. Complete focused history and physical exam and determine an acute coronary syndrome suggestive of heart attack.
      b. Obtain approval from medical direction, either on-line or off-line.
      c. Be sure patient is alert and oriented.
      d. If chewable baby aspirin is available, have patient chew one 160 mg tablet followed by swallowing another 160 mg tablet. If no chewable aspirin available, have patient swallow one 160 mg to one 325 mg tablet.
      e. Reassess patient and record vital signs.
    7. Action
      a. Decreases ability of platelets to clump together.
    8. Side effects
      a. Stomach irritation
      b. Heartburn
      c. Nausea/vomiting
    9. Reassessment
      a. Conduct an ongoing assessment.
      b. Record any changes and findings.
  B. Nitroglycerin (pp. 427–431) **(Fig. 14-11, pp. 430–431)**
    1. Medication name
      a. Generic
        (1) Nitroglycerin

    b. Trade
        (1) Nitrobid®
        (2) Nitrolingual® Spray
        (3) Nitrostat®

2. Indications (must have all of the following criteria)
    a. Exhibits signs and symptoms of chest pain
    b. Has physician-prescribed nitroglycerin
    c. Has on-line or off-line authorization by medical direction

3. Contraindications
    a. Hypotension or blood pressure below 90 mmHg systolic
    b. Head injury
    c. Infants and children
    d. Patient has already taken three doses prior to EMT arrival
    e. Patient has recently taken Viagra®

4. Medication form
    a. Tablet
    b. Sublingual spray

5. Dosage
    a. One dose, repeat in 3–5 minutes if no relief, BP > 90, and authorized by medical direction up to a maximum of three doses

6. Administration (**Fig. 14-10, pp. 429–430**)
    a. Complete focused history and physical exam.
    b. Have patient sit or lie supine.
    c. Stress baseline vitals to ensure a blood pressure above 90 mmHg systolic.
    d. Contact medical direction if no standing orders.
    e. Ensure right medication, right patient, right route, right dose, patient alert and responsive.
    f. Check expiration date of nitroglycerin.
    g. Question patient on last dose administration, effects, and ensure understanding of route of administration.
    h. Ask patient to lift tongue and place tablet or spray dose under tongue (while wearing BSI gloves) or have patient place tablet or spray under tongue.
    i. Have patient keep mouth closed (without swallowing) until dissolved and absorbed.
    j. Recheck blood pressure within 2 minutes.
    k. Record activity, time, dose, and response.
    l. Perform reassessment.

7. Actions
    a. Dilates blood vessels
    b. Decreases workload of heart
    c. Decreases cardiac oxygen demand
        (1) Side effects
    d. Hypotension
    e. Headache
    f. Pulse rate changes

8. Reassessment strategies
    a. Monitor blood pressure
    b. Ask patient about effect on pain relief
    c. Seek medical direction before readministration

Point to Emphasize

After receiving nitroglycerin, patients may report headaches or dizziness. These are normal side effects.

Point of Interest

AEDs may soon be as common as fire extinguishers in public places. For example, American Airlines has placed AEDs aboard many of its aircraft.

Slides/Videos

Brady Skill Series: EMT-B, "Automated External Defibrillator"

☑

Teaching Tip

If possible, bring a variety of AEDs to class and demonstrate their similarities and differences.

Point of Interest

Studies show that the person most likely to receive inadvertent defibrillation is the AED operator. *Be careful!*

Reading/Reference
Hazinski, M.F., "Saving Lives Through Public Access Defibrillation," *Emergency Medical Services,* Sept. 2001.

Reading/Reference
Erich, J., "AEDs Aplenty: What does Their Proliferation Mean for EMS?" *EMS Magazine,* Feb. 2005.

      d. Monitor airway and breathing. If breathing is inadequate, begin positive-pressure ventilation with supplemental oxygen.

      e. If drug has no effect, consult with medical direction before readministration.

      f. Record reassessment findings.

V. Summary: assessment and care (p. 433) **(Figs. 14-12a, p. 432, Fig. 14-12b, p. 433; and Fig. 14-13, p. 434)**

VI. Cardiac compromise and cardiac arrest (pp. 433–435)

  A. Chain of survival (pp. 433, 435) **(Fig. 14-14, p. 435)**

    1. Early access

    2. Early CPR

    3. Early defibrillation

    4. Early advanced life support

VII. Automated external defibrillation and cardiopulmonary resuscitation (pp. 435–441) **(Table 14-1, p. 423)**

  A. Rationale for AED use (pp. 435–436)

    1. The most frequent initial rhythm in sudden cardiac arrest is ventricular fibrillation

    2. The most effective treatment for terminating ventricular fibrillation is electrical defibrillation

    3. The probability of successful defibrillation is directly related to the time from fibrillation to defibrillation.

      a. Defibrillation within 3-5 minutes

      b. ALS within 8 minutes

    4. Ventricular fibrillation will, without prompt or appropriate treatment, degenerates into asystole

  B. Importance of current CPR and AED standards (pp. 436–437)

    1. "Push hard and push fast" will help avoid compressions that are delivered either too slow or too shallow.

    2. The ratio of 30:2 minimizes interruptions to compressions for pulse checks and ventilations, which have been shown to be detrimental to blood flow especially to the head.

    3. Compressions delivered prior to defibrillation in unwitnessed cardiac arrest helps ensure the heart is better perfused, making defibrillation more successful.

    4. Resuming chest compression following defibrillation is desirable since rarely will a perfusing rhythm be evident by a pulse check immediately after defibrillation.

    5. In VF SCA cases, the provision of CPR as described above can double or triple the chance of survival (as opposed to defibrillation alone).

  C. Types of defibrillators (pp. 437–438) **(Fig. 14-15, p. 438)**

    1. Advantages of AEDs

      a. Speed of operation

      b. Safer, more effective delivery

      c. More efficient monitoring

    2. Fully automated

      a. Operates without action by EMT, except to turn on power. (No longer sold)

    3. Semi-automated

      a. Uses a computer voice synthesizer to advise EMT as to the steps to take based upon its analysis of the patient's cardiac rhythm.

  D. Analysis of cardiac rhythms (pp. 438–440) **(Fig. 14-16, p. 439)**

    1. Ventricular fibrillation (VF or V-Fib)

  a. 50% to 60% of cardiac arrests

  b. Most common rhythm the AED defibrillates

 2. Ventricular tachycardia (V-Tach)

  a. AED will respond, usually when heart rate exceeds 180 beats per minute

  b. Some V-Tach patients remain responsive and are not appropriate candidates for defibrillation.

 3. Asystole

  a. Defibrillation is not appropriate.

 4. Pulseless electrical activity (PEA)

  a. Defibrillation is not appropriate.

E. When and when not to use the AED (pp. 440–441) **(Fig. 14-17, p. 440)**

 1. Nontraumatic cardiac arrest patients older than 1 year of age

 2. <1 year

  a. Do not use the AED

 3. Pediatric AEDs preferred in children 1-8 years of age

 4. Use adult AED in patients over 8 years of age

 5. Witnessed arrest or <4 minutes since arrest

  a. Attach AED and follow instruction

 6. Unwitnessed arrest or >5 minutes since arrest

  a. Perform 2 minutes (approximately 5 cycles of 30 compressions to 2 ventilation) before attaching the AED

VIII. Recognizing and treating cardiac arrest (pp. 441–447)

A. Assessment and care: cardiac arrest (p. 441)

 1. Scene size-up and initial assessment

  a. Patients under 1 year of age (infants and neonates)

   (1) Begin or resume CPR

   (2) Transport as rapidly as possible

   (3) Contact ALS backup and hospital medical direction for further orders

  b. Patients 1–8 years of age

   (1) Begin or resume CPR for at least 5 cycles of 30:2 (approximately 2 minutes) prior to AED application if the cardiac arrest was not witnessed

   (2) If the cardiac arrest was witnessed by the EMT, immediately apply the AED and proceed with the AED protocol

   (3) Request ALS support to provide advanced cardiac life support, if this has not already been done

   (4) The reason that CPR is typically performed

   (5) If and when the AED is used for this age group, use the dose attenuating circuit if possible so as to provide the correct dose of energy

  c. Patients over 8 years of age

   (1) Rapidly consider if the "down time" of the patient has been less than 4 minutes, or greater than 4–5 minutes

   (2) For patients with a witnessed arrest, or a down time of less than 4 minutes

    (a) Immediately apply the AED

   (3) If the down time is greater than 4–5 minutes

    (a) 5 cycles of CPR (30:2) should be provided prior to AED application

B. Focused history and physical exam (p. 441)

 1. Unresponsiveness to verbal and painful stimuli

2. No breathing

3. No pulse

C. Emergency medical care (pp. 442–446)

    1. Follow the appropriate steps of cardiopulmonary resuscitation and automated external defibrillation

    2. Performing defibrillation (**Fig 14-18, p. 442**)

        a. Take standard (body substance isolation) precautions.

        b. Perform an initial assessment of the patient (**Fig. 14–19a, p. 443**).

            (1) If the patient is over 1 year of age and is found to be in cardiac arrest, decide to either resume CPR or apply the AED according to the patient's age and the estimated "down time."

        c. If the patient is less than 1 year of age or is a victim of trauma, do not apply the AED unless directed by local protocol and medical direction

        d. Begin or resume CPR while the AED is readied for operation (**Figures 14–19b and 14–19c, p. 443**)

        e. Attach the adhesive monitoring-defibrillation pads to the cables

        f. Apply the two defibrillation pads to the patient's bared chest following the AED manufacturer's instructions (**Figure 14–19d, p. 443; Fig. 14-20a, p. 444; Fig. 14-20c, p. 445**).

        g. Turn on power to the AED.

        h. Older AED models have a tape recorder to record the cardiac arrest resuscitation events. If the AED is equipped with a tape recorder, begin your narrative

        i. When the AED enters its analysis mode, stop any ongoing CPR and say "Clear!" making sure that no one is touching the patient

        j. Begin analysis of the patient's heart rhythms (**Fig. 14–19e, p. 444**)

        k. If the AED indicates "Deliver Shock," make sure that everyone is clear of the patient by visually checking all personnel and stating, "I'm clear, you're clear, everyone is clear" (**Fig. 14–19f, p. 444**)

        l. After the first 2 minutes of CPR, pause to check the patient's pulse for no longer than 10 seconds

            (1) If the pulse is present, check the breathing:

                (a) If the patient is breathing adequately, deliver oxygen at 15 lpm by a nonrebreather mask and transport.

            (2) If the patient is not breathing adequately

                (a) Provide positive pressure ventilation with supplemental oxygen attached to the ventilation device and transport

            (3) If no pulse is present, reanalyze the rhythm

        m. After delivering the second shock, if indicated, resume CPR and transport as soon as possible

            (1) The EMT may have standing orders to deliver a third shock if necessary prior to transport. Consult with medical control.

        n. A "No Shock" message can mean one of three things

            (1) The patient you thought was pulseless has a pulse after all

(2) The formerly pulseless patient has now regained a pulse

(3) The patient is pulseless but the AED is detecting a nonshockable rhythm

(4) If the pulse is present, check the breathing:

  (a) If the patient is breathing adequately, deliver

  (b) oxygen at 15 lpm by a nonrebreather mask and transport.

(5) If the patient is not breathing adequately

  (a) Provide positive pressure ventilation with supplemental oxygen attached to the ventilation device and transport

o. Transport after a total of two (or three) shocks are delivered (with an intervening period of CPR) or a total of two (or three) "No Shock" messages are received

(1) If V-Fib persists after second or third shock, contact medical direction to request additional defibrillatory shocks with CPR between until a "No Shock" advisory is received or the patient regains a pulse

(2) A patient who is in cardiac arrest and is suspected of being hypothermic (having a low body temperature) should receive only one shock before immediate transport

3. Use of the AED by a single EMT

  a. Perform the initial assessment.

  b. Verify that the patient is unresponsive, with no breathing and no pulse.

  c. Leave the patient's side briefly to call EMS and get the AED.

  d. If the "down time" was under 4–5 minutes in the adult or witnessed in the child, attach the AED's external monitoring/defibrillation pads.

  (1) If not, perform 2 minutes of CPR (5 cycles of 30:2 compressions/ventilations first)

  e. Turn on the AED and initiate rhythm analysis.

  f. Deliver the first shock as the AED indicates.

  g. Leave the patient to call for help from EMS dispatch only when one of these occurs

  (1) The AED gives a "No Shock" message.

  (2) You detect a pulse in the patient.

  (3) You have delivered two shocks.

  (4) Other help arrives.

4. Using a fully automated AED

5. Transporting the cardiac arrest patient

  a. The patient regains a pulse

  b. A total of two (or three) shocks have been delivered (according to your local protocol).

  c. The AED has given either two or three consecutive "No Shock" messages (each separated by 2 minutes of CPR).

D. Transporting a patient with a pulse (pp. 446–447)

  1. Check the patient's airway and provide oxygen at 15 lpm by nonrebreather mask if the patient's breathing is adequate, or provide positive pressure ventilation with supplemental oxygen if the patient's breathing is inadequate.

2. Since most cardiac arrest victims vomit, have suction ready for use and clear the airway of any obstructions or fluids.

3. Secure the patient to a stretcher and transfer him to the ambulance. If you regained a pulse while still on scene, the patient should be placed on a backboard so that compressions would be more effective if the cardiac arrest would recur en route to the medical facility.

4. Consider the most efficient way of getting ACLS to the patient. Consult with dispatch and medical direction and consider rendezvousing with an ALS unit en route or awaiting arrival of the ALS unit if that will get the patient advanced care more rapidly.

5. Continue to keep the AED attached to the patient during transport. Remember to stop the emergency vehicle if rhythm analysis is occurring or to deliver any shocks.

6. If you have not already done so, perform the focused history and physical exam en route.

7. Perform an ongoing assessment every 5 minutes.

8. If the patient shows no pulse or breathing, then follow these steps

    a. Stop the vehicle, turning off the motor.

    b. Start CPR if the AED is not immediately available.

    c. When the AED is ready, stop CPR and initiate rhythm analysis.

    d. Deliver another singular shock if warranted. Then resume 2 minutes of CPR prior to checking a pulse. Deliver a second shock if there is no pulse and the AED advises another shock is warranted. If no shocks are indicated, perform CPR again for 2 minutes, then reanalyze until two or three "No Shock" messages have been received.

    e. Continue resuscitation as per local protocol.

    f. Continue transport.

  E. Transporting a patient without a pulse (p. 447)

  F. Providing for advanced cardiac life support (p. 447)

  G. Summary: assessment and care (p. 447) **(Fig, 14-21, p. 448)**

IX. Special considerations for the AED (pp. 447–448) **(Fig. 14-22, p. 449)**

  A. Safety considerations (pp. 447–448)

    1. Electrical conductors

      a. Water

      b. Metal

    2. Transdermal medication patch

    3. Surgically implanted pacemaker or defibrillator

    4. Excessive hair

  B. AED maintenance (pp. 448–451) **(Fig. 14-23, p. 450)**

  C. Training and skills maintenance (p. 451)

  D. Medical direction (p. 451)

    1. Medical direction's involvement

      a. Making sure that the EMS system has all necessary links in the AHA Chain of Survival

      b. Overseeing all levels of EMTs

      c. Reviewing the continual competency skill review program

      d. Engaging in an audit and/or quality improvement program

On the Net

AED Instructor Foundation. http://www.aedinstructorfoundation.org

On the Net

Public Access Defibrillation League. http://www.padl.org

On the Net

For the latest from the American Heart Association, go to: www.americanheart.org

ENRICHMENT (OPTIONAL)

The following sections contain information that is valuable as background for the EMT, but that goes substantially beyond the U.S. Department of Transportation's EMT-Basic National Standard Curriculum.

On the Net
Ischemic Heart Disease.
http://medlib.med.utah.edu/WebPath/TUTORIAL/MYOCARD/MYOCARD.html

CASE STUDY FOLLOW-UP

Ask a student volunteer to read the Case Study that begins on page 414 of the textbook. You may wish to use the following questions to engage students in a discussion of the Case Study Follow-up that begins on page 460 of the textbook. Provide missing information and clarify ideas as needed.

Q1. During your initial assessment, what signs and symptoms indicate that Mr. Antak is a possible cardiac compromise patient?

A1. *Sudden onset of crushing chest pain; pale, cool, slightly moist skin.*

Q2. Why can the EMTs assist the patient with administration of nitroglycerin?

A2. *The patient shows signs and symptoms of chest pain; he has physician-prescribed nitroglycerin tablets with him; and medical direction gives on-line approval for administration.*

Q3. How is the nitroglycerin administered?

A3. *Sublingually. The EMT instructs the patient to open his mouth, lift his tongue, and then let the tablet dissolve under his tongue.*

IN REVIEW

Assess students' ability to apply what they have just learned by discussing the Review Questions on page 462 in the textbook.

Q1. Define the cardiovascular system.

A1. *The cardiovascular system is made up of the heart, blood vessels, and blood. It brings oxygen and nutrients to and takes carbon dioxide and other wastes away from body cells. (p. 415)*

Q2. Explain the exchange that takes place between the capillaries and the body's cells.

A2. *Oxygen and nutrients pass into the cells through the walls of the capillaries. Carbon dioxide and wastes pass from the cells into the blood to be carried away for excretion from the body. (pp. 415–417)*

Q3. Define perfusion and shock (hypoperfusion).

A3. *Perfusion is adequate delivery of oxygen and nutrients to the cells. Shock (hypoperfusion) is depressed delivery of oxygen and nutrients to the cells caused by inadequate circulation of the blood through the capillaries. (p. 420)*

Q4. Name the common signs and symptoms of cardiac compromise.

A4. *The common signs and symptoms of cardiac compromise are chest pain (or pain in the neck, jaw, arm, back, or epigastric region); sweating; difficulty in breathing; anxiety; feelings of impending doom; abnormal pulse or blood pressure; and nausea or vomiting. (pp. 425–426)*

Q5. Describe the standard emergency medical treatment for patients with signs and symptoms of cardiac compromise.

A5. *The standard emergency medical treatment for a patient with signs and symptoms of cardiac compromise is as follows: (1) Administer oxygen at 15 liters per minute by nonrebreather mask. (2) Reassure the patient and place in a position of comfort. (3) Assist in administering prescribed nitroglycerin if authorized by medical direction. (4) Administer aspirin, if authorized by medical direction. (5) Consider ALS backup. Transport promptly. Apply pulse oximeter. (pp. 426–427)*

Q6. Explain the dosage of aspirin in a cardiac emergency and how it is administered.

A6. *The dosage of aspirin is 160 mg to 325 mg as soon as possible after the onset of the chest discomfort and symptoms of heart attack. It is recommended that 160 mg of baby aspirin be chewed, and a second 160 mg of aspirin be swallowed. If no chewable baby aspirin is available, the patient should swallow the aspirin. (p. 428)*

Q7. Explain under what conditions the administration of nitroglycerin is indicated.

A7. *Nitroglycerin is indicated when all of the following conditions are met: (1) The patient exhibits signs or symptoms of chest pain. (2) The patient has physician-prescribed nitroglycerin. (3) Approval has been obtained from medical direction. (pp. 430–431)*

Q8. List the four links in the AHA chain of survival.

A8. *The four links in the AHA chain of survival are early access, early CPR, early defibrillation, and early advanced life support. (pp. 434, 435)*

Q9. Name and describe the heart rhythms that might benefit from defibrillation.

A9. *Ventricular fibrillation is the condition in which defibrillation is most often used. Defibrillation is also sometimes appropriate for patients with ventricular tachycardia, a very rapid heart rhythm. (pp. 438–440)*

Q10. Explain the major difference between automated external defibrillation and manual defibrillation.

A10. *The major difference between automated external defibrillation and manual defibrillation is as follows: The AED analyzes the heart rhythms and determines if administration of a shock is appropriate. In manual defibrillation, the operator must analyze the rhythms himself and decide when to administer a shock. (pp. 437–438)*

Q11. Describe patients for whom use of the AED is appropriate and those for whom it is not.

A11. *AED is intended for adult patients in nontraumatic cardiac arrest. It is not appropriate for children under 8 years old or for patients in whom trauma preceded cardiac arrest. (p. 440)*

Q12. Explain how delivery of CPR is coordinated with use of the AED.

A12. *CPR is coordinated with use of the AED as follows: If CPR is in progress when EMTs arrive on the scene, it should be halted to permit verification of lack of pulse and breathing. CPR should be begun or resumed while the AED is being set up. It should be halted during rhythm analysis and the delivery of shocks. It should be provided for up to 1 minute between sets of three stacked shocks. If the machine delivers a "No shock" message but the patient has no pulse, it should be provided for 1 minute before another rhythm analysis. It should also be provided if the patient has no pulse after delivery of two sets of three stacked shocks or the machine gives three consecutive "No shock" messages. (pp. 442–445)*

Q13. Name the procedures an EMT should follow in dealing with an adult patient with no pulse.

A13.
- *Take body substance isolation precautions.*
- *Perform an initial assessment of the patient.*
- *Begin or resume CPR while the AED is readied for operation.*
- *Attach the adhesive monitoring-defibrillation pads to the cables.*
- *Turn on power to the AED.*
- *Apply the two defibrillation pads to the patient's bared chest.*
- *When the AED enters its analysis mode, stop any ongoing CPR and say "Clear!"*

- *Begin analysis of the patient's heart rhythms.*
- *If the AED indicates "Deliver Shock," make sure that everyone is clear of the patient by visually checking all personnel and stating "I'm clear, you're clear, everyone is clear."*
- *Resume CPR for 2 minutes (or five sets of 30:2 compressions/ventilations).*
- *After the first 2 minutes of CPR, pause to check the patient's pulse for no longer than 10 seconds.*
  - *If the pulse is present, check the breathing.*
  - *If the patient is breathing adequately, deliver oxygen at 15 lpm by a nonrebreather mask and transport.*
  - *If the patient is not breathing adequately, provide positive-pressure ventilation with supplemental oxygen attached to the ventilation device and transport.*
  - *If no pulse is present, reanalyze the rhythm. If indicated, provide a second shock in the manner described in step 10. If the AED gives a "No Shock" message, proceed to Step 13.*
- *After delivering the second shock, resume CPR and transport as soon as possible.*
- *A "No Shock" message can mean one of three things: The patient you thought was pulseless has a pulse after all, or the formerly pulseless patient has now regained a pulse, or finally the patient is pulseless but the AED is detecting a nonshockable rhythm. If the machine gives a "No Shock" message after any rhythm analysis, check the patient's pulse and breathing.*
  - *If the pulse is present, check the breathing.*
  - *If the patient is breathing adequately, deliver oxygen at 15 lpm by a nonrebreather mask and transport.*
  - *If the patient is not breathing adequately, provide positive-pressure ventilation with supplemental oxygen and transport.*
- *Transport after a total of two (or three) shocks are delivered (with an intervening period of CPR) or a total of two (or three) "No Shock" messages are received.*
- *If V-Fib persists after second or third shock, contact medical direction to request additional defibrillatory shocks with CPR between until a "No Shock" advisory is received or the patient regains a pulse. (pp. 442–449)*

Q14. Explain the basic steps to follow if a resuscitated patient goes back into cardiac arrest during transport.

A14. *The basic steps to follow if a resuscitated patient goes back into cardiac arrest during transport are: Stop the vehicle, turning off the motor. Start CPR if the AED is not immediately ready. When the AED is ready, stop CPR and initiate rhythm analysis. Deliver as many as three shocks if indicated. Then check the pulse and resume CPR for 1 minute if there is no pulse. Deliver a second set of three stacked shocks if indicated. If no shocks are indicated, perform CPR for 1 minute, then reanalyze for up to three "No Shock" messages. Continue resuscitation as per local protocol. Continue transport. (pp. 446–447)*

©2008 by Pearson Education, Inc.
Prehospital Emergency Care, 8th ed.

CRITICAL THINKING

Assess students' ability to respond to real-life emergency situations by discussing the Critical Thinking questions on page 463 in the textbook.

Q1. What assessment findings indicate that this patient is indeed in cardiac arrest?

A1. *Since the patient is unresponsive, is not breathing, and has no pulse, he is in cardiac arrest.*

Q2. Which components of the Chain of Survival have already been met?

A2. *This patient has already benefited from early access to the EMS system through 911 and early CPR.*

Q3. Why is this patient a candidate for immediate versus delayed AED use?

A3. *Since this patient's cardiac arrest was witnessed, and CPR was being performed upon your arrival, and you arrived on the scene within four minutes of the cardiac arrest, the AED should be applied as soon as it is available. If the patient was in cardiac arrest for greater than 4 to 5 minutes, and no CPR was being performed upon your arrival, you would first perform 5 cycles of CPR (approximately 2 minutes) prior to applying the AED.*

Q4. What cardiac rhythm is this patient most likely going to show?

A4. *This patient will most likely show a ventricular fibrillation rhythm. It is the most common rhythm associated with sudden out-of-hospital cardiac arrest. The rhythm will quickly deteriorate to asystole within minutes without proper treatment.*

Q5. What is the compression/ventilation ratio going to be for this patient?

A5. *Those performing CPR on this patient should use a ratio of 30 compressions to 2 ventilations.*

Q6. If the AED indicates that no shock is warranted, what should the next action of the care providers be?

A6. *If the AED indicates that no shock is warranted, the rescuers should resume CPR for 5 cycles (approximately 2 minutes) and then reanalyze the patient's rhythm.*

SKILLS DEMONSTRATION AND PRACTICE

Activity 1: Arrange for use of a vacant classroom, which will serve as a station for practice of initial assessment skills. You will need the type of AED used by your EMS system and a shockable mannequin. Invite an EMT to serve as teaching assistant. Briefly discuss his or her role before class.

Divide students into teams of two. If the number of students does not divide equally by two, it is acceptable to have one group of three. Direct the first team to the station, explaining that after the teaching assistant has demonstrated the skills needed to use an AED, each partner, in turn, will practice his or her own skills. While the other teams are waiting for their turn, instruct them to practice their CPR skills on the CPR mannequins.

Visit the station to monitor progress of demonstration and practice. Also, circulate among the students practicing their CPR skills, remarking on good technique, and offering instruction or encouragement, as appropriate. When each team has completed practice, tell students to return to the classroom.

Activity 2: Arrange for use of a vacant classroom, which will serve as a station for practice of initial assessment skills. You will need the type of AED used by your EMS system and a shockable mannequin. Invite an EMT to serve as teaching assistant. Briefly discuss his or her role before class.

Divide students into teams of two. If the number of students does not divide equally by two, it is acceptable to have one group of three. Direct the first team to the station, explaining that after the teaching assistant has demonstrated the skills needed to use an AED, each partner, in turn, will practice his or her own skills. While the other teams are waiting for their turn, instruct them to practice their CPR skills on the CPR mannequins.

Visit the station to monitor progress of demonstration and practice. Also, circulate among the students practicing their CPR skills, remarking on good technique, and offering instruction or encouragement, as appropriate. When each team has completed practice, tell students to return to the classroom.

PRACTICE SCENARIO

Have students apply what they have just learned to a real-life situation encountered by EMS personnel by enacting the following role. Invite two volunteers to play the role of EMTs and one to be the patient.

Begin the practice by taking the two EMT players outside the classroom.

Provide them with a complete jump kit containing BSI equipment, oxygen equipment, a portable suction unit, and a stretcher. Describe the following situation to them:

You have been dispatched to a residence at 34 Congress Street, where a 49-year-old male (female) is complaining of chest pain. I will call you to the "scene" to deal with this situation in a little while.

Return to the classroom and describe the scenario below to the patient and the class and give the patient simulated nitroglycerin and aspirin tablets (small breath mints).

Your name is Phil (or Phyllis) Getz. About 20 minutes ago, while you were hammering the last spindles on the side of your new deck, you began to have severe chest pain. At first, you thought you'd overdone it by carrying too many spindles at once, so you stopped to rest. Nothing has made the pain better or worse; you are still short of breath. You describe the pain as "tightness" radiating from your chest to your jaw. You rate the pain as an 8 on a 1-to-10 scale of pain. You have a history of angina and high blood pressure. You have a prescription for nitroglycerin and have already taken one tablet.

Tell the patient to take his or her place and to start role-playing. Dispatch the EMTs to the scene. Allow the role play to progress naturally. Intervene only if the players seem to be at a loss for what to do.

If the EMTs call medical direction, respond to them and ask for a medical radio report. If the report is appropriate and the EMT team requests permission to assist the patient with the administration of nitroglycerin and aspirin, give permission for them to do so. End the play when the EMTs have prepared the patient for transport to the ambulance.

When the role play has ended, discuss the following points:

- What did the EMTs do well?
- What, if anything, should they have done differently?

You may wish to divide students into pairs and direct them to take turns administering simulated nitroglycerin and aspirin tablets to each other.

ASSIGNMENTS

Assign students to read Chapter 15, "Altered Mental Status and Diabetic Emergencies," before the next class. Also ask them to complete Chapter 14 of the Workbook.

EVALUATION

Chapter Quiz Distribute copies of the Chapter Quiz provided in Handout 14-2 to evaluate student understanding of this chapter. Remind students not to refer to their textbooks or notes while taking the quiz.

Test Manager You may wish to create a custom-tailored test using Prentice Hall *TestGen for Prehospital Emergency Care, Eighth Edition* to evaluate student understanding of this chapter.

Online Test Preparation (for students and instructors) Additional test preparation is available through *EMT Achieve: Basic Test Preparation* at http://www.prenhall.com/EMTAchieve. Instructors can also monitor student mastery online.

REINFORCEMENT

Handouts If classroom discussions or performance on the quiz indicates that some students have not fully mastered the chapter content, you may wish to assign some or all of the Reinforcement Handouts for this chapter.

TECH EXTRAS

Brady Skills Series EMT-B Videos/CD Have your students watch the skills come to life on either VHS or CD-ROM.

PowerPoint Presentation (for instructors) The PowerPoint material developed for this chapter offers useful reinforcement of chapter content.

Student CD A wide variety of material on this CD-ROM will reinforce and also expand student knowledge and skills.

Companion Website (for students) Additional review quizzes and links to EMS resources will contribute to further reinforcement of this chapter. Please visit http://www.prenhall.com/mistovich.

Reading/Reference
Textbook, pp. 464–490

Workbook
Chapter 14 Activities

Chapter Quiz
Handout 14-2

TestGen
Chapter 14 Test

Online Test Preparation
Send your students to
http://www.prenhall.com/
EMTAchieve

Handouts 14-3 to 14-10
Reinforcement Activities

**Brady Skills Series
EMT-B Videos/CD**
Visual Reinforcement

**PowerPoint
Presentation**
Chapter 14

Student CD
Chapter 14

Companion Website
http://www.prenhall.com/
mistovich

OBJECTIVES CHECKLIST

Cognitive		Date Mastered
4-3.1	Describe the structure and function of the cardiovascular system.	
4-3.2	Describe the emergency medical care of the patient experiencing chest pain/discomfort.	
4-3.3	List the indications for automated external defibrillation (AED).	
4-3.4	List the contraindications for automated external defibrillation.	
4-3.5	Define the role of the EMT-Basic in the emergency cardiac care system.	
4-3.6	Explain the impact of age and weight on defibrillation.	
4-3.7	Discuss the position of comfort for patients with various cardiac emergencies.	
4-3.8	Establish the relationship between airway management and the patient with cardiovascular compromise.	
4-3.9	Predict the relationship between the patient experiencing cardiovascular compromise and basic cardiac life support.	
4-3.10	Discuss the fundamentals of early defibrillation.	
4-3.11	Explain the rationale for early defibrillation.	
4-3.12	Explain that not all chest pain patients result in cardiac arrest and do not need to be attached to an automated external defibrillator.	
4-3.13	Explain the importance of prehospital ACLS intervention if it is available.	
4-3.14	Explain the importance of urgent transport to a facility with Advanced Cardiac Life Support if it is not available in the prehospital setting.	
4-3.15	Discuss the various types of automated external defibrillators.	
4-3.16	Differentiate between the fully automated and the semi-automated defibrillator.	
4-3.17	Discuss the procedures that must be taken into consideration for standard operations of the various types of automated external defibrillators.	
4-3.18	State the reasons for ensuring that the patient is pulseless and apneic, when using the automated external defibrillator.	
4-3.19	Discuss the circumstances that may result in inappropriate shocks.	
4-3.20	Explain the considerations for interruption of CPR when using the automated external defibrillator.	
4-3.21	Discuss the advantages and disadvantages of automated external defibrillators.	
4-3.22	Summarize the speed of operation of automated external defibrillation.	
4-3.23	Discuss the use of remote defibrillation through adhesive pads.	
4-3.24	Discuss the special considerations for rhythm monitoring.	

4-3.25	List the steps in the operation of the automated external defibrillator.	
4-3.26	Discuss the standard of care that should be used to provide care to a patient with persistent ventricular fibrillation and no available ACLS.	
4-3.27	Discuss the standard of care that should be used to provide care to a patient with recurrent ventricular fibrillation and no available ACLS.	
4-3.28	Differentiate between the single rescuer and multirescuer care with an automated external defibrillator.	
4-3.29	Explain the reasons for pulses not being checked between shocks with an automated external defibrillator.	
4-3.30	Discuss the importance of coordinating ACLS trained providers with personnel using automated external defibrillators.	
4-3.31	Discuss the importance of post-resuscitation care.	
4-3.32	List components of post-resuscitation care.	
4-3.33	Explain the importance of frequent practice with the automated external defibrillator.	
4-3.34	Discuss the need to complete the Automated Defibrillator: Operator's Shift Checklist.	
4-3.35	Discuss the role of the American Heart Association in the use of automated external defibrillation.	
4-3.36	Explain the role medical direction plays in the use of automated external defibrillation.	
4-3.37	State the reasons why a case review should be completed following the use of the automated external defibrillator.	
4-3.38	Discuss the components that should be included in a case review.	
4-3.39	Discuss the goal of quality improvement in automated external defibrillation.	
4-3.40	Recognize the need for medical direction of protocols to assist in the emergency medical care of the patient with chest pain.	
4-3.41	List the indications for the use of nitroglycerin.	
4-3.42	State the contraindications and side effects for the use of nitroglycerin.	
4-4.43	Define the function of all controls on an automated external defibrillator, and describe event documentation and battery defibrillator maintenance.	

Affective		**Date Mastered**
4-3.44	Defend the reasons for obtaining initial training in automated external defibrillation and the importance of continuing education.	
4-3.45	Defend the reason for maintenance of automated external defibrillators.	
4-3.46	Explain the rationale for administering nitroglycerin to a patient with chest pain or discomfort.	

Psychomotor		Date Mastered
4-3.47	Demonstrate the assessment and emergency medical care of a patient experiencing chest pain/discomfort.	
4-3.48	Demonstrate the application and operation of the automated external defibrillator.	
4-3.49	Demonstrate the maintenance of an automated external defibrillator.	
4-3.50	Demonstrate the assessment and documentation of patient response to the automated external defibrillator.	
4-3.51	Demonstrate the skills necessary to complete the Automated Defibrillator: Operator's Shift Checklist.	
4-3.52	Perform the steps in facilitating the use of nitroglycerin for chest pain or discomfort.	
4-3.53	Demonstrate the assessment and documentation of patient response to nitroglycerin.	
4-3.54	Practice completing the prehospital care report for patients with cardiac emergencies.	

©2008 by Pearson Education, Inc.
Prehospital Emergency Care, 8th ed.

CHAPTER 14 QUIZ

Write the letter of the best answer in the space provided.

_____ 1. The valve located between the right atrium and the right ventricle that prevents blood from returning to the right atrium is the _____ valve.
   A. mitral   **C.** tricuspid
   B. aortic   **D.** bicuspid

_____ 2. The right atrium receives dexoygenated blood from the inferior and superior _____, the largest veins in the body.
   A. aorta   **C.** pulmonary arteries
   B. vena cava   **D.** pulmonary veins

_____ 3. The electrical impulse that causes the heart to contract is generated in the right atrium at the
   A. bundle of His.   **C.** sinoatrial node.
   B. Purkinje fibers.   **D.** atrioventricular node.

_____ 4. The arteries that branch off the base of the aorta and supply the heart with oxygen-rich blood are called _____ arteries.
   A. pulmonary   **C.** carotid
   B. posterior tibial   **D.** coronary

_____ 5. Blood components respond to injury by forming a clot, or _____, in order to stop bleeding.
   A. plasma   **C.** platelet
   B. thrombus   **D.** plaque

_____ 6. The delivery of oxygen and nutrients from the blood, through the thin capillary walls into the cells, and the removal of carbon dioxide and other waste products, is known as
   A. hypoperfusion.   **C.** metabolism.
   B. shock.   **D.** perfusion.

_____ 7. In cases involving a patient complaining of chest pain and/or difficulty breathing, the EMT should suspect
   A. cardiac problems.   **C.** tracheal deviation.
   B. trauma.   **D.** hypovolemia.

_____ 8. While patients with known cardiac problems may take a variety of medications, the most commonly prescribed medication is
   A. nitroglycerin.   **C.** epinephrine.
   B. Lasix.   **D.** Digoxin.

_____ 9. If a patient experiences no relief after one dose of nitroglycerin, another dose may be administered after 3 to 5 minutes if authorized by medical direction, to a maximum of _____ doses.
   A. three   **C.** two
   B. five   **D.** six

_____ **10.** Because nitroglycerin lowers blood pressure, it must not be given to a patient whose systolic blood pressure is lower than _____ mmHg.
  A. 130   **C.** 100
  B. 120   **D.** 90

_____ **11.** One contraindication to the administration of nitroglycerin is the patient's
  A. recent ingestion of Viagra®.   **C.** excessive respiratory efforts.
  B. use of aspirin.   **D.** extremity injury.

_____ **12.** The condition known as _____ occurs when a portion of the heart muscle dies because of the lack of an adequate supply of oxygenated blood.
  A. angina pectoris   **C.** acute myocardial infarction
  B. hypertension   **D.** pulmonary edema

_____ **13.** The tiny blood vessels that connect arterioles to venules are
  A. valves.   **C.** capillaries.
  B. arteries.   **D.** veins.

_____ **14.** The measured force exerted during the contraction of the heart is the _____ blood pressure.
  A. systolic   **C.** diastolic
  B. systemic   **D.** myocardial

_____ **15.** A common side effect of the administration of nitroglycerin is
  A. headache.   **C.** altered mental status.
  B. hypovolemia.   **D.** diaphoresis.

_____ **16.** During cardiac arrest, instead of smooth contractions, the heart shows a different type of electrical activity, most commonly the uncoordinated twitchings known as
  A. asystole.   **C.** ventricular fibrillation.
  B. ventricular tachycardia.   **D.** atrial fibrillation.

_____ **17.** Cardiac arrest in children is most often the result of
  A. hypoxia.   **C.** trauma.
  B. bradycardia.   **D.** ventricular fibrillation.

_____ **18.** In cases of _____, the heart has a rhythm, but is so weakened that it fails to pump, or it does not respond to the electrical activity, or there is so much blood loss that there is nothing to pump.
  A. asystole   **C.** pulseless electrical activity
  B. ventricular fibrillation   **D.** ventricular tachycardia

_____ **19.** The absence of electrical activity and pumping action in the heart is called
  A. pulseless electrical activity.   **C.** ventricular fibrillation.
  B. ventricular tachycardia.   **D.** asystole.

_____ **20.** After receiving a "No Shock" message and if no pulse is present, the EMT should
  A. check breathing.   **C.** resume CPR.
  B. "Deliver Shock."   **D.** reanalyze.

_____ **21.** The normal maximum total number of shocks that the EMT can deliver without approval from medical direction is
  A. 2–3.   **C.** 8–9.
  B. 5–6.   **D.** 11–12.

_____22. EMTs may use AEDs under the authority of the
- **A.** medical director's license.
- **B.** American Heart Association.
- **C.** Red Cross.
- **D.** Paramedic Supervisor.

_____23. The second wave form of the ECG that represents the contraction of the ventricles and the main contraction of the heart is called the
- **A.** QRS complex.
- **B.** P wave.
- **C.** T wave.
- **D.** PR interval.

_____24. The first link in the American Heart Association's chain of survival in cardiac arrest cases is early
- **A.** access.
- **B.** CPR.
- **C.** defibrillation.
- **D.** advanced care.

_____25. To be considered for application of the AED, an unresponsive patient must be
- **A.** pulseless and diaphoretic.
- **B.** pulseless and apneic.
- **C.** apneic and hypoglycemic.
- **D.** diaphoretic and hypoxic.

_____26. The rhythm for which the AED most commonly delivers shocks is
- **A.** ventricular fibrillation.
- **B.** ventricular tachycardia.
- **C.** pulseless electrical activity.
- **D.** asystole.

_____27. If you detect no pulse and no breathing after the AED has delivered a shock, you should
- **A.** reanalyze.
- **B.** reshock up to two times.
- **C.** perform 2 minutes of CPR.
- **D.** perform 1 minute of CPR.

_____28. The first step after taking BSI precautions in assessing a patient in cardiac arrest is to
- **A.** perform a focused physical exam.
- **B.** attach the AED.
- **C.** perform an initial assessment.
- **D.** obtain a SAMPLE history.

_____29. If at any time an EMT gets a "No Shock" message on the AED and determines that the patient has a pulse, he or she should
- **A.** deliver three more shocks.
- **B.** resume CPR.
- **C.** check the patient's breathing.
- **D.** begin immediate transport.

_____30. Use of an AED would be indicated for all of the following cardiac-arrest patients *except*
- **A.** 10-year-old child.
- **B.** 98-pound teenager.
- **C.** 73-year-old woman.
- **D.** 40-year-old trauma victim.

IN THE FIELD

Read the following real-life situation. Then answer the questions that follow.

You and your EMT partner respond to a call at the Wilson Corporation. The dispatcher reports a conscious male about 50 years of age complaining of chest pain. When you arrive at the scene, the patient's secretary leads you into an office. There you see a man sitting on the sofa next to his desk. He is alert with labored respirations. He is pale and diaphoretic. Your pulse check reveals a weak and rapid radial pulse, and you note his skin to be cool and moist to the touch. He is complaining of a squeezing tightness in the center of his chest.

1. What should be your first action in providing emergency medical care?

2. During the focused history and physical exam, you determine that the patient has a history of heart disease and has physician-prescribed nitroglycerin. What actions must you take prior to assisting the patient with his prescribed medication?

3. What reassessment steps should follow the administration of nitroglycerin?

Student's Name _____

CHAPTER 14 REVIEW

Write the word or words that best complete each sentence in the space provided.

1. An unresponsive patient with no respiration and no pulse is in _____

   _____.

2. The _____ are the top two chambers on each side of the heart.

3. The blood in the left atrium is ejected through the _____ valve and into
   the left ventricle upon contraction of the heart.

4. The most common symptom of cardiac compromise is _____

   _____.

5. As an EMT, you should not take the time to try to _____ the type or cause
   of a cardiac emergency.

6. _____ can be administered as either a sublingual tablet or a sublingual

   spray.

7. The three drugs that an EMT may administer to a cardiac patient, with the approval of medical

   direction, are _____, _____, and

   _____.

8. The aim of administering nitroglycerin is to _____ the blood vessels in the

   heart.

9. If the responsive patient with chest pain is breathing adequately, administer oxygen at

   _____ liters per minute via a(n) _____ mask.

10. In general, the EMT's emergency treatment of patients with heart failure or an acute myocardial

    infarction will not _____.

11. Several components of blood are involved in clot formation. They are:

    _____, _____, and

    _____.

12. The _____ pressure represents the pressure exerted against the arterial

    walls during relaxation of the left ventricle.

13. If a patient experiences no relief after one dose of nitroglycerin, another dose may be administered

after _____ to _____ minutes if authorized by

medical direction, to a maximum of _____ doses.

14. The heart contains specialized contractile tissue as well as conductive tissue, known as the

_____ _____ _____,

which allows it to generate electrical impulses.

15. The circulatory, or cardiovascular, system has three major components: the

_____, the _____

_____, and the _____.

16. _____ _____ occurs when the heart, for any of a

variety of reasons, is not pumping effectively or at all, and no pulses can be felt.

17. _____ is the procedure of sending an electrical current through the chest

to convert a heart that is in an abnormal and lethal rhythm with no pulse to a rhythm with a pulse.

18. In the chain of survival, defibrillation within _____

_____ is the critical factor in determining survival of cardiac arrest.

19. Whichever type of AED your service has chosen to use, always follow local protocols and

_____ _____ for maintenance.

20. _____ _____ is a disorganized cardiac rhythm

that produces no pulse or cardiac output.

21. _____ _____ is a very fast heart rhythm that is

generated in the ventricle instead of the sinoatrial node in the atrium.

22. _____ is the absence of electrical activity and pumping action in the heart.

23. Ideally, at least two EMTs should be present when defibrillation is to be performed with a semi-

automated AED—one to operate the _____, the other to perform

_____.

24. Whenever you have a cardiac-arrest patient, contact dispatch and request

_____ backup as soon as you can without delaying the start of

defibrillation.

25. The _____ is a graphic representation of the heart's electrical activity as

detected from the chest wall surface.

26. In a normally functioning heart, the heart's electrical impulse is generated from the
_____ node.

27. The most effective treatment for ventricular fibrillation is electrical _____.

28. The role of _____ is to perform certain interventions to increase the
possibility of successful defibrillation or to administer medications to keep the patient from going
back into cardiac arrest.

29. The AED should only be applied to patients who are _____,
_____, and _____.

30. People whose conduction systems cannot sustain a regular and effective cardiac rhythm on their own
often receive surgically implanted cardiac _____.

31. The two types of "shockable rhythms" for an AED unit are _____
_____ and _____ _____.

32. Always alert people to move away from the patient by saying _____ in a
loud voice before beginning a rhythm analysis or delivering a shock.

33. Do not attach an AED if a patient is younger than _____ years or has
sustained _____ before collapse.

34. If at any time you get a "No Shock" message and determine that the patient has a pulse, check the
patient's _____.

35. Remember to _____ _____ and
_____ _____ with compressions so that the brain
and heart can still receive blood flow during the arrest management.

CARDIAC EMERGENCIES: LISTING

1. List seven signs and symptoms often associated with cardiac compromise.

2. List six emergency care steps for patients experiencing cardiac compromise.

3. List the three conditions that must be met before assisting a patient with the administration of nitroglycerin.

4. List the five contraindications to the administration of nitroglycerin.

5. List three trade names of nitroglycerin.

©2008 by Pearson Education, Inc.
Prehospital Emergency Care, 8th ed.

CARDIAC EMERGENCIES: MATCHING

Write the letter of the term in the space next to the appropriate description below.

_____ 1. Major artery of the upper arm

_____ 2. Major artery of the thigh

_____ 3. Major artery in the neck

_____ 4. The force exerted during circulation of the blood against the arterial walls

_____ 5. Smallest artery, leading to a capillary

_____ 6. Smallest vein, leading from a capillary

_____ 7. Breastbone, located in the center of the chest

_____ 8. The two major veins that carry oxygen-depleted blood back to the heart

_____ 9. Depressed delivery of oxygen and nutrients to the cells resulting from inadequate circulation of blood through the capillaries

_____ 10. A fatty deposit within an artery

_____ 11. Force exerted against the arterial walls during relaxation of the left ventricle of the heart

_____ 12. The specialized contractile and conductive tissue of the heart that generates electrical impulses and causes the heart to beat

_____ 13. Major artery that starts at the left ventricle and carries oxygen-rich blood to the body

_____ 14. Network of arteries supplying the heart with blood

_____ 15. Medication often prescribed for patients with a history of heart problems for the relief of chest pain

_____ 16. One of the two lower chambers of the heart

_____ 17. Type of blood vessel that carries blood away from the heart

_____ 18. Component of the blood essential to the formation of blood clots

_____ 19. One of the two upper chambers of the heart

_____ 20. Tiny blood vessel connecting arterioles to venules, site of gas and nutrient exchange

A. aorta

B. arteriole

C. artery

D. atrium

E. blood pressure

F. brachial artery

G. capillary

H. cardiac conduction system

I. carotid artery

J. coronary arteries

K. diastolic pressure

L. femoral artery

M. hypoperfusion

N. nitroglycerin

O. plaque

P. platelets

Q. sternum

R. venae cavae

S. ventricle

T. venule

REINFORCEMENT

NITROGLYCERIN

Write in the missing information on the medication flash card below, and save the completed card for future reference.

Nitroglycerin

Medication Names

  1. Generic: _____

  2. Trade: _____

Indications

  1. _____

  2. _____

  3. _____

Contraindications

  1. _____

  2. _____

  3. _____

  4. _____

  5. _____

Medication Form:

Dosage:

Actions

  1. _____

  2. _____

  3. _____

Side Effects

  1. _____

  2. _____

  3. _____

ASPIRIN
— ■ —

Write in the missing information on the medication flash card below, and save the completed card for future reference.

Aspirin

Medication Names

1. Generic: _____

2. Trade: _____

Indications

1. _____

2. _____

3. _____

Contraindications

1. _____

2. _____

3. _____

4. _____

5. _____

Medication Form:

Dosage:

Actions

1. _____

2. _____

3. _____

Side Effects

1. _____

2. _____

3. _____

REINFORCEMENT

AED BASICS: LISTING

1. List the two types of automated external defibrillators.

2. List the rhythms that an AED will detect for which no shock is indicated.

3. List the rhythms that an AED will recognize as shockable.

4. List the four elements in the American Heart Association's chain of survival.

REINFORCEMENT

ORGANIZING AED USE

Place the following actions in the correct sequence by writing 1 next to the action that should be done first, 2 next to the action that should be done next, and so on.

_____ Reanalyze rhythm after 2 minutes of CPR.

_____ Apply the AED.

_____ Second rescuer should begin or resume CPR.

_____ Initiate analysis of rhythm.

_____ Take BSI precautions.

_____ Start narrative of event.

_____ Check pulse and breathing. If no pulse, continue CPR for 2 minutes.

_____ Stop CPR and instruct everyone to clear the patient.

_____ Assess airway, breathing, and pulse, stopping CPR if necessary.

_____ If shock advised, clear patient and deliver shock. If no shock advised, perform CPR for 2 minutes.

Cardiac Emergencies

Review of Circulatory System

Heart

Vessels

Blood

Cardiac Conduction System

Blood Pressure

Inadequate Circulation

Cardiac Compromise and Acute Coronary Syndromes

Assessment and Care

Nitroglycerin

Aspirin

Disease Process of Acute Coronary Syndromes

Conditions That May Cause Cardiac Emergencies

Angina Pectoris

Acute Myocardial Infarction

Heart Failure

Automated External Defibrillation

Cardiac Arrest

The Chain of Survival

- Early access
- Early CPR
- Early defibrillation
- Early ALS

HANDOUT 14-2: Chapter 14 Quiz

1. C	9. A	17. A	25. B
2. B	10. D	18. C	26. A
3. C	11. A	19. D	27. C
4. D	12. C	20. C	28. C
5. B	13. C	21. A	29. C
6. D	14. A	22. A	30. D
7. A	15. A	23. A	
8. A	16. C	24. A	

HANDOUT 14-3: In the Field

1. Administer oxygen at 15 liters per minute via a nonrebreather mask.
2. (a) Assess the patient's blood pressure. Systolic blood pressure must be greater than 90 mmHg. (b) Obtain order from medical direction either on-line or off-line. (c) Check the medication to ensure that it is prescribed to the patient, that it is the proper medication, and that it has not expired.
3. (a) Reassess blood pressure within 2 minutes. (b) Question patient about the effect of the medication on relief of pain. (c) Record your actions, patient's response, and reassessment findings.

HANDOUT 14-4: Chapter 14 Review

1. cardiac arrest
2. atria
3. mitral (bicuspid)
4. chest pain
5. diagnose
6. Nitroglycerin
7. oxygen, nitroglycerin, aspirin
8. dilate
9. 15, nonrebreather
10. differ
11. platelets, thrombin, fibrin
12. diastolic
13. 3, 5, 3
14. cardiac conduction system
15. heart, blood vessels, blood
16. Cardiac arrest
17. Defibrillation
18. 5 minutes
19. manufacturer's recommendations
20. Ventricular fibrillation
21. Ventricular tachycardia
22. Asystole
23. AED, CPR
24. ACLS
25. electrocardiogram (ECG or EKG)
26. sinoatrial (SA)
27. defibrillation
28. ALS (Advanced Life Support)

29. pulseless, apneic, unresponsive
30. pacemakers
31. ventricular fibrillation, ventricular tachycardia
32. CLEAR!
33. 1, trauma
34. breathing
35. push hard, push fast

HANDOUT 14-5: Cardiac Emergencies: Listing

1. Any seven: pain or discomfort in any of the following areas: chest, neck, jaw, arm, or back; epigastric pain; sudden onset of sweating; cool, pale skin; difficulty breathing; lightheadedness or dizziness; anxiety or irritability; feelings of impending doom; abnormal or irregular pulse rate; abnormal blood pressure; nausea and/or vomiting.
2. (1) Administer oxygen at 15 liters per minute via a nonrebreather mask. (2) Decrease the anxiety of the patient by providing calm reassurance and placing him or her in a position of comfort. (3) Assist the patient who has physician-prescribed nitroglycerin. (4) Administer aspirin, if medical direction orders it. (5) Consider calling for ALS backup; initiate early transport. (6) Apply pulse oximeter.
3. (1) The patient exhibits signs or symptoms of chest pain. (2) The patient has physician-prescribed nitroglycerin. (3) The EMT has received approval from medical direction, either on-line or off-line, to give the medication.
4. (1) The patient's baseline blood pressure is below 90 mmHg systolic. (2) The patient has a suspected head injury. (3) The patient is an infant or a child. (4) Three doses have already been taken by the patient. (5) The patient has recently taken Viagra®.
5. Nitrostat®, Nitrobid®, Nitrolingual® Spray

HANDOUT 14-6: Cardiac Emergencies: Matching

1. F	6. T	11. K	16. S
2. L	7. Q	12. H	17. C
3. I	8. R	13. A	18. P
4. E	9. M	14. J	19. D
5. B	10. O	15. N	20. G

HANDOUT 14-7: Nitroglycerin (completion)

Medication Names:
1. Generic: nitroglycerin
2. Trade: Nitrostat®, Nitrobid®, Nitrolingual® Spray

Indications:
1. Patient exhibits signs or symptoms of chest pain.
2. Patient has physician-prescribed nitroglycerin.
3. The EMT has received approval from medical direction, either on-line or off-line, to give the medication.

Contraindications:
1. Patient's baseline blood pressure is below 90 mmHg.
2. Patient has a suspected head injury.
3. Patient is an infant or a child.
4. Patient has already taken three doses.
5. Patient has already taken Viagra®.

Medication Form:
Tablet, sublingual spray

Dosage:
One tablet or one spray under the tongue. This dose may be repeated in 3–5 minutes if (1) the patient experiences no relief; (2) the blood pressure remains above 90 mmHg systolic; and (3) medical direction gives authorization. The total dose is three tablets or sprays, including what the patient took prior to the arrival of EMS.

Action:
1. Dilates blood vessels
2. Decreases workload of the heart
3. Decreases cardiac oxygen demand

Side Effects:
1. Headache
2. Drop in blood pressure
3. Changes in pulse rate as the body compensates for changes in blood vessel size.

HANDOUT 14-8: Aspirin (completion)

Medication Names:
1. Generic: aspirin
2. Trade: ASA, Bayer, Ecotrin, St. Joseph's, Bufferin

Indications:
1. Patient exhibits chest discomfort suggestive of heart attack.
2. Medical direction has given approval, either on-line or off-line.

Contraindications:
A known allergy or hypersensitivity to aspirin

Medication Form:
tablet

Dosage:
160 mg to 325 mg as soon as possible after onset of symptoms

Action:
Decreases ability of platelets to clump together

Side Effects:
1. Stomach irritation
2. Heartburn
3. Nausea/vomiting

HANDOUT 14-9: AED Basics: Listing

1. Fully automated AEDs; semi-automated AEDs
2. Asystole, pulseless electrical activity
3. Ventricular fibrillation, ventricular tachycardia
4. Early access, early CPR, early defibrillation, early advanced care

HANDOUT 14-10: Organizing AED Use

Correct numerical order reading from top to bottom: 10, 4, 3, 7, 1, 5, 9, 6, 2, 8

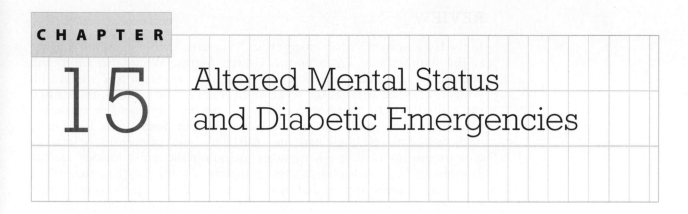

15 Altered Mental Status and Diabetic Emergencies

This chapter covers portions of Lesson 4-4 and Lesson 4-10 of the U.S. Department of Transportation's EMT-Basic National Standard Curriculum.

OBJECTIVES

Numbered objectives are from the U.S. Department of Transportation EMT-Basic National Standard Curriculum. Asterisked objectives, if any, pertain to material that is supplemental to the DOT curriculum. Page numbers in parentheses refer to pages in the textbook.

Cognitive

4-4.1 Identify the patient taking diabetic medications with altered mental status and the implications of a diabetes history. (pp. 469–476)

4-4.2 State the steps in the emergency medical care of the patient taking diabetic medicine with an altered mental status and a history of diabetes. (pp. 470–476)

4-4.3 Establish the relationship between airway management and the patient with altered mental status. (pp. 466, 468, 475, 484, 486, 488)

4-4.4 State the generic and trade names, medication forms, dose, administration, action, and contraindications for oral glucose. (pp. 475–476)

4-4.5 Evaluate the need for medical direction in the emergency medical care of the diabetic patient. (pp. 472, 474, 475, 487, 488)

* State the steps in the emergency care of the patient with an altered mental status and an unknown history. (p. 468)

Affective

4-4.6 Explain the rationale for administering oral glucose. (p. 474)

Psychomotor

4-4.7 Demonstrate the steps in the emergency medical care for the patient taking diabetic medicine with an altered mental status and a history of diabetes.

4-4.8 Demonstrate the steps in the administration of oral glucose.

4-4.9 Demonstrate the assessment and documentation of patient response to oral glucose.

4-4.10 Demonstrate how to complete a prehospital care report for patients with diabetic emergencies.

Total Teaching Time
105 minutes

Resources Needed
- Scored Chapter 14 Quizzes
- Oral glucose product most commonly used in your EMS system
- Tongue depressors

Additional Resources
Larmon/Davis, *Basic Life Support Skills*

Elling, *EMT Achieve: Basic Test Preparation*

Limmer/Mistovich/O'Keefe, *Audio Lecture & Study Guide: EMT*

Mistovich/Kuvlesky, *SUCCESS! for the EMT, Second Edition*

REVIEW

In the last lesson, "Cardiac Emergencies," students learned that heart disease is the number one killer in the United States. While the EMT will occasionally be called to a patient who is in cardiac arrest, or to a patient who goes into cardiac arrest at the scene or en route to the hospital, more often the call will be to a responsive patient who has signs and symptoms—particularly chest pain—that may be caused by heart disease. The EMT must be prepared to treat all patients with signs and symptoms of cardiac compromise as cardiac emergencies including the most serious cardiac problem of all—cardiac arrest, the complete cessation of heartbeat. Not every cardiac arrest is preceded by chest pain, nor do all patients with chest pain proceed to cardiac arrest, but for those who do, rapid intervention is vital. Without it, such patients will almost surely die. In cases of cardiac arrest, the actions of properly trained and equipped EMTs can make the difference between life and death.

Distribute the scored quizzes from the last class. Go over each question on the quiz and handle any concerns students may have about the answers.

INTRODUCTION TO CHAPTER 15

Handout 15-1
Chapter 15 Objectives Checklist

Chapter 15, "Altered Mental Status and Diabetic Emergencies," is the fourth lesson in Module 4. An altered mental status is a condition in which the patient displays a change in his normal mental state that may range from disorientation to complete unresponsiveness. Significant decreases in the mental status can lead to serious airway and breathing compromise. Therefore, it is important for the EMT to recognize and provide emergency care for patients who exhibit an altered mental status.

Diabetes mellitus is a disease that frequently causes changes in the patient's mental status due to alterations in the blood sugar level. There are several million people in the United States who have been diagnosed with diabetes and, as the population ages, the incidence of diabetes will also increase. Unfortunately, several million other Americans have diabetes mellitus but have yet to be diagnosed. Many times, their first indication of having the disease may be an incident of altered mental status such as disorientation or even loss of consciousness.

Prompt recognition and appropriate emergency care of a patient who has an altered mental status, in addition to a history of diabetes that is controlled by medication, is necessary.

Distribute the Chapter 15 Objectives Checklist and give students a few minutes to look it over. Then briefly paraphrase the objectives for this lesson in your own words.

LECTURE

Lecture Master 15
You may wish to display Lecture Master 15 when presenting the lecture to the class.

The following suggested lecture outline is based on the Department of Transportation's EMT-Basic National Standard Curriculum. In some places, the DOT curriculum has been rearranged or expanded upon so that it is more complete or easier for the student to understand. The page numbers in parentheses refer to pages in the textbook. The parenthetical references in dark, heavy type are to figures, tables, and scans in the textbook.

©2008 by Pearson Education, Inc.
Prehospital Emergency Care, 8th ed.

I. Assessment and care—Altered mental status patient with an unknown history (pp. 465–469)

  A. Scene size-up (p. 466)

    1. Medical or trauma?

    2. Look for medications, alcohol, drugs.

    3. If more than one patient, suspect gas or poison.

  B. Initial assessment (p. 466)

    1. Pay particular attention to airway and breathing.

  C. Focused history and physical exam (pp. 466–468)

    1. SAMPLE history

    2. Baseline vital signs

    3. Physical exam

      a. Head

      b. Pupils

      c. Mouth and oral mucosa

      d. Chest

      e. Breath sounds

      f. Abdomen

      g. Lower and upper extremities

      h. Posterior body

      i. Blood glucose level

  D. Emergency medical care (pp. 468)

    1. Maintain spinal stabilization, if trauma suspected.

    2. Maintain patent airway.

    3. Suction secretions, blood, and vomitus.

    4. Maintain oxygen therapy.

    5. Be prepared to assist ventilation.

    6. Position the patient.

    7. Transport.

  E. Conditions that may cause altered mental status in patient with unknown history (pp. 468) **(Table 15-1, p. 468)**

    1. Shock

    2. Poisoning or drug overdose

    3. Post-seizure

    4. Infection

    5. Traumatic head injury

    6. Inadequate airway or breathing

    7. Alcohol intoxication

    8. Stroke

    9. Diabetes

II. Assessment and care—Patient with altered mental status with a history of diabetes (pp. 469–474)**(Fig. 15-1, p. 469; Figs. 15-8, 15-9, pp. 477–479)**

  A. Scene size-up (p. 470)

  B. Initial assessment (p. 470) **(Fig. 15-2, p. 470)**

  C. Focused history and physical exam (pp. 470–473)

    1. Signs and symptoms **(Fig. 15-3, p. 471)**

      a. Rapid onset of altered mental status

        (1) After missing a meal on a day the patient took prescribed insulin

        (2) After vomiting a meal on a day the patient took prescribed insulin

        (3) After an unusual exercise or physical work episode

        (4) May occur with no identifiable predisposing factor

Point of Interest

Diabetes is the sixth leading cause of death by disease. Also, high blood pressure affects 60–65 percent of people with diabetes.

On the Net

Assessment and treatment of altered mental status. http://www.moondragon. org/ems/alteredmental. html

On the Net

For more on diabetes from the National Institute of Diabetes and Digestive and Kidney Diseases of the National Institutes of Health, go to: www. niddk.nih.gov

On the Net

American Diabetes Association. http://www.diabetes.org

    b. Intoxicated appearance, staggering, slurred speech to complete unresponsiveness

    c. Elevated heart rate

    d. Cool, moist skin

    e. Hunger

    f. Seizures

    g. Insulin in refrigerator or other diabetes medications found at scene

    h. Uncharacteristic or bizarre behavior, combativeness

    i. Anxiousness or restlessness

    j. Bruising at insulin inject sites on abdomen

    k. Elderly patients—signs similar to those of stroke

    l. Blood glucose reading of <60 mg/dL (**Table 15-2, p. 472; Fig. 15-4, p. 473**)

  2. Dissemination of the episode

  3. Onset

  4. Duration

  5. Evidence of trauma

  6. Interruptions

  7. Seizures

  8. Fever

  9. Baseline vital signs

  10. Ensure known history of diabetes

    a. Medical identification device (**Fig. 15-2, p. 470**)

    b. Ask about (look for) medications

      (1) Insulin (Humulin®, Novolin®, Iletin®, Semilente®)

      (2) Diabanese®

      (3) Glucamide®

      (4) Orinase®

      (5) Micronase®

      (6) Diabeta®

      (7) Tolinase®

      (8) Glucotrol®

      (9) Humalog®

      (10) Glucophage®

      (11) Glynase®

    c. Determine

      (1) Last meal

      (2) Last medication dose

      (3) Any related illnesses

D. Emergency medical care (pp. 474)

  1. Establish and maintain an open airway.

  2. If breathing is adequate

    a. Administer oxygen by nonrebreather mask at 15 liters per minute.

  3. If breathing is inadequate

    a. Provide positive pressure ventilations with supplemental oxygen.

  4. Determine if patient is alert enough to swallow.

    a. If so, administer oral glucose. (**Figs. 15-5 through 15-7, pp. 474–476**)

  5. Transport.

E. Ongoing assessment (pp. 474)

  1. Reassessment of mental status to see if medication has had an effect.

  2. Retesting of blood glucose level.

Reading/Reference
Stewart, C., "New Trends in Diabetes Management," *EMS Magazine*, Nov. 2001.

III. Medication (pp. 474–476)
  A. Oral glucose (pp. 474–476)
    1. Medication name
      a. Generic
        (1) Glucose, oral
      b. Trade
        (1) Glutose®
        (2) Insta-glucose®
    2. Indications
      a. Altered mental status
      b. Known history of diabetes controlled by medication
      c. Ability to swallow the medication
    3. Contraindications
      a. Unresponsiveness
      b. Inability to swallow
    4. Medication form
      a. Gel, in toothpaste-type tubes
    5. Dosage
      a. One tube
    6. Administration
      a. Obtain order from medical direction, either on-line or off-line.
      b. Ensure signs and symptoms of altered mental status with a known history of diabetes, controlled by medication.
      c. Obtain blood glucose reading, if allowed.
      d. Ensure patient is conscious and can swallow and protect the airway.
      e. Administer glucose. **(Figs. 15-5 through 15-7, pp. 474–476)**
        (1) Between cheek and gum
        (2) Place on tongue depressor between cheek and gum.
      f. Perform ongoing assessment.
    7. Actions
      a. Increases blood sugar
    8. Side effects
      a. None when given properly.
      b. May be aspirated by the patient without a gag reflex.
    9. Reassessment strategies
      a. If patient loses consciousness or seizes, remove tongue depressor from mouth.
      b. Check to see if medication has had an effect.
      c. Recheck blood glucose level.

⦿

Point to Emphasize

It does not matter if the diabetic patient is hypoglycemic or hyperglycemic. "Sugar for everyone" is the rule of thumb. Don't spend time trying to diagnose. Treat the patient instead.

ENRICHMENT (OPTIONAL) ├──────────────■

The following sections contain information that is valuable as background for the EMT, but that goes substantially beyond the U.S. Department of Transportation's EMT-Basic National Standard Curriculum.

IV. Understanding diabetic emergencies (pp. 476–482)
  A. Glucose (sugar) (pp. 477–480)
  B. Hormones that control blood glucose levels (p. 480)
    1. Insulin
    2. Glucagon
    3. Other hormones

    C. Normal metabolism and glucose regulation (pp. 480–481)
       (Fig. 15-10, p. 481)
    D. Diabetes mellitus (DM) (pp. 481–482) **(Fig. 15-11, p. 483)**
V. Emergencies related to diabetes mellitus (pp. 482–488)
  (Table 15-3, p. 486)
    A. Hypoglycemia (pp. 482–484)
      1. Overview of the disease process
      2. Assessment
      3. Emergency medical care
    B. Hyperglycemia (p. 484)
      1. Overview of the disease process
      2. Assessment
      3. Emergency medical care
    C. Hyperglycemic condition: diabetic ketoacidosis (DKA)
      (pp. 484–487)
      1. Overview of the disease process
      2. Assessment
      3. Emergency medical care
    D. Hyperglycemic condition: hyperglycemic hyperosmolar
      nonketotic syndrome (HHNS) (pp. 487–488)
      1. Overview of the disease process
      2. Assessment
      3. Emergency medical care

CASE STUDY FOLLOW-UP

Ask a student volunteer to read the Case Study that begins on page 465 of the textbook. You may wish to use the following questions to engage students in a discussion of the Case Study Follow-up that begins on page 488 of the textbook. Provide missing information and clarify ideas as needed.

Q1. What are the indications that Mr. Bennet has an altered mental status?

A1. *A neighbor said he had been acting strangely and talking but not making sense. He responds to questions with mumbled words, seems disoriented, and does not know his name, where he is, who his neighbor is, or what day it is.*

Q2. How do you determine that Mr. Bennet's altered mental status might be a result of his diabetes?

A2. *His neighbor mentions he has a "sugar problem," and there is a bottle of insulin in the refrigerator.*

Q3. What authorization do you have to administer oral glucose to a patient with probable diabetes-related altered mental status?

A3. *Standing orders from medical direction.*

Q4. How does administration of the oral glucose affect Mr. Bennet?

A4. *Mr. Bennet begins to respond more quickly to commands and questions. He remembers his name and where he is. His airway is clear and breathing remains adequate. His pulse rate decreases to 86/minute, and his skin becomes less pale, dryer, and warmer. By the time of arrival at the hospital, Mr. Bennet is alert and oriented to person, place, and time. He has no complaints and appears in no distress.*

Assess students' ability to apply what they have just learned by discussing the Review Questions on page 490 in the textbook.

Q1. Describe the emergency medical care for a patient with an altered mental status and no known history of diabetes.

A1. *Emergency medical care for a patient with altered mental status and no known history of diabetes is as follows: Maintain spinal stabilization if trauma is suspected. Maintain an open airway, suction as needed, be prepared to assist ventilations, maintain oxygen therapy, position the patient on the left side, and transport. (p. 468)*

Q2. Name the common signs and symptoms of a patient with an altered mental status who has a diabetic history.

A2. *Common signs and symptoms of a patient with an altered mental status and a history of diabetes include rapid onset of altered mental status; appearance of intoxication (staggering, slurred speech to complete unresponsiveness); elevated heart rate; cool, moist skin; hunger; seizure activity; uncharacteristic or bizarre behavior; combativeness; anxiousness or restlessness; bruising at insulin injection sites on abdomen; in the elderly, weakness or paralysis that mimic stroke; blood glucose reading of < 60 mg/dL. (pp. 470–472)*

Q3. Describe the emergency medical care for a patient who has an altered mental status and has a history of diabetes that is controlled by medication.

A3. *Emergency medical care for a patient with altered mental status and history of diabetes controlled by medication is as follows: Establish and maintain an open airway; provide high-flow oxygen; determine that the patient is alert enough to swallow; administer oral glucose in accordance with on-line or off-line orders from medical direction; transport. (p. 474)*

Q4. Explain why airway management is a major concern in the patient with an altered mental status.

A4. *Airway management is a major concern because a patient with altered mental status may not have or may lose the ability to maintain an open airway. (pp. 477–478)*

Q5. Name the indications for oral glucose.

A5. *Indications for oral glucose are an altered mental status, a history of diabetes controlled by medication, and the ability to swallow. (p. 475)*

Q6. Name the contraindications for oral glucose.

A6. *Contraindications for oral glucose are unresponsiveness or inability to swallow. (p. 475)*

Q7. Describe two methods of administering oral glucose.

A7. *Oral glucose may be administered by squeezing the contents of the tube between the patient's cheek and gum, or squeezing the contents of the tube onto the end of a tongue depressor, then placing the tongue depressor between the patient's cheek and gum. Only a small amount at a time should be placed in the patient's mouth. The area between cheek and gum may be lightly massaged to disperse the gel and increase absorption. (pp. 475–476)*

Q8. Describe the role of medical direction in emergency care for the diabetic patient.

A8. *Oral glucose may be administered only on the orders of medication direction, either on-line or as an off-line standing order or protocol. (p. 475)*

CRITICAL THINKING

Assess students' ability to respond to real-life emergency situations by discussing the Critical Thinking questions on page 490 in the textbook.

Q1. What emergency care would you provide during the initial assessment?

A1. *During the initial assessment of this patient, the EMTs should open the patient's airway with the head-tilt, chin-lift maneuver and initiate high concentration oxygen therapy. The use of airway adjuncts could also be considered at this time.*

Q2. Based on the signs, what condition do you suspect the patient is experiencing?

A2. *This patient is most likely suffering from hypoglycemia. This field impression is based on information from the history and physical exam findings. The patient's prescription for Novolin, which is an injectable form of insulin, provides a medical history of Type I diabetes mellitus. The physical exam reveals pale, cool, clammy skin; tachycardia; and an altered mental status, all of which are consistent with hypoglycemia.*

Q3. What other assessment procedures would be helpful to you regarding this patient?

A3. *It would be tremendously helpful to check the patient's blood glucose level with a glucose meter.*

Q4. What would you expect the blood glucose reading to be in the patient?

A4. *Based on this patient's presentation, the blood glucose reading would most likely be 60 mg/dL or less.*

Q5. Why is the onset of the altered mental status significant in this patient?

A5. *The fact that the patient's altered mental status developed rapidly, coupled with her current presentation and medical history, is a definite indication that the patient's blood glucose level is a factor in her condition. Patients who experience hypoglycemic events typically present with a rapid onset of an altered mental status.*

SKILLS DEMONSTRATION AND PRACTICE

Demonstrate use of the oral glucose product most commonly used in your EMS system.

Divide students into teams of two. Have students administer oral glucose to one another. Observe practice and provide assistance, if necessary.

Caution: Do not allow administration of oral glucose to students with diabetes.

ASSIGNMENTS

Assign students to read Chapter 16, "Stroke," before the next class. Also ask them to complete Chapter 15 of the Workbook.

EVALUATION

Chapter Quiz Distribute copies of the Chapter Quiz provided in Handout 15-2 to evaluate student understanding of this chapter. Remind students not to refer to their textbooks or notes while taking the quiz.

Test Manager You may wish to create a custom-tailored test using Prentice Hall *TestGen for Prehospital Emergency Care, Eighth Edition* to evaluate student understanding of this chapter.

Online Test Preparation (for students and instructors) Additional test preparation is available through *EMT Achieve: Basic Test Preparation* at http://www.prenhall.com/EMTAchieve. Instructors can also monitor student mastery online.

REINFORCEMENT

Handouts If classroom discussions or performance on the quiz indicates that some students have not fully mastered the chapter content, you may wish to assign some or all of the Reinforcement Handouts for this chapter.

TECH EXTRAS

Brady Skills Series EMT-B Videos/CD Have your students watch the skills come to life on either VHS or CD-ROM.

PowerPoint Presentation (for instructors) The PowerPoint material developed for this chapter offers useful reinforcement of chapter content.

Student CD A wide variety of material on this CD-ROM will reinforce and also expand student knowledge and skills.

Companion Website (for students) Additional review quizzes and links to EMS resources will contribute to further reinforcement of this chapter. Please visit http://www.prenhall.com/mistovich.

Reading/Reference
Textbook, pp. 491–509

Workbook
Chapter 15 Activities

Chapter Quiz
Handout 15-2

TestGen
Chapter 15 Test

Online Test Preparation
Send your students to http://www.prenhall.com/EMTAchieve

Handouts 15-3 to 15-6
Reinforcement Activities

Brady Skills Series EMT-B Videos/CD
Visual Reinforcement

PowerPoint Presentation
Chapter 15

Student CD
Chapter 15

Companion Website
http://www.prenhall.com/mistovich

OBJECTIVES

OBJECTIVES CHECKLIST

Cognitive		Date Mastered
4-4.1	Identify the patient taking diabetic medications with altered mental status and the implications of a diabetes history.	
4-4.2	State the steps in the emergency medical care of the patient taking diabetic medicine with an altered mental status and a history of diabetes.	
4-4.3	Establish the relationship between airway management and the patient with altered mental status.	
4-4.4	State the generic and trade names, medication forms, dose, administration, action, and contraindications for oral glucose.	
4-4.5	Evaluate the need for medical direction in the emergency medical care of the diabetic patient.	
*	State the steps in the emergency care of the patient with an altered mental status and an unknown history.	

Affective		Date Mastered
4-4.6	Explain the rationale for administering oral glucose.	

Psychomotor		Date Mastered
4-4.7	Demonstrate the steps in the emergency medical care for the patient taking diabetic medicine with an altered mental status and a history of diabetes.	
4-4.8	Demonstrate the steps in the administration of oral glucose.	
4-4.9	Demonstrate the assessment and documentation of patient response to oral glucose.	
4-4.10	Demonstrate how to complete a prehospital care report for patients with diabetic emergencies.	

CHAPTER 15 QUIZ

Write the letter of the best answer in the space provided.

_____ **1.** Insulin can best be described as a(n)
- **A.** amino acid.
- **B.** hormone.
- **C.** blood sugar.
- **D.** platelet.

_____ **2.** The organ(s) responsible for the production of insulin is (are) the
- **A.** liver.
- **B.** kidneys.
- **C.** pancreas.
- **D.** spleen.

_____ **3.** All of the following are signs or symptoms commonly associated with a diabetic emergency *except*
- **A.** an elevated heart rate.
- **B.** combativeness.
- **C.** seizure activity.
- **D.** hot, dry skin.

_____ **4.** The simple form of sugar that is the body's main source of energy is
- **A.** insulin.
- **B.** glucose.
- **C.** adrenalin.
- **D.** diabanese.

_____ **5.** Glucose is administered in the form of a
- **A.** tablet.
- **B.** liquid for injection.
- **C.** suspension.
- **D.** gel.

_____ **6.** Use the following memory aid to gather a history from a patient with an altered mental status
- **A.** SAMPLE.
- **B.** AVPU.
- **C.** START.
- **D.** DCAP-BTLS.

_____ **7.** The type of diabetes that requires a patient to inject insulin daily is
- **A.** Type I.
- **B.** Type II.
- **C.** "maturity-onset diabetes."
- **D.** diabetic ketoacidosis.

_____ **8.** If a patient has excessive thirst, breath with a fruity odor, and warm, dry skin, you would suspect
- **A.** hypoglycemia.
- **B.** epilepsy.
- **C.** hyperglycemia.
- **D.** cerebral edema.

_____ **9.** All of the following are medications often taken by diabetics *except*
- **A.** Glynase®.
- **B.** Humalog®.
- **C.** nitroglycerin.
- **D.** Orinase®.

_____ **10.** For the EMT to administer oral glucose, the patient must meet all of the following criteria *except*
- **A.** an altered mental status.
- **B.** a baseline blood pressure that is greater than 90 mmHg systolic.
- **C.** a history of diabetes controlled by medication.
- **D.** the ability to swallow.

_____ **11.** Proper administration of oral glucose usually produces
- **A.** headache.
- **B.** bradycardia.
- **C.** diaphoresis.
- **D.** no side effects.

_____ **12.** What action does oral glucose take in the bloodstream?
- **A.** decreases blood sugar
- **B.** increases blood sugar
- **C.** decreases insulin level
- **D.** increases insulin level

_____ **13.** If you are in doubt as to whether the patient is suffering from an emergency related to hypoglycemia or hyperglycemia, err to benefit the patient and
- **A.** allow the patient to drink.
- **B.** withhold liquids from the patient.
- **C.** administer oral glucose.
- **D.** withhold oral glucose.

_____ **14.** Which of the following is a contraindication to the administration of oral glucose?
- **A.** history of diabetes
- **B.** altered mental status
- **C.** trauma
- **D.** unresponsiveness

_____ **15.** Patients with an altered mental status and without suspected spinal injury should be transported in what position?
- **A.** shock
- **B.** lateral recumbent
- **C.** prone
- **D.** supine

IN THE FIELD

Read the following real-life situation. Then answer the questions that follow.

You and your partner are dispatched at 1015 to the Riverside Apartments on Montgomery Drive, Apartment 323, for an unconscious male. Upon your arrival, the patient's excited wife meets you at the door. As she leads you to the kitchen, she explains that her husband, who is diabetic, has not been feeling well and stayed home from work today due to nausea and vomiting. While they were sitting at the kitchen table, he suddenly passed out and she immediately called 9-1-1. As you enter the kitchen, you see a male patient in his late 50s slumped in a kitchen chair. Your initial assessment reveals that the patient is unresponsive, bradypneic (10 breaths per minute), with a weak and rapid radial pulse and pale, cool, and clammy skin.

1. What condition do these signs and symptoms suggest?

2. In addition to a SAMPLE history, what additional questions would you ask the patient's wife?

3. Is oral glucose indicated for this patient? Why or why not?

4. What additional emergency medical care would you provide to this patient?

CHAPTER 15 REVIEW

Write the word or words that best complete each sentence in the space provided.

1. The body's main source of energy is _____.

2. The hormone secreted by the pancreas that is needed to promote the movement of glucose from the blood into the cells is known as _____.

3. When there is a(n) _____ of insulin, glucose cannot enter the cells; instead, it remains in the bloodstream, causing a high level of glucose in the blood, a condition known as _____.

4. When a diabetic's insulin level is too high, too much sugar enters the cells and not enough sugar remains in the blood, a condition called _____.

5. _____ _____ is the medication of choice in the emergency medical care of the diabetic patient with an altered mental status.

6. Assess and document the mental status of a diabetic patient using the _____ scale.

7. As an alternative to squeezing small portions of the tube of oral glucose into the patient's mouth, the EMT could use a(n) _____ _____.

8. Type _____ diabetes typically develops in adulthood and is controlled by diet, exercise, oral medications, and, in severe cases, with insulin.

9. _____ _____ is a disease characterized by an altered relationship between glucose and insulin.

10. If no mechanism of injury is apparent, you would suspect that a patient's altered mental status is a result of a(n) _____.

11. Never administer oral glucose to a patient who cannot swallow or who is _____.

12. For a patient with an altered mental status, repeat the ongoing assessment every _____ _____.

13. The most common sign of hypoglycemia is a(n) _____ _____.

©2008 by Pearson Education, Inc.
Prehospital Emergency Care, 8th ed.

14. An altered mental status from hypoglycemia will typically have a(n) _____

onset.

15. A patient may take as long as _____ minutes before showing improvement

from receiving oral glucose.

REINFORCEMENT

DIABETIC EMERGENCIES: LISTING

1. List five medications often taken by diabetics.

2. List nine signs and symptoms associated with a diabetic emergency.

3. List the three indications for administering glucose to a diabetic patient.

4. List the four steps in the administration of glucose.

REINFORCEMENT

ORAL GLUCOSE

Write in the missing information on the medication flash card below and save the completed card for future reference.

Oral Glucose

Medication Names

  1. Generic: _____

  2. Trade: _____

Indications

  1. _____

  2. _____

  3. _____

Contraindications

  1. _____

  2. _____

Medication Form:

Dosage: _____

Actions _____

  1. _____

  2. _____

Side Effects

  1. _____

  2. _____

Lecture Master 15

Altered Mental Status and Diabetic Emergencies

Altered Mental Status— Unknown History
Assessment and Care

Conditions That May Cause AMS

Altered Mental Status— History of Diabetes
Assessment and Care

Blood Glucose Meter

Oral Glucose

HANDOUT 15-2: Chapter 15 Quiz

1. B	**5.** D	**9.** C	**13.** C
2. C	**6.** A	**10.** B	**14.** D
3. D	**7.** A	**11.** D	**15.** B
4. B	**8.** C	**12.** B	

HANDOUT 15-3: In the Field

1. A diabetic emergency
2. Did the patient take his medication today? Did the patient eat (or skip any) meals today or yesterday?
3. Oral glucose is not indicated. Unresponsiveness (inability to swallow) is a contraindication to the administration of oral glucose.
4. Monitor and maintain open airway, administer oxygen by nonrebreather mask at 15 liters per minute, and transport.

HANDOUT 15-4: Chapter 15 Review

1. glucose
2. insulin
3. lack, hyperglycemia
4. hypoglycemia
5. Oral glucose
6. AVPU
7. tongue depressor
8. II (two)
9. Diabetes mellitus
10. illness
11. unresponsive
12. 5 minutes
13. altered mental status
14. sudden (rapid)
15. 20

HANDOUT 15-5: Diabetic Emergencies: Listing

1. Any five of the following: Insulin, Humulin®, Novolin®, Iletin®, Semilente®, Diabanese®, Glucamide®, Orinase®, Micronase®, Diabeta®, Glynase®, Tolinase®, Glucotrol®, Humalog®, Glucophage®

2. Any nine: rapid onset of altered mental status, intoxicated appearance, tachycardia, cool and moist skin, hunger, seizures, uncharacteristic or bizarre behavior, combativeness, anxiety or restlessness, bruising at insulin injection sites, weakness or paralysis (especially in the elderly), blood glucose < 60 mg/dL
3. An altered mental status, a history of diabetes controlled by medication, the ability to swallow the medication
4. Obtain order from medical direction. Ensure the signs and symptoms are consistent with an altered mental status associated with a history of diabetes controlled by medication. Ensure patient is responsive and able to swallow the medication and protect his airway. Administer the oral glucose by either squeezing small portions of the tube into the mouth or via a tongue depressor between the check and gum.

HANDOUT 15-6: Oral Glucose (completion)

Medication Names:
1. Generic: Oral glucose
2. Trade: Glutose®, Insta-glucose®

Indications:
1. Altered mental status
2. History of diabetes controlled by medication
3. Ability to swallow the medication

Contraindications:
1. Unresponsive patient
2. Patient unable to swallow the medication.

Medication Form:
Gel, in toothpaste-type tubes

Dosage:
The typical dosage is one tube.

Actions:
1. Increases blood sugar level
2. Increases sugar available to the brain

Side Effects:
None, when administered properly

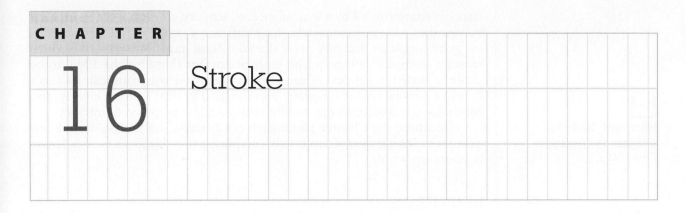

16 Stroke

This chapter contains information that is valuable as background for the EMT but that goes substantially beyond the U.S. Department of Transportation's EMT-Basic National Standard Curriculum.

OBJECTIVES

The asterisked objectives pertain to material that is supplemental to the DOT curriculum. Page numbers in parentheses refer to pages in the textbook.

Cognitive

* * Describe the assessment of the patient with an altered mental status and a loss of speech, sensory, or motor function. (pp. 495–502)
* * List the common signs and symptoms of a nontraumatic brain injury. (pp. 494–501, 503)
* * Describe the emergency care for a patient with an altered mental status and a loss of speech, sensory, or motor function. (pp. 501–502, 504)
* * Describe the conditions most likely to cause altered mental status with a loss of speech, sensory, or motor function. (pp. 493–494, 502, 504, 506–507)

REVIEW

In the last lesson, "Altered Mental Status and Diabetic Emergencies," students learned that diabetes mellitus is a disease that frequently causes changes in the patient's mental status due to alterations in the blood sugar level. There are several million people in the United States who have been diagnosed with diabetes and, as the population ages, the incidence of diabetes will also increase. Unfortunately, several million others have diabetes mellitus but have yet to be diagnosed. Many times their first indication of having the disease may be an incident of altered mental status such as disorientation or even loss of consciousness. Prompt recognition and appropriate emergency care of a patient who has an altered mental status, in addition to a history of diabetes that is controlled by medication, is necessary. Distribute the scored quizzes from the last class. Go over each question on the quiz and handle any concerns students may have about the answers.

INTRODUCTION TO CHAPTER 16

Chapter 16, "Stroke," is the fifth chapter in Module 4. In this chapter, students will learn how to assess and treat patients whose altered mental

Total Teaching Time
125 minutes

Resources Needed
* Scored Chapter 17 Quizzes
* Guest who has had a stroke that was managed by the EMS system

Additional Resources
Larmon/Davis, *Basic Life Support Skills*

Elling, *EMT Achieve: Basic Test Preparation*

Limmer/Mistovich/ O'Keefe, *Audio Lecture & Study Guide: EMT*

Mistovich/Kuvlesky, *SUCCESS! for the EMT, Second Edition*

status is accompanied by a loss of speech, sensory, or motor function. This frequently occurs in patients who have suffered a stroke. Stroke, however, is only one condition that may cause altered mental status with a loss of speech, sensory, or motor function. The most important thing for the EMT to be aware of is that, regardless of cause, these signs and symptoms can lead to a blocked airway and inadequate breathing. The EMT must closely and continuously monitor airway and breathing and be prepared to intervene.

Distribute the Chapter 16 Objectives Checklist and give students a few minutes to look it over. Then briefly paraphrase the objectives for this lesson in your own words.

LECTURE

The following suggested lecture outline is based on the Department of Transportation's EMT-Basic National Standard Curriculum. In some places, the DOT curriculum has been rearranged or expanded upon so that it is more complete or easier for the student to understand. The page numbers in parentheses refer to pages in the textbook. The parenthetical references in dark, heavy type are to figures, tables, and scans in the textbook.

ACUTE STROKE: ALTERED SPEECH, SENSORY FUNCTION, MOTOR FUNCTION, OR MENTAL STATUS

I. **Neurological deficit resulting from stroke** (pp. 492–502) **(Figs. 16-9 and 16-10, pp. 503–505)**
  A. Acute stroke (pp. 492–494)
   1. Overview of the disease process **(Fig. 16-1, p. 494)**
     a. Ischemic stroke
      (1) Thrombotic stroke
      (2) Embolic stroke
     b. Hemorrhagic stroke
  B. Transient ischemic attack (TIA) (pp. 494–495)
  C. Assessment and care (pp. 495–502)
   1. Scene size-up
     a. Trauma or medical condition?
      (1) Signs of mechanism of injury
      (2) Alcohol, drugs, or drug paraphernalia
      (3) Where patient is found and how dressed
      (4) Bucket or ice pack near patient
   2. Initial assessment
     a. Airway and breathing are priorities.
     b. Assess responsiveness carefully.
   3. Focused history and physical exam **(Fig. 16-2, p. 497; Fig. 16-3, p. 497)**
     a. Unresponsive patient
      (1) Physical exam
        (a) Rapid assessment
      (2) Baseline vitals
        (a) Pay particular attention to blood pressure.
        (b) Repeat every 5 minutes.
      (3) SAMPLE history
     b. Responsive patient
      (1) SAMPLE history
        (a) If patient can't speak, use yes/no questions and gestures or motions.
        (b) Be very alert to complaints of headache.

Handout 16-1
Chapter 16 Objectives Checklist

Lecture Master
You may wish to display Lecture Master 16 when presenting the lecture to the class.

Point of Interest
A stroke strikes every minute in America. Four of five American families will be affected by stroke during their lifetime.

On the Net
For more on stroke and the National Stroke Association, go to: www.stroke.org

On the Net
Brain Attack Center. www.umm.edu/mbac/

Slides/Videos
"Cerebral Events," *Pulse*, Mar. 2001.

Reading/Reference
Nordberg, M. "Is Prehospital Care Killing Stroke Patients?" *EMS Magazine*, Nov 2005

On the Net
Transient ischemic attack. www.healthhubs.com/tia/

        (2) Physical exam

           (a) Rapid assessment

        (3) Baseline vitals

           (a) Pay particular attention to blood pressure.

           (b) Repeat every 5 minutes.

    c. Cincinnati Prehospital Stroke Scale (**Fig. 16-4, p. 498**)

    d. Los Angeles Prehospital Stroke Screen (**Fig. 16-5, p. 498**)

  4. Signs and symptoms (**Fig. 16-6, p. 500**)

    a. Altered mental status

    b. Paralysis or weakness, especially to one side of the body

    c. Numbness on one side of the body

    d. Speech disturbances

    e. Loss of bowel or bladder control

    f. Unequal pupils

    g. Loss of vision in one or both eyes

    h. Double vision or other visual disturbances

    i. Eyes turned away from paralyzed side

    j. Nausea and vomiting

    k. Severe headache

    l. Seizure activity

    m. Stiff neck

    n. Sensor or receptive aphasia

    o. Expressive or motor aphasia

    p. Incoordination of extremities on one side

    q. Poor balance, clumsiness, ataxia

    r. Hearing loss to one side

    s. Light or sound sensitivity

    t. Vertigo

  5. Emergency medical care (**Figs. 16-7, p. 501 and 16-8, p. 502**)

    a. Maintain a patent airway.

    b. Suction secretions and vomitus.

    c. Be prepared to assist ventilation.

    d. Maintain oxygen therapy.

    e. Position the patient.

    f. Protect any paralyzed extremities.

    g. Transport.

  6. Detailed physical exam

  7. Ongoing assessment

    a. Every 5 minutes

ENRICHMENT (OPTIONAL)

The following sections contain information that is valuable as background for the EMT, but that goes substantially beyond the U.S. Department of Transportation's EMT-Basic National Standard Curriculum

II. Causes of stroke (pp. 502–507)(**Fig. 16-11, pp. 506–507**)

  A. Ischemic strokes

    1. Thrombosis

    2. Embolism

  B. Hemorrhagic strokes

CASE STUDY FOLLOW-UP

Ask a student volunteer to read the Case Study that begins on page 492 of the textbook. You may wish to use the following questions to engage students in a discussion of the Case Study Follow-up that begins on page 508 of the textbook. Provide missing information and clarify ideas as needed.

Q1. During your scene size-up, what odors do you notice and what might those odors indicate?

A1. *The smell of urine and feces might indicate loss of bladder and bowel control.*

Q2. During your initial assessment, what do you note about Mrs. Stein's speech and face?

A2. *Her speech is severely slurred, and her face is pulled and drooping on the right side.*

Q3. What does your rapid physical assessment of Mrs. Stein reveal?

A3. *Her head shows no evidence of trauma. Her pupils are equal and reactive, but she has obvious facial droop to the right side. Her chest is rising and falling symmetrically and the breath sounds are equal bilaterally. Her abdomen is soft and no tenderness or rigidity is noted. Her pelvis is stable with no tenderness on palpation. Mrs. Stein is able to obey commands, and a check of strength in all four extremities reveals she has good left hand grip strength, but grip strength on the right is absent and strength in her left foot is good, but is again absent on the right. The posterior of her body shows no abnormalities. There are no medical identification tags.*

Q4. What does your detailed physical exam reveal about Mrs. Stein's condition?

A4. *Pupils are equal and reactive. Mrs. Stein's speech remains excessively slurred and garbled. She does not respond to a deep pinch to her right hand or foot. There is no movement on the right side of her body.*

Q5. What care do you continue providing to Mrs. Stein that may help alleviate her condition?

A5. *Administration of oxygen at 15 liters per minute.*

IN REVIEW

Assess students' ability to apply what they have just learned by discussing the Review Questions on page 509 in the textbook.

Q1. Explain why the airway and breathing must be closely monitored in a patient with an altered mental status or stroke.

A1. *Airway and breathing must be closely monitored in a patient with an altered mental status or stroke because these patients often lose the ability to protect the airway. They can lose the gag reflex and become unable to swallow. Injury to the brain also often results in inadequate breathing. (pp. 495–496)*

Q2. List several signs and symptoms of stroke.

A2. *Signs and symptoms include altered mental status; paralysis or weakness on one side of body; numbness or loss of sensation on one side of body; speech disturbances; loss of bladder or bowel control; unequal pupils; loss of vision in one or both eyes; double vision; eyes turned away from paralyzed side of body; nausea and vomiting; severe headache; seizures; stiff neck; inability to understand what is being said; inability to form words to talk; uncoordinated extremities, usually on one side; poor balance, clumsiness, difficulty walking; hearing loss to one side; light or sound sensitivity; vertigo (pp. 500–501)*

Q3. List the steps in the emergency care of the patient suffering from an altered mental status or stroke.

A3. *Steps in the emergency care of the patient suffering from an altered mental status or stroke are as follows: (1) Maintain a patent airway. (2) Suction as needed. (3) Assist with ventilations as needed. (4) Maintain oxygen therapy. (5) Position the patient—unresponsive patient on left side; responsive patient with chest and head elevated. (6) Protect paralyzed extremities. (7) Transport to a stroke center. (pp. 501–502)*

Q4. Compare and contrast stroke and TIA with regard to signs and symptoms, how they progress, and emergency medical care.

A4. *Stroke and TIA have similar signs and symptoms, but with TIA the signs and symptoms will disappear within 24 hours, most commonly within minutes, while the signs and symptoms of stroke will worsen or not improve. Emergency medical care is the same for both conditions. (pp. 493–495)*

CRITICAL THINKING

Assess students' ability to respond to real-life emergency situations by discussing the Critical Thinking questions on page 509 in the textbook.

Q1. What is the oxygenation status of the patient?

A1. *Although there are no other indications that his breathing is in any way inadequate, the pulse oximeter reading is 92% on room air. A SpO_2 reading of less than 95% should alert you to hypoxia.*

Q2. How would you manage the oxygenation status of the patient?

A2. *This patient would benefit from the application of a nonrebreather mask with 15 lpm of supplemental oxygen. The nonrebreather mask is appropriate in this situation because the patient has an adequate respiratory rate and adequate tidal volume. If either the respiratory rate or tidal volume becomes inadequate, you would immediately begin positive pressure ventilation.*

Q3. What type of stroke do you suspect the patient suffered?

A3. *Based on the sudden onset of obvious stroke symptoms, no further deterioration in the patient's condition, the irregular heart rate, and the fact that the patient is alert and oriented, the EMTs should suspect an ischemic stroke.*

Q4. What signs and symptoms would cause you to believe the patient suffered a stroke?

A4. *The patient's slurred speech, facial droop, arm drift and unilateral (one sided) weakness, coupled with an elevated blood pressure, irregularly irregular heart rhythm, and normal blood glucose reading indicate a stroke.*

Q5. How would you manage the patient?

A5. *Apply a nonrebreather mask with supplemental oxygen set at a rate of 15 lpm, place him in the lateral recumbent position on the gurney (or in a position of comfort if he insists), and transport.*

Q6. What is the significance of the pulse rhythm?

A6. *The patient's irregularly irregular pulse, which indicates an atrial fibrillation rhythm, is a common risk factor for stroke. This finding, when added to the other signs and symptoms, helps to verify that this patient is most likely suffering from a stroke.*

GUEST PRESENTATION AND DIALOG

Arrange to have as a guest someone who has actually experienced a stroke. In advance of today's presentation, discuss briefly with the guest any objectives or goals you may have for this visit. *Note:* The guest should be emotionally and physically recovered enough to share comfortably his or her experience. Also, consider providing an honorarium to the guest in appreciation for his or her contributions.

Before introducing the guest to students, inform them that they will have an opportunity to ask questions following the presentation. You may wish to suggest that students write down any questions that come to mind as their guest is sharing his or her stroke experience. Introduce the day's guest.

When the presentation concludes, invite students with questions to direct them, in turn, to their guest. Deflect questions that are too personal and provide clarification if any questions are beyond the medical knowledge of the guest.

ASSIGNMENTS

Assign students to read Chapter 17, "Seizures and Syncope," before the next class. Also ask them to complete Chapter 16 of the Workbook.

EVALUATION

Chapter Quiz Distribute copies of the Chapter Quiz provided in Handout 16-2 to evaluate student understanding of this chapter. Remind students not to refer to their textbooks or notes while taking the quiz.

Test Manager You may wish to create a custom-tailored test using Prentice Hall *TestGen for Prehospital Emergency Care, Eighth Edition* to evaluate student understanding of this chapter.

Online Test Preparation (for students and instructors) Additional test preparation is available through *EMT Achieve: Basic Test Preparation* at http://www.prenhall.com/EMTAchieve. Instructors can also monitor student mastery online.

REINFORCEMENT

Handouts If classroom discussions or performance on the quiz indicates that some students have not fully mastered the chapter content, you may wish to assign some or all of the Reinforcement Handouts for this chapter.

Reading/Reference
Textbook, pp. 510–524

Workbook
Chapter 16 Activities

Chapter Quiz
Handout 16-2

TestGen
Chapter 16 Test

Online Test Preparation
Send your students to
http://www.prenhall.com/
EMTAchieve

Handouts 16-3 to 16-5
Reinforcement Activities

TECH EXTRAS

Brady Skills Series EMT-B Videos/CD Have your students watch the skills come to life on either VHS or CD-ROM.

PowerPoint Presentation (for instructors) The PowerPoint material developed for this chapter offers useful reinforcement of chapter content.

Student CD A wide variety of material on this CD-ROM will reinforce and also expand student knowledge and skills.

Companion Website (for students) Additional review quizzes and links to EMS resources will contribute to further reinforcement of this chapter. Please visit http://www.prenhall.com/mistovich.

Brady Skills Series EMT-B Videos/CD
Visual Reinforcement

PowerPoint Presentation
Chapter 16

Student CD
Chapter 16

Companion Website
http://www.prenhall.com/mistovich

OBJECTIVES *(vertical, left margin)*

OBJECTIVES CHECKLIST

Cognitive	Date Mastered
* Describe the assessment of the patient with an altered mental status and a loss of speech, sensory, or motor function.	
* List the common signs and symptoms of a nontraumatic brain injury.	
* Describe the emergency care for a patient with an altered mental status and a loss of speech, sensory, or motor function.	
* Describe the conditions most likely to cause altered mental status with a loss of speech, sensory, or motor function.	

CHAPTER 16 QUIZ

Write the letter of the best answer in the space provided.

_____ **1.** Altered mental status and the inability to speak or feel sensation or move are all signs and symptoms of

    A. trauma.
    B. neurological deficit.
    C. embolism.
    D. diabetes mellitus.

_____ **2.** The most common nontraumatic brain injury is

    A. seizure.
    B. hypoxia.
    C. stroke.
    D. hypothermia.

_____ **3.** Paralysis that affects both lower extremities is called

    A. paraplegia.
    B. quadriplegia.
    C. monoplegia.
    D. hemiplegia.

_____ **4.** The process of clot formation is referred to as

    A. lordosis.
    B. thrombosis.
    C. embolism.
    D. hemorrhagia.

_____ **5.** All of the following are signs and symptoms of a neurological deficit resulting from nontraumatic brain injury *except*

    A. severe headache.
    B. paralysis.
    C. unequal pupils.
    D. fever.

_____ **6.** The medical term for loss of speech is

    A. aphasia.
    B. anesthesia.
    C. plegia.
    D. paralysis.

_____ **7.** Because of its similarity to a heart attack, a stroke is also referred to as a

    A. brain attack.
    B. heart stroke.
    C. brain arrhythmia.
    D. brain infarction.

_____ **8.** The major focus in emergency care of the nontraumatic patient with no history of diabetes and a loss of speech, sensory, or motor function is to provide the patient with

    A. oral glucose.
    B. insulin.
    C. oxygen.
    D. epinephrine.

_____ **9.** Most commonly, the signs and symptoms of a transient ischemic attack last for approximately

    A. 48 hours.
    B. 30–60 minutes.
    C. 15 minutes.
    D. 1–3 hours.

_____ **10.** If the possible stroke emergency patient is unable to protect her own airway because of a reduction in her mental status, she should be placed in what position?

    A. shock
    B. left lateral recumbent
    C. prone
    D. Trendelenberg

IN THE FIELD

Read the following real-life situation. Then answer the questions that follow.

The emergency medical dispatcher sends you to the Eagan residence on 1705 Altura Avenue. Upon arrival, the patient's grandson leads you and your partner into the living room. You observe a female patient in her late 60s or early 70s sitting on the sofa. The patient appears confused and is slurring her speech.

Your partner introduces herself and then completes a quick physical assessment. The patient exhibits drooping facial muscles and right-sided paralysis. Her pupils are unequal in size. Vital signs include a pulse rate of 120 and blood pressure of 160/80 mmHg.

1. What condition do these signs and symptoms suggest?

2. What emergency care measures should you take with this patient?

3. How would you transport this patient?

CHAPTER 16 REVIEW

Write the word or words that best complete each sentence in the space provided.

1. The term _____ _____ is defined as any deficiency in the functioning of the brain or nervous system.

2. Because the _____ controls breathing rate and depth, it is very possible to find inadequate breathing or unusual breathing patterns in a patient who presents with signs of stroke.

3. Diabetics who are _____ may show signs and symptoms very similar to those of a stroke patient, especially if the patient is elderly.

4. Though the EMT may rule out trauma at the scene, it is important to note if the patient has suffered a(n) _____ _____ within the last few weeks.

5. When collecting the SAMPLE history, it is especially important to note if the possible stroke patient complained of a(n) _____ prior to becoming unresponsive.

6. When the possible stroke patient cannot move a paralyzed extremity, it is vital that the EMT _____ the paralyzed extremity from _____.

7. After the EMT performs a rapid assessment of a possible stroke patient, it is appropriate to perform a(n) _____ _____ _____ if the patient's condition and time permit.

8. If a stroke occurs on the left side of the brain, the damage is noticeable on the _____ side of the body.

9. Most commonly, the signs and symptoms of a(n) _____ _____ _____ last less than 15 minutes.

10. Drugs that can reverse the consequences of stroke must be administered to certain stroke patients within _____ _____ of the first sign or symptom.

REINFORCEMENT

STROKE: LISTING

1. List four questions that will guide your emergency care of the possible stroke patient.

2. List seven of the common signs and symptoms of neurological deficit resulting from nontraumatic brain injury.

3. List the six steps in the emergency medical care of the patient with an altered mental status or a loss of speech, sensory, or motor function.

4. List three of the medical conditions that predispose a patient to a stroke.

LECTURE MASTER 16

Stroke

Neurological Deficit Resulting from Stroke
Acute Stroke

Overview of the Disease Process

- Stroke
- Transient ischemic attack (TIA)

Scene Size-up

Initial Assessment

Focused History and Physical Exam

Signs and Symptoms

Emergency Medical Care

Detailed Physical Exam

Ongoing Assessment

Causes of Stroke

Ischemic Stroke

Hemorrhagic Stroke

HANDOUT 16-2: Chapter 16 Quiz

1.	B	**4.**	B	**7.**	A	**9.**	C
2.	C	**5.**	D	**8.**	C	**10.**	B
3.	A	**6.**	A				

HANDOUT 16-3: In the Field

1. Stroke
2. Maintain a patent airway. Be prepared to assist ventilations. Maintain oxygen therapy, and transport.
3. Supine, with the head and chest elevated

HANDOUT 16-4: Chapter 16 Review

1. neurological deficit
2. brain
3. hypoglycemic
4. head injury
5. headache
6. protect, injury
7. detailed physical exam
8. right
9. transient ischemic attack
10. 3 hours

HANDOUT 16-5: Stroke: Listing

1. Any four: When did the symptoms begin? Is there any recent history of trauma to the head? Does the patient have a history of previous stroke? Was there any seizure activity noted prior to your arrival? What was the patient doing at the time of onset of signs and symptoms? Does the patient have a history of diabetes? Has the patient complained of a headache or stiff neck? Has the patient complained of dizziness, nausea, vomiting, or weakness? Has the patient experienced any slurred speech?

2. Any seven: altered mental status; paralysis; numbness; speech disturbances; loss of bladder/bowel control; unequal pupils; loss of vision; vision disturbances; eyes turned away from paralyzed side; nausea and vomiting; severe headache; seizure activity; stiff neck; inability to understand what is being said; inability to form words; uncoordinated extremities; poor balance, clumsiness, ataxia; hearing loss to one side; light or sound sensitivity; vertigo.

3. Maintain a patent airway, suction secretions and vomitus, be prepared to assist ventilation, maintain oxygen therapy, position the patient, protect any paralyzed extremities; rapid transport to a stroke center.

4. Atherosclerosis, heart disease, and/or hypertension

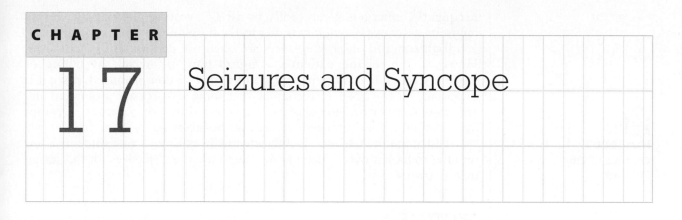

CHAPTER

17 Seizures and Syncope

This chapter contains information that is valuable as background for the EMT but that goes substantially beyond the U.S. Department of Transportation's EMT-Basic National Standard curriculum.

OBJECTIVES

The asterisked objectives pertain to material that is supplemental to the DOT curriculum. Page numbers in parentheses refer to pages in the textbook.

Cognitive

* Explain the assessment and emergency care for a seizing patient. (pp. 512–517, 518–519)
* Recognize the common signs and symptoms of a generalized seizure. (pp. 516–517)
* Recognize signs and symptoms of status epilepticus. (p. 513)
* Identify various conditions that cause seizures. (pp. 511–512)
* Recognize the common signs and symptoms of syncope. (pp. 517, 519)
* Differentiate between syncope and seizures. (pp. 517, 519)

REVIEW

In the last lesson, "Stroke," students learned how to assess and treat patients whose altered mental status is accompanied by a loss of speech, sensory, or motor function. This frequently occurs in patients who have suffered a stroke. Stroke, however, is only one condition that may cause altered mental status with a loss of speech, sensory, or motor function. The most important thing for the EMT to be aware of is that, regardless of the cause, this set of signs and symptoms can lead to a blocked airway and inadequate breathing. The EMT must closely and continuously monitor the airway and breathing and be prepared to intervene.

Distribute the scored quizzes from the last class. Go over each question on the quiz and handle any concerns students may have about the answers.

INTRODUCTION TO CHAPTER 17

Chapter 17, "Seizures and Syncope," is the sixth lesson in Module 4. A seizure is a sudden discharge of electrical activity in the brain that can lead to unusual behavior, from staring spells to gross muscle spasm. Most (but not all) seizure activity is accompanied by an altered mental status. Tell students that many seizures are self-limiting and last only 2 to 3 minutes. As a result, the seizure will have stopped by the time EMS arrives on the scene.

Total Teaching Time
115 minutes

Resources Needed
- Scored Chapter 16 Quizzes
- Complete jump kit containing BSI equipment, oral glucose, a tongue depressor, and refusal form
- Oxygen equipment
- Portable suction unit
- Wheeled stretcher
- Epilepsy medical identification device
- Moulage to simulate a contusion on the forehead

Additional Resources
Larmon/Davis, *Basic Life Support Skills*

Elling, *EMT Achieve: Basic Test Preparation*

Limmer/Mistovich/ O'Keefe, *Audio Lecture & Study Guide: EMT*

Mistovich/Kuvlesky, *SUCCESS! for the EMT, Second Edition*

Frequently, emergency care will consist of assisting the patient during recovery and transporting him or her to the hospital. Though quite dramatic and frightening to observe, seizures are often not dangerous in themselves. However, the seizing patient can injure him- or herself by falling or thrashing around, and the patient's airway can be compromised. Also, it is important for the EMT to recognize that some seizures are prolonged and are associated with life-threatening conditions or injuries. Prompt intervention in the prolonged seizure may be lifesaving.

Distribute the Chapter 17 Objectives Checklist and give students a few minutes to look it over. Then briefly paraphrase the objectives for this lesson in your own words.

LECTURE

The following suggested lecture outline is based on the Department of Transportation's EMT-Basic National Standard Curriculum. In some places, the DOT curriculum has been rearranged or expanded upon so that it is more complete or easier for the student to understand. The page numbers in parentheses refer to pages in the textbook. The parenthetical references in dark, heavy type are to figures, tables, and scans in the textbook.

SEIZURES AND SYNCOPE

I. **Seizure** (pp. 511–517)
  A. Sudden, temporary alteration in behavior caused by massive electrical discharge in group of nerve cells in brain (p. 511)
  B. Causes (pp. 511–512)
    1. Epilepsy
      a. Most common cause of seizure
    2. Other causes—injury or medical condition (**Table 17–1, p. 512**)
      a. High fever
      b. Infections
      c. Poisoning
      d. Hypoglycemia
      e. Hyperglycemia
      f. Head trauma
      g. Shock
      h. Hypoxia
      i. Stroke
      j. Drug or alcohol withdrawal
      k. Dysrhythmias
      l. Hypertension
      m. Pregnancy complications
      n. Blood electrolyte imbalance
      o. Idiopathic
  C. Assessment and care (pp. 512–517) (**Fig. 17-5, pp. 518–519**)
    1. Scene size-up
      a. Signs of trauma
      b. Prescription medication associated with epilepsy (**Table 17-2, p. 515**)
      c. Guide seizing patient's motions—protect patient. (**Fig. 17-1, p. 513**)
    2. Initial assessment

![Handout icon]
Handout 17-1
Chapter 17 Objectives Checklist

● ➤
Lecture Master
You may wish to display Lecture Master 17 when presenting the lecture to the class.

On the Net
For more on epilepsy and the Epilepsy Foundation, go to: www.efa.org

On the Net
Information about seizure disorders. http://www. neurology channel.com/ seizures/

  a. Closely assess patency of airway and adequacy of breathing and circulation.

  b. Act to provide patent airway and ventilation, if necessary. (**Fig. 17-2, p. 513**)

 3. Focused history and physical exam (**Fig. 17-3, p. 514**)

 4. Signs and symptoms (**Fig. 17-4, p. 516**)

  a. Aura

  b. Loss of consciousness

  c. Tonic phase (muscle rigidity)

  d. Hypertonic phase (extreme rigidity with hyperextension of back)

  e. Clonic phase (convulsion)

  f. Postictal phase (recovery)

 5. Emergency medical care (**Fig. 17-6, p. 520**)

  a. Position the patient.

  b. Maintain a patent airway.

  c. Suction.

  d. Assist breathing.

  e. Prevent injury to patient.

  f. Maintain oxygen therapy.

  g. Transport

 6. Ongoing assessment

II. Syncope (pp. 517–519)

 A. Sudden and temporary loss of consciousness due to temporary lack of blood flow to brain. (p. 517)

 B. Usually begins in standing position. (p. 519)

 C. Patient remembers feeling faint. (p. 519)

 D. Patient becomes on responsive almost immediately (p. 519)

 E. Skin is usually pale and moist. (p. 519)

 F. Emergency care (p. 519)

  1. Conduct initial assessment, focused history, and physical exam.

  2. Place patient in supine position.

  3. Provide reassurance.

  4. If other signs and symptoms are present, provide oxygen via nonrebreather mask.

  5. Assess vital signs.

  6. Consult with medical direction.

  7. Ongoing assessment

ENRICHMENT (OPTIONAL)

The following sections contain information that is valuable as background for the EMT, but that goes substantially beyond the U.S. Department of Transportation's EMT-Basic National Standard Curriculum

III. Types of seizures (pp. 519–522)

 A. Generalized tonic-clonic seizure (grand mal)—discussed above (p. 521)

 B. Simple partial seizure (p. 521)

  1. Jerky muscle activity in one part of the body

  2. Patient awake and aware

  3. May not require emergency care; check medical direction.

 C. Complex partial seizure (pp. 521–522)

  1. One- to 2-minute duration

  2. Patient has blank stare, seems dazed.

On the Net
Frequently asked questions about syncopal episodes. http://www.ninds.nih.gov/health_and_medical/disorders/syncope_doc.htm

Point to Emphasize
Maintaining an open airway is the priority in patients suffering from a seizure. After a seizure has stopped, suction the patient and administer supplemental oxygen.

3. Patient does not respond to commands or show personality change.
4. Reassure patient, protect him or her, check with medical direction.

D. Absence (petit mal) seizure (p. 522)
1. Most common in children
2. Blank stare, blinking, chewing motion, lack of attention
3. No emergency care needed; recommend medical evaluation.

E. Febrile seizure (p. 522)
1. Most common in infants and children
2. Caused by high fever
3. Short in duration
4. May not require emergency care, but assume such seizures are serious.

CASE STUDY FOLLOW-UP

Ask a student volunteer to read the Case Study that begins on page 511 of the textbook. You may wish to use the following questions to engage students in a discussion of the Case Study Follow-up that begins on page 522 of the textbook. Provide missing information and clarify ideas as needed.

Q1. How does Firefighter Demarco protect the patient while she is seizing?

A1. *Firefighter Demarco cradles her head to protect it from striking the hard floor and maintains an airway with a jaw thrust.*

Q2. According to the patient's sister, what is the usual seizure pattern of the patient?

A2. *Carmen gets an unusual taste in her mouth, then goes unconscious, seizes for usually less than 5 minutes, and then becomes very tired and weak.*

Q3. How does Carmen feel after the seizure?

A3. *Like she just did aerobics for 3 hours. She feels totally exhausted, like sleeping. She also feels embarrassed.*

Q4. What steps should be taken when Carmen refuses transport?

A4. *Check with medical direction and have Carmen and her sister, as witness, sign the refusal of treatment form.*

IN REVIEW

Assess students' ability to apply what they have just learned by discussing the Review Questions on page 524 in the textbook.

Q1. Explain why the airway is frequently compromised in the actively seizing or postictal patient.

A1. *The airway is frequently compromised in postictal or actively seizing patients due to their altered mental status, which is frequently associated with airway obstruction due to secretions, blood, vomitus, or the patient's inability to keep the tongue from blocking the airway. (pp. 513–514)*

Q2. List pertinent questions to ask the seizure patient, relatives, or bystanders during the SAMPLE history.

A2. *Questions to ask during the SAMPLE history include the following:*

- *Was the patient awake during the seizures?*
- *Was the muscle activity a twitching or jerking motion? Isolated to one part of the body or generalized?*
- *When did the seizure start? How long did it last?*
- *Did the patient experience an aura before the seizure?*
- *Did the patient hit his head or fall? Bite his tongue or mouth? Lose bowel or bladder control?*
- *Is there any recent history of fever, headache, or stiff neck?*
- *Is the patient allergic to any medications?*
- *What medications does the patient take? Did the patient take his seizure medication as prescribed?*
- *Does the patient have a history of epilepsy, previous seizures, diabetes, stroke, or heart disease?*
- *When was the last time the patient suffered a seizure?*
- *Was this a typical type of seizure for him to suffer?*
- *When did the patient last have something to eat or drink?*
- *What was the patient doing immediately prior to the seizure activity? (p. 515)*

Q3. Name the five stages of a generalized tonic-clonic seizure and the signs and symptoms associated with each one.

A3. *The five stages of a generalized tonic-clonic seizure and their signs and symptoms are the following:*

- *Aura (sensory experience that warns of a seizure, such as a feeling, an odor, a sound, a taste, or a visual experience)*
- *Tonic phase (becomes unresponsive, falls to ground, muscle rigidity)*
- *Hypertonic phase (extreme muscular rigidity with hyperextension of the back)*
- *Clonic phase (convulsions, possible loss of bowel or bladder control)*
- *Postictal phase (return of awareness, exhaustion, possible headache or weakness to one side, gradual recovery) (pp. 516–517)*

Q4. Describe the emergency care steps recommended for treating a generalized seizure.

A4. *Emergency care steps for a generalized seizure are the following:*

- *Place patient in lateral recumbent (recovery) position.*
- *Maintain a patent airway (if status epilepticus, positive pressure ventilations with supplemental oxygen).*
- *Suction.*
- *Assist breathing (oxygen at 15 liters per minute by nonrebreather mask or positive pressure ventilations with supplemental oxygen as appropriate).*
- *Prevent injury to the patient during seizure.*
- *Maintain oxygen therapy.*
- *Transport. (p. 517)*

Q5. Define status epilepticus and describe how you would care for a patient who is in status epilepticus.

A5. *Status epilepticus is seizures that last more than 10 minutes or occur consecutively without an intervening period of responsiveness. It is a dire emergency requiring aggressive airway management, positive-pressure ventilation with supplemental oxygen, and immediate transport. (p. 513)*

Q6. List the common conditions or injuries that may cause seizures.

A6. *Common conditions or injuries that may cause seizures include high fever, infections, poisoning, hypoglycemia, hyperglycemia, head trauma, shock, hypoxia, stroke, drug or alcohol withdrawal, dysrhythmias, hypertension, and complications of pregnancy. Seizures may also be idiopathic (cause unknown). (pp. 511–512)*

Q7. Define and describe syncope and explain how you can distinguish it from a seizure.

A7. *Syncope is fainting, a sudden and temporary loss of consciousness. It differs from seizure in the following ways: Syncope usually occurs when the patient is standing up; the patient remembers feeling faint; recovery is rapid; the skin may be pale and moist. (pp. 517, 519)*

CRITICAL THINKING

Assess students' ability to respond to real-life emergency situations by discussing the Critical Thinking questions on page 524 in the textbook.

Q1. How would you manage the airway in this patient?

A1. *Open the patient's mouth, immediately suction until it is clear, and establish an airway using a jaw-thrust technique; consider inserting a nasopharyngeal or oropharyngeal airway. If the teeth are clenched shut, insert a nasopharyngeal airway. If the mouth is open or the jaw is flaccid, insert an oropharngeal airway.*

Q2. Would spinal injury management be a consideration?

A2. *Since the mechanism of this patient's injury could have also caused a spinal injury, the care of this patient should include appropriate spinal immobilization techniques. This may be somewhat difficult to perform with an actively seizing patient.*

Q3. What type of seizure do you suspect the patient is experiencing?

A3. *Based on the situation presented, the EMTs should suspect a reactive, also known as a secondary, generalized tonic-clonic seizure.*

Q4. What do you suspect as the cause of the seizure?

A4. *The trauma to the patient's head and subsequent brain injury is the most likely cause of the seizure activity.*

Q5. What emergency care would you provide for the patient?

A5. *The EMT should establish initial manual in-line stabilization of the spine, open and secure the patient's airway, suction the blood and vomitus, provide positive pressure ventilation with supplemental oxygen connected to the ventilation device, perform a rapid trauma assessment, and manage any other life-threatening injuries. The EMTs* *should then secure the patient using appropriate spinal immobilization equipment and begin immediate transport.*

PRACTICE SCENARIO

Give students the opportunity to apply what they have learned to a real-life situation encountered by EMS personnel by conducting a role play. Ask for two volunteers to play the role of EMTs who are responding to a 9-1-1 call and one volunteer to be the patient.

Begin with the two EMTs. Take them outside the classroom and provide them with a complete jump kit containing BSI equipment, oral glucose, a tongue depressor, and refusal form; oxygen equipment; a portable suction unit; and a stretcher. Then describe the following scenario to them:

It is evening rush hour in the city. You are dispatched to a "person having a fit" at a subway station. You should respond appropriately to what you find there. The emphasis of the scene is on dealing with altered mental status. However, you should utilize all the skills you have learned to date. We will call you to the scene in just a minute. When you return to the classroom, describe the following scenario to the patient and the rest of the class:

It is evening rush hour in the city. You are a 30-year-old professional with epilepsy. Unfortunately, you were so busy today that you forgot to take your Dilantin®. You were in the subway waiting to take the train home. Suddenly, you saw strange colors, which is what you always experience before you have a seizure. You have a brief seizure, which you, of course, do not remember. You hit your head on the subway platform when the seizure started. When you come to, the EMTs are with you. You are disoriented at first. You are very embarrassed. You gradually become more oriented. There is a small bruise on your forehead that hurts a little bit. Resist their offer to take you to the hospital, but you may change your mind if they are persuasive enough. Provide the patient with an epilepsy medical identification device and apply moulage to simulate a contusion on the forehead. Tell the patient to take his or her place and to start acting. Call the EMTs back into the classroom.

Allow the role play to progress naturally. Intervene only if the players seem to be at a loss for what to do. End the play when the EMTs have prepared the patient for transport to the ambulance or have obtained a signed refusal form.

With the entire class, discuss the following questions:

- What did the EMTs do well?
- What, if anything, should they have done differently?

ASSIGNMENTS

Assign students to read Chapter 18, "Allergic Reaction and Anaphylaxis," before the next class. Also ask them to complete Chapter 17 of the Workbook.

EVALUATION

Chapter Quiz Distribute copies of the Chapter Quiz provided in Handout 17-2 to evaluate student understanding of this chapter. Remind students not to refer to their textbooks or notes while taking the quiz.

Reading/Reference
Textbook, pp. 525–546

Workbook
Chapter 17 Activities

Chapter Quiz
Handout 17-2

TestGen
Chapter 17 Test

Online Test Preparation
Send your students to
http://www.prenhall.com/
EMTAchieve

Handouts 17-3 to 17-5
Reinforcement Activities

**Brady Skills Series
EMT-B Videos/CD**
Visual Reinforcement

**PowerPoint
Presentation**
Chapter 17

Student CD
Chapter 17

Companion Website
http://www.prenhall.com/
mistovich

Test Manager You may wish to create a custom-tailored test using Prentice Hall *TestGen for Prehospital Emergency Care, Eighth Edition* to evaluate student understanding of this chapter.

Online Test Preparation (for students and instructors) Additional test preparation is available through *EMT Achieve: Basic Test Preparation* at http://www.prenhall.com/EMTAchieve. Instructors can also monitor student mastery online.

REINFORCEMENT

Handouts If classroom discussions or performance on the quiz indicates that some students have not fully mastered the chapter content, you may wish to assign some or all of the Reinforcement Handouts for this chapter.

TECH EXTRAS

Brady Skills Series EMT-B Videos/CD Have your students watch the skills come to life on either VHS or CD-ROM.

PowerPoint Presentation (for instructors) The PowerPoint material developed for this chapter offers useful reinforcement of chapter content.

Student CD A wide variety of material on this CD-ROM will reinforce and also expand student knowledge and skills.

Companion Website (for students) Additional review quizzes and links to EMS resources will contribute to further reinforcement of this chapter. Please visit http://www.prenhall.com/mistovich.

OBJECTIVES CHECKLIST

Cognitive	Date Mastered
* Explain the assessment and emergency care for a seizing patient.	
* Recognize the common signs and symptoms of a generalized seizure.	
* Recognize signs and symptoms of status epilepticus.	
* Identify various conditions that cause seizures.	
* Recognize the common signs and symptoms of syncope.	
* Differentiate between syncope and seizures.	

CHAPTER 17 QUIZ

Write the letter of the best answer in the space provided.

_____ 1. A sudden and temporary alteration in brain function caused by massive electrical discharge in a group of nerve cells in the brain is called
    A. a convulsion
    B. a seizure.
    C. postictal activity.
    D. dysrhythmias.

_____ 2. The chronic brain disorder that is characterized by recurrent seizures is called
    A. the aura.
    B. CVA.
    C. epilepsy.
    D. postictal activity.

_____ 3. All of the following are common causes of seizures *except*
    A. shock.
    B. hypoxia.
    C. infection.
    D. lactose.

_____ 4. The period following a seizure in which the patient may be unresponsive, extremely sleepy, weak, and disoriented is called the
    A. grand mal state.
    B. postictal state.
    C. tonic phase.
    D. clonic phase.

_____ 5. Many patients will tell the EMT that they knew they were going to seize because of the
    A. tonic phase.
    B. postictal state.
    C. clonic phase.
    D. aura.

_____ 6. The period of a seizure when the patient's muscles become contracted and tense with arching of the back is called the
    A. tonic phase.
    B. postictal state.
    C. clonic phase.
    D. aura.

_____ 7. The period of a seizure when muscles spasm and then relax, producing violent and jerky activity, is called the
    A. clonic phase.
    B. tonic phase
    C. aura
    D. postictal state

_____ 8. A life-threatening condition characterized by a patient's seizing for over 10 minutes or consecutive seizures without an intermittent period of consciousness is called
    A. a grand mal seizure.
    B. a convulsion.
    C. status epilepticus.
    D. epilepsy.

_____ 9. A sudden and temporary loss of consciousness is called
    A. epilepsy.
    B. a convulsion.
    C. syncope.
    D. seizure.

_____ 10. The type of seizure most common in children between 6 months and 6 years old that is caused by high fever is called a(n) _____ seizure.
    A. absence (petit mal)
    B. febrile
    C. grand mal
    D. complex partial

_____11. A type of seizure most common in children, which is characterized by a blank stare, lasting only a few seconds, and beginning and ending abruptly, is called a(n) _____ seizure.

    A. complex partial   **C.** Jacksonian

    B. focal sensory   **D.** absence (petit mal)

_____12. If a patient's seizures last longer than 10 minutes, the EMT should begin

    A. endotracheal intubation.   **C.** positive-pressure ventilations.

    B. CPR.   **D.** AED use.

_____13. All of the following are common medications used in the treatment of epilepsy _except_

    A. Dilantin®.   **C.** insulin.

    B. Mysoline®.   **D.** phenobarbital.

_____14. The term for weakness on one side of the body is

    A. aphasia.   **C.** hemiparalysis.

    B. dysphasia.   **D.** hemiparesis.

_____15. Usually, a postictal patient should be placed in the _____ position.

    A. Trendelenburg   **C.** lateral recumbent

    B. Fowler's   **D.** prone

IN THE FIELD

Review the following real-life situation. Then answer the questions that follow.

You and your partner are dispatched to the local mall for a man having a seizure. Upon your arrival, you are greeted by a mall security guard who reports that your patient was noted walking alone through the mall when he suddenly fell to the ground and began having a "convulsion." The guard tells you that the episode must have lasted about 6 or 7 minutes. Your patient is a male, approximately 30 years old, who is in a semi-sitting position next to a water fountain. He appears to be breathing adequately and is conscious, although a bit dazed.

1. What type of seizure did the security guard describe to you?

2. In what stage of the seizure is the patient upon your arrival? How long should this stage last?

3. What emergency care measures should you take with this patient?

4. What should you do if the patient states that this is normal for him and he doesn't want to go to the hospital?

CHAPTER 17 REVIEW

Write the word or words that best complete each sentence in the space provided.

1. A(n) _____ is a sudden and temporary alteration in brain function caused by massive electrical discharge in a group of nerve cells in the brain.

2. A common cause of seizures is _____, a chronic brain disorder characterized by recurrent seizures.

3. The _____ state follows the seizure and is the recovery period for the patient.

4. Seizure activity that is related to an injury or a medical condition may be an ominous sign of _____ _____ or even permanent brain damage.

5. You cannot force a patient to accept transport or treatment, but you do need to _____ the call.

6. If the patient is talking normally, it indicates a(n) _____ airway and _____ breathing.

7. A patient who suffers seizures that last more than 10 minutes or seizures that occur consecutively without a period of responsiveness between them is considered to be in _____ _____.

8. Perform a(n) _____ _____ if the patient is postictal and still has an altered mental status or if she does not have a past medical history of epilepsy or seizures.

9. The _____ serves as a warning that a seizure is going to begin and involves some type of sensory perception by the patient.

10. _____ is a sudden and temporary loss of consciousness.

11. The EMT should place the syncopal patient in the _____ position to allow for improved blood flow to the brain.

12. _____ seizures, caused by high fever, are most common in young children.

13. The EMT needs to be aware that medical conditions such as _____ _____ and _____ may be confused with a seizure or may produce a seizure.

14. A seizing patient's movements should be _____ rather than

_____ in order to prevent further injury.

15. The EMT should gather a(n) _____ history from the responsive seizure

patient, relatives, and/or bystanders.

SEIZURES AND SYNCOPE: LISTING

1. List five common causes of seizures.

2. List seven steps in the emergency medical care for a seizing patient.

3. List the stages or phases of a seizure.

4. List four steps of emergency medical care for a syncope patient.

LECTURE MASTER 17

Seizures and Syncope

Seizure
Scene Size-up

Initial Assessment

Focused History and Physical Exam

Emergency Medical Care

Ongoing Assessment

Syncope
Assessment and Care

Types of Seizures
Generalized Tonic-Clonic (Grand Mal)

Simple Partial Seizure

Complex Partial Seizure

Absence (Petit Mal) Seizure

Febrile Seizure

©2008 by Pearson Education, Inc.
Prehospital Emergency Care, 8th ed.

CHAPTER 17 ANSWER KEY

HANDOUT 17-2: Chapter 17 Quiz

1. B	**5.** D	**9.** C	**13.** C
2. C	**6.** A	**10.** B	**14.** D
3. D	**7.** A	**11.** D	**15.** C
4. B	**8.** C	**12.** C	

HANDOUT 17-3: In the Field

1. A generalized tonic-clonic seizure or grand mal seizure
2. Postictal state, 10–30 minutes
3. Position the patient in a lateral recumbent position, maintain oxygen therapy, transport.
4. You must contact medical direction (follow local protocol).

HANDOUT 17-4: Chapter 17 Review

1. seizure
2. epilepsy
3. postictal
4. brain injury
5. document
6. open, adequate
7. *status epilepticus*
8. rapid assessment
9. aura
10. Syncope
11. supine
12. Febrile
13. heart attack, stroke
14. guided, restrained
15. sample

HANDOUT 17-5: Seizures and Syncope: Listing

1. Any five: high fever; infection; poisoning; hypoglycemia; hyperglycemia; head injury; shock; hypoxia; stroke; drug or alcohol withdrawal; dysrhythmias; hypertension; pregnancy complications; idiopathic causes
2. Position the patient. Maintain a patent airway. Suction. Assist breathing. Prevent injury to the patient. Maintain oxygen therapy. Transport.
3. Aura; tonic phase; hypertonic phase; clonic phase; postictal state.
4. Conduct an initial assessment and focused history and physical exam. Place the patient in the supine position. Administer oxygen at 15 liters per minute via nonrebreather mask. Assess vital signs.

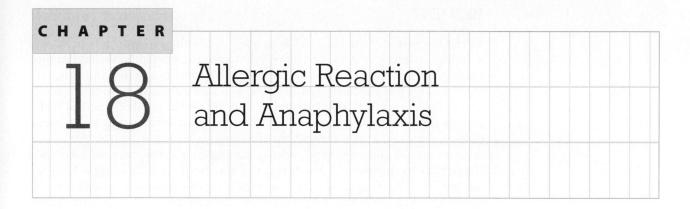

18 Allergic Reaction and Anaphylaxis

This chapter covers Lesson 4-5 and portions of Lesson 4-10 of the U.S. Department of Transportation's EMT-Basic National Standard Curriculum.

OBJECTIVES

Numbered objectives are from the U.S. Department of Transportation EMT-Basic National Standard Curriculum. Asterisked objectives, if any, pertain to material that is supplemental to the DOT curriculum. Page numbers in parentheses refer to pages in the textbook.

Cognitive

4-5.1 Recognize the patient experiencing an allergic reaction. (pp. 529–533)

4-5.2 Describe the emergency medical care of the patient with an allergic reaction. (pp. 533–543)

4-5.3 Establish the relationship between the patient with an allergic reaction and airway management. (pp. 530, 535, 536)

4-5.4 Describe the mechanism of allergic response and implications for airway management. (pp. 526–529, 530, 535, 536)

4-5.5 State the generic and trade names, medication forms, dose, administration, action, and contraindications for the epinephrine auto-injector. (p. 542–543)

4-5.6 Evaluate the need for medical direction in the emergency medical care of the patient with an allergic reaction. (pp. 534, 542)

4-5.7 Differentiate between the general category of those patients having an allergic reaction and those patients having an allergic reaction and requiring immediate medical care, including immediate use of an epinephrine auto-injector. (pp. 526–533, 534)

Affective

4-5.8 Explain the rationale for administering epinephrine using an auto-injector. (pp. 536, 538)

Psychomotor

4-5.9 Demonstrate the emergency medical care of the patient experiencing an allergic reaction.

4-5.10 Demonstrate the use of an epinephrine auto-injector.

4-5.11 Demonstrate the assessment and documentation of the patient response to an epinephrine injection.

4-5.12 Demonstrate proper disposal of equipment.

4-5.13 Demonstrate completing a prehospital care report for patients with allergic emergencies.

Total Teaching Time
120 minutes

Resources Needed

- Scored Chapter 17 Quizzes
- Epinephrine auto-injector
- Complete jump kit containing BSI equipment
- Pediatric epinephrine auto-injector
- Oxygen equipment
- Portable suction unit
- Stretcher

Additional Resources

Larmon/Davis, *Basic Life Support Skills*

Elling, *EMT Achieve: Basic Test Preparation*

Limmer/Mistovich/O'Keefe, *Audio Lecture & Study Guide: EMT*

Mistovich/Kuvlesky, *SUCCESS! for the EMT, Second Edition*

REVIEW

In the last lesson, "Seizures and Syncope," students learned that a seizure is a sudden alteration in mental status that causes unusual behavior ranging from briefly staring into space to falling to the floor with gross muscle spasms. Many seizures are self-limiting and last only 2 to 3 minutes. Most often, the seizure will have stopped by the time EMS is called and the EMT arrives on the scene; emergency care will consist of assisting the patient during recovery and transporting him or her to the hospital. Although seizures can be quite dramatic and frightening to observe, they are often not dangerous in themselves. However, the seizing patient can injure him- or herself by falling or thrashing around, and the patient's airway can be compromised. Also, it is important for the EMT to recognize that some seizures are prolonged and are associated with life-threatening conditions or injuries. Prompt intervention for the prolonged seizure may be lifesaving. Distribute the scored quizzes from the last class. Go over each question on the quiz and handle any concerns students may have about the answers.

INTRODUCTION TO CHAPTER 18

Chapter 18, "Allergic Reaction and Anaphylaxis," is the seventh lesson of Module 4. Allergic reactions can occur at any time and to anyone. A wide variety of substances can produce such reactions. Foods, medications, insect stings—even exercise—are common causes. An allergic reaction may be as mild as a runny nose or small skin rash or so severe that the airway closes and blood pressure becomes dangerously low. Point out to students that as EMTs their ability to recognize promptly and to manage effectively a severe allergic reaction in a patient may prevent deterioration in the patient's condition and even save the life of the patient.

Distribute the Chapter 18 Objectives Checklist and give students a few minutes to look it over. Then briefly paraphrase the objectives for this lesson in your own words.

LECTURE

The following suggested lecture outline is based on the Department of Transportation's EMT-Basic National Standard Curriculum. In some places, the DOT curriculum has been rearranged or expanded upon so that it is more complete or easier for the student to understand. The page numbers in parentheses refer to pages in the textbook. The parenthetical references in dark, heavy type are to figures, tables, and scans in the textbook.

ALLERGIC REACTION

I. Allergic reaction (pp. 526–536)**(Figs. 18-3, 18-4, pp. 535–537)**
   A. Definition (pp. 526–527)
      1. Misdirected and excessive response by the immune system to a foreign substance or allergen
   B. Sensitization (pp. 527–528) **(Fig. 18-1, p. 528)**
   C. Anaphylactoid reaction (pp. 528–529)
   D. Possible causes (p. 529)
      1. Insect bites/stings
         a. Bees, wasps, etc.
      2. Food
         a. Nuts, crustaceans, peanuts, etc.

Handout 18-1
Chapter 18 Objectives Checklist

Lecture Master
You may wish to display Lecture Master 20 when presenting the lecture to the class.

Point of Interest
Anaphylaxis causes 100–500 deaths per year. These numbers are declining, however, due to better recognition and treatment.

Point of Interest
In 1992, British doctors at Oxford discovered that there is one "allergy" gene causing hay fever, asthma, and eczema. One in three people carry the gene, showing varying degrees of symptoms.

On the Net
Info on insect-sting allergies, signs and symptoms, and treatment. www.healthsquare.com

3. Plants

4. Medications **(Tables 18-1 and 18-2, p. 529)**

5. Others

E. Assessment findings may include (pp. 529–533) **(Fig. 18-2a, p. 531)**

  1. Skin

    a. Patient may state he or she has a warm tingling feeling in the face, mouth, chest, feet, and hands.

    b. Itching

    c. Hives **(Fig. 18-2b and 18-2c, p. 531)**

    d. Red skin (flushing)

    e. Swelling to face, neck, hands, feet, and/or tongue

  2. Respiratory system

    a. Patient may state he or she feels a tightness in the throat/chest.

    b. Cough

    c. Rapid breathing

    d. Labored breathing

    e. Noisy breathing

    f. Hoarseness (losing the voice)

    g. Stridor

    h. Wheezing (audible without stethoscope)

  3. Cardiac

    a. Increased heart rate

    b. Decreased blood pressure

  4. Generalized findings

    a. Itchy, watery eyes

    b. Headache

    c. Sense of impending doom

    d. Runny nose

  5. Decreasing mental status

  6. Assessment findings that reveal shock (hypoperfusion) or respiratory distress indicate the presence of a severe allergic reaction.

F. Relationship to airway management (p. 534)

  1. These patients may initially present with airway/respiratory compromise or airway/respiratory compromise may develop as the allergic reaction progresses.

  2. The airway should be managed according to the principles identified in the airway management lesson presented earlier. (See Chapter 7.)

G. Emergency medical care (pp. 533–536)

  1. Patient has come in contact with substance that caused past allergic reaction and complains of respiratory distress or exhibits signs and symptoms of shock (hypoperfusion). **(Table 18-3, p. 534)**

    a. Perform initial assessment.

    b. Perform focused history and physical exam.

      (1) History of allergies?

      (2) What was patient exposed to?

      (3) How was patient exposed?

      (4) What effects?

      (5) Progression

      (6) Interventions

    c. Assess baseline vital signs and SAMPLE history.

    d. Administer oxygen if not already done in the initial assessment.

Point to Emphasize

For a patient to be in anaphylaxis, he or she must have either respiratory distress or signs and symptoms of shock (hypoperfusion).

Point to Emphasize

Most fatalities occur within the first 30 minutes following exposure to an allergen, so act quickly!

Point to Emphasize

Airway management is the top priority for patients with a severe allergic reaction. Apply oxygen at 15 lpm. If the patient is not breathing adequately, provide artificial ventilations.

e. Determine if patient has prescribed preloaded epinephrine available. Facilitate administration of preloaded epinephrine.

    f. Contact medical direction.

    g. Record and reassess in 2 minutes.

    h. Record reassessment findings.

    i. If patient does not have epinephrine auto-injector available, transport immediately.

2. Patient has contact with substance that causes allergic reaction without signs of respiratory distress or shock (hypoperfusion).

    a. Continue with focused assessment.

    b. Patient not wheezing or without signs of respiratory compromise or hypotension should not receive epinephrine.

II. Medications (pp. 536–543)

  A. Epinephrine auto-injector (pp. 536–543) **(Fig. 18-5, p. 538; Fig. 18-8, pp. 542–543)**

    1. Medication name

      a. Generic

        (1) epinephrine

      b. Trade

        (1) Adrenalin®

    2. Indications—must meet the following three criteria:

      a. Patient exhibits the assessment findings of a severe allergic reaction including respiratory distress and/or shock.

      b. Medication is prescribed for this patient by a physician.

      c. Medical direction authorizes use for this patient.

    3. Contraindications

      a. None when used in a life-threatening situation

    4. Medication form

      a. Liquid administered via an automatically injectable needle and syringe system

    5. Dosage

      a. Adult

        (1) One adult auto-injector (0.3 mg)

      b. Infant and child

        (1) One infant/child auto-injector (0.15 mg)

    6. Administration **(Fig. 18-6, p. 539; Fig. 18-7, pp. 540–541)**

      a. Obtain order from medical direction, either on-line or off-line.

      b. Obtain patient's prescribed auto-injector. Ensure that:

        (1) Prescription is written for the patient experiencing allergic reactions.

        (2) Medication has not expired and is not discolored (if able to see).

      c. Remove safety cap from the auto-injector.

      d. Place tip of auto-injector against the patient's thigh.

        (1) Lateral portion of the thigh

        (2) Midway between the waist and the knee

      e. Push the injector firmly against the thigh until the injector activates.

      f. Hold the injector in place until the medication is injected.

      g. Record activity and time.

    h. Dispose of injector in biohazard container.
  7. Actions
    a. Dilates the bronchioles
    b. Constricts blood vessels
  8. Side effects
    a. Increased heart rate
    b. Pallor
    c. Chest pain
    d. Headache
    e. Nausea
    f. Vomiting
    g. Excitability, anxiousness
    h. Dizziness
  9. Reassessment strategies
    a. Transport
    b. Continue focused assessment of airway, breathing, and circulatory status
      (1) Patient condition continues to worsen.
        (a) Decreasing mental status
        (b) Increasing breathing difficulty
        (c) Decreasing blood pressure
        (d) Obtain medical direction
          i. Additional dose of epinephrine
        (e) Treat for shock (hypoperfusion)
        (f) Prepare to provide positive-pressure ventilation with supplemental oxygen
        (g) Prepare to initiate Basic Cardiac Life Support measures—CPR, AED.
      (2) Patient condition improves. Provide supportive care.
        (a) Continue oxygen therapy
        (b) Treat for shock (hypoperfusion), if necessary

CASE STUDY FOLLOW-UP

Ask a student volunteer to read the Case Study that begins on page 526 of the textbook. You may wish to use the following questions to engage students in a discussion of the Case Study Follow-up that begins on page 544 of the textbook. Provide missing information and clarify ideas as needed.

Q1. What does your initial assessment indicate about the patient?

A1. *The patient, who is dressed in jogging clothes, appears to be having difficulty breathing. There are redness and hives on his face and neck. The patient is alert and scratching his arms and legs. He responds to questions in one- or two-word phrases with gasps for breath in between. He states, "I—can't—breathe—and—I itch—all over." Stridor is evident as he inhales. Audible wheezes are heard on inhalation and exhalation. His breathing is labored at a rate of 28 per minute. The radial pulse is barely palpable and is estimated at a rate of approximately 130 per minute. The skin is dry and warm to the touch.*

Q2. How does John describe his pertinent past medical history?

A2. *He indicates that he is allergic to yellow-jacket stings. He has a prescribed epinephrine auto-injector in a "fanny pack" around his waist. He suffered a similar reaction about 2 years ago, after which his family physician prescribed the auto-injector. His last reaction was so* *severe that he had to have an endotracheal tube and spent several days in the hospital. He states that the signs, symptoms, and intensity of this reaction are very similar to those of the last one.*

Q3. How does John describe the onset of this illness?

A3. *John states, "I was—jogging on the—trail—when I—felt a sting—in—my left leg. I—ran out of—the woods—to the road. I—felt my—throat—closing and I—began to itch badly." John estimates that it was about 3 minutes from the time of the sting to the onset of signs and symptoms of the reaction.*

Q4. How do you check the epinephrine auto-injector before and after you contact medical direction and receive permission to use it?

A4. *Before contacting medical direction, the epinephrine auto-injector is checked to ensure that it is John's and has not expired. When medical direction gives permission to use the auto-injector, the prescription and expiration date are rechecked and the injector is studied for discoloration or sediment.*

Q5. How does John respond to the epinephrine? What normal side effects does he experience?

A5. *His breathing is much less labored, and the wheezing significantly decreases. He feels much better, although, as a normal side effect, he feels nervous and his heart is pounding hard.*

IN REVIEW

Assess students' ability to apply what they have just learned by discussing the Review Questions on page 546 in the textbook.

Q1. Explain the meaning of sensitization in relation to allergic reaction.

A1. *Sensitization is the process by which antibodies are produced to seek out and destroy a foreign substance or antigen. These antibodies cause allergic reaction with later exposures to the substance. (For this reason, allergic reactions are not usually produced on first exposure to a substance.) (pp. 527–528)*

Q2. List the four routes through which an allergen can be introduced into the body.

A2. *An allergen can be introduced into the body by injection, ingestion, inhalation, or contact. (p. 529)*

Q3. List the major categories of common causes of allergic reaction and give examples of each category.

A3. *Major categories of common causes of allergic reaction, with examples, are the following: (1) venom from bites or stings: wasps, hornets, yellow jackets, fire ants, deer flies, gnats, horseflies, mosquitoes, cockroaches, spiders, miller moths, snakes; (2) foods: peanuts, other nuts, milk, eggs, shellfish, whitefish, food additives, chocolate, cottonseed oil, berries; (3) plants: pollen from many plants, especially ragweed and grasses; (4) medications: penicillin, other antibiotics, local anesthetics, aspirin, seizure medications, muscle relaxants, nonsteroidal anti-inflammatory agents, vitamins, insulin, tetanus and diphtheria toxoids; (5) other substances: latex, glue; (6) exercise: especially likely to cause allergic reaction when certain foods have been ingested close to the time of exercise. (p. 529)*

Q4. Describe the airway complications that may occur in anaphylaxis and the appropriate management of them.

A4. *Airway complications that may occur in anaphylaxis and appropriate management are as follows: Swelling of the upper airway at the level of the larynx may threaten to close off the patient's air flow. Inserting an airway adjunct will not help relieve the obstruction since it is at the level of the larynx. It may be necessary to provide positive-pressure ventilation to force the air past the swollen upper airway. Tracheal intubation may be required. (pp. 530–531)*

Q5. List the common signs and symptoms of allergic reaction and anaphylaxis in relation to the following body systems/categories: skin, respiratory system, cardiovascular system, central nervous system, gastrointestinal system, genitourinary system, generalized signs and symptoms.

A5. *The common signs and symptoms of allergic reaction and anaphylaxis are the following:*

Skin: warm, tingling feeling in the face, mouth, chest, feet, and hands (early); intense itching, especially of hands and feet (hallmark symptom); hives (hallmark sign); red, flushed skin; swelling to the face, lips, neck, hands, feet, and tongue; cyanosis in severe cases.

Respiratory system: "lump in the throat"; tightness in the chest; high-pitched cough; tachypnea (increased breathing rate); labored, noisy breathing; hoarseness or impaired ability to talk; excessive amounts of mucus coughed up; partially or completely occluded airway; difficulty in breathing.

Cardiovascular system: tachycardia (increased heart rate); hypotension (decreased blood pressure); irregular pulse; absent radial pulse (severe shock).

Central nervous system: increased anxiety; unresponsiveness; disorientation; restlessness; seizures; headache.

Gastrointestinal system: nausea/vomiting; abdominal cramping; diarrhea; difficulty in swallowing; loss of bowel control.

Genitourinary system: urgency to urinate; cramping of the uterus.

Generalized signs/symptoms: itchy, watery eyes; runny or stuffy nose; sense of impending doom; complaints of "not feeling well"; general weakness or discomfort. (pp. 532–533)

Q6. Name the two key categories of signs and symptoms of a severe allergic reaction (anaphylaxis).

A6. *The two key categories of signs and symptoms of a severe allergic reaction (anaphylaxis) are: (1) respiratory compromise—airway occlusion; breathing difficulty or inadequate breathing with possible wheezing, stridor, or crowing; and (2) shock (hypoperfusion)—absent or weak pulses; rapid heartbeat; decreased blood pressure; deteriorating mental status. (pp. 527–528)*

Q7. Describe the difference in emergency medical treatment for (a) a mild allergic reaction, and (b) a severe allergic reaction (anaphylaxis).

A7. *(a) The emergency medical care for a mild allergic reaction is to maintain an open airway, provide oxygen, and transport the patient as soon as possible. Monitor for progression to anaphylaxis. (b) The emergency medical care for a severe allergic reaction (anaphylaxis) is the following: (1) Maintain a patent airway. (2) Suction any* *secretions. (3) Maintain oxygen therapy. (4) Assist ventilations with positive pressure ventilation, if necessary. (5) Administer epinephrine by prescribed auto-injector on orders from medical direction. (6) Consider requesting ALS back-up. (7) Initiate early transport. (p. 536)*

Q8. List the indications and contraindications for the epinephrine auto-injector.

A8. *The indications for the epinephrine auto-injector are as follows (all of the following criteria must be met): The patient exhibits signs and symptoms of a severe allergic reaction (anaphylaxis), including respiratory distress and/or shock; the medication is prescribed to the patient; and there is an on-line or off-line order from medical direction for administration. Contraindications: none for a life-threatening allergic reaction. (p. 542)*

Q9. Describe the method of administration of the epinephrine auto-injector.

A9. *To administer the epinephrine by auto-injector, do the following: (1) Obtain an order from medical direction, either on-line or off-line. (2) Obtain the patient's prescribed auto-injector, making sure the prescription is written for the patient and has not expired, become discolored, or contain particulates or sediments. (3) Remove the safety cap. (4) Place the tip of the auto-injector against the lateral thigh midway between waist and knee. (5) Push the injector against the thigh until the spring-loaded needle is deployed and the medication is injected. (6) Hold the auto-injector in place until all of the medication has been injected. (7) Dispose of the auto-injector in a biohazard container. (8) Record that epinephrine was administered, the dose, and time of administration. (pp. 542–543)*

Q10. Describe the actions and possible side effects of the epinephrine auto-injector.

A10. *The actions of the epinephrine auto-injector are as follows: constricts blood vessels to improve blood pressure, reduces the leakage from the blood vessels, relaxes smooth muscle in the lungs, stimulates the heartbeat, and works to reverse swelling and hives. The possible side effects are increased heart rate, pale skin, dizziness, chest pain, headache, nausea and vomiting, excitability, and anxiousness. (p. 543)*

CRITICAL THINKING

Assess students' ability to respond to real-life emergency situations by discussing the Critical Thinking questions on page 546 in the textbook.

Q1. What is causing the airway compromise in the patient?

A1. *This patient's airway compromise is due to edema of the upper airway. The edema is a result of the released and circulating chemical mediators from MAST cells and basophils that cause the capillaries to become more permeable and leak.*

Q2. What is causing the respiratory distress?

A2. *The bronchioles are constricted (decreased in diameter) and the mucosal lining of the inside of the bronchiole swells. Both cause a reduction in the diameter of the airway, resulting in an increase in the*

©2008 by Pearson Education, Inc.
Prehospital Emergency Care, 8th ed.

*resistance. This makes it much more difficult for the patient to move
air through the bronchioles and into the alveoli, leading to poor gas
exchange and hypoxia.*

Q3. How would you manage the airway and ventilation?

A3. *The EMTs should open the airway using a head-tilt chin-lift maneuver
and begin assisting this patient's respirations with a BVM and 15 lpm
of supplemental oxygen connected to the BVM reservoir. Understand
that providing ventilations may be difficult due to the swelling of the
patient's airway. You may feel significant resistance when squeezing
the bag of the BVM due to the high airway resistance created by the
bronchoconstriction and mucosal swelling.*

Q4. What would explain the low blood pressure?

A4. *The circulating chemical mediators cause the vessels to dilate. This will
decrease the resistance in the vessel and result in a reduction in blood
pressure. Also, the capillaries are leaking, leading to volume loss. Both
combined will produce a decreased blood pressure and hypoperfusion.*

Q5. What emergency care would you provide to the patient?

A5. *Manage both the airway and breathing by providing positive pressure
ventilations with a BVM and supplemental oxygen, call for ALS
assistance, and immediately prepare for transport. If you carry an
epinephrine auto-injector on the ambulance, you should administer it
to the patient.*

Q6. What criteria would you use to determine the need for the
administration of epinephrine?

A6. *The patient's allergic reaction must be causing respiratory compromise
(respiratory distress, stridor, or wheezing) or shock (weak pulses,
decreasing mental status, or low blood pressure) before epinephrine
would be indicated.*

Q7. What are the side effects of epinephrine?

A7. *The side effects of epinephrine are increased heart rate; pale, cool,
clammy skin; dizziness; headache; palpitations; excitability and
anxiousness; chest pain; and nausea and vomiting.*

Q8. What type of reaction is the patient suffering from?

A8. *Based on the patient's presentation, vital signs, and oral intake history,
it can safely be assumed that the patient is suffering from a severe
allergic (anaphylactic) reaction. More specifically, since the patient
had a reaction to a medication on first time exposure and was not
sensitized, the patient experienced an anaphylactoid reaction.*

PRACTICE SCENARIO

Give students the opportunity to apply what they have learned to a real-life
situation encountered by EMS personnel.

Introduce the role play by reviewing with students the signs and
symptoms of an anaphylactic reaction. Also explore reasons that these
reactions are potentially more serious in a child than in an adult. Next,
explain to students that they are going to view a recreation of an allergic
emergency involving a child. Ask for four volunteers: two to play the role of

EMTs who are responding to a 9-1-1 call, one to be the housekeeper, and one to be the patient.

Begin by taking the two EMT players outside the classroom. Provide them with a complete jump kit containing BSI equipment, oxygen equipment, a pediatric epinephrine auto-injector, a portable suction unit, and a stretcher. Describe the following situation to them:

You are dispatched to a home in the suburbs. The dispatcher says that the patient is a child who is having trouble breathing. You should act appropriately on whatever conditions you find at the scene. The emphasis of the scene is on dealing with allergic reactions. However, you should utilize all the skills you have learned to date.

Tell them you will call them to the scene shortly.

When you return to the classroom, ask the housekeeper and the patient to come to the front of the classroom. Describe the following situation to them and the class:

It is early afternoon. After kindergarten, 5-year-old Roberta arrives home and is greeted by the housekeeper, Paul. After Roberta changes clothes, Paul allows her to play outside. Half an hour later Roberta runs back into the house, wailing and screaming that she has been stung by a bee. Paul scrapes the stinger from the child's skin as he learned to do in first-aid class and comforts Roberta. Strangely, she becomes too quiet. Paul observes that Roberta is drowsy and that she is having trouble breathing. As far as Paul knows, Roberta is healthy, takes no medicines, and has no allergies. He is concerned that something might be wrong with the child, so rather than take her to her pediatrician, Dr. Jones, he quickly calls 9-1-1.

Be sure that the patient and housekeeper understand what they are to do. Then, have them take their places and begin acting. Call the EMTs back into the classroom. Allow the role play to progress naturally. Provide appropriate vital signs and other objective information about the patient if the EMTs assess this information. Intervene only if the players seem to be at a loss for what to do. End the play when the EMTs have prepared the patient for transport to the ambulance.

With the entire class, discuss the following questions:

- What did the EMTs do well?

- What, if anything, should they have done differently?

ASSIGNMENTS

Assign students to read Chapter 19, "Poisoning Emergencies," before the next class. Also ask them to complete Chapter 18 of the Workbook.

EVALUATION

Chapter Quiz Distribute copies of the Chapter Quiz provided in Handout 18-2 to evaluate student understanding of this chapter. Remind students not to refer to their textbooks or notes while taking the quiz.

Test Manager You may wish to create a custom-tailored test using Prentice Hall *TestGen for Prehospital Emergency Care, Eighth Edition* to evaluate student understanding of this chapter.

Online Test Preparation (for students and instructors) Additional test preparation is available through *EMT Achieve: Basic Test Preparation* at

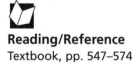

Reading/Reference
Textbook, pp. 547–574

Workbook
Chapter 18 Activities

Chapter Quiz
Handout 18-2

TestGen
Chapter 18 Test

http://www.prenhall.com/EMTAchieve. Instructors can also monitor student mastery online.

REINFORCEMENT

Handouts If classroom discussions or performance on the quiz indicates that some students have not fully mastered the chapter content, you may wish to assign some or all of the Reinforcement Handouts for this chapter.

TECH EXTRAS

Brady Skills Series EMT-B Videos/CD Have your students watch the skills come to life on either VHS or CD-ROM.

PowerPoint Presentation (for instructors) The PowerPoint material developed for this chapter offers useful reinforcement of chapter content.

Student CD A wide variety of material on this CD-ROM will reinforce and also expand student knowledge and skills.

Companion Website (for students) Additional review quizzes and links to EMS resources will contribute to further reinforcement of this chapter. Please visit http://www.prenhall.com/mistovich.

Online Test Preparation
Send your students to
http://www.prenhall.com/
EMTAchieve

Handouts 18-3 to 18-7
Reinforcement Activities

**Brady Skills Series
EMT-B Videos/CD**
Visual Reinforcement

**PowerPoint
Presentation**
Chapter 18

Student CD
Chapter 18

Companion Website
http://www.prenhall.com/
mistovich

OBJECTIVES

OBJECTIVES CHECKLIST

Cognitive		Date Mastered
4-5.1	Recognize the patient experiencing an allergic reaction.	
4-5.2	Describe the emergency medical care of the patient with an allergic reaction.	
4-5.3	Establish the relationship between the patient with an allergic reaction and airway management.	
4-5.4	Describe the mechanism of allergic response and implications for airway management.	
4-5.5	State the generic and trade names, medication forms, dose, administration, action, and contraindications for the epinephrine auto-injector.	
4-5.6	Evaluate the need for medical direction in the emergency medical care of the patient with an allergic reaction.	
4-5.7	Differentiate between the general category of those patients having an allergic reaction and those patients having an allergic reaction and requiring immediate medical care, including immediate use of an epinephrine auto-injector.	

Affective		Date Mastered
4-5.8	Explain the rationale for administering epinephrine using an auto-injector.	

Psychomotor		Date Mastered
4-5.9	Demonstrate the emergency medical care of the patient experiencing an allergic reaction.	
4-5.10	Demonstrate the use of an epinephrine auto-injector.	
4-5.11	Demonstrate the assessment and documentation of the patient response to an epinephrine injection.	
4-5.12	Demonstrate proper disposal of equipment.	
4-5.13	Demonstrate completing a prehospital care report for patients with allergic emergencies.	

CHAPTER 18 QUIZ

Write the letter of the best answer in the space provided.

_____ **1.** A severe form of allergic reaction is called
    A. an allergen.   **C.** epinephrine.
    B. anaphylaxis.   **D.** an immune reaction.

_____ **2.** Harmless to most individuals, allergens are foreign substances that cause an abnormal immune system response known as
    A. mitosis.   **C.** an allergic reaction.
    B. hypotoxemia.   **D.** an immune response.

_____ **3.** An EMT who notices that his hands are red and itchy after a call may be experiencing an allergic reaction to
    A. latex gloves.   **C.** exercise.
    B. talcum powder.   **D.** heat exposure.

_____ **4.** Signs and symptoms of an allergic reaction include all of the following *except*
    A. itching.   **C.** decreased blood pressure.
    B. increased appetite.   **D.** watery eyes.

_____ **5.** A sign of a severe allergic reaction is
    A. runny nose.   **C.** mild edema.
    B. cyanosis.   **D.** malaise.

_____ **6.** The dose of epinephrine that should be given to an adult suffering severe allergic reaction is _____ mg.
    A. 0.3   **C.** 0.05
    B. 0.5   **D.** 0.15

_____ **7.** Epinephrine is most commonly administered as a(n)
    A. tablet.   **C.** prescribed inhaler.
    B. gel.   **D.** auto-injector.

_____ **8.** When administered as a medication, epinephrine will accomplish all of the following *except*
    A. constrict blood vessels.   **C.** relax the bronchioles.
    B. lower blood pressure.   **D.** stimulate the heartbeat.

_____ **9.** The dose of epinephrine that should be given to infants/children is _____ mg.
    A. 0.5   **C.** 0.15
    B. 0.3   **D.** 0.05

_____ **10.** If the patient's condition improves following the administration of epinephrine, you should
    A. perform ongoing assessment.   **C.** initiate CPR.
    B. administer a second dose.   **D.** connect the AED.

IN THE FIELD

Review the following real-life situations. Then answer the questions that follow.

The patient is an 8-year-old boy with a known history of allergies and asthma. His mother tells you that she administered his EpiPen® 5 minutes before your arrival. However, you believe that she gave it incorrectly. "He pulled away when I tried to give the shot," explains the mother. "I saw some of the medicine form a mist in the air."

You examine the arm where the mother says that she gave the injection, but find no puncture mark. The child's distress has worsened since your arrival, and he now seems barely conscious.

"I have three more EpiPens®," offers the mother.

1. What action(s) should you take at this time?

Your next patient is an unconscious construction worker named Fred. "He had barely started to work with some fiberglass insulation when he fainted," explains one of his coworkers.

You ask the coworkers more questions and find out that Fred was sneezing and coughing just before he fainted. They also noticed that he was using a handkerchief to wipe his watery eyes and runny nose. "He usually wears a respiratory mask on the job site," adds one of the coworkers, "but he forgot to bring it today."

Upon conducting a physical examination of the patient, you find a Medic Alert tag indicating that Fred has a number of allergies. His vital signs include a blood pressure of 70/42 and a weak pulse of 136. During your initial assessment, the foreman hands you an EpiPen® kit. "I found this in Fred's lunch box," he says. "Will it help?"

2. What action(s) should you take at this time?

©2008 by Pearson Education, Inc.
Prehospital Emergency Care, 8th ed.

CHAPTER 18 REVIEW

Write the word or words that best complete each sentence in the space provided.

1. An abnormal or excessive response of the body's immune system to a foreign material is called a(n) _____ _____.

2. Foreign substances recognized by the cells of the immune system and eventually destroyed by the body's response are called _____.

3. A severe form of an allergic reaction is called _____ _____.

4. Antibodies are proteins that search for the antigen, combine with it, and then help to destroy it in a process known as _____.

5. _____ from insect bites or stings, especially of wasps, hornets, yellow jackets, and fire ants, may cause an allergic reaction and anaphylaxis.

6. Red, itchy, possibly raised blotches on the skin are known as _____.

7. Management of the airway during anaphylaxis may require _____ _____, the placement of a tube in the trachea to facilitate breathing.

8. When administered as a medication, epinephrine will _____ blood vessels to improve the patient's _____ _____.

9. A spring-loaded needle and syringe with a single dose of epinephrine is known as a(n) _____-_____.

10. The correct dose of epinephrine for an adult is _____ mg; for a child, it is _____ mg.

REINFORCEMENT

ALLERGIC REACTIONS: TRUE OR FALSE

Indicate if the following statements are true or false by writing T or F in the space provided.

_____ 1. Generally, an individual must come into contact with an allergen more than once for an anaphylactic reaction to occur.

_____ 2. Antibodies are proteins that search for an antigen, combine with it, and destroy it.

_____ 3. After 15 to 20 minutes, a patient suffering an allergic reaction has little risk of slipping into anaphylactic shock.

_____ 4. During an allergic reaction, you can expect to discover a higher-than-average blood pressure.

_____ 5. Epinephrine auto-injectors may not be administered to unconscious patients.

_____ 6. Epinephrine has no contraindications when used in a life-threatening situation.

_____ 7. A possible side effect of epinephrine use is chest pain.

_____ 8. Some anaphylactic reactions require repeated doses of epinephrine before the allergic reaction stops.

_____ 9. The two key categories of signs and symptoms that specifically indicate anaphylaxis are respiratory compromise and shock.

_____ 10. A patient experiencing an allergic reaction with no signs of respiratory distress or shock should receive epinephrine.

REINFORCEMENT

RECOGNIZING SIGNS AND SYMPTOMS OF ANAPHYLAXIS

Place a check mark in front of the signs and symptoms commonly associated with anaphylaxis or anaphylactic shock.

_____ increased pulse

_____ constipation

_____ decreased respirations

_____ increased appetite

_____ vomiting

_____ altered mental status

_____ flushed skin

_____ absent radial and/or pedal pulses

_____ diarrhea

_____ decreased pulse

_____ increased respirations

_____ decreased blood pressure

_____ feeling of impending doom

_____ stridor

EPINEPHRINE AUTO-INJECTOR

Write in the missing information on the medication flash card below, and save the completed card for future reference.

Epinephrine Auto-Injector

Medication Names

  1. Generic _____

  2. Trade _____

Indications

  1. _____

  2. _____

  3. _____

Contraindications

_____

_____

Medication Form: _____

Dosage: _____

Actions

  1. _____

  2. _____

  3. _____

  4. _____

Side Effects

  1. _____

  2. _____

  3. _____

  4. _____

  5. _____

  6. _____

  7. _____

LECTURE MASTER 18

Allergic Reaction

Physiology of an Allergic Reaction
Causes of Allergic Reaction
Routes

Substances
Assessment and Care
Scene Size-Up

Initial Assessment

Focused History and Physical Exam

Emergency Medical Care

Ongoing Assessment
Epinephrine Auto-Injector

HANDOUT 18-2: Chapter 18 Quiz

1. B	**4.** B	**7.** D	**9.** C
2. C	**5.** B	**8.** B	**10.** A
3. A	**6.** A		

HANDOUT 18-3: In the Field

1. Sample response: Immediately establish contact with medical direction. Inform them of the situation and request permission to administer a second dose of the medication or to provide additional instructions. All remaining EpiPens® should be taken on the ambulance. It may be necessary to request an ALS intercept on this call.

2. Sample response: Complete all steps in the initial assessment. Ensure that a member of the EMT team is managing BVM ventilation or intubation if local protocols allow. Call for an ALS intercept or begin rapid transport as soon as possible. Because the patient is unconscious and in shock, he meets the criteria for use of epinephrine. Contact medical direction if required to do so. Make sure that the medication in the EpiPen® kit belongs to the patient, that it is not expired, and that it is clear and colorless. After using the auto-injector, dispose of it in the appropriate biohazard container. Record the time of administration and reassess vital signs.

HANDOUT 18-4: Chapter 18 Review

1. allergic reaction
2. allergens
3. anaphylactic shock
4. sensitization
5. Venom
6. hives
7. tracheal intubation
8. constrict, blood pressure
9. auto-injector
10. 0.3, 0.15

HANDOUT 18-5: Allergic Reactions: True or False

1. T	**4.** F	**7.** T	**9.** T
2. T	**5.** F	**8.** T	**10.** F
3. F	**6.** T		

HANDOUT 18-6: Recognizing Signs and Symptoms of Anaphylaxis

Check marks should appear before all of the following conditions: increased pulse; vomiting; altered mental status; flushed skin; absent radial and/or pedal pulses; diarrhea; increased respirations; decreased blood pressure; feeling of impending doom; stridor

HANDOUT 18-7: Epinephrine Auto-Injector (completion)

Medication Name:
1. Generic—epinephrine
2. Trade—Adrenalin® (EpiPen® and EpiPen Jr.® as auto-injectors)

Indications:
1. Patient exhibits signs and symptoms of anaphylaxis, including respiratory distress and/or shock.
2. Medication is prescribed to the patient.
3. EMT has received order approving use from medical direction, either on-line or off-line.

Contraindications:
None in a life-threatening situation

Medication Form:
Liquid drug in auto-injector

Dosage:
Adult (>66 lbs.)—0.3 mg. Infant and child (<66 lbs.)—0.15 mg.

Actions:
1. Constricts blood vessels to improve blood pressure
2. Reduces leakage from blood vessels
3. Relaxes smooth muscle in the bronchioles to improve breathing; stimulates heartbeat
4. Works to reverse swelling and hives

Side Effects:
1. Increased heart rate
2. Pallor
3. Dizziness
4. Chest pain
5. Headache
6. Nausea and vomiting
7. Excitability and anxiousness

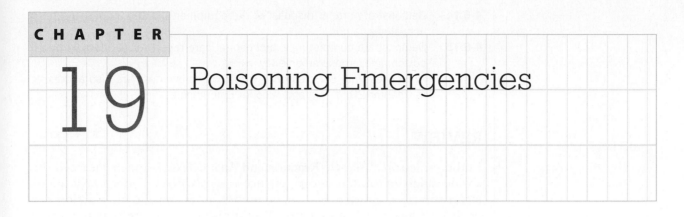

19 Poisoning Emergencies

This chapter covers portions of Lesson 4-6 and Lesson 4-10 of the U.S. Department of Transportation's EMT-Basic National Standard Curriculum.

OBJECTIVES

Numbered objectives are from the U.S. Department of Transportation EMT-Basic National Standard Curriculum. Asterisked objectives, if any, pertain to material that is supplemental to the DOT curriculum. Page numbers in parentheses refer to pages in the textbook.

Cognitive

4-6.1   List various ways that poisons enter the body. (p. 549)

4-6.2   List signs/symptoms associated with poisoning. (pp. 553, 559, 560–561, 562)

4-6.3   Discuss the emergency medical care for the patient with possible overdose. (pp. 553–555, 559, 561, 562–564)

4-6.4   Describe the steps in the emergency medical care for the patient with suspected poisoning. (pp. 553–555, 559, 561, 562–564)

4-6.5   Establish the relationship between the patient suffering from poisoning or overdose and airway management. (pp. 551–564, 568–571)

4-6.6   State the generic and trade names, indications, contraindications, medication form, dose, administration, actions, side effects, and re-assessment strategies for activated charcoal. (p. 556–557)

4-6.7   Recognize the need for medical direction in caring for the patient with poisoning or overdose. (pp. 551, 554, 555, 556, 562, 571)

Affective

4-6.8   Explain the rationale for administering activated charcoal. (p. 554–555)

4-6.9   Explain the rationale for contacting medical direction early in the prehospital management of the poisoning or overdose patient. (pp. 551, 554, 555, 556, 562, 571

Psychomotor

4-6.10   Demonstrate the steps in the emergency medical care for the patient with possible overdose.

4-6.11   Demonstrate the steps in the emergency medical care for the patient with suspected poisoning.

4-6.12   Perform the necessary steps required to provide a patient with activated charcoal.

4-6.13   Demonstrate the assessment and documentation of patient response.

Total Teaching Time
120 minutes

Resources Needed
- Scored Chapter 18 Quizzes
- Activated charcoal kit
- Complete jump kit containing BSI equipment and a patient refusal form
- Oxygen equipment
- Portable suction unit
- Stretcher
- Flour to simulate powdered insecticide

Additional Resources
Larmon/Davis, *Basic Life Support Skills*

Elling, *EMT Achieve: Basic Test Preparation*

Limmer/Mistovich/ O'Keefe, *Audio Lecture & Study Guide: EMT*

Mistovich/Kuvlesky, *SUCCESS! for the EMT, Second Edition*

4-6.14   Demonstrate proper disposal of the equipment for the administration of activated charcoal.

4-6.15   Demonstrate completing a prehospital care report for patients with a poisoning/overdose emergency.

Objectives from DOT lesson 4-6 relating to overdose are also addressed in Chapter 20, "Drug and Alcohol Emergencies."

REVIEW

In the last lesson, "Allergic Reaction and Anaphylaxis," students learned that a wide variety of substances can produce such reactions. Foods, medications, insect stings—even exercise—are common causes. An allergic reaction may be as mild as a runny nose or small skin rash or so severe that the airway closes and blood pressure becomes dangerously low. Because the reactions are often hard to predict and their consequences potentially life-threatening, it is important for the EMT to be prepared to recognize promptly and to manage effectively severe allergic reaction in a patient. Delay in emergency care can easily lead to deterioration in the patient's condition and even to death. Distribute the scored quizzes from the last class. Go over each question on the quiz and handle any concerns students may have about the answers.

INTRODUCTION TO CHAPTER 19

Chapter 19, "Poisoning Emergencies," is the eighth lesson of Module 4. Each year in the United States, thousands of people die or become extremely ill from suicidal or accidental poisoning. Most calls to poison control centers involve children, especially toddlers who get into and swallow poisonous substances while exploring their environment. Most poisonings occur at home and involve painkillers or other drugs, cleaning substances, and cosmetics. In addition, poisonings result from exposure to industrial chemicals, pesticides, and other substances encountered in the workplace or outdoor environment. When EMS is promptly called and the appropriate assessment, emergency care, and transport are provided, most cases of poisoning can have a successful outcome.

Distribute the Chapter 19 Objectives Checklist and give students a few minutes to look it over. Then briefly paraphrase the objectives for this lesson in your own words.

LECTURE

The following suggested lecture outline is based on the Department of Transportation's EMT-Basic National Standard Curriculum. In some places, the DOT curriculum has been rearranged or expanded upon so that it is more complete or easier for the student to understand. The page numbers in parentheses refer to pages in the textbook. The parenthetical references in dark, heavy type are to figures, tables, and scans in the textbook.

POISONING EMERGENCIES

I. Poisons and routes of exposure (pp. 548–551)
  A. Routes of exposure (pp. 548–551) **(Fig. 19-1, p. 550)**
    1. Ingestion
    2. Inhalation

Handout 19-1
Chapter 19 Objectives Checklist

● ➤

Lecture Master
You may wish to display Lecture Master 19 when presenting the lecture to the class.

Point to Emphasize
Like an astute detective, the EMT must use all senses (except taste) to gather information about poisonings from the scene.

©2008 by Pearson Education, Inc.
Prehospital Emergency Care, 8th ed.

    3. Injection

    4. Absorption

  B. Airway and breathing management (p. 551)

    1. No matter what poison or route, EMT should:

      a. Establish and/or maintain a patent airway.

      b. Determine whether breathing is adequate or inadequate.

      c. Provide positive-pressure ventilation for inadequate breathing or oxygen via nonrebreather for adequate breathing

    2. Poisoning patient can deteriorate quickly, so continuous ongoing assessment is necessary.

  C. Antidotes (p. 551)

    1. Definition

      a. Substance that can neutralize a poison or toxic substance or its effects.

    2. Available only for a small number of poisons.

    3. Treatment of a poisoning patient usually toward prevention of absorption and management of signs and symptoms.

II. Assessment and emergency care (pp. 551–565) **(Figs. 19-12, and 19-13, pp. 563–565)**

  A. Ingested poison (pp. 551–555)

    1. Important questions to ask:

      a. What substance?

      b. Was any alcohol ingested with the substance?

      c. When did patient ingest poison? or When was patient exposed to it?

      d. Over what time period?

      e. How much was ingested?

      f. What interventions were performed?

      g. Does patient have psychiatric history suggesting a possible suicide attempt?

      h. Does patient have an underlying illness, allergy, chronic drug use, or addiction?

      i. How much does the patient weigh?

    2. Signs and symptoms **(Fig.19-2, p. 553)**

      a. History of ingestion

      b. Swelling of mucous membranes of mouth

      c. Nausea, vomiting

      d. Diarrhea

      e. Altered mental status

      f. Abdominal pain, tenderness, distention

      g. Chemical burns or stains around mouth or throat **(Fig. 19-3, p. 554)**

      h. Painful swallowing

      i. Unusual breath or body odors

      j. Respiratory distress

      k. Altered heart rate

      l. Altered blood pressure

      m. Dilated or constricted pupils

      n. Warm and dry or cool and moist skin

    3. Emergency medical care

      a. Remove pills, tablets, or fragments with gloves from patient's mouth, as needed, without injuring oneself.

Teaching Tip

Ask students if they have ever encountered poisoning accidents. What was the substance? How did it enter the body? How did they determine what caused the poisoning? What did they do?

Teaching Tip

Contact the local Poison Control Center and request to have a representative speak to the class.

On the Net

For the American Association of Poison Control Centers, go to: www.aapcc.org

Point to Emphasize

With the millions of potential poisons available, it makes little sense to memorize those that require the use of activated charcoal. Instead, always consult with medical direction to determine whether the use of activated charcoal is appropriate.

On the Net

Great information about the signs and symptoms of various drugs and alcohol. Slang dictionary also quite helpful. http://www. addictions.org/signs.htm

b. Consult medical direction—activated charcoal. (**Fig. 19-4, p. 555**)

    c. Bring all containers, bottles, labels, etc., of poison agents to receiving facility.

4. Activated charcoal (**Fig. 19-5, pp. 556–557**)

    a. Medication name

        (1) Generic

            (a) Activated charcoal

        (2) Trade

            (a) SuperChar

            (b) InstaChar

            (c) Actidose

            (d) LiquiChar

            (e) Others

    b. Indications

        (1) Poisoning by mouth and orders from medical direction

    c. Contraindications

        (1) Altered mental status

        (2) Ingestion of acids or alkalies

        (3) Unable to swallow

        (4) Cyanide overdose

    d. Medication form

        (1) Premixed in water, frequently available in plastic bottle containing 12.5 grams activated charcoal

        (2) Powder should be avoided in field

    e. Dosage

        (1) Adults and children: 1 gram activated charcoal/kg of body weight

        (2) Usual adult dose: 30–100 grams

        (3) Usual infant/child dose: 12.5–25 grams

    f. Administration (**Fig. 19-6, p. 557**)

        (1) Obtain order from medical direction either on-line or off-line.

        (2) Container must be shaken thoroughly.

        (3) Since medication looks like mud, patient may need to be persuaded to drink it.

        (4) A covered container and a straw may improve patient compliance, since the patient cannot see the medication this way.

        (5) If patient takes a long time to drink the medication, the charcoal will settle and will need to be shaken or stirred again.

        (6) Record activity and time.

        (7) If patient vomits, ask medical direction to authorize one repeat of dose.

    g. Actions

        (1) Binds to certain poisons and prevents them from being absorbed into the body

        (2) Not all brands of activated charcoal are the same; some bind much more poison than others, so consult medical direction about the brand to use.

    h. Side effects

        (1) Black stools

        (2) Some patients, particularly those who have ingested poisons that cause nausea, may vomit.

       (3) If the patient vomits, the dose should be repeated once.
    i. Reassessment strategies
       (1) Be prepared for the patient to vomit or further deteriorate.
B. Inhaled poisons (pp. 555–559)
  1. Signs and symptoms
    a. History of inhalation of toxic substance
    b. Difficulty breathing
    c. Chest pain or tightness
    d. Cough, stridor, wheezing, crackles
    e. Hoarseness, oral or pharyngeal burns
    f. Dizziness
    g. Headache, often severe
    h. Confusion
    i. Seizures
    j. Altered mental status
    k. Cyanosis
    l. Respiratory rate faster or slower than normal
    m. Nausea, vomiting
    n. Paint on lips, indicating "huffing"
    o. Respiratory tract burns
       (1) Singed nasal hairs
       (2) Soot in sputum
       (3) Soot in throat
  2. Emergency medical care
    a. Have trained rescuers remove patient from poisonous environment. **(Fig. 19-7, p. 558)**
    b. Ensure an open airway and give oxygen if not already done in the initial assessment. **(Fig. 19-8, p. 559)**
    c. Bring all containers, bottles, labels, etc., of poison agents to receiving facility.
C. Toxic injection (pp. 559–561 and Chapter 20, "Drug and Alcohol Emergencies," and Chapter 22, "Environmental Emergencies") **(Fig. 19-9, p. 560)**
  1. Signs and symptoms
    a. Weakness, dizziness
    b. Chills, fever
    c. Nausea, vomiting
    d. High or low blood pressure
    e. Pupillary changes
    f. Needle tracks
    g. Pain at site of injection
    h. Trouble breathing
    i. Abnormal skin vitals
    j. Possible paralysis
    k. Swelling and redness at injection site
  2. Emergency medical care
    a. Airway and oxygen
    b. Be alert for vomiting
    c. Bring all containers, bottles, labels, etc., of poison agents to receiving facility
D. Absorbed poisons (pp. 561–562)
  1. Signs and symptoms
    a. History of exposure
    b. Liquid or powder on patient's skin

       c. Burns

       d. Itching and/or irritation

       e. Swelling

       f. Redness

    2. Emergency medical care

       a. Skin

         (1) Remove contaminated clothing while protecting oneself from contamination.

         (2) Powder

           (a) Brush powder off patient, then continue as for other absorbed poisons. **(Fig. 19-10, p. 562)**

         (3) Liquid

           (a) Irrigate with clean water for at least 20 minutes (and continue en route to facility, if possible).

       b. Eye

         (1) Irrigate with clean water away from affected eye for at least 20 minutes and continue en route to facility, if possible. **(Fig. 19-11, p. 562)**

ENRICHMENT (OPTIONAL)

The following sections contain information that is valuable as background for the EMT, but that goes substantially beyond the U.S. Department of Transportation's EMT-Basic National Standard Curriculum.

  III. **Common poisons** (pp. 566–571)

    A. Food poisoning (p. 566)

      1. General information

      2. Signs and symptoms

      3. Emergency medical care

    B. Carbon monoxide (pp. 566–567)

      1. General information

      2. Signs and symptoms

      3. Emergency medical care

    C. Cyanide (pp. 567–568)

      1. General information

      2. Signs and symptoms

      3. Emergency medical care

    D. Acids and alkalis (pp. 568–569)

      1. General information

      2. Signs and symptoms

      3. Emergency medical care

    E. Hydrocarbons (p. 569)

      1. General information

      2. Signs and symptoms

      3. Emergency medical care

    F. Methanol (wood alcohol) (pp. 569–570)

      1. General information

      2. Signs and symptoms

      3. Emergency medical care

    G. Isopropanol (isopropyl alcohol) (p. 570)

      1. General information

      2. Signs and symptoms

      3. Emergency medical care

H. Ethylene glycol (pp. 570–571)
    1. General information
        a. First Stage: Neuorological
        b. Second Stage: Cardiopulmonary
        c. Third Stage: Renal
    2. Signs and symptoms
    3. Emergency medical care
I. Poisonous plants (p. 571)
    1. General information
    2. Signs and symptoms
    3. Emergency medical care
IV. Poison control centers (p. 571)
    A. Can assist EMTs via toll-free telephone (p. 571)
    B. Check with medical direction before and after calling (p. 571)

CASE STUDY FOLLOW-UP

Ask a student volunteer to read the Case Study that begins on page 548 of the textbook. You may wish to use the following questions to engage students in a discussion of the Case Study Follow-up that begins on page 572 of the textbook. Provide missing information and clarify ideas as needed.

Q1. Why does your partner gather some of the leaves, stems, roots, and dirt at the scene?

A1. *They may provide information about Sophie's condition.*

Q2. Why do you sweep Sophie's mouth with your gloved hand?

A2. *To help ensure that Sophie's airway remains open as well as to find evidence of what she has taken into her mouth.*

Q3. What appears to be the poison ingested by Sophie?

A3. *Philodendron leaves and soil.*

Q4. What medication does the poison control center authorize? How do you administer it to Sophie?

A4. *The center calls for administration of activated charcoal with a dose of 1 gram/kg of activated charcoal, or 16 grams, since Sophie's weight is 35 pounds (16 kg). The activated charcoal is administered to Sophie in a plastic child's cup with a covered lid, and the dose and time of administration are noted.*

IN REVIEW

Assess students' ability to apply what they have just learned by discussing the Review Questions on page 573 in the textbook.

Q1. Explain why children are frequent victims of poisoning.

A1. *Children are frequent victims of poisoning because they get into things as they explore their environment. (p. 548)*

Q2. List the four ways poisons enter the body.

A2. *Poisons enter the body via ingestion, inhalation, injection, or absorption. (p. 549)*

Q3. Describe the relationship between poisoning and airway management.

A3. *Poisonings of all types may affect the patient's airway by causing damage or swelling of airway passages or by causing vomiting. (p. 551)*

Q4. Describe the main ways of determining if a poisoning has taken place.

A4. *The main ways of determining if a poisoning has taken place are through clues gathered from the environment (e.g., empty bottles, spilled chemicals, overturned plants) and from information provided by the patient or others at the scene. (The signs and symptoms of poisoning are similar to those for many other medical conditions.) (pp. 549–550)*

Q5. Describe the general emergency medical care steps for a poisoning or overdose patient.

A5. *The emergency medical care steps for a poisoning or overdose patient are as follows: Take BSI and safety precautions. Establish and maintain a patent airway; administer oxygen; be prepared to assist ventilations; position the patient (on left side if altered mental status; on spine board if spinal injury is suspected; otherwise in position of comfort); contact poison control center and/or medical direction for treatment; bring bottles, labels, plant parts, vomitus, or other evidence of the poisonous substance to the hospital; consider ALS; transport. (p. 551)*

Q6. Give the indications, contraindications, dosage, and administration steps for the administration of activated charcoal.

A6. *The indications for activated charcoal are as follows: a patient who has ingested poisons by mouth, upon orders from medical direction. Contraindications: patients who have an altered mental status, patients who have swallowed acids or alkalies, patients who are unable to swallow, patients with a cyanide overdose. Dosage: Unless directed otherwise by medical direction, give both adults and children 1 gram of activated charcoal per kilogram of body weight. The usual adult dose is 30–100 grams. The usual dose for infants and children is 12.5–25 grams. Administration: Obtain an order from medical direction, either on-line or off-line. Use a covered container and straw to improve patient compliance. Shake the container thoroughly before administering. If patient takes a long time to drink the medication, shake it again. Record the time and patient response. If the patient vomits, notify medical direction to authorize one repeat of the dose. (pp. 556–557)*

Q7. List the general emergency care steps for an ingested poison.

A7. *The emergency care steps for an ingested poison are as follows: (1) Ensure a patent airway. (2) Remove pills, tablets, or fragments with gloves from patient's mouth. (3) Administer oxygen or assist ventilations, if needed. (4) Prevent further injury. (5) Consult medical direction regarding administration of activated charcoal. (6) Bring all containers, bottles, labels, etc., of poison agents to receiving facility. (pp. 553–554)*

Q8. List the general emergency care steps for inhaled poisons.

A8. *The emergency care steps for inhaled poisons are as follows: (1) Have trained rescuers remove patient from poisonous environment and bring into fresh air. (2) Place patient in a supine position or position of comfort. (3) Ensure a patent airway and administer oxygen or begin* *ventilations with supplemental oxygen. (4) Bring all containers, bottles, labels, etc., of poison agents to receiving facility. (p. 559)*

Q9. List the general emergency care steps for injected poisons.

A9. *The emergency care steps for injected poisons are as follows: (1) Ensure a patent airway and administer oxygen or begin ventilations with supplemental oxygen. (2) Be alert for vomiting. (3) In cases of bites or stings, protect yourself from injury and the patient from repeated injection. (4) Bring all containers, bottles, labels, etc., of poison agents to receiving facility. (p. 561)*

Q10. List the general emergency care steps for absorbed poisons (a) to the skin and; (b) to the eye.

A10. *The emergency care steps for absorbed poisons are as follows: (a) To the skin: Remove contaminated clothing from patient while protecting yourself from contamination. Brush powder off patient if poison is dry. If liquid, irrigate with clean water for at least 20 minutes. Monitor airway and respiratory status and give oxygen and positive pressure ventilation, if necessary. (b) To the eye: Irrigate with clean water for at least 20 minutes and continue en route to facility, if possible. (p. 562)*

CRITICAL THINKING

Assess students' ability to respond to real-life emergency situations by discussing the Critical Thinking questions on page 574 in the textbook.

Q1. Why was it a good idea to allow the fire department to access the home first?

A1. *Fire department personnel are specifically trained and equipped for structure entries and subsequent safety evaluations; most ambulance personnel are not. The fire department has the proper personal protective equipment to make a safe entry and remove the patient. If you and your partner were to enter, both of you may have been overcome by the toxic fumes.*

Q2. What is the underlying mechanism for poisoning in this patient?

A2. *This patient was apparently poisoned by the fumes and carbon monoxide present in the home, which would have both been inhaled. Carbon monoxide interferes with the binding of oxygen on hemoglobin. This reduces the delivery of oxygen to the cells and makes the patient hypoxic.*

Q3. What is the single greatest intervention you could provide for this patient?

A3. *Since the etiology of the problem is with an inadequate amount of oxygen binding with hemoglobin, the most important treatment is to provide the highest concentration of oxygen possible. If the patient is breathing adequately, apply a nonrebreather mask at 15 lpm. If breathing is inadequate, it is necessary to provide positive pressure ventilation with supplement oxygen connected to the ventilation device delivering the highest possible concentration of oxygen.*

Q4. Given this type of poisoning, why is the pulse oximeter of little use?

A4. *The pulse oximeter reads the color of the hemoglobin in the blood. Red hemoglobin is attached with oxygen. Typically, a greater amount of red hemoglobin indicates better saturated hemoglobin with oxygen. Carbon* *monoxide, when attached to hemoglobin molecules, will cause the hemoglobin to turn bright red. The pulse oximeter reads the bright red hemoglobin as being saturated with oxygen; whereas it really has carbon monoxide attached. Carbon monoxide can not be used by the cells. The pulse oximeter provides a falsely high reading due to the extreme red color of the hemoglobin resulting from carbon monoxide attachment. The patient could have a SpO_2 reading of 100% and be severely hypoxic.*

Q5. What would be the basic tenets of care the patient should receive?

A5. *This patient should initially be moved at least 150 feet from the poisonous environment, receive positive pressure ventilations with high-concentration supplemental oxygen, and rapid transport to an appropriate facility.*

PRACTICE SCENARIO

Give students an opportunity to apply what they have learned to a real-life situation encountered by EMS personnel by enacting a role play. Ask two volunteers to play the role of EMTs who are responding to a 9-1-1 call, one volunteer to be a bystander, and one volunteer to be the patient.

Begin by taking the two EMT players outside the classroom. Provide them with a complete jump kit containing BSI equipment, oxygen equipment, a portable suction unit, and a stretcher. A patient refusal form should also be included in the jump kit. Then describe the following situation to them:

You are dispatched to a local farm. The dispatcher says that the patient is a farmhand who has poisoned himself with an insecticide. You should act appropriately on what you find there. The emphasis of the scene is on dealing with poisons. However, you should utilize all the skills you have learned to date. You will be called to the scene in just a minute. Return to the classroom and have the bystander and the patient come to the front of the classroom. Describe the following situation to them and the class:

Ted, a farmhand, accidentally spilled some powdered insecticide in the shed. He tried to clean it up before his boss, Mr. Murdoch, saw it. He used his hands. When he was almost done, Mr. Murdoch discovered him. Like always, Mr. Murdoch got upset—not because Ted spilled the insecticide, but because he used unsafe methods to clean it up. So Mr. Murdoch called 9-1-1. When the EMTs arrive, Ted insists that he has brushed off all the powder, feels fine, and doesn't want to go to the hospital. However, Ted may change his mind if the EMTs are persuasive enough.

Decide who will play each role. (Names may be changed depending on the gender of actors.) Dust the patient's hands and pants with a small amount of flour to simulate powdered insecticide. Next, direct the patient and the bystander to take their places and to start acting. Then, call the EMTs back into the classroom.

Allow the role play to progress naturally. Provide appropriate vital signs and other objective information about the patient if the EMTs assess this information. Intervene only if the players seem to be at a loss for what to do.

End the play when the EMTs have prepared the patient for transport to the ambulance or obtained a signed patient refusal form.

With the entire class, discuss the following:

■ What did the EMTs do well?

■ What, if anything, should they have done differently?

©2008 by Pearson Education, Inc.
Prehospital Emergency Care, 8th ed.

ASSIGNMENTS

Assign students to read Chapter 20, "Drug and Alcohol Emergencies," before the next class. Also ask them to complete Chapter 19 of the Workbook.

EVALUATION

Chapter Quiz Distribute copies of the Chapter Quiz provided in Handout 19-2 to evaluate student understanding of this chapter. Remind students not to refer to their textbooks or notes while taking the quiz.

Test Manager You may wish to create a custom-tailored test using Prentice Hall *TestGen for Prehospital Emergency Care, Eighth Edition* to evaluate student understanding of this chapter.

Online Test Preparation (for students and instructors) Additional test preparation is available through *EMT Achieve: Basic Test Preparation* at http://www.prenhall.com/EMTAchieve. Instructors can also monitor student mastery online.

REINFORCEMENT

Handouts If classroom discussions or performance on the quiz indicates that some students have not fully mastered the chapter content, you may wish to assign some or all of the Reinforcement Handouts for this chapter.

TECH EXTRAS

Brady Skills Series EMT-B Videos/CD Have your students watch the skills come to life on either VHS or CD-ROM.

PowerPoint Presentation (for instructors) The PowerPoint material developed for this chapter offers useful reinforcement of chapter content.

Student CD A wide variety of material on this CD-ROM will reinforce and also expand student knowledge and skills.

Companion Website (for students) Additional review quizzes and links to EMS resources will contribute to further reinforcement of this chapter. Please visit http://www.prenhall.com/mistovich.

Reading/Reference
Textbook, pp. 575–594

Workbook
Chapter 19 Activities

Chapter Quiz
Handout 19-2

TestGen
Chapter 19 Test

Online Test Preparation
Send your students to
http://www.prenhall.com/
EMTAchieve

Handouts 19-3 to 19-7
Reinforcement Activities

**Brady Skills Series
EMT-B Videos/CD**
Visual Reinforcement

**Powerpoint
Presentation**
Chapter 19

Student CD
Chapter 19

Companion Website
http://www.prenhall.com/
mistovich

OBJECTIVES

OBJECTIVES CHECKLIST

Cognitive		Date Mastered
4-6.1	List various ways that poisons enter the body.	
4-6.2	List signs/symptoms associated with poisoning.	
4-6.3	Discuss the emergency medical care for the patient with possible overdose.	
4-6.4	Describe the steps in the emergency medical care for the patient with suspected poisoning.	
4-6.5	Establish the relationship between the patient suffering from poisoning or overdose and airway management.	
4-6.6	State the generic and trade names, indications, contraindications, medication form, dose, administration, actions, side effects, and reassessment strategies for activated charcoal.	
4-6.7	Recognize the need for medical direction in caring for the patient with poisoning or overdose.	

Affective		Date Mastered
4-6.8	Explain the rationale for administering activated charcoal.	
4-6.9	Explain the rationale for contacting medical direction early in the prehospital management of the poisoning or overdose patient.	

Psychomotor		Date Mastered
4-6.10	Demonstrate the steps in the emergency medical care for the patient with possible overdose.	
4-6.11	Demonstrate the steps in the emergency medical care for the patient with suspected poisoning.	
4-6.12	Perform the necessary steps required to provide a patient with activated charcoal.	
4-6.13	Demonstrate the assessment and documentation of patient response.	
4-6.14	Demonstrate proper disposal of the equipment for the administration of activated charcoal.	
4-6.15	Demonstrate completing a prehospital care report for patients with a poisoning/overdose emergency.	

CHAPTER 19 QUIZ

Write the letter of the best answer in the space provided.

_____ **1.** Any substance—liquid, solid, or gas—that impairs health or causes death by its chemical action when it enters the body or comes into contact with the skin is called a(n)
   A. allergen.   **C.** antigen.
   B. poison.   **D.** caustic.

_____ **2.** The most common poisons ingested by children include all of the following *except*
   A. fertilizers.   **C.** cleaning products.
   B. plants.   **D.** toiletries.

_____ **3.** Carbon monoxide is an example of an _____ poison.
   A. ingested   **C.** absorbed
   B. inhaled   **D.** injected

_____ **4.** When treating an absorbed poisoning patient, if the poison is a liquid, you should irrigate all parts of the patient's body for at least _____ minutes.
   A. 5   **C.** 20
   B. 10   **D.** 45

_____ **5.** Use of activated charcoal is indicated in some cases of _____ poisoning.
   A. injected   **C.** absorbed
   B. inhaled   **D.** ingested

_____ **6.** Activated charcoal is administered in the form of a(n)
   A. tablet.   **C.** gel.
   B. suspension.   **D.** inhaler.

_____ **7.** All of the following are trade names for activated charcoal *except*
   A. SuperChar.   **C.** Liqui-Char.
   B. CharCoal.   **D.** Actidose.

_____ **8.** The usual dose of activated charcoal for an adult is
   A. 12.5–25 grams.
   B. 3 grams/kg of body weight.
   C. 30–100 grams.
   D. 10 grams/kg of body weight.

_____ **9.** In treating cases of inhaled poisons, the drug of first choice is
   A. activated charcoal.   **C.** glucose.
   B. syrup of ipecac.   **D.** oxygen.

_____ **10.** The most common sources of injected poisons are
   A. drugs.   **C.** plants.
   B. bites and stings.   **D.** over-the-counter medications.

IN THE FIELD

Read the following real-life situation. Then answer the questions that follow.

The emergency medical dispatcher sends you to a residence at 7290 Riverside. The young woman who placed the 9-1-1 call is waiting for you on the doorstep, even though the day is chilly.

The woman reports that she dropped by the house to visit her friend Randy Johnson and saw through the window that he was passed out on the couch. The door was unlocked, so she went in to try to wake him but couldn't. She tells you, "I wanted to stay and help him, but I just started feeling so bad. I felt sick to my stomach and my head hurt, almost like there was a band around it. Then I remembered that Randy had been having trouble with his furnace and was using a kerosene heater until he could get the furnace fixed. So I was afraid maybe something was wrong with the heater and came outside and called 9-1-1 from my cell phone. What's going on?"

1. Based on your scene size-up, what answer would you give the woman?

2. What action(s) would you take?

©2008 by Pearson Education, Inc.
Prehospital Emergency Care, 8th ed.

CHAPTER 19 REVIEW

Write the word or words that best complete each sentence in the space provided.

1. The ingestion of poisonous plants is an extremely common poisoning emergency, especially in

   _____.

2. Protect the ingested poison patient from aspiration by placing him or her, if possible, in the

   _____ _____ position.

3. In some cases of ingested poisoning, medical direction will order administration of

   _____ _____.

4. Unless directed otherwise by medical direction, give both adults and children

   _____ _____ of activated charcoal per

   _____ of body weight.

5. Activated charcoal absorbs poisons in the stomach, prevents their _____ by

   the body, and enhances their elimination from the body.

6. _____ _____ poisoning is the leading cause of

   death among people who inhale smoke from fires.

7. Any treatment recommended by the poison control center should be discussed with

   _____ _____ before it is administered to the

   patient.

8. If poison has been splashed into the eye, _____ the affected eye with clean

   water for at least _____ _____.

9. No matter what else is done regarding poisoning treatment, if the _____

   and _____ are not maintained, the patient will die.

POISONING: LISTING

1. List the four ways that poisons can enter the body.

2. List nine questions that should be asked during assessment of a patient with ingested poisoning.

3. List four contraindications for administration of activated charcoal.

4. List the emergency care steps for treating patients with inhaled poisoning.

©2008 by Pearson Education, Inc.
Prehospital Emergency Care, 8th ed.

POISONING: MATCHING

Write the letter of the type of poisoning next to the appropriate scenario below.

A. ingested poisoning
B. inhaled poisoning
C. absorbed poisoning
D. injected poisoning

_____ **1.** You are called to a suburban home to assist an 18-year-old male who has been found on the floor of his bathroom. He has a reduced pulse rate and reduced rate of breathing. His pupils are constricted to pinpoint size. He seems very sleepy and unresponsive. There is a constricting band tied around his upper arm. You find a hypodermic needle behind a clothes hamper.

_____ **2.** A 19-year-old male farm worker stumbles while carrying an open drum of pesticides. The powder spills all over his clothes and body. Within minutes, a stinging, burning sensation spreads across his hands, arms, neck, and face. "It's like being on fire," he tells another farm worker. "Get some help fast!"

_____ **3.** A 38-year-old woman collapses on the floor of her garage while cleaning out her car. She had left the car idling so that she could listen to her favorite radio station without running down the battery. By the time her husband discovers her, the woman is barely breathing. He rushes to call an EMS unit.

_____ **4.** A 45-year-old man in extreme pain from a recent back operation decides to double his self-administered dosage of Demerol. By the end of the day, he feels extremely lethargic and is sweating profusely. His pupils look pinpoint in size. Sensing trouble, his teenage son calls the nearest ambulance service.

ACTIVATED CHARCOAL

Write in the missing information on the medication flash card below, and save the completed card for future reference.

Activated Charcoal

Medication Names

  1. Generic: _____

  2. Trade: _____

Indications

_____

_____

_____

Contraindications

  1. _____

  2. _____

  3. _____

  4. _____

Medication Form: _____

Dosage: _____

Actions

_____

_____

Side Effects

  1. _____

  2. _____

©2008 by Pearson Education, Inc.
Prehospital Emergency Care, 8th ed.

LECTURE MASTER 19

Poisoning Emergencies

Poisons and Routes of Exposure

Managing the Poisoning Patient

Antidotes

Ingested Poisons

Assessment and Care

Activated Charcoal

Inhaled Poisons

Assessment and Care

Injected Poisons

Assessment and Care

Absorbed Poisons

Assessment and Care

Common Poisons

Poison Control Centers

HANDOUT 19-2: Chapter 19 Quiz

1. B	**4.** C	**7.** B	**9.** D
2. A	**5.** D	**8.** C	**10.** B
3. B	**6.** B		

HANDOUT 19-3: In the Field

1. Sample response: "It is likely that your friend may have been overcome by carbon monoxide fumes from the heater."
2. Sample response: If you are trained and have proper gear, enter the room to remove the patient. (If not, call medical direction for instructions and request a fire department rescue unit.) Remember that you have two patients, the woman and her friend. Prioritize treatment, with the advice of medical direction. After the unconscious patient has been removed, establish an open airway and administer oxygen at 15 liters per minute via nonrebreather mask or begin ventilations with supplemental oxygen. Also administer oxygen therapy to the woman. Provide transport to the hospital, paying particular attention to the patients' airways and breathing.

HANDOUT 19-4: Chapter 19 Review

1. children
2. lateral recumbent
3. activated charcoal
4. 1 gram, kg
5. absorption
6. Carbon monoxide
7. medical direction
8. irrigate, 20 minutes
9. airway, breathing

HANDOUT 19-5: Poisoning: Listing

1. Ingestion, inhalation, absorption, injection
2. Was any substance ingested? Was alcohol ingested with the substance? When did the patient ingest the poison? Over what time period was the substance ingested? How much of the substance was taken? Has anyone attempted to treat the poisoning? Does the patient have a psychiatric history that may suggest a possible suicide attempt? Does the patient have an underlying medical illness, allergy, chronic drug use, or addiction? How much does the patient weigh?

3. Altered mental status, ingestion of acids or alkalies, inability to swallow, cyanide overdose
4. Get the patient out of the toxic environment as quickly as possible. Place the patient in a supine position or position of comfort. As soon as possible, administer oxygen by nonrebreather mask. Start positive-pressure ventilation with supplemental oxygen immediately if the patient is not breathing or has inadequate breathing. Bring all containers, bottles, labels, or other clues about the poisoning agent to the receiving facility.

HANDOUT 19-6: Poisoning: Matching

1. D	**2.** C	**3.** B	**4.** A

HANDOUT 19-7: Activated Charcoal (completion)

Medication Name:
1. Generic: activated charcoal
2. Trade: SuperChar, InstaChar, Actidose, Actidose-Aqua, Liqui-Char, Charcoaid

Indications:
Upon orders from medical direction, administer to a patient who has ingested poisons by mouth.

Contraindications:
1. Patient has altered mental status.
2. Patient has swallowed acids or alkalies.
3. Patient is unable to swallow.
4. Patient has cyanide overdose.

Medication Form:
(1) Premixed powder in water, shaken into a suspension.
(2) Powder—to be avoided in field.

Dosage:
Usually 1 gram per kilogram of body weight for both adults and children.

Actions:
Absorbs poisons in the stomach; prevents absorption of poisons by the body; enhances elimination of poisons from the body

Side Effects:
1. Blackening of stools
2. Vomiting

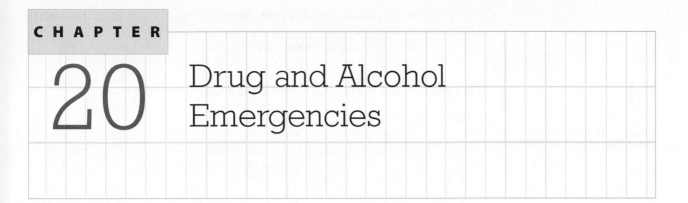

20 Drug and Alcohol Emergencies

This chapter covers portions of Lesson 4-6 and Lesson 4-10 of the U.S. Department of Transportation's EMT-Basic National Standard Curriculum.

OBJECTIVES

Numbered objectives are from the U.S. Department of Transportation EMT-Basic National Standard Curriculum. Asterisked objectives, if any, pertain to material that is supplemental to the DOT curriculum. Page numbers in parentheses refer to pages in the textbook.

Cognitive

4-6.3   Discuss emergency medical care for the patient with possible overdose. (pp. 582–583, 585)

    *   Describe the steps in the assessment of a drug or alcohol overdose patient. (pp. 577, 579–584)

    *   Explain how to determine if an emergency is drug or alcohol related. (pp. 577, 579–584)

    *   List six factors that may make a drug or alcohol emergency life-threatening. (pp. 579–580)

    *   Discuss the signs and symptoms that indicate a drug or alcohol emergency. (pp. 581–582)

    *   Discuss techniques for managing a violent drug or alcohol patient. (p. 583)

Psychomotor

4-4.10   Demonstrate the steps in the emergency medical care for the patient with possible overdose.

Additional objectives from DOT Lesson 4-4 are addressed in Chapter 19, "Poisoning Emergencies."

REVIEW

In the last lesson, "Poisoning Emergencies," students learned that thousands of people die or become extremely ill from suicidal or accidental poisoning. Most calls to poison control centers involve children, especially toddlers who get into and swallow poisonous substances while exploring their environment. Most poisonings occur at home and involve painkillers or other drugs, cleaning substances, and cosmetics. In addition, poisonings result from exposure to industrial chemicals, pesticides, and other substances encountered in the workplace or outdoor environment. When EMS is promptly called and the appropriate assessment, emergency care, and

Total Teaching Time
95 minutes

Resources Needed
- Scored Chapter 19 Quizzes
- Complete jump kit, including BSI equipment and a patient refusal form
- Oxygen equipment
- Portable suction unit
- Stretcher

Additional Resources
Larmon/Davis, *Basic Life Support Skills*

Elling, *EMT Achieve: Basic Test Preparation*

Limmer/Mistovich/ O'Keefe, *Audio Lecture & Study Guide: EMT*

Mistovich/Kuvlesky, *SUCCESS! for the EMT, Second Edition*

transport are provided, cases of poisoning can have a successful outcome. Distribute the scored quizzes from the last class. Go over each question on the quiz and handle any concerns students may have about the answers.

INTRODUCTION TO CHAPTER 20

Chapter 20, "Drug and Alcohol Emergencies," is the ninth chapter in Module 4. Drugs and alcohol are abused by a variety of people in a number of ways. In general, the emergency management steps learned in Chapter 19, "Poisoning Emergencies," are applicable to treating patients in most alcohol and drug emergencies. However, the EMT needs to be aware of special problems associated with drug or alcohol emergencies. For instance, it is likely that drug or alcohol overdose patients will have injured themselves, so they may have to be treated for trauma as well. Students should also be aware that patients under the influence of, or withdrawing from, alcohol or drugs can be difficult to manage, behaving in an aggressive or even violent manner and posing threats to the EMT's safety.

For the EMT, the primary concern in managing drug and alcohol emergencies will be to protect his or her own safety, maintain an open airway, treat for life-threatening conditions, and offer calm, nonjudgmental assistance.

Distribute the Chapter 20 Objectives Checklist and give students a few minutes to look it over. Then briefly paraphrase the objectives for this lesson in your own words.

LECTURE

The following suggested lecture outline is based on the Department of Transportation's EMT-Basic National Standard Curriculum. In some places, the DOT curriculum has been rearranged or expanded upon so that it is more complete or easier for the student to understand. The page numbers in parentheses refer to pages in the textbook. The parenthetical references in dark, heavy type are to figures, tables, and scans in the textbook.

DRUG AND ALCOHOL EMERGENCIES

I. Nature of drug and alcohol emergencies (pp. 576–577) **(Fig. 20-1, p. 576) (Table 20-1, pp. 578–579)**
    A. Overdose (p. 576)
    B. Withdrawal (p. 576)
II. Assessment and care (pp. 577–583) **(Fig. 20-4, pp. 584–585; Fig. 20-5, p. 586)**
    A. Scene size-up (p. 577)
        1. Potential for violence
        2. Need for BSI precautions
        3. Physical evidence of drug or alcohol abuse
    B. Initial assessment (pp. 579–580)
        1. Recheck mental status every 5 minutes.
        2. Focus on airway and breathing.
        3. Indications of life-threatening drug or alcohol emergency (high-priority patient) **(Fig. 20-2, p. 580)**
            a. Unresponsiveness
            b. Inadequate breathing
            c. Fever
            d. Abnormal heart rate (slow, fast, weak, irregular)

Handout 20-1
Chapter 20 Objectives Checklist

● ➤

Lecture Master
You may wish to display Lecture Master 20 when presenting the lecture to the class.

Point to Emphasize
Like an astute detective, the EMT must look for information in the area immediately around the patient (and in the patient's pockets) for evidence of drug or alcohol use (e.g., empty or partially filled pill bottles or boxes, syringes, empty liquor bottles, prescriptions, hospital discharge orders, or physician's notes) that might help to identify what drug the patient has taken.

☑

Teaching Tip
Ask students if they have ever encountered drug or alcohol overdoses. What was the substance? How did it enter the body? What did they do?

On the Net
For the American Association of Poison Control Centers, go to: www.aapcc.org

Point to Emphasize
In drug and alcohol emergencies, the goals are to identify and treat the loss of vital functions caused by the drug, not the specific effects of the drug itself.

©2008 by Pearson Education, Inc.
Prehospital Emergency Care, 8th ed.

  e. Vomiting with altered mental status

  f. Seizures

 C. Focused history and physical exam. (pp. 580–582)
  (Fig. 20-3, p. 581)

  1. Signs and symptoms

   a. Can vary widely

   b. Depends on abused substance

 D. Emergency medical care (pp. 582–583)

  1. Establish and maintain a patent airway; concurrently establish spinal stabilization if the patient is unresponsive or has suffered an injury.

  2. Administer oxygen at 15 liters per minute by nonrebreather mask or positive-pressure ventilation with supplemental oxygen, as needed.

  3. If the uninjured patient is unresponsive place in recovery position.

  4. Maintain proper body temperature.

  5. Assess blood glucose level.

  6. Restrain patient only if necessary.

 E. Ongoing assessment (pp. 582–583)

III. Managing a violent drug or alcohol patient (p. 583)

 A. Talk-down technique (not to be used with PCP users) (p. 583)

  1. Make the patient feel welcome.

  2. Identify yourself clearly. **(Fig. 20-6, p. 587)**

  3. Reassure the patient that his or her condition is caused by the drug and will not last forever.

  4. Help the patient verbalize what is happening to him or her.

  5. Reiterate simple and concrete statements.

  6. Forewarn the patient about what will happen as the drug begins to wear off.

  7. Once the patient has been calmed, transport.

ENRICHMENT (OPTIONAL)

The following sections contain information that is valuable as background for the EMT, but that goes substantially beyond the U.S. Department of Transportation's EMT-Basic National Standard Curriculum.

IV. Drug withdrawal (pp. 583, 587)

 A. Drug users develop tolerance, dependency. (p. 583)

 B. Withdrawal signs and symptoms usually peak at 48 to 72 hours after stopping drug use. (p. 587)

 C. May cause seizures or deterioration in patient's mental status (p. 587)

V. The alcoholic syndrome (pp. 587–589)

 A. Background (pp. 587–588) **(Fig. 20-7, p. 588)**

  1. Both problem drinking and true addiction

  2. Alcoholics prone to injuries or medical conditions brought on by drinking

 B. The withdrawal syndrome (pp. 583, 587–588) **(Fig. 20-8, p. 590)**

  1. Stage 1

   a. Within 8 hours

   b. Nausea, insomnia, sweating, tremors

  2. Stage 2

   a. Within 8 to 72 hours

   b. Worsening of Stage 1 symptoms plus hallucinations

Teaching Tip

If possible, obtain a tape of an actual situation in which a talk-down technique is used with a patient who is experiencing a "bad trip." Protect the identities of the individuals involved.

Reading/Reference

Guttenberg, M., & Aseda, G., "Under the Influence," *JEMS,* Aug. 2002.

On the Net

Behavior characteristics associated with substance abuse and links to individual substance information. http://www.addictions.org/signs.htm

Teaching Tip

Have a street drug expert address the class on different drugs in the area and paraphernalia associated with drug use.

Teaching Tip

Contact the local Alcoholics Anonymous and request to have a representative speak to the class.

Point to Emphasize

Before treating a victim suspected of cocaine intoxication, always take body substance isolation precautions to prevent the spread of Hepatitis B, HIV, and other infectious diseases.

    3. Stage 3
      a. Within 48 hours
      b. Major seizures
    4. Stage 4
      a. Delirium tremens
  C. Delirium tremens (p. 589)
    1. Severe confusion
    2. Loss of memory
    3. Tremors
    4. Restlessness and irritability
    5. Extremely high fever
    6. Dilated pupils
    7. Profuse sweating
    8. Insomnia
    9. Nausea and vomiting
    10. Diarrhea
    11. Hallucinations
    12. Tachycardia
VI. **Special considerations for PCP and cocaine** (pp. 589–591)
  A. PCP (p. 589)
  B. Cocaine (p. 589)
  C. Signs and symptoms of PCP or cocaine abuse (p. 591)
    1. Extreme agitation
    2. Involuntary eye movements
    3. Unresponsiveness to pain
    4. Severe muscular rigidity
    5. Excessive bronchial and oral secretions
    6. Hypertension
    7. Decreased urinary output
    8. Seizures
    9. Respiratory depression or arrest
    10. Vivid visual hallucinations
    11. Cardiac problems
    12. Aortic dissection
    13. Stroke or intracranial hemorrhage
    14. Severe headache
    15. Respiratory problems
    16. Neurological problems
    17. Psychiatric problems
  D. Emergency care
VII. **Huffing** (p. 591)
  A. Chemicals
  B. Paints
  C. Freon
  D. Gas propellants
  E. Glue
VIII. **Methamphetamines** (p. 592)

CASE STUDY FOLLOW-UP

Ask a student volunteer to read the Case Study that begins on page 576 of the textbook. You may wish to use the following questions to engage students in a discussion of the Case Study Follow-up that begins on page 592 of the textbook. Provide missing information and clarify ideas as needed.

Q1. Why do you consider the need for spinal immobilization of the patient?

A1. *Because the cut to the head indicates the possibility of trauma.*

Q2. What clue do you have that alcohol may be involved?

A2. *The smell of alcohol on the patient's breath.*

Q3. How is the patient prepared for extrication from his car?

A3. *By first applying a cervical spine immobilization collar and then immobilizing him to a KED vest for extrication to a long backboard.*

Q4. What care do you provide to Mr. Lynch en route to the emergency department?

A4. *Reassessment of his mental status, monitoring of vitals, preparation for vomiting, administration of oxygen with close monitoring of his airway, and provision of emotional support.*

IN REVIEW

Assess students' ability to apply what they have just learned by discussing the Review Questions on page 593 in the textbook.

Q1. Describe how you can determine whether a patient's condition is alcohol or drug related.

A1. *To determine whether a patient's condition is alcohol or drug related, (1) Note clues such as bottles or needles at the scene and, with a gloved hand, check the patient's mouth for signs of partially dissolved pills or tablets. (2) Smell the patient's breath for traces of alcohol. (3) Ask friends, family members, or bystanders what they know about the incident. (p. 577)*

Q2. Outline the special safety precautions you need to take for a drug or alcohol emergency.

A2. *Safety precautions for a drug or an alcohol emergency include scene size-up, calling for police backup, BSI precautions, leaving the patient an escape route, ensuring your own escape route, leaving the scene if you discover the patient is armed, keeping scissors and other equipment and supplies away from the patient's reach, and restraints, if necessary. (p. 577)*

Q3. List the six indicators that a drug or alcohol patient is a high priority for transport.

A3. *The six indicators that a drug or an alcohol patient is a high priority for transport are as follows: (1) unresponsiveness, (2) inadequate breathing, (3) fever, (4) abnormal heart rate (slow, fast, weak, or irregular), (5) vomiting with an altered mental status, and (6) seizures. (pp. 579–580)*

Q4. Explain why the signs and symptoms of alcohol- and drug-related emergencies vary so widely.

A4. *The signs and symptoms of alcohol- and drug-related emergencies vary so widely depending on the amount and kind of drug or mixture of drugs that were taken. (pp. 581–582)*

Q5. List the emergency care steps for an alcohol or drug emergency.

A5. *The emergency care steps for an alcohol or a drug emergency are as follows: (1) Establish and maintain a clear airway. (2) Administer oxygen and provide ventilations with supplemental oxygen as needed. (3) Position the patient. (4) Maintain proper body temperature. (5) Assess blood glucose level. (6) Restrain the patient only if necessary. (p. 582)*

CRITICAL THINKING

Assess students' ability to respond to real-life emergency situations by discussing the Critical Thinking questions on page 594 in the textbook.

Q1. What is the nature of illness surrounding this patient's complaints?

A1. *The nature of this patient's illness is poisoning. The specific type of poisoning is by inhalation.*

Q2. How is the chemical involved in this emergency gaining access to the bloodstream?

A2. *The chemicals that the patient was inhaling (or "huffing") are gaining access to his bloodstream through the alveolar/capillary exchange in the lungs.*

Q3. What could be some adverse physiological effects had the patient been able to engage in the activity longer?

A3. *Long-term or overdose "huffing" can result in memory loss, delirium, glazed eyes, slurred speech, drowsiness, swollen mucous membranes, hallucinations, confusion, unsteady gait, seizures, erratic heart beat, and even death.*

Q4. Describe the care necessary for this patient in order of priority.

A4. *For this patient the EMTs should initiate oxygen therapy with a nonrebreather mask and high-concentration oxygen, maintain the body temperature, and transport the patient to the appropriate facility.*

PRACTICE SCENARIO

Give students an opportunity to apply what they have learned to a real-life situation encountered by EMS personnel by performing a role play. Ask two volunteers to play the role of EMTs who are responding to a 9-1-1 call—one volunteer to be a friend and one volunteer to be the patient.

Begin by taking the two EMT players outside the classroom. Provide them with a complete jump kit containing BSI equipment, oxygen equipment, a portable suction unit, and a stretcher. A patient refusal form should also be included in the jump kit. Then describe the following situation to them:

You are dispatched to a residence in an affluent neighborhood. The dispatcher says that the patient is a 47-year-old woman who is experiencing a "bad trip" after mixing drugs and alcohol. When you arrive, you should respond appropriately to what you find at the scene. The emphasis of the scene is on managing a violent drug or alcohol patient. However, you should utilize all the skills you have learned to date. You will be called to the scene in just a minute.

Return to the classroom and have the bystander and the patient come to the front of the classroom. Describe the following situation to them and the class:

Lil, a 47-year-old computer whiz, recently lost her job. Lil is currently on medication for her depression, and she doesn't usually drink to excess. However, today she started drinking at 3:00 P.M. Jan, her friend and next door neighbor, came over about 5:15 P.M. after hearing a thud on the wall, followed by the sound of breaking glass and then sobbing. One wine bottle is broken on the floor; a second one—nearly empty—is on the cocktail table. When Jan suggests she take Lil to the hospital, Lil refuses. She says that she took a few extra pills, so she'll be fine in a little while. Afraid that Lil has seriously overdosed, Jan calls 9-1-1 from the bedroom phone. When the EMTs arrive, Lil is sobbing uncontrollably at the kitchen table. She insists that she is OK, and states that she doesn't want to go to the hospital. However, Lil may change her mind if the EMTs are able to convince her.

Decide who will play each role. (Names may be changed depending on the gender of actors.) Next, direct the patient and the friend to take their places and to start acting. Then, call the EMTs back into the classroom. Allow the role play to progress naturally. Intervene only if the players seem to be at a loss for what to do.

End the play when the EMTs have prepared the patient for transport to the ambulance or obtained a signed patient refusal form.

With the entire class, discuss the following:

- What did the EMTs do well?
- What, if anything, should they have done differently?

ASSIGNMENTS

Assign students to read Chapter 21, "Acute Abdominal Pain," before the next class. Also ask them to complete Chapter 20 of the Workbook.

EVALUATION

Chapter Quiz Distribute copies of the Chapter Quiz provided in Handout 20-2 to evaluate student understanding of this chapter. Remind students not to refer to their textbooks or notes while taking the quiz.

Test Manager You may wish to create a custom-tailored test using Prentice Hall *TestGen for Prehospital Emergency Care, Eighth Edition* to evaluate student understanding of this chapter.

Online Test Preparation (for students and instructors) Additional test preparation is available through *EMT Achieve: Basic Test Preparation* at http://www.prenhall.com/EMTAchieve. Instructors can also monitor student mastery online.

REINFORCEMENT

Handouts If classroom discussions or performance on the quiz indicates that some students have not fully mastered the chapter content, you may wish to assign some or all of the Reinforcement Handouts for this chapter.

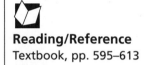

Reading/Reference
Textbook, pp. 595–613

Workbook
Chapter 20 Activities

Chapter Quiz
Handout 20-2

TestGen
Chapter 20 Test

Online Test Preparation
Send your students to http://www.prenhall.com/EMTAchieve

Handouts 20-3 to 20-6
Reinforcement Activities

Brady Skills Series EMT-B Videos/CD
Visual Reinforcement

PowerPoint Presentation
Chapter 20

Student CD
Chapter 20

Companion Website
http://www.prenhall.com/mistovich

TECH EXTRAS

Brady Skills Series EMT-B Videos/CD Have your students watch the skills come to life on either VHS or CD-ROM.

PowerPoint Presentation (for instructors) The PowerPoint material developed for this chapter offers useful reinforcement of chapter content.

Student CD A wide variety of material on this CD-ROM will reinforce and also expand student knowledge and skills.

Companion Website (for students) Additional review quizzes and links to EMS resources will contribute to further reinforcement of this chapter. Please visit http://www.prenhall.com/mistovich.

OBJECTIVES CHECKLIST

Cognitive	Date Mastered
4-6.3 Discuss the emergency medical care for the patient with possible overdose.	
* Describe the steps in the assessment of a drug or alcohol overdose patient.	
* Explain how to determine if an emergency is drug or alcohol related.	
* List six factors that may make a drug or alcohol emergency life-threatening.	
* Discuss the signs and symptoms that indicate a drug or alcohol emergency.	
* Discuss techniques for managing a violent drug or alcohol patient.	

Psychomotor	Date Mastered
4-4.10 Demonstrate the steps in the emergency medical care for the patient with possible overdose.	

CHAPTER 20 QUIZ

Write the letter of the best answer in the space provided.

_____ 1. The self-administration of drugs (or of a single dose) in a manner that is not in accord with approved medical or social patterns is called
     A. an overdose.   **C.** withdrawal.
     B. drug abuse.   **D.** dependence.

_____ 2. All of the following are examples of stimulants and appetite depressants *except*
     A. heroin.   **C.** methylphenidate.
     B. caffeine.   **D.** cocaine.

_____ 3. From the time it is ingested, alcohol is completely absorbed from the stomach and intestinal track within _____ hours.
     A. 4   **C.** 5
     B. 2   **D.** 3

_____ 4. All of the following are signs and symptoms of CNS stimulant abuse *except*
     A. bradycardia.   **C.** increased blood pressure.
     B. dilated pupils.   **D.** tachypnea.

_____ 5. The technique that can help reduce the patient's anxiety, panic, depression, or confusion is called
     A. CISD.   **C.** psychological supportive care.
     B. psychological assessment.   **D.** talk-down.

_____ 6. All of the following are common signs and symptoms of drug withdrawal *except*
     A. confusion.   **C.** profuse sweating.
     B. bradypnea.   **D.** abdominal cramping.

_____ 7. A common underlying psychiatric disorder associated with alcoholism is
     A. paranoia.   **C.** syncope.
     B. schizophrenia.   **D.** Wernicke-Korsakoff syndrome.

_____ 8. Alcohol withdrawal syndrome is characterized by all of the following signs and symptoms *except*
     A. insomnia.   **C.** hypoxia.
     B. seizures.   **D.** anorexia.

_____ 9. The last stage of alcohol withdrawal is a severe, life-threatening condition with a mortality rate of approximately 5–15 percent. It is called
     A. hallucinations.   **C.** insomnia.
     B. CNS depression.   **D.** delirium tremens.

_____ 10. One of the basic steps in the emergency care of the drug-, substance-, or alcohol-abuse patient is administration of
     A. oxygen.   **C.** insulin.
     B. epinephrine.   **D.** activated charcoal.

IN THE FIELD

Read the following real-life situation. Then answer the question that follows.

You are called to Charlie's Pub for a man acting "bizarrely." It is just after midnight, and you and your partners were sleeping at the time you were called out. En route, you ask dispatch if the police are either en route or already on-scene. The dispatcher informs you that they are en route with an ETA of 10 minutes.

When you arrive, you find a 35-year-old man sitting next to a parked truck. He states that he is "not hurt," but he cannot tell you the day, time, or even what month it is. Upon questioning, the bartender says that the man got to the bar about one hour before and only had a "couple of drinks."

The patient smells of alcohol and states, "I've had a couple of vodka tonics." Almost in the same breath, the patient takes out a knife and begins stabbing holes in the tire next to him, yelling, "Leave me alone or I'll kill everyone I see including myself!"

1. What action(s) should you take with this patient?

CHAPTER 20 REVIEW

Write the word or words that best complete each sentence in the space provided.

1. Alcohol is classified as a type of drug called a(n) _____

   _____ _____ depressant.

2. _____ are prone to a wide variety of illnesses ranging from cirrhosis of the

   liver to peritonitis.

3. CNS depressant drugs typically cause _____ pupils, while narcotics cause

   _____ pupils.

4. _____ are CNS depressants that are derived from opium (opiates) or

   synthetic (opioids).

5. Emergencies associated with hallucinogens and marijuana are usually more

   _____ than _____.

6. A habitual drug user may develop a(n) _____ to a drug, in which larger

   doses are required to produce the desired effects.

7. Physical or psychological _____ occurs when the patient experiences a

   strong need to use a drug repeatedly.

8. One of the most serious disorders associated with alcoholism is _____

   _____ syndrome, a chronic brain syndrome resulting from the toxic effect

   of alcohol on the central nervous system combined with malnutrition.

9. _____ _____ occurs after a period of abstinence

   from the drug or alcohol to which a person's body has become accustomed.

10. One of the most dangerous hallucinogens is _____, which is known as

    PCP and at least 46 other names.

©2008 by Pearson Education, Inc.
Prehospital Emergency Care, 8th ed.

DRUG AND ALCOHOL EMERGENCIES: LISTING

1. List five narcotic and opiate/opioid depressants that are commonly abused.

2. List six signs and symptoms that indicate a high-priority substance-abuse patient.

3. List five common signs and symptoms characteristic of the use of volatile inhalants.

4. List the five emergency care steps provided to the drug-, substance-, or alcohol-abuse patient.

5. List the seven steps of the talk-down technique.

DRUG AND ALCOHOL EMERGENCIES: TRUE OR FALSE

Indicate if the following statements are true or false by writing T or F in the space provided.

_____ **1.** A patient's withdrawal from alcohol or drugs is not as serious an emergency as an overdose.

_____ **2.** Cocaine is a common narcotic depressant.

_____ **3.** Amphetamines are examples of commonly abused stimulants and appetite depressants.

_____ **4.** Alcohol ingestion, even in smaller doses, is a major factor in drug overdoses, homicides, burns, and general trauma.

_____ **5.** The heart rate may be decreased or rapid and weak when CNS stimulants have been used.

_____ **6.** Hallucinogens are sometimes called psychedelic drugs.

_____ **7.** The talk-down technique can help reduce the anxiety of a patient known to have used PCP.

_____ **8.** Alcohol emergencies are usually related to alcoholic syndrome.

_____ **9.** Alcoholics often do not eat right, their health deteriorates, and they are more prone to illness.

_____ **10.** The first stage of alcohol withdrawal occurs within 48 hours and is characterized by major seizures.

LECTURE MASTER 20

Drug and Alcohol Emergencies

Definitions

Commonly Used Drugs

Assessment and Care

   Scene Size-up

   Initial Assessment

   Focused History and Physical Exam

   Common Signs and Symptoms of Substance Abuse

   Emergency Care

Managing a Violent Drug or Alcohol Patient

   The Talk-Down Technique

Enrichment

   Drug Withdrawal

   Alcoholic Syndrome

   Withdrawal Syndrome

   Special Considerations for PCP and Cocaine

HANDOUT 20–2: Chapter 20 Quiz

1. B	**4.** A	**7.** B	**9.** D
2. A	**5.** D	**8.** C	**10.** A
3. B	**6.** B		

HANDOUT 20–3: In the Field

1. This is a patient who has become both violent and suicidal. The key factor here is that all EMTs should wait for the police to arrive and then examine the patient after he has been subdued and restrained.

HANDOUT 20–4: Chapter 20 Review

1. central nervous system
2. Alcoholics
3. dilated, pinpoint
4. Narcotics
5. psychological, physical
6. tolerance
7. dependence
8. Wernicke-Korsakoff
9. Withdrawal syndrome
10. phencyclidine

HANDOUT 20–5: Drug and Alcohol Emergencies: Listing

1. Codeine, heroin, methadone, morphine, and opium
2. Unresponsiveness, inadequate breathing, abnormal heart rate, vomiting with an altered mental status, seizures, and fever
3. Any five of the following: excitement, euphoria, drunkenness, aggressiveness, depression, headache, drowsiness, nausea, swollen mucous membranes of the nose and mouth, glazed eyes, slurred speech, hallucinations, incoordination, erratic pulse and blood pressures, and seizures
4. Establish and maintain an airway. Administer oxygen. Position the patient to help protect the airway. Maintain the body temperature. Restrain the patient only if necessary.
5. Make the patient feel welcome. Identify yourself clearly. Reassure the patient that his or her condition is caused by the drug and will not last forever. Help the patient verbalize what is happening to him or her. Reiterate simple and concrete statements. Forewarn the patient about what will happen as the drug begins to wear off. Once the patient has been calmed, transport.

HANDOUT 20–6: Drug and Alcohol Emergencies: True or False

1. F	**4.** T	**7.** F	**9.** T
2. F	**5.** F	**8.** T	**10.** F
3. T	**6.** T		

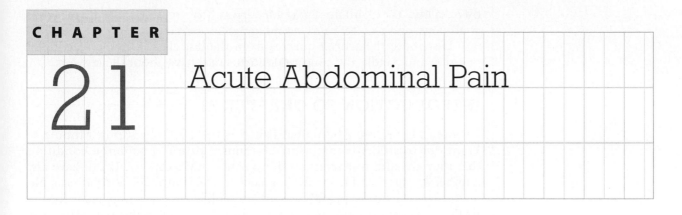

21 Acute Abdominal Pain

This chapter contains information that is valuable as background for the EMT but that goes substantially beyond the U.S. Department of Transportation's EMT-Basic National Standard curriculum.

OBJECTIVES

Numbered objectives are from the U.S. Department of Transportation's EMT-Basic National Standard Curriculum. Asterisked objectives, if any, pertain to material that is supplemental to the DOT curriculum. Page numbers refer to pages in the textbook.

Cognitive

* * Describe the structure and function of the organs contained within the abdominal cavity. (pp. 596–598)
* * Define the term acute abdomen. (p. 598)
* * Describe the assessment of a patient with acute abdominal pain. (pp. 601–605, 606, 607)
* * Describe the signs and symptoms of acute abdominal pain. (p. 605)
* * Discuss the appropriate emergency medical care for a patient with acute abdominal pain. (pp. 605–606, 607)
* * Discuss possible causes of acute abdominal pain. (pp. 607, 609–611)

Psychomotor

* * Demonstrate assessment and examination techniques used for acute abdominal pain.
* * Demonstrate appropriate emergency medical care for acute abdominal pain.

REVIEW

In the last lesson, "Drug and Alcohol Emergencies," students learned that drugs and alcohol are abused by a variety of people in a number of ways. In general, the emergency management steps learned in Chapter 19, "Poisoning Emergencies," are applicable to treating patients in most alcohol and drug emergencies. However, the EMT needs to be aware of special problems associated with drug and alcohol emergencies. For instance, it is likely that drug or alcohol overdose patients will have injured themselves, so they may need to be treated for trauma as well. Point out that patients under the influence of, or withdrawing from, alcohol or drugs can be difficult to manage, behaving in an aggressive or even violent manner, and posing threats to the safety of EMTs. Remind students that, as EMTs, their primary concern in managing drug and alcohol emergencies will be to protect their

Total Teaching Time
120 minutes

Resources Needed
* Scored Chapter 20 Quizzes
* Complete jump kit, including BSI equipment and a patient refusal form
* Oxygen equipment
* Portable suction unit
* Stretcher and blankets

Additional Resources
Larmon/Davis, *Basic Life Support Skills*

Elling, *EMT Achieve: Basic Test Preparation*

Limmer/Mistovich/O'Keefe, *Audio Lecture & Study Guide: EMT*

Mistovich/Kuvlesky, *SUCCESS! for the EMT, Second Edition*

own safety, to maintain an open airway, to treat for life-threatening conditions, and to offer calm, nonjudgmental assistance.

Distribute the scored quizzes from the last class. Go over each quiz question and handle any concerns students may have about the answers.

INTRODUCTION TO CHAPTER 21

Chapter 21, "Acute Abdominal Pain," is the 10th chapter in Module 4. Point out to students that acute abdominal pain is a common condition that they are sure to encounter during their EMS careers. It can have any number of causes and may often signal a very serious medical condition. No matter what the cause, in all cases of abdominal pain it is important for the EMT to assess for life-threatening conditions, to make the patient as comfortable as possible, to administer oxygen, and to get the patient to the hospital quickly.

Distribute the Chapter 21 Objectives Checklist, and give students a few minutes to look it over. Then briefly paraphrase the objectives for this lesson in your own words.

LECTURE

The following suggested lecture outline is based on the Department of Transportation's EMT-Basic National Standard Curriculum. In some places, the DOT curriculum has been rearranged or expanded upon so that it is more complete or easier for the student to understand. The page numbers in parentheses refer to pages in the textbook. The parenthetical references in dark, heavy type are to figures, tables, and scans in the textbook.

ACUTE ABDOMINAL PAIN

I. Abdominal structure and function (pp. 596–598)
  A. Site of vital organs for digestion and excretion (p. 596) **(Fig. 21-1, p. 597; Tables 21-1, p. 598 and 21-2, p. 599)**
  B. Reference points (pp. 597–598) **(Fig. 21-2, p. 597)**
    1. Left upper quadrant (LUQ)
    2. Right upper quadrant (RUQ)
    3. Right lower quadrant (RLQ)
    4. Left lower quadrant (LLQ)
II. Acute abdominal pain (pp. 598–601)
  A. Causes of abdominal pain (pp. 598–599)
  B. Types of abdominal pain (pp. 599–600) **(Fig. 21-3, p. 600)**
  C. Peritonitis (pp. 600–601) **(Fig. 21-4, p. 602)**
III. Assessment and care (pp. 601–607) **(Fig. 21-8, pp. 606–607; Fig. 21-9, p. 608)**
  A. Scene size-up (p. 601)
    1. Look for threats to you, patient, and other personnel.
    2. Take body substance isolation (BSI) precautions.
    3. Look for mechanism of injury to rule out trauma.
    4. Heed clues to patient's condition (type and smell of bleeding; location of patient).
  B. Initial assessment (pp. 601–602)
    1. Look for guarded position. **(Fig. 21-5, p. 603)**
    2. Ensure that patient has patent airway and adequate breathing.
    3. Be alert for vomiting and possible aspiration.
    4. Assess circulation.

Handout 21-1

Chapter 21 Objectives Checklist

On the Net

Assessing acute abdominal pain. www.physsportsmed .com/issues/1996/04_96/ bergman.htm

On the Net

Charts and basic descriptions to help assess abdominal pain. www. doctorupdate.net/du_ toolkit/s_sorters/s3.html

On the Net

Frequently asked questions about acute abdominal pain and its causes. www.vh.org/pediatric/ patient/pediatrics/cqqa/ abdominalpain.html

Lecture Master
You may wish to display Lecture Master 21 when presenting this lesson.

©2008 by Pearson Education, Inc.
Prehospital Emergency Care, 8th ed.

5. Look for signs of shock (hypoperfusion).
6. Categorize as a transport priority if patient meets any of the following criteria:
   a. Poor general appearance
   b. Unresponsive
   c. Responsive, not following commands
   d. Shock (hypoperfusion)
   e. Severe pain

C. Focused history and physical exam (pp. 602–605) **(Fig. 21-5, p. 604)**
1. Look for guarded position. **(Fig. 21-5, p. 603)**
2. Observe whether the patient is restless or quiet.
3. Inspect patient's abdomen.
4. Gently palpate each abdominal quadrant—quadrant with pain last.
5. Assess abdomen for softness, rigidity, tenderness, masses.
6. Ask patient if there is pain in other areas.
7. Document quadrant in which pain is located.
8. Markle test

D. Signs and symptoms (p. 605)
1. Pain or tenderness
2. Anxiety and fear
3. Guarded position
4. Rapid and shallow breathing
5. Rapid pulse
6. Blood pressure changes
7. Nausea, vomiting, and/or diarrhea
8. Rigid abdomen
9. Distended abdomen
10. Other signs and symptoms associated with shock
11. Signs of internal bleeding

E. Emergency medical care (pp. 605–606)
1. Keep the airway patent.
2. Place the patient in the position of comfort.
3. Administer oxygen at 15 liters per minute via a nonrebreather mask. **(Fig. 21-7, p. 605)**
4. Never give anything by mouth.
5. Calm and reassure the patient.
6. If signs and symptoms of hypoperfusion are present, treat for shock. (See Chapter 27, "Bleeding and Shock.")
7. Initiate a quick and efficient transport.

F. Ongoing assessment (p. 606)
1. Perform ongoing assessment during transport.
2. Document and record all vital signs.

IV. **Conditions that may cause acute abdominal pain** (pp. 606–607)
A. Appendicitis (p. 607)
1. Inflammation of the appendix
2. Common signs and symptoms of appendicitis
   a. Abdominal pain or cramping
   b. Nausea and vomiting
   c. Low-grade fever and chills
   d. Lack of appetite (anorexia)
   e. Abdominal guarding
B. Pancreatitis (pp. 607, 609)
1. Inflammation of the pancreas
2. Common signs and symptoms of pancreatitis
   a. Nausea and vomiting

Slides/Videos
Slide presentation related to abdominal pain in female patients. www.uphs.upenn.edu/fampract/Presentations/abpain/

Point to Emphasize
Definitive care for the patient with acute abdominal pain is hospitalization and, possibly, surgery. Never spend extended time at the scene trying to diagnose the patient.

Point to Emphasize
Never give a patient with acute abdominal pain anything by mouth.

b. Abdominal tenderness and distention

   c. Severe abdominal pain with radiation from the umbilicus (navel) to the back and shoulders

   d. Extreme cases will have fever, rapid pulse, and signs of shock.

C. Cholecystitis (p. 609)

   1. Inflammation of the gallbladder

   2. Common signs and symptoms of cholecystitis

   a. Sudden onset of abdominal pain located from middle of upper quadrants (epigastric area) to RUQ areas

   b. Pain present more commonly at night and associated with ingestion of fatty foods

   c. Tenderness upon palpation of RUQ

   d. Low-grade fever

   e. Nausea and vomiting (contents may be greenish)

D. Intestinal obstruction (p. 609)

   1. Blockage of the inside of the intestines

   2. Common signs and symptoms of intestinal obstruction

   a. Moderate to severe abdominal pain, depending on location of obstruction, generally described as crampy

   b. Nausea and vomiting

   c. Constipation (difficulty in moving bowels)

   d. Abdominal distention

E. Hernia (p. 609)

   1. Protrusion or thrusting forward of a portion of the intestine through an opening or weakness in the abdominal wall

   2. Common signs and symptoms of hernia

   a. Sudden onset of abdominal pain, usually after heavy lifting or straining

   b. Fever

   c. Rapid pulse

   d. Others similar to intestinal obstruction

F. Ulcer (p. 609)

   1. Open wound or sore within the digestive tract

   2. Common signs and symptoms of ulcer

   a. Sudden onset of abdominal pain in LUQ and epigastric area, usually described as a burning or gnawing type pain before meals or during stressful events

   b. Nausea and vomiting (in some cases may vomit blood)

   c. Signs and symptoms of shock in cases of massive bleeding

   d. Peritonitis with rigid abdomen in cases of perforation or bleeding

G. Esophageal varices (p. 610) **(Fig. 21-10, p. 610)**

   1. Bulging, engorgement, or weakening of the blood vessels of the lining of the lower esophagus

   2. Common signs and symptoms of esophageal varices

   a. Vomiting of large amounts of bright red blood

   b. Absence of pain or tenderness in abdomen

   c. Rapid pulse

   d. Breathing difficulty

   e. Pale, cool, clammy skin

   f. Other signs and symptoms of shock

   g. Yellowing (jaundice) of the skin or sclera of eyes due to liver disease

H. Abdominal aortic aneurysm (AAA) (pp. 610–611) **(Fig. 21-11, p. 610)**

    1. Weakened, ballooned, and enlarged area of the wall of the abdominal aorta

    2. Common signs and symptoms of AAA

        a. Gradual onset of lower lumbar and abdominal pain. Rupture associated with sudden onset of severe, constant, abdominal pain

        b. Pain

            (1) Usually described as a "tearing" pain

            (2) May radiate to lower back, flank, or pelvis.

        c. Possible nausea and vomiting

        d. Mottled or spotty abdominal skin

        e. Pale, cool, clammy, and possibly cyanotic skin in legs due to decreased blood supply and perfusion

        f. Absent or decreased femoral or pedal pulses

        g. If the abdomen is soft, a pulsating abdominal mass may be felt. If the aneurysm has burst, the abdomen will be rigid and tender.

I. Vomiting and diarrhea (p. 611)

CASE STUDY FOLLOW-UP

Ask a student to volunteer to read the Case Study that begins on page 596 of the textbook. You may wish to use the following questions to engage students in a discussion of the Case Study Follow-up that begins on page 611 of the textbook. Provide missing information and clarify ideas as needed.

Q1. What does the patient's mother tell you about the patient's condition when you arrive?

A1. *That her son Doug has had a fever for the last couple of days and that he woke up that morning saying his "stomach hurt real bad."*

Q2. During your initial assessment, in what position do you find Doug?

A2. *The boy is lying on his left side, curled up, and holding his stomach.*

Q3. During your focused history, what do you find out about Doug's abdominal pain?

A3. *The pain began this morning around 5 o'clock; nothing makes the pain better but laying flat makes it worse; the pain is a dull cramping and is located around the navel, radiating down to the RLQ; Doug says it is "the worst stomach pain" he has ever had; and it has been constant since early this morning.*

Q4. What does your physical exam of Doug reveal about his abdominal pain?

A4. *That his abdomen is soft but tender to palpation in the RLQ with some guarding.*

Q5. What diagnosis of Doug's condition is eventually made at the hospital?

A5. *Appendicitis.*

IN REVIEW

Assess students' ability to apply what they have learned by discussing the Review Questions on page 612 in the textbook.

Q1. List the organs contained within the abdominal cavity.

A1. *The organs contained within the abdominal cavity are stomach, duodenum, small intestine, large intestine, liver, gallbladder, spleen, pancreas, kidneys, bladder. (The kidneys are actually located behind the lining of the abdominal cavity.) (pp. 596–597)*

Q2. Using the umbilicus as a reference point, name the quadrants of the abdominal cavity and the organs you would expect to find in each quadrant.

A2. *The quadrants of the abdominal cavity and the organs in each are as follows: Left upper quadrant (LUQ) contains most of the stomach, the spleen, the pancreas, and part of the large intestine. The left kidney is behind the abdominal lining. Right upper quadrant (RUQ) contains most of the liver, the gallbladder, and part of the large intestine. The right kidney is behind the abdominal lining. Right lower quadrant (RLQ) contains the appendix and part of the large intestine. Left lower quadrant (LLQ) contains part of the large intestine. (p. 597)*

Q3. List the signs and symptoms of acute abdomen.

A3. *The signs and symptoms of acute abdomen are pain or tenderness; anxiety and fear; guarded position; rapid and shallow breathing; rapid pulse; low or high blood pressure; nausea, vomiting, diarrhea; rigid abdomen; distended abdomen; signs/symptoms of shock; signs of internal bleeding. (p. 605)*

Q4. List the factors that would make you consider a patient who is suffering abdominal pain as a priority for transport.

A4. *Factors for high transport priority are: poor general appearance; unresponsive; responsive, not following commands; shock (hypoperfusion); severe pain. (p. 602)*

Q5. Describe the general guidelines for conducting a physical examination of a patient with acute abdominal pain.

A5. *To conduct a physical examination of a patient with acute abdominal pain, do the following: Determine if the patient is restless or quiet and whether pain is increased upon movement; inspect the abdomen to determine if it is distended; gently palpate the abdominal quadrant, most painful area last; assess whether the abdomen feels soft or rigid: if rigid, determine if guarding is involuntary or voluntary; assess whether the abdomen is tender or nontender; note any masses; ask if there is pain in other body areas; document the quadrant in which any pain is located. (pp. 602–605)*

Q6. Outline the steps for emergency medical care of a patient with acute abdominal pain.

A6. *The steps for emergency medical care of a patient with acute abdominal pain are as follows: (1) Keep the airway patent. (2) Place the patient in a position of comfort. (3) Administer oxygen at 15 liters per minute via a nonrebreather mask. (4) Do not give anything by mouth. (5) Calm and reassure the patient. (6) Treat for shock if signs*

©2008 by Pearson Education, Inc.
Prehospital Emergency Care, 8th ed.

of hypoperfusion are present. (7) Initiate a quick and efficient transport. (pp. 605–606)

CRITICAL THINKING

Assess students' ability to respond to real-life emergency situations by discussing the Critical Thinking questions on page 613 in the textbook.

Q1. What emergency care would you provide during the initial assessment?

A1. *The respiratory rate and tidal volume are adequate; thus, the EMTs should initiate oxygen therapy with a nonrebreather mask and high-concentration oxygen.*

Q2. What assessment findings would lead you to suspect the patient is experiencing an acute abdomen?

A2. *The patient's complaint of severe abdominal pain, growing much more severe in the past several days, along with vomiting blood and having black, tarry stools are definite indications of acute abdominal distress.*

Q3. What are the vital signs indicating?

A3. *The patient's vital signs indicate that the patient is experiencing shock (hypoperfusion). The systolic blood pressure is decreased, the pulse pressure is narrow, the heart rate is elevated, and the skin is pale, cool, and clammy. Also, the patient is alert but sluggish to respond to commands.*

Q4. Based on the assessment findings and history information, what might the patient be suffering from?

A4. *This patient is most likely suffering from a perforated ulcer, which is bleeding into his stomach, digestive tract, and abdominal cavity (causing peritonitis).*

Q5. What is the significance of the bowel movement findings?

A5. *The black, tarry stools indicate bleeding in the patient's upper digestive tract.*

PRACTICE SCENARIO

Give students an opportunity to apply what they have learned to a real-life situation encountered by EMS personnel by performing a role play. Ask two volunteers to play the role of EMTs who are responding to a 9-1-1 call—one volunteer to be a store owner, and one volunteer to be the patient.

Begin by taking the two EMT players outside the classroom. Provide them with a complete jump kit containing BSI equipment, oxygen equipment, a portable suction unit, and a stretcher. A patient refusal form should also be included in the jump kit. Then describe the following situation to them:

You are dispatched to a small "mom-and-pop" store in a central city neighborhood at noon time. The dispatcher says that the patient is a woman in her 60s who is complaining of stomach pain. When you arrive, you should respond appropriately to what you find at the scene. You should utilize all the skills you have learned to date with the patient. You will be called to the scene in just a minute.

Return to the classroom and have the bystander and the patient come to the front of the classroom. Describe the following situation to them and the class:

Erica, a 63-year-old homeless woman, has been vomiting since early this morning. She now reports some stomach pain and is experiencing labored, heavy breathing. She also has a bruise on her forehead from a fall 2 days before. She has had a bad headache ever since. Just before the EMTs arrive, she vomits a large amount of bright red blood in the corner of the store. The storeowner knows Erica and is aware that she has a history of drinking heavily. The storeowner is the person who placed the call to 9-1-1.

Decide who will play each role. (Names may be changed depending on the gender of actors.) You may wish to use moulage to simulate the volunteer playing Erica to show a contusion on the forehead and coffee-ground-like emesis around the mouth. Next, direct the patient and the friend to take their places and to start acting. Then, call the EMTs back into the classroom.

Allow the role play to progress naturally. Intervene only if the players seem to be at a loss for what to do. Be prepared to supply the following assessment information: Breathing—10 breaths per minute; pulse—110; mental status—responsive, but increasingly disoriented; skin—pale, cool, diaphoretic; BP—60/40. The patient's neck veins are flat. Her abdomen is rigid and tender to palpation.

End the play when the EMTs have prepared the patient for transport to the ambulance.

With the entire class, discuss the following:

- What did the EMTs do well?
- What, if anything, should they have done differently?

ASSIGNMENTS

Assign students to read Chapter 22, "Environmental Emergencies," before the next class. Also ask them to complete Chapter 21 of the Workbook.

EVALUATION

Chapter Quiz Distribute copies of the Chapter Quiz provided in Handout 21-2 to evaluate student understanding of this chapter. Remind students not to refer to their textbooks or notes while taking the quiz.

Test Manager You may wish to create a custom-tailored test using Prentice Hall *TestGen for Prehospital Emergency Care, Eighth Edition* to evaluate student understanding of this chapter.

Online Test Preparation (for students and instructors) Additional test preparation is available through *EMT Achieve: Basic Test Preparation* at http://www.prenhall.com/EMTAchieve. Instructors can also monitor student mastery online.

REINFORCEMENT

Handouts If classroom discussions or performance on the quiz indicates that some students have not fully mastered the chapter content, you may wish to assign some or all of the Reinforcement Handouts for this chapter.

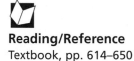

Reading/Reference
Textbook, pp. 614–650

Workbook
Chapter 21 Activities

Chapter Quiz
Handout 21-2

TestGen
Chapter 21 Test

Online Test Preparation
Send your students to http://www.prenhall.com/EMTAchieve

Handouts 21-3 to 21-6
Reinforcement Activities

TECH EXTRAS

Brady Skills Series EMT-B Videos/CD Have your students watch the skills come to life on either VHS or CD-ROM.

PowerPoint Presentation (for instructors) The PowerPoint material developed for this chapter offers useful reinforcement of chapter content.

Student CD A wide variety of material on this CD-ROM will reinforce and also expand student knowledge and skills.

Companion Website (for students) Additional review quizzes and links to EMS resources will contribute to further reinforcement of this chapter. Please visit http://www.prenhall.com/mistovich.

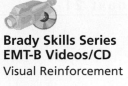

Brady Skills Series EMT-B Videos/CD
Visual Reinforcement

PowerPoint Presentation
Chapter 21

Student CD
Chapter 21

Companion Website
http://www.prenhall.com/mistovich

OBJECTIVES

OBJECTIVES CHECKLIST

Cognitive	Date Mastered
* Describe the structure and function of the organs contained within the abdominal cavity.	
* Define the term acute abdomen.	
* Describe the assessment of a patient with acute abdominal pain.	
* Describe the signs and symptoms of acute abdominal pain.	
* Discuss the appropriate emergency medical care for a patient with acute abdominal pain.	
* Discuss possible causes of acute abdominal pain.	

Psychomotor	Date Mastered
* Demonstrate assessment and examination techniques used for acute abdominal pain.	
* Demonstrate appropriate emergency medical care for acute abdominal pain.	

CHAPTER 21 QUIZ

Write the letter of the best answer in the space provided.

_____ 1. All of the following vital organs are located in the abdominal cavity *except* the
  A. stomach.   **C.** lungs.
  B. gallbladder.   **D.** abdominal aorta.

_____ 2. Pain that is felt in a body part removed from its point of origin is called _____ pain.
  A. referred   **C.** radiating
  B. ghost   **D.** provoked

_____ 3. In the abdominal cavity there is a pear-shaped sac that holds bile, which aids in the digestion of fats. It is called the
  A. duodenum.   **C.** pancreas.
  B. spleen.   **D.** gallbladder.

_____ 4. An abdominal wall muscle contraction that the patient cannot control, resulting from inflammation of the peritoneum, is called involuntary
  A. rigidity.   **C.** protecting.
  B. guarding.   **D.** posturing.

_____ 5. A protrusion or thrusting forward of a portion of the intestine through an opening or weakness in the abdominal wall is called
  A. appendicitis.   **C.** cholecystitis.
  B. ulceration.   **D.** hernia.

_____ 6. Sudden onset of severe, constant abdominal pain that may radiate to lower back, flank, or pelvis and is usually described as a "tearing" pain is a common symptom of a(n)
  A. abdominal aortic aneurysm. **C.** ulcer.
  B. appendicitis.   **D.** hernia.

_____ 7. The sac-like structure that acts as a reservoir for the urine received from the kidneys is the
  A. spleen.   **C.** liver.
  B. bladder.   **D.** pancreas.

_____ 8. One of the basic steps in emergency care of acute abdominal pain is
  A. giving the patient water.
  B. administration of oxygen.
  C. administering activated charcoal.
  D. keeping the patient standing.

_____ 9. Inflammation of the gallbladder is commonly associated with the presence of
  A. ulcers.   **C.** a hernia.
  B. pancreatitis.   **D.** gallstones.

_____ 10. Ingestion of alcohol or large amounts of food is a common trigger for
  A. hernias.   **C.** pancreatitis.
  B. ulcers.   **D.** esophageal varices.

IN THE FIELD

Read the following real-life situation. Then answer the questions that follow.

You are dispatched to a local apartment complex for a patient complaining of severe abdominal pain. Upon your arrival, you evaluate the scene for hazards and note none. You are met at the door by a woman who leads you to a bedroom where a 35-year-old male is sitting on the edge of the bed with his knees bent and arms crossed over his abdomen. Your patient is alert and oriented to person, place, and time. His breathing is noted to be heavy but unlabored. Your partner starts the patient on oxygen at 15 liters per minute via a nonrebreather mask. The patient's radial pulse is weak and rapid, and skin is cool, moist, and clammy. The patient complains of abdominal cramping to his right lower abdomen as well as nausea, fever, and chills over the past few hours.

1. What emergency care steps should you take with this patient?

CHAPTER 21 REVIEW

Write the word or words that best complete each sentence in the space provided.

1. It is helpful to reference the abdomen by dividing it into quarters, or quadrants, using the

   _____ as the central reference point.

2. The _____ _____ quadrant contains part of the

   large intestine and the female reproductive organs.

3. A person with an acute abdomen generally appears very ill and will assume a(n)

   _____ _____ with his knees drawn up and his

   hands clenched over his abdomen.

4. Pancreatitis, or inflammation of the _____, may cause severe pain in the

   middle of the upper quadrants (epigastric area) of the abdomen.

5. _____ are open wounds or sores within the digestive tract, usually in the

   stomach or the beginning of the small intestine.

6. _____ _____ are a bulging, engorgement, or

   weakening of the blood vessels in the lining of the lower part of the esophagus.

7. _____ and _____ are symptoms of the acute

   abdomen as well as of the common stomach flu.

8. The abdominal cavity is located _____ the diaphragm and extends to the

   _____ of the pelvis.

9. The lining of the abdominal cavity is called the _____.

10. The large vessels inside the abdominal cavity are the _____

    _____ and the _____

    _____ _____.

REINFORCEMENT

ACUTE ABDOMINAL PAIN: LISTING

1. List the five criteria that categorize the acute abdomen patient as a priority for transport.

2. List the seven emergency care steps for a patient with acute abdominal pain.

3. List five common conditions that may cause acute abdominal pain.

©2008 by Pearson Education, Inc.
Prehospital Emergency Care, 8th ed.

Acute Abdominal Pain: True or False

Indicate if the following statements are true or false by writing T or F in the space provided.

_____ **1.** It is possible to use the ribs as a reference point when assessing the abdominal cavity.

_____ **2.** The appendix is located in the RLQ (right lower quadrant).

_____ **3.** Many EMTs have found that patients who are experiencing abdominal bleeding are likely to faint.

_____ **4.** When assessing a patient with acute abdominal pain, the physical exam should focus only on the abdomen.

_____ **5.** Decreasing blood pressure, increasing heart rate, and pale, cool, moist skin are indicators of hypoperfusion (shock).

_____ **6.** The EMT should never extend scene time trying to determine the exact cause of acute abdominal pain.

_____ **7.** Appendicitis is not life-threatening and can be treated easily.

_____ **8.** Ulcers are associated with a breakdown of the lining that normally protects the intestine from the digestive fluids contained inside the digestive tract.

_____ **9.** Giving the acute abdominal pain patient a glass of milk is generally a good way of easing the pain.

_____ **10.** An abdominal aortic aneurysm can rupture and is one of the most lethal causes of abdominal pain.

Acute Abdominal Pain

Abdominal Structure and Function

Abdominal Quadrants

Types of Abdominal Structures

Acute Abdominal Pain

Causes

Types: Visceral, Parietal, Referred

Assessment and Care

Scene Size-up

Initial Assessment

Focused History and Physical Exam

- SAMPLE History
- Signs and Symptoms

Emergency Medical Care

Conditions That Cause Acute Abdominal Pain

CHAPTER 21 ANSWER KEY

HANDOUT 21-2: Chapter 21 Quiz

1. C	**4.** B	**7.** B	**9.** D
2. A	**5.** D	**8.** B	**10.** C
3. D	**6.** A		

HANDOUT 21-3: In the Field

1. Continue with the focused history and physical exam. Obtain a SAMPLE history and baseline vital signs and perform a rapid physical exam. As this patient is presenting with signs and symptoms of hypoperfusion (shock), he is a high-priority patient and transport should be initiated as soon as possible. Throughout your physical exam and transport, the patient should be placed in a position of comfort.

HANDOUT 21-4: Chapter 21 Review

1. navel (umbilicus)
2. left lower
3. guarded position
4. pancreas
5. Ulcers
6. Esophageal varices
7. Vomiting, diarrhea
8. below, top
9. peritoneum
10. abdominal aorta, interior vena cava

HANDOUT 21-5: Acute Abdominal Pain: Listing

1. Poor general appearance; unresponsive; responsive, but not following commands; shock (hypoperfusion); severe pain.
2. Keep the airway patent. Place the patient in a position of comfort. Administer oxygen at 15 liters per minute via a nonrebreather mask. *Never give anything by mouth.* Calm and reassure the patient. If signs and symptoms of hypoperfusion are present, treat for shock. Initiate a quick and efficient transport.
3. Any five: appendicitis; pancreatitis; cholecystitis; intestinal obstruction; hernia; ulcer; esophageal varices; abdominal aortic aneurysm; vomiting and diarrhea.

HANDOUT 21-6: Acute Abdominal Pain: True or False

1. F	**4.** F	**7.** F	**9.** F
2. T	**5.** T	**8.** T	**10.** T
3. T	**6.** T		

This chapter covers portions of Lessons 4-7 and Lesson 4-10 of the U.S. Department of Transportation's EMT-Basic National Standard Curriculum.

OBJECTIVES

Numbered objectives are from the U.S. Department of Transportation's EMT-Basic National Standard Curriculum. Asterisked objectives, if any, pertain to material that is supplemental to the DOT curriculum. Page numbers refer to pages in the textbook.

Cognitive

4-7.1   Describe the various ways that the body loses heat. (pp. 616–618)

4-7.2   List the signs and symptoms of exposure to cold. (pp. 619–630, 631)

4-7.3   Explain the steps in providing emergency medical care to a patient exposed to the cold. (pp. 627–629, 632)

4-7.4   List the signs and symptoms of exposure to heat. (pp. 630, 632–636, 639)

4-7.5   Explain the steps in providing emergency medical care to a patient exposed to heat. (pp. 637–638, 640)

4-7.8   Discuss the emergency medical care of bites and stings. (pp. 638–640, 642)

Psychomotor

4-7.9   Demonstrate the assessment and emergency medical care of a patient with exposure to cold.

4-7.10 Demonstrate the assessment and emergency medical care of a patient with exposure to heat.

4-7.12 Demonstrate completing a prehospital care report for patients with environmental emergencies.

Additional objectives from DOT Lesson 4-7 are addressed in Chapter 23, "Drowning and Diving Emergencies."

REVIEW

In the last lesson, "Acute Abdominal Pain," students learned that abdominal pain is a common condition that they are sure to encounter during their EMS careers. Remind students that abdominal pain can have any number of causes and may often signal a very serious medical condition. Summarize by telling students that no matter what the cause, in all cases of abdominal pain it is important that they assess life-threatening conditions, make the patient as comfortable as possible, administer oxygen, and get the patient to the

Total Teaching Time
180 minutes

Resources Needed
- Scored Chapter 21 Quizzes
- Complete jump kit containing BSI equipment
- Oxygen equipment
- Portable suction unit
- Stretcher and blankets

Additional Resources
Larmon/Davis, *Basic Life Support Skills*

Elling, *EMT Achieve: Basic Test Preparation*

Limmer/Mistovich/ O'Keefe, *Audio Lecture & Study Guide: EMT*

Mistovich/Kuvlesky, *SUCCESS! for the EMT, Second Edition*

hospital quickly. Distribute the scored quizzes from the last class. Go over each quiz question and handle any concerns students may have about the answers.

INTRODUCTION TO CHAPTER 22

Chapter 22, "Environmental Emergencies," is the 11th chapter in Module 4. Tell students that a number of situations that they may face as an EMT are termed "environmental emergencies." These conditions are brought on or worsened by some element or combination of elements in the patient's natural surroundings. Such emergencies can arise from interaction with the climate, as in exposure to excessive heat or cold. They can also be brought on by contact with creatures living in the environment, as in the bites or stings of snakes or spiders. Remind students that because environmental emergencies often occur in isolated areas that do not have ready access to a hospital emergency department, it is important that they learn how to assess and provide on-scene or en route emergency medical care for patients affected by environmental emergencies.

Distribute the Chapter 22 Objectives Checklist, and give students a few minutes to look it over. Then briefly paraphrase the objectives for this lesson in your own words.

LECTURE

The following suggested lecture outline is based on the Department of Transportation's EMT-Basic National Standard Curriculum. In some places, the DOT curriculum has been rearranged or expanded upon so that it is more complete or easier for the student to understand. The page numbers in parentheses refer to pages in the textbook. The parenthetical references in dark, heavy type are to figures, tables, and scans in the textbook.

ENVIRONMENTAL EMERGENCIES

I. **Heat and cold emergencies** (pp. 615–619)
   A. Regulation of temperature: how the body produces and conserves heat (pp. 615–619)
      1. When heat gained exceeds heat lost
         a. Hyperthermia (high body core temperature)
      2. Hyperthermia is most common in high air temperature and humidity and little or no breeze
   B. Regulation of temperature: how the body cools itself (pp. 615–619)
      1. When heat lost exceeds heat gained
         a. Hypothermia (low body core temperature)
      2. Causes of heat loss (**Fig. 22-1, p. 617**)
         a. Radiation
         b. Convection (**Fig. 22-2, p. 618**)
         c. Conduction
         d. Evaporation
         e. Respiration
      3. When treating patients with hypothermia, the EMT must be aware of the methods of heat loss to prevent further heat loss.

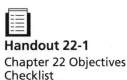

Handout 22-1
Chapter 22 Objectives Checklist

Lecture Master
You may wish to display Lecture Master 22 when presenting this lecture to the class.

Slides/Videos
"Outdoor Emergencies," *Pulse,* Sept. 2001.

Reading/Reference
Werfel, P., "Caught Cold," *JEMS,* Apr. 2001.

On the Net
Cold emergencies, frostbite, frostnip, and hypothermia. www.emergencymedicaled .com

Reading/Reference
Brown-Guard, D., "Freezing to Death: Prehospital Management of Frostbite and Hypothermia," *Emergency Medical Services,* Nov. 1999.

II. Exposure to cold (pp. 619–630)

    A. Generalized hypothermia—generalized cold emergency (pp. 619–621)

      1. Mortality as high as 87 percent

      2. Thermal control lost once body temperature lowered to 95°F.

      3. Coma occurs when body's core temperature reaches approximately 79°F.

      4. Death can occur within 2 hours of first signs and symptoms.

      5. Signs and symptoms of generalized hypothermia (**Fig. 22-3, p. 620**)

        a. Core temperature 95°F to 98°F (35°C to 37°C)

          (1) Cold, pale skin

          (2) Alert and shivering

          (3) Poor muscle coordination

          (4) Rapid breathing

          (5) Rapid heart rate

        b. Core temperature 90°F to 95°F (32°C to 35°C)

          (1) Cold, waxy skin

          (2) Puffy face, possibly pink

          (3) Confusion

          (4) Muscle rigidity, no shivering

          (5) Slow heart rate

       c. Core temperature 86°F to 90°F (30°C to 32°C)

          (1) Dilated pupils

          (2) Diminished reflexes

          (3) Stupor or coma

          (4) Rigid muscles

          (5) Slow breathing rate

          (6) Hypotension

          (7) Slow heart rate

       d. Core temperature 82°F to 86°F (28°C to 30°C)

          (1) Fixed, dilated pupils

          (2) Coma

          (3) Flaccid muscles

          (4) Slow respiration

          (5) Slow or rapid heart rate

          (6) Possible cardiac arrest

       e. Core temperature 68°F to 82°F (20° C to 28°C)

          (1) Cyanosis

          (2) Fixed, dilated pupils

          (3) Unresponsiveness

          (4) Barely detectable vital signs

          (5) Irregular pulse

          (6) Cardiac arrest

      6. Predisposing factors (**Fig. 22-4, p. 621**)

        a. Cold environment

          (1) Can occur in temperatures as high as 65°F depending on chill factor.

          (2) Wetness always compounds the problem.

        b. Age

          (1) Very young

            (a) Small size with large skin surface area

            (b) Small muscle mass (poor or absent shivering response)

            (c) Inability to use adaptive behaviors (moving to a warm environment)

              (d) Less body fat
        (2) Very old
              (a) Impaired recognition of cold
              (b) Diminished basal metabolism
              (c) Poor connection of blood vessels in
                  extremities
              (d) Less body fat
     c. Medical conditions
        (1) Recent surgery
        (2) Shock (hypoperfusion)
        (3) Head injury
        (4) Burns
        (5) Generalized infection
        (6) Spinal-cord injuries
        (7) Thyroid gland disorders
        (8) Diabetic conditions such as hypoglycemia
     d. Drugs/poisons
  7. Stages of hypothermia (**Fig. 22-5, p. 622**)
  8. Immersion hypothermia (**Fig. 22-6, p. 622**)
     a. Result of lowering of body temperature due to
        immersion in cold or cool water
     b. Body temperature drops to water temperature within
        10 minutes.
     c. Death can occur within a few minutes when water
        temperature is 50°F or lower.
     d. First priority: get patient out of water, out of wet
        clothing, and into warm environment.
  9. Urban hypothermia
     a. External
     b. Internal
B. Local cold injury (pp. 621–623)
  1. Commonly called "frostbite" (freezing of body tissues)
  2. Often accompanied by generalized hypothermia
  3. Occurs when ice crystals form between skin cells and expand
     as they extract fluid from the cells
  4. Obstructs circulation
  5. Tends to occur on feet, hands, ears, nose, and cheeks
  6. Predisposing factors
     a. Any kind of trauma suffered by people injured in cold
        weather
     b. Extremes of age
     c. Tight or tightly laced footwear
     d. Use of alcohol during exposure to cold
     e. Wet clothing
     f. High altitudes
     g. Loss of blood
     h. Arteriosclerosis
  7. Stages of local cold injury (**Fig. 24-7, p. 623**)
     a. Early or superficial cold injury
        (1) Usually involves tips of ears, nose, cheekbones,
            tips of toes and fingers, and chin
        (2) Patient usually unaware of injury
        (3) As exposure time lengthens or temperature drops,
            patient loses feeling and sensation in affected area.
        (4) Skin may begin to turn waxy gray or yellow.
        (5) Skin remains soft but cold to the touch.

On the Net
Info on water hypothermia
and treatment.
www.walrus.com

(6) Normal skin color does not return on palpation.

(7) Patient may report tingling sensation as area rewarms.

b. Late or deep cold injury—extreme emergency that can result in permanent tissue loss (**Fig. 22-8, p. 624**)

(1) Involves both the skin and the tissue beneath it

(2) Skin is white, waxy

(3) Palpation reveals firm to completely solid frozen feeling

(4) Injury may involve whole hand or foot

(5) Swelling and blisters filled with clear or straw-colored fluid

(6) Area becomes blotchy or mottled with colors from white to purple to grayish-blue as area thaws

C. Assessment and care: cold-related emergency (pp. 623–630) (**Figs. 22-13, pp. 631–632 and 22-14, p. 633**)

1. Scene size-up

a. Ensure personal safety and safety of the EMT-Basic crew.

b. Consider how the characteristics of the scene may have affected the patient and how the patient interacted with the environment before EMS arrival.

2. Initial assessment

a. Closely assess airway, especially in unresponsive patient.

b. Be prepared to provide positive-pressure ventilation with supplemental oxygen if breathing is inadequate.

c. Patient breathing adequately

(1) Administer oxygen, warmed and humidified if possible, by a nonrebreather mask at 15 liters per minute.

d. Check carotid and radial pulses

e. Pulse absent

(1) Begin chest compression with artificial ventilation.

f. Note skin color and condition.

(1) Early

(a) Skin may appear red

(2) Late

(a) Skin changes to pale, then cyanotic, then gray

(3) As condition progresses, skin will become firm and cold to the touch.

3. Focused history and physical exam

a. Remove patient from cold environment.

b. Conduct exam in back of warmed ambulance.

c. Patient responding

(1) SAMPLE history

(2) Document complaints of pain and other symptoms.

(3) Determine if patient is using any medications, especially drugs that might depress the central nervous system or cause blood vessels to dilate.

(4) Determine last food intake.

(5) Determine what patient was doing prior to incident.

(6) Determine how long patient was exposed to cold environment.

Point of Interest
The abdomen is the last place to get cold. A cold abdomen, upon palpation, means profound hypothermia.

        (7) Perform rapid assessment if trauma is suspected or if patient complains of pain in several areas of the body.
        (8) Assess extremities for local cold injuries.
        (9) Perform motor assessment
    d. Patient unresponsive
        (1) Perform rapid assessment.
        (2) Gather SAMPLE history from family and bystanders.
4. Signs and symptoms of generalized hypothermia (**Fig. 22-9, p. 626**)
    a. Cool abdominal skin
    b. Decreasing mental status
        (1) Amnesia, memory lapses, incoherence
        (2) Mood changes
        (3) Impaired judgment
        (4) Reduced ability to communicate
        (5) Dizziness
        (6) Vague, slow, slurred, thick speech
        (7) Drowsiness progressing even to unresponsiveness to verbal or painful stimuli
    c. Decreasing motor and sensory function correlating with the degree of hypothermia
        (1) Joint and/or muscle stiffness; muscle rigidity as hypothermia progresses; stiff or rigid posture
        (2) Lack of coordination
        (3) Apparent exhaustion or inability to get up after rest
        (4) Uncontrollable fits of shivering at first; little or no shivering as hypothermia progresses
        (5) Reduced sensation or loss of sensation
    d. Changing vital signs
        (1) Respiratory changes
        (2) Changes in pulse
        (3) Changes in skin color
            (a) Red in early stages
            (b) Pale and then cyanotic in later stages
            (c) Gray, waxen, hard skin that is cold to the touch in latest stages
        (4) Slowly responding pupils
        (5) Low to absent blood pressure
5. Emergency medical care for generalized hypothermia
    a. Basic principles
        (1) Preventing further heat loss
        (2) Rewarming patient as quickly and as safely as possible
        (3) Staying alert for complications
    b. Steps to follow
        (1) Remove from cold environment.
        (2) Handle extremely gently.
        (3) Administer oxygen via nonrebreather mask at 15 liters per minute if not already done as part of initial assessment.
        (4) Patient goes into cardiac arrest

> **(a)** Provide only one set of defibrillation shocks if the AED is available or, if necessary, begin CPR.
>
> **(5)** Patient alert and responding
>> **(a)** Actively rewarm.
>>> **(i)** Wrapping in warm blankets
>>> **(ii)** Turning up heat in patient compartment of the ambulance
>>> **(iii)** Placing heat packs or hot water bottles in patient's groin, armpits, and on chest (**Fig. 22-10, p. 628**)
>>
>> **(b)** Applying heat slowly and gently; never immersing in tub of hot water or placing in hot shower
>> **(c)** Checking patient often to ensure that you are not burning patient's skin with rewarming techniques
>
> **(6)** Patient is unresponsive
>> **(a)** Use only passive rewarming (**Fig. 22-11, p. 628**)
>>> **(i)** Wrap patient in blankets.
>>> **(ii)** Turn up heat in patient compartment of ambulance
>>
>> **(b)** Seek medical direction
>> **(c)** Follow local protocol
>
> **(7)** Do not allow patient to eat or drink stimulants.
> **(8)** Never rub or massage patient's arms or legs.
> **(9)** Transport as quickly as possible.

6. Emergency medical care for immersion hypothermia
   a. Instruct patient to make least effort needed to stay afloat until you reach him.
   b. Lift patient from water in a horizontal or supine position to prevent vascular collapse.
   c. Remove patient's wet clothing carefully and gently.
   d. Continue treatment as for generalized hypothermia.
7. Signs and symptoms of early or superficial local cold injury
   a. Blanching of the skin (when palpated, normal color does not return)
   b. Loss of feeling and sensation in injured area
   c. Continued softness of skin in injured area and in tissue beneath it
   d. Tingling sensation during rewarming
8. Signs and symptoms of late or deep local cold injury
   a. White, waxy skin
   b. A firm to frozen feeling when skin is palpated
   c. Swelling
   d. Blisters
   e. Flushed skin with areas of purple and blanching or mottled and cyanotic skin if partially or wholly thawed
9. Emergency medical care for local cold injury
   a. Remove patient immediately from cold environment.
   b. Never initiate thawing procedures if there is any danger of refreezing.
   c. Administer oxygen at 15 liters per minute by nonrebreather mask.

d. Prevent further injury to the injured part.
e. If patient has an early or superficial injury
   (1) Carefully remove any jewelry or wet or restrictive clothing, but if clothing is frozen to skin, leave it in place.
   (2) Immobilize affected extremity.
   (3) Cover affected skin with dressings or dry clothing.
   (4) Never rub or massage affected skin.
   (5) Never reexpose affected skin to the cold.
   (6) No part of injured extremity should be in direct contact with a hard surface.
f. If patient has late or deep injury
   (1) Carefully remove any jewelry or wet or restrictive clothing, but if clothing is frozen to skin, leave it in place.
   (2) Cover affected skin with dressings or dry clothing.
   (3) Do not break any blisters or treat them with salve or ointment.
   (4) Do not rub or massage affected skin.
   (5) Never apply heat to rewarm the skin.
   (6) Do not allow patient to walk on an injured extremity.
g. Steps for rewarming frozen tissue
   (1) Extremely painful for patient; medical direction may want patient to take an analgesic to help relieve pain during process.
   (2) Immerse affected tissue in a warm water bath. **(Fig. 22-11, p. 630)**
   (3) Monitor water to make sure that it stays at an even temperature.
   (4) Continuously stir the water to keep heat evenly distributed and constant.
   (5) Keep tissue in warm water until it is soft and color and sensation return to it.
   (6) Dress the area with dry, sterile dressings.
   (7) Elevate the affected extremity.
   (8) Protect the warmed part against refreezing.
   (9) Transport as soon as possible.
10. Conduct a detailed physical exam if time and patient's condition permit.
11. Ongoing assessment

III. **Exposure to heat** (pp. 630–638)
A. Stages of hyperthermia (pp. 630–634)
   1. Heat cramps
      a. Is least serious form of heat-related injury
      b. Manifest as muscle cramps or spasms thought to result from body losing too much salt during sweating
   2. Heat exhaustion
      a. Disturbance of body's blood flow
      b. Resulting in a mild state of shock brought on by pooling of blood in vessels just below skin, which causes blood to flow away from major organs
      c. Is brought on by extreme physical exertion in a hot, humid environment

Reading/Reference
Criss, E., "Rewarming Techniques Compared," *JEMS*, July 2000.

On the Net
Heat emergencies: heat stroke, heat exhaustion, heat cramps. www.survivalcenter.com/firstaid/heat.htm

      d. Occurs when large quantities of salt and water lost by profuse sweating are not replaced; blood circulation diminishes, affecting the brain, heart, and lungs

      e. Signs and symptoms

        (1) Normal to cool skin temperature

        (2) Skin either pale or ashen gray

        (3) Patient sweaty

  3. Heat stroke

      a. Life-threatening medical emergency with mortality ranging from 20–70 percent

      b. May arise when patient suffering heat exhaustion does not seek a cool environment, does not stop physical activity, and does not replace lost fluid

      c. Occurs when body's heat-regulating mechanisms break down and become unable to cool the body sufficiently

      d. Because no cooling takes place, the body stores increasingly more heat, heat-producing mechanisms speed up, and eventually brain cells are damaged, causing permanent disability or death.

      e. Signs and symptoms

        (1) Hot, red skin

        (2) Either moist or dry skin (about half victims sweat whereas about half cease to sweat)

B. Factors predisposing to hyperthermia (p. 634)

  1. Climate (hot temperatures; high humidity)

  2. Exercise and strenuous activity **(Fig. 22-15, p. 634)**

  3. Age (elderly and infants—extremes of age)

  4. Preexisting illnesses and conditions

      a. Heart disease

      b. Kidney disease

      c. Cerebrovascular disease

      d. Parkinson's disease

      e. Thyroid gland disorders

      f. Skin diseases, including eczema, scleroderma, and healed burns

      g. Dehydration

      h. Obesity

      i. Infections or other conditions that cause fever

      j. Fatigue

      k. Diabetes

      l. Malnutrition

      m. Alcoholism

      n. Mental retardation

      o. Certain drugs

        (1) Alcohol, cocaine, diuretics, barbiturates, hallucinogens, and medications that hamper sweating

C. Assessment and care: heat-related emergency (pp. 634–638)

  1. Scene size-up

      a. Scan the scene for evidence that patient is suffering from heat-related emergency.

      b. Consider the ambient temperature and humidity. **(Fig. 22-16, p. 635)**

      c. Look for clues to patient's activities prior to the incident.

Slides/Videos
"The Skill of Survival—Desert Regio. . . a guide to hot weather survival," Alan Madison Productions

    d. Note person's clothing (jogging shorts, bicycling attire, etc.).

    e. Note location of patient (closed vehicle on a hot day; closed, uncooled dwelling).

    f. Look for medications or drugs.

    g. Recognize your own limits and protect yourself from overexposure to heat by dressing appropriately and drinking enough water to stay hydrated.

2. Initial assessment

    a. Gather general impression of patient.

    b. Determine whether patient is dressed inappropriately for the hot environment.

    c. Assess patient's mental status; may range from alert and oriented to completely unresponsive.

    d. Be aware that mental status may deteriorate as condition worsens.

    e. Assess airway and breathing; provide oxygen at 15 liters per minute by nonrebreather mask if mental status alters or continues to deteriorate.

    f. If breathing is inadequate, begin positive-pressure ventilation with supplemental oxygen.

    g. Assess pulse: radial pulse may be weak and rapid or absent depending on the level of dehydration.

    h. Consider the patient with altered mental status and hot skin a priority patient.

3. Focused history and physical exam

    a. Move patient to a cool environment as quickly as possible.

    b. Responsive patient

        (1) SAMPLE history

        (2) Modify the OPQRST to gather additional information about some symptoms.

        (3) Pay particular attention to medications the patient may be taking.

        (4) Determine patient's last oral intake, especially consumption of water and other liquids.

        (5) Get a description of events that preceded the incident.

        (6) Conduct a focused medical assessment, targeting areas of complaint gathered during the SAMPLE history.

        (7) Take baseline vital signs.

    c. Unresponsive patient

        (1) Conduct a rapid medical assessment, take baseline vital signs, and then gather the SAMPLE history from family or bystanders.

4. Signs and symptoms of generalized hyperthermia (Fig. 22-17, p. 636)

    a. Muscle cramps

    b. Weakness and exhaustion

    c. Dizziness or faintness

    d. Rapid pulse that is usually strong at first but becomes weak

    e. Initial deep, rapid breathing that becomes shallow and weak as damage progresses

    f. Headache

©2008 by Pearson Education, Inc.
Prehospital Emergency Care, 8th ed.

      g. Seizures

      h. Loss of appetite, nausea, or vomiting

      i. Altered mental status, possibly unresponsiveness

      j. Moist, pale skin with normal-to-cool temperature or hot, dry, or moist skin

   5. Emergency medical care for a heat emergency patient with moist, pale, normal-to-cool skin

      a. Move patient to a cool place.

      b. Administer oxygen at 15 lpm via nonrebreather mask.

      c. Remove as much of patient's clothing as you can.

      d. Cool patient by applying cold, wet compresses and/or by fanning lightly. (**Fig. 22-18, p. 637**)

      e. Place patient in a supine position and raise patient's feet and legs 8 to 12 inches.

      f. If the patient is fully responsive and not nauseated, have him drink cool water.

      g. If the patient is unresponsive or has altered mental status or is vomiting, do *not* give fluids.

      h. Transport when the patient—

        (1) Is unresponsive or has altered mental status

        (2) Is vomiting or is nauseated and will not drink fluids

        (3) Has a history of medical problems

        (4) Has a temperature above 101°F

        (5) Has a rising temperature

        (6) Does not respond to therapy (symptoms do not improve)

   6. Emergency medical care for a heat emergency patient with hot skin, moist or dry

      a. Remove patient from source of heat and place in a cool environment.

      b. Remove as much of the patient's clothing as is possible or reasonable.

      c. Administer oxygen at 15 liters per minute via nonrebreather mask.

      d. Immediately begin to cool patient. (**Fig. 22-19, p. 637**)

        (1) Pour cool water over patient.

        (2) Place cold packs in patient's groin, at each side of neck, in armpits, and behind each knee to cool the large surface blood vessels.

        (3) Wrap a wet sheet that has been soaked in cool water around patient.

        (4) Fan patient aggressively or direct an electric fan at patient.

        (5) Keep patient's skin wet to promote cooling.

        (6) Use slower cooling if patient starts to shiver (Shivering produces heat.)

      e. Be prepared to manage seizures or prevent aspiration of vomitus.

      f. Transport immediately, continuing to administer oxygen and cooling methods during transport.

   7. Ongoing assessment

  D. Summary: assessment and care—heat emergency (p. 638) (**Figs. 22-20, pp. 639–640 and 22-21, p. 641**)

IV. Bites and stings (pp. 638–642)

  A. Snakebites less common than insect bites and stings (p. 638)

◆

Slides/Videos
"Insect Bites and Stings,"
Pulse, Sept. 2001.

B. Insect bites minor unless patient has allergic reaction (p. 638)

C. Anaphylactic shock is a life-threatening emergency (p. 638)

D. Assessment and care: bites and stings (pp. 638–642)

1. Scene size-up
   a. First priority is to protect yourself and your partner.
   b. Pause and look and listen for swarming bees or hornets before going to patient's side.
   c. When you get to the patient's side, scan the ground carefully, looking for snakes, anthills, or openings to underground yellow jacket nests.
   d. Be alert to the fact that insects may have become trapped in the patient's clothing.
   e. Once your safety is ensured, look around scene for evidence of what may have bitten or stung the patient.

2. Initial assessment
   a. Gather general impression of patient and his mental status.
   b. Be especially alert when assessing the airway and breathing.

3. Focused history and physical exam
   a. If you detect signs of anaphylactic shock, continue with assessment and emergency medical care as described in Chapter 18, "Allergic Reaction."
   b. If the patient displays the more common signs and symptoms of reaction to bites and stings, continue with the assessment as described in the section on injected poisons in Chapter 19, "Poisoning Emergencies," and then provide the appropriate emergency medical care.

4. Signs and symptoms of anaphylactic shock
   a. Hives
   b. Flushing
   c. Upper airway obstruction
   d. Faintness
   e. Dizziness
   f. Generalized itching
   g. Generalized swelling, including eyelids, lips, tongue
   h. Difficulty swallowing
   i. Shortness of breath, wheezing, or stridor
   j. Labored breathing
   k. Abdominal cramps
   l. Confusion
   m. Loss of responsiveness
   n. Convulsions
   o. Hypotension (low blood pressure)

5. Emergency medical care for anaphylactic shock
   a. Maintain a patent airway.
   b. Administer epinephrine by a prescribed auto-injector with permission from medical direction.
   c. Consider calling for advanced life support.
   d. Initiate early transport.

6. General signs and symptoms of a bite or sting
   a. History of bite (snake or spider) or sting (insect, scorpion, or marine animal)
   b. Pain—often intermediate and severe or burning
   c. Redness or other discoloration around bite

d. Swelling around the bite, sometimes gradually spreading
   e. Weakness or faintness
   f. Dizziness
   g. Chills
   h. Fever
   i. Nausea or vomiting
   j. Bite marks
   k. Stinger
7. Emergency medical care for a bite or sting
   a. Remove stinger, if present, by gently scraping against it.
   b. Wash area around bite or sting.
   c. Remove any jewelry or other constricting objects.
   d. Lower the injection site slightly below the level of the patient's heart.
   e. Apply a cold pack to an insect bite or sting; do not apply cold to snakebites or injuries inflicted by marine animals.
   f. Consult medical direction and follow local protocols regarding the use of a constricting band in the treatment of snakebite.
   g. Observe the patient carefully for the signs and symptoms of an allergic reaction.
   h. Keep the patient calm, limit his physical activity, and keep him warm.
   i. If the patient shows any signs of allergic reaction, transport immediately.
8. Ongoing assessment
   a. Monitor the patient's airway, breathing, and circulation carefully.
   b. Be prepared to provide emergency care for anaphylactic shock.

ENRICHMENT (OPTIONAL)

The following sections contain information that is valuable as background for the EMT, but that goes substantially beyond the U.S. Department of Transportation's EMT-Basic National Standard Curriculum.

   V. Myxedema coma (pp. 642–643)
      A. Overview of disease process (pp. 642–643)
      B. Emergency care (p. 643)
   VI. Lightning strike injuries (pp. 643–645)
      A. Overview of lightning strike disease process (pp. 643–644)
      B. Assessment (pp. 644–645) **(Fig. 22-22, p. 644)**
      C. Emergency medical care (p. 645)
   VII. Snakebite (pp. 645–646)
      A. Characteristics of snakebites (p. 645) **(Figs. 22-23, p. 645 and 22-24, p. 646)**
      B. Factors that determine the severity of snakebite (pp. 645–646)
      C. Emergency medical care same as general emergency care for bites and stings (p. 646)
   VIII. Insect bites and stings (pp. 646–647)
      A. Local reactions rarely serious or life-threatening (p. 646)
      B. Allergic reactions serious and may be life-threatening (p. 646)
      C. Black widow spider (p. 646)

Point of Interest
There are 2,600 black widow spider bites reported each year, over half of which have severe reactions. The black widow is the leading cause of spider-related deaths in the United States.

D. Brown recluse spider (pp. 646–647) **(Fig. 22-25, p. 646)**
E. Scorpion (p. 647)
F. Fire ant (p. 647)
G. Tick (p. 647) **(Fig. 22-26, p. 647)**
H. Marine life bites and stings (p. 647)

CASE STUDY FOLLOW-UP

Ask a student volunteer to read the Case Study that begins on page 615 of the textbook. You may wish to use the following questions to engage the students in a discussion of the Case Study Follow-up that begins on page 648 of the textbook. Provide missing information and clarify ideas as needed.

Q1. What indications do you receive that Mrs. Rector is disoriented?

A1. *Mrs. Rector appears to be disoriented to time as she says, "I should have taken out the garbage tomorrow. Is that Thursday? But I hadn't taken it out yesterday."*

Q2. During your focused physical exam, what sign suggests that Mrs. Rector is experiencing generalized hypothermia?

A2. *The skin on Mrs. Rector's abdomen is cool to the touch.*

Q3. What sign suggests that Mrs. Rector is experiencing local cold injury?

A3. *She has no sensation in her toes. The skin is soft but very cold to the touch and normal skin color does not return after palpation.*

Q4. How do you rewarm Mrs. Rector?

A4. *With passive rewarming, by covering her with an additional warm, dry blanket and moving her to the previously warmed-up patient compartment of the ambulance.*

Q5. As a result of the rewarming, of what does Mrs. Rector complain?

A5. *Pain in her feet.*

IN REVIEW

Assess the students' ability to apply what they have just learned by discussing the Review Questions on page 650 in the textbook.

Q1. Name the five processes through which the body loses heat.

A1. *The five processes though which the body loses heat are radiation, convection, conduction, evaporation, and respiration. (pp. 617–618)*

Q2. Explain the difference between hypothermia and hyperthermia.

A2. *In hypothermia, a person's body loses more heat than it produces or gains, leading to a reduced core temperature. In hyperthermia, a person's body produces or gains more heat than it loses, leading to an increased core temperature. (pp. 618–619)*

Q3. List the signs and symptoms of generalized hypothermia.

A3. *The signs and symptoms of generalized hypothermia are cool or cold skin temperature; decreasing motor and sensory function; and vital signs changes including rapid breathing, rapid pulse, slowly responding pupils, skin color from red to blue or pale, and low blood pressure. (pp. 625–627)*

Q4. Explain the steps in treatment of a patient suffering from a local cold injury.

A4. *The steps in treatment of a patient suffering from local cold injury are as follows: Remove the patient from the cold environment; protect the injured area; administer oxygen at 15 liters per minute via nonrebreather mask if not already begun; remove patient's wet or restrictive clothing; immobilize the affected extremity; cover it; do not rub, massage, or reexpose it to the cold; in cases of later or deep local cold injury, do not permit the patient to walk on the extremity. (p. 629)*

Q5. Explain the treatment of the patient suffering from a heat emergency.

A5. *The treatment of a patient suffering from a heat emergency is as follows: Move the patient from a hot environment to a cooler one; administer oxygen at 15 liters per minute via nonrebreather mask; remove or loosen patient's clothing; cool the patient by applying cold, wet compresses and/or by fanning; place the patient in a supine position with feet and legs elevated 8 to 12 inches; if medical direction approves and the patient is responsive and not vomiting, give one-half glassful of cool water every 15 minutes. In patients with hot and moist or dry skin, efforts at cooling should be aggressive, with the use of cool packs, wet sponges or towels, and stronger fanning. Do not give liquids, but transport immediately. (pp. 637–638)*

Q6. List conditions that would predispose a patient to experience a cold emergency.

A6. *Conditions that would predispose a patient to experience a cold emergency are cold environment, age (very young or old), preexisting medical conditions, drugs, and poisons. (pp. 619, 621–622)*

Q7. List conditions that would predispose a patient to experience a heat emergency.

A7. *Conditions that would predispose a patient to experience a heat emergency are a hot, humid environment; exercise and strenuous activity; extremes in age; preexisting illnesses and medical conditions; use of certain drugs or medications. (p. 634)*

Q8. Explain the difference between active and passive rewarming.

A8. *Active rewarming is a technique of aggressively applying heat to warm a patient's body. Active rewarming includes the following techniques: wrapping the patient in warmed blankets; placing heat packs and hot water bottles on the patient's groin, in the armpits, and on the chest, and turning up the heat in the patient compartment of the ambulance. Passive rewarming is taking measures to prevent further heat loss and giving the patient's body the optimum chance to rewarm itself. Passive rewarming can include wrapping the patient in blankets and turning up the heat in the patient compartment of the ambulance. (pp. 627–628)*

Q9. Explain some of the effects of a lightning strike on the nervous, cardiac, respiratory, and musculoskeletal system, as well as the skin, eyes, and ears.

A9. *Nervous system: altered mental status; retrograde amnesia; anterograde amnesia; weakness; pain, tingling, and numbness; pale, cool, and clammy skin; temporary paralysis; dizziness; loss of pupillary function; seizures. Cardiac system: asystole or ventricular fibrillation; irregular pulse. Respiratory system: apnea. Skin: burns, including* *linear burns, feathering, punctuate burns, and thermal burns. Musculoskeletal system: dislocations, fractures. Eyes: unequal pupils, drooping eyelids. Ears: ruptured tympanic membrane, tinnitis, deafness. (pp. 643–645)*

Q10. Explain the emergency medical care for the lightning strike patient.

A10. *Emergency medical care for the lightning strike patient includes: ensure scene safety; establish in-line manual stabilization of the patient's head and neck; establish an airway if the patient has an altered mental status; if the patient is in cardiac arrest, perform CPR, apply an AED, and provide aggressive ventilation with a high concentration of oxygen. If the patient has a pulse but no or inadequate breathing, begin aggressive positive-pressure ventilation with supplemental oxygen; immobilize the patient to a backboard; transport while continuously monitoring the patient's condition. (p. 645)*

Q11. List the signs and symptoms associated with stings and bites.

A11. *Signs and symptoms associated with stings and bites include a history of the bite, pain, redness, swelling, weakness, dizziness, chills, fever, nausea, vomiting, bite marks, and a stinger embedded in the tissue. Be alert for signs and symptoms of developing anaphylactic shock. (p. 642)*

Q12. Explain the general emergency medical care for a patient suffering from a bite or sting.

A12. *The general emergency care for a patient suffering from a bite or sting is as follows: Remove the stinger, if still present, by gently scraping against it. Wash the area, and remove any jewelry or other constricting objects. Lower the injection site slightly below the heart. Apply a cold pack to an insect bite or sting but not to snakebites or marine-life stings; apply a constricting band for snakebite if advised by medical direction or local protocol. Observe and provide care for allergic reaction if it develops; keep the patient calm, limit the patient's physical activity, and keep the patient warm. Transport. (p. 642)*

CRITICAL THINKING

Assess students' ability to respond to real-life emergency situations by discussing the Critical Thinking questions on page 650 in the textbook.

Q1. Does this call initially present as one with an environmental concern?

A1. *The initial circumstances of this call wouldn't necessarily indicate that environmental factors would be an issue. One would assume that since the patient is inside the residence, he would not be prone to an environmental emergency.*

Q2. What is the patient's initial emergency that rendered the patient susceptible to an evironmental emergency?

A2. *The wet, naked patient fell while getting out of the shower and, based on the instability and pain found during the assessment, probably fractured or dislocated his hip. This kept the patient from being able to move from the cold tile floor. Also, the patient was wet and was not wearing any clothing. The cold floor would cool the patient through the mechanism of conduction. Heat is being transferred from the patient's body to the cold tile floor. As the water evaporates from the patient, it takes the absorbed warmth from the skin, cooling him further. Also, the patient has no protection offered by clothes to reduce the radiation of* *heat from his body to the environment. Clothes will insulate the body and keep warm air trapped inside. Without this protection, the patient radiates heat to the cooler air temperature.*

Q3. What would you expect to find regarding the patient's core temperature with the tympanic thermometer?

A3. *This patient's core temperature would most likely be below normal due to the mechanisms of cooling already noted.*

Q4. How might your treatment of this patient change, given a disturbance in his core temperature?

A4. *The EMTs would have to do several things differently because of the decrease in the patient's core temperature. The first is that it would be a high priority to move the patient from the floor and to prevent any further heat loss. Second, they would need to be exceedingly gentle while moving the patient in order to prevent a cardiac dysrhythmia. Finally, they would need to keep the patient in the supine position while moving him from the floor to the wheeled stretcher and during transport. It is important to provide passing rewarming. This would be accomplished by wrapping the patient in blankets and turning the heat in the back of the ambulance on high.*

Q5. Describe the factors that contributed to the potential change in the patient's core temperature.

A5. *The patient's advanced age and traumatic injury along with being naked, wet, and lying on a cold tile floor in an air-conditioned building would definitely have contributed to the change in the patient's core temperature.*

ROLE PLAY

Tell students that they will now have the chance to apply what they have learned through role-playing a real-life situation encountered by EMS personnel. Call for four volunteers—two to play the roles of EMTs responding to a 9-1-1 call, one to be a bystander, and one to be the patient.

Take the two EMT volunteers outside the classroom and provide them with a complete jump kit containing BSI equipment, oxygen equipment, a portable suction unit, and a stretcher. Also provide blankets. Describe the following situation to them:

You are dispatched to a country park on a dew-drenched summer morning. The dispatcher said that the patient was bitten by a snake. You should act appropriately on what you find there. The emphasis of the scene is in dealing with environmental emergencies. However, you should use all the skill you have learned to date.

Reenter the classroom, first telling the two EMT volunteers to wait in the hallway until you call them to the scene in just a minute. Ask the bystander and the patient volunteers to come to the front of the classroom. Decide who is going to play each role, and then describe the following situation to the volunteers and to the class in general:

You (the patient) were power-walking in a country park on a dew-drenched summer morning. With your headphones on and your gaze straight ahead, you were not paying much attention to the cross-country trail you were on. You apparently stepped on a snake of some sort and it bit you on your unprotected lower leg. You yelled in fright and the snake slithered off. Hearing your yell, a park officer (the bystander) galloped up on

Reading/Reference
Textbook, pp. 651–668

Workbook
Chapter 22 Activities

Chapter Quiz
Handout 22-2

TestGen
Chapter 22 Test

Online Test Preparation
Send your students to
http://www.prenhall.com/
EMTAchieve

Handouts 22-3 to 22-5
Reinforcement Activities

**Brady Skills Series
EMT-B Videos/CD**
Visual Reinforcement

**PowerPoint
Presentation**
Chapter 22

Student CD
Chapter 22

Companion Website
http://www.prenhall.com/
mistovich

horseback a moment later. The officer called for an ambulance, then directed you to lie quietly on the ground until the ambulance arrived. When the ambulance arrives, you are feeling chilled, even though your leg is burning.

Tell the patient and the bystander to take their places and to start acting. Call the EMTs back into the classroom at the appropriate time. Allow the role play to progress naturally. Provide appropriate vital signs and other objective information about the patient if the EMTs assess this information. Intervene only if the players seem to be at a loss for what to do.

Critique the role play with the class by asking the following questions:

- What did the EMTs do well?
- What, if anything, should they have done differently?

ASSIGNMENTS

Assign students to read Chapter 23, "Drowning and Diving Emergencies," before the next class. Also ask them to complete Chapter 22 of the Workbook.

EVALUATION

Chapter Quiz Distribute copies of the Chapter Quiz provided in Handout 22-2 to evaluate student understanding of this chapter. Remind students not to refer to their textbooks or notes while taking the quiz.

Test Manager You may wish to create a custom-tailored test using Prentice Hall *TestGen for Prehospital Emergency Care, Eighth Edition* to evaluate student understanding of this chapter.

Online Test Preparation (for students and instructors) Additional test preparation is available through *EMT Achieve: Basic Test Preparation* at http://www.prenhall.com/EMTAchieve. Instructors can also monitor student mastery online.

REINFORCEMENT

Handouts If classroom discussions or performance on the quiz indicates that some students have not fully mastered the chapter content, you may wish to assign some or all of the Reinforcement Handouts for this chapter.

TECH EXTRAS

Brady Skills Series EMT-B Videos/CD Have your students watch the skills come to life on either VHS or CD-ROM.

PowerPoint Presentation (for instructors) The PowerPoint material developed for this chapter offers useful reinforcement of chapter content.

Student CD A wide variety of material on this CD-ROM will reinforce and also expand student knowledge and skills.

Companion Website (for students) Additional review quizzes and links to EMS resources will contribute to further reinforcement of this chapter. Please visit http://www.prenhall.com/mistovich.

OBJECTIVES CHECKLIST

Cognitive		Date Mastered
4-7.1	Describe the various ways that the body loses heat.	
4-7.2	List the signs and symptoms of exposure to cold.	
4-7.3	Explain the steps in providing emergency medical care to a patient exposed to the cold.	
4-7.4	List the signs and symptoms of exposure to heat.	
4-7.5	Explain the steps in providing emergency medical care to a patient exposed to heat.	
4-7.8	Discuss the emergency medical care of bites and stings.	

Psychomotor		Date Mastered
4-7.9	Demonstrate the assessment and emergency medical care of a patient with exposure to cold.	
4-7.10	Demonstrate the assessment and emergency medical care of a patient with exposure to heat.	
4-7.12	Demonstrate completing a prehospital care report for patients with environmental emergencies.	

EVALUATION

CHAPTER 22 QUIZ

Write the letter of the best answer in the space provided.

_____ 1. Water chill, which occurs when clothing or the body gets wet, is an example of
  A. conduction. C. radiation.
  B. convection. D. evaporation.

_____ 2. Wind chill, which occurs when currents of air pass over the body, is an example of
  A. conduction. C. radiation.
  B. convection. D. evaporation.

_____ 3. All of the following are signs and symptoms of hypothermia *except*
  A. agitation and hyperactivity.
  B. shivering in early stages.
  C. loss of motor coordination.
  D. cool abdominal skin temperature.

_____ 4. In providing emergency care steps for the hypothermic patient who is alert and responsive, an EMT should
  A. passively rewarm the extremities.
  B. provide the patient with stimulants.
  C. get the patient to walk around.
  D. actively rewarm the patient.

_____ 5. Rough handling of a patient with hypothermia may result in
  A. apnea. C. blood clots.
  B. ventricular fibrillation. D. seizures.

_____ 6. Superficial local cold injuries are sometimes referred to as
  A. "white nose." C. hyperthermia.
  B. frost touch. D. frostbite.

_____ 7. All the following are signs and symptoms you might expect to find in a heat emergency patient with hot, dry skin *except*
  A. rapid, shallow breathing. C. dilated pupils.
  B. generalized weakness. D. heavy perspiration.

_____ 8. To rapidly cool a patient with a hyperthermic emergency, apply ice packs to the neck, groin, and
  A. wrists. B. armpits.
  C. knees. D. ankles.

_____ 9. The mildest form of hyperthermia is called
  A. heat exhaustion. C. heat stroke.
  B. heat cramps. D. fever.

_____ **10.** All of the following are factors that put a patient at risk for generalized hyperthermia *except*

    A. environment.   **C.** age.

    B. diet.   **D.** drugs and poisons.

_____ **11.** Hot skin that is either dry or moist represents

    A. a dire emergency.   **C.** heat cramps.

    B. heat exhaustion.   **D.** a stable patient.

IN THE FIELD

Read the following real-life situation. Then answer the questions that follow.

It is an overcast March afternoon when you are dispatched to a call for a woman who has fallen at 45 Standish Street. The temperature is in the 30s, with gusty winds. Banks of dirty snow from last week's storm still line the streets and sidewalks.

1. What might the information from dispatch plus the weather conditions lead you to expect at this call?

2. A police car is on the scene when you arrive. The officers assure you that the scene is safe. One officer says he'll lead you to the patient, who has fallen in a snowdrift near the garbage can next to the garage. Given what you know of the situation to this point and given that the police are on the scene, what step might you take to prepare for this patient before leaving the ambulance?

3. Behind the house, you see a woman apparently in her 60s, lying just off an icy set of steps in a snow bank. She is wearing only a housecoat and slippers. What injury possibilities do these circumstances suggest? What actions should you take before proceeding further in your assessment?

4. As you proceed, you discover that the woman is not alert, but does respond inappropriately to loudly spoken questions. She is not shivering, and the skin on her abdomen is cool to the touch. She has a blood pressure of 102/60, a heart rate of 60, and a respiration rate of 14. Her skin is pale, cool, and firm to the touch. What do these findings indicate? How should you proceed?

CHAPTER 22 REVIEW

Write the word or words that best complete each sentence in the space provided.

1. The mechanism of _____ causes body heat to be lost through direct contact.

2. The process of _____ causes cold air molecules that are in immediate contact with the skin to be warmed.

3. The most significant mechanism of heat loss is _____, which involves the transfer of heat from the surface of one object to the surface of another without physical contact.

4. Most radiant heat loss occurs from a person's _____, _____, and _____.

5. The process in which a liquid or solid changes to a vapor is called _____.

6. _____ causes loss of body heat as a result of exhaled warm air.

7. When cooling affects the entire body, a problem known as _____ _____ develops.

8. Application of an external heat source to the body is known as _____ _____.

9. _____ _____ is taking measures to prevent further heat loss and giving the patient's body the optimum chance to rewarm itself.

10. _____ _____ _____ results from the freezing of body tissue.

11. Another name for late or deep local cold injuries is _____.

12. Heat-related emergencies are grouped under the name _____.

13. The patient with a(n) _____ _____ _____, who also has hot skin, should be considered a priority patient.

14. Always transport a hyperthermic patient with hot skin that is _____ or _____.

15. Apply a(n) _____ _____ to an insect bite or sting to help relieve pain and swelling.

16. Do not apply cold to bites of _____ or to injuries inflicted by

 _____ _____.

17. The _____ _____ _____

 is characterized by a shiny black body, thin legs, and a crimson red marking on its abdomen, usually

 in the shape of an hourglass or two triangles.

18. The _____ _____ gets its name from the intense,

 fiery, burning pain its bite causes.

19. The two classes of poisonous snakes in the United States are _____

 _____ and _____ _____.

20. Soaking the affected area in _____ water for 30 minutes or throughout

 transport will help break down venom from a marine bite or sting.

ENVIRONMENTAL EMERGENCIES: TRUE OR FALSE

Indicate if the following statements are true or false by writing T or F in the space provided.

_____ **1.** Shivering is one of the body's compensatory mechanisms.

_____ **2.** Water chill, which happens when the body or clothes get wet, is an example of convectional cooling.

_____ **3.** Administering a drink of alcohol is an effective way to reduce the effects of hypothermia.

_____ **4.** In all cases of hypothermia, an EMT should begin active rewarming with the extremities.

_____ **5.** If clothing is frozen to the skin, it should be left in place.

_____ **6.** All heat emergency patients should be allowed to drink cool water.

_____ **7.** A patient with hot skin that is either moist or dry represents a dire medical emergency.

_____ **8.** Snakebites are relatively uncommon, and the number of people who die from them each year is extremely small.

_____ **9.** Black widow spider bites are the leading cause of death from spider bites in the United States.

_____ **10.** The bite of the brown recluse spider is a serious medical condition that usually does not heal and may require surgical repair.

Environmental Emergencies

Heat and Cold Emergencies
Regulation of Temperature

Exposure to Cold
Generalized Hypothermia

Immersion

Hypothermia

Local Cold Injury

Assessment and Care for
Generalized Hypothermia

Assessment and Care for
Immersion Hypothermia

Assessment and Care for Local
Cold Injury

Exposure to Heat
Hyperthermia

Assessment and Care

- Patient with moist, pale,
  normal-to-cool skin
- Patient with hot skin, dry or
  moist

Bites and Stings
Assessment and Care

Enrichment
Lightning Strike Injuries

Assessment and Care

Snakebite

- Coral snakes
- Pit vipers

Insect Bites and Stings
- Black widow spiders
- Brown recluse spiders
- Scorpions
- Fire ants
- Ticks

Marine Life Bites and Stings

CHAPTER 22 ANSWER KEY

HANDOUT 22-2: Chapter 22 Quiz

1. A	**4.** D	**7.** D	**10.** B
2. B	**5.** B	**8.** B	**11.** A
3. A	**6.** D	**9.** B	

HANDOUT 22-3: In the Field

1. The fall coupled with the cold conditions should at least suggest the possibility of hypothermia.

2. Because you suspect the possibility of hypothermia and because police are present to secure the vehicle, you could leave the motor running and the heat turned up to high in the patient compartment.

3. The circumstances make the possibility of hypothermia even higher. In addition, because the woman is in her 60s and has suffered a fall, you would want to take in-line manual stabilization as a precaution. To try to protect her from the cold, you would, while maintaining manual stabilization, log roll her onto her side and slip a blanket under her before proceeding with the assessment. You will also want to immobilize her to a long board before transport.

4. Your findings indicate severe hypothermia. This is a priority patient. You should load the patient into the ambulance to prevent further heat loss (taking precautions noted above). Handle the patient as gently as possible to prevent the potential cardiac dysrhythmia, ventricular fibrillation. You should ensure an open airway and provide oxygen at 15 liters per minute (warmed and humidified, if possible) via nonrebreather mask. Wrap her in blankets and transport immediately.

HANDOUT 22-4: Chapter 22 Review

1. conduction
2. convection
3. radiation
4. neck, head, feet
5. evaporation
6. Respiration
7. generalized hypothermia
8. active rewarming
9. Passive rewarming
10. Local cold injury
11. frostbite
12. hyperthermia
13. altered mental status
14. moist, dry
15. cold pack
16. snakes, marine life
17. black widow spider
18. fire ant
19. pit vipers, coral snakes
20. hot

HANDOUT 22-5: Environmental Emergencies: True or False

1. T	**4.** F	**7.** T	**9.** T
2. F	**5.** T	**8.** T	**10.** T
3. F	**6.** F		

©2008 by Pearson Education, Inc.
Prehospital Emergency Care, 8th ed.

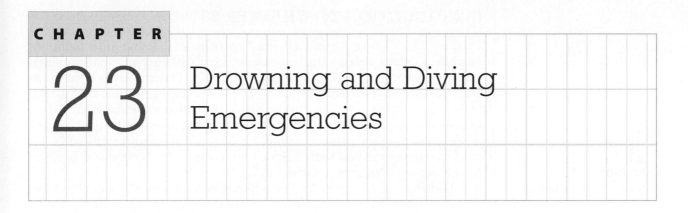

CHAPTER

23 | Drowning and Diving Emergencies

This chapter covers portions of Lesson 4-7 and Lesson 4-10 of the U.S. Department of Transportation's EMT-Basic National Standard Curriculum.

OBJECTIVES

Numbered objectives are from the U.S. Department of Transportation's EMT-Basic National Standard Curriculum. Asterisked objectives, if any, pertain to material that is supplemental to the DOT curriculum. Page numbers refer to pages in the textbook.

Cognitive

4-7.6 Recognize the signs and symptoms of water-related emergencies. (pp. 655, 657–658, 664–665)

4-7.7 Describe the complications of drowning. (pp. 653–654, 655–658)

Psychomotor

4-7.11 Demonstrate the assessment and emergency medical care of a drowning patient.

4-7.12 Demonstrate completing a prehospital care report for patients with environmental emergencies.

Additional objectives from DOT Lesson 4-7 are addressed in Chapter 22, "Environmental Emergencies."

REVIEW

In the last lesson, students learned that a number of situations faced by EMTs are termed "environmental emergencies." These are conditions brought on or worsened by some element or combination of elements in the patient's natural surroundings. Such emergencies can arise from interaction with the climate, as in exposure to excessive cold or heat. They can also be brought on by contact with creatures living in the environment, as in the bites or stings of snakes, spiders and insects, or marine animals. Because environmental emergencies often occur in isolated areas without ready access to a hospital emergency department, it is important that the EMT learn how to assess and provide on-scene or en route emergency medical care for patients affected by environmental emergencies.

Distribute the scored quizzes from the last class. Go over each quiz question, and handle any concerns students may have about the answers.

Total Teaching Time
85 minutes

Resources Needed
- Scored Chapter 22 Quizzes
- Guest who has had a drowning experience that was managed by the EMS system. The guest should be emotionally and physically recovered enough to comfortably share his or her experience. Consider providing an honorarium to the guest in appreciation for contribution.

Additional Resources
Larmon/Davis, *Basic Life Support Skills*

Elling, *EMT Achieve: Basic Test Preparation*

Limmer/Mistovich/ O'Keefe, *Audio Lecture & Study Guide: EMT*

Mistovich/Kuvlesky, *SUCCESS! for the EMT, Second Edition*

INTRODUCTION TO CHAPTER 23

Chapter 23, "Drowning and Diving Emergencies," is the 12th lesson of Module 4. Water-related incidents make up a category of environmental emergencies posing special challenges for EMTs. Patients in such incidents often sustain life-threatening injuries. They need emergency medical care as rapidly as possible. But the circumstances in which patients receive their injuries may expose medical personnel attempting to assist them to the risk of injury. Caring for patients in such circumstances requires of EMTs not only emergency medical skills but also the ability to recognize and avoid or reduce potential hazards at the scene.

Distribute the Chapter 23 Objectives Checklist and give students a few minutes to look it over. Then briefly paraphrase the objectives for this lesson in your own words.

LECTURE

The following suggested lecture outline is based on the Department of Transportation's EMT-Basic National Standard Curriculum. In some places, the DOT curriculum has been rearranged or expanded upon so that it is more complete or easier for the student to understand. The page numbers in parentheses refer to pages in the textbook. The parenthetical references in dark, heavy type are to figures, tables, and scans in the textbook.

DROWNING AND DIVING EMERGENCIES

I. **Water-related emergencies** (pp. 652–660)
   A. Drowning (pp. 653–656)
      1. An incident in which someone is submersed or immersed in a liquid that results in a primary reparatory impairment. **(Fig. 23-1, p. 654)**
      2. Major causes
         a. Getting exhausted in the water
         b. Losing control and getting swept into water that is too deep
         c. Losing a support (such as a sinking boat)
         d. Getting trapped or entangled while in the water
         e. Using drugs or alcohol before getting in the water
         f. Suffering seizures while in the water
         g. Using poor judgment while in the water
         h. Suffering hypothermia
         i. Suffering trauma
         j. Having a diving accident
      3. Safety measures in water-related emergencies
         a. Basic rule
            (1) Unless the water emergency occurs in open, shallow water that has a stable, uniform bottom, never go out into the water to attempt a rescue unless you meet all of the following criteria
         b. You are a good swimmer.
         c. You are specially trained in water-rescue techniques.
         d. You are wearing a personal flotation device.
         e. You are accompanied by other rescuers.
      4. Responsive patient close to shore
         a. Use reach, throw, row, go strategy **(Fig. 23-2, p. 656)**
      5. Unresponsive patient or out of reach with a line

    a. Row to patient in boat. (**Fig. 23-3, p. 656**)
    b. Wade to patient.
    c. Swim to patient.
    d. Use a float board.
  6. Possible spine injury
    a. Suspect a spine injury if swimmer may have been in a diving accident or struck by a boat, water skier, surfboard, or other object.
    b. Suspect a spine injury in any unresponsive swimmer, especially one in shallow, warm water.
    c. If a suspected spine injury, support the back and stabilize the head and neck as other care is given.
B. Resuscitation (pp. 656–657)
  1. Mammalian diving reflex
    a. Reflex that can prevent death in a cold water (below 70° F or 21° C) submersion
    b. When the face is submerged in cold water
      (1) Breathing is inhibited.
      (2) Heart rate slows.
      (3) Blood vessels throughout most of body constrict.
      (4) Blood flow to heart and brain is maintained. (The colder the water, the more oxygen is diverted to the heart and brain.)
    c. Reflex more pronounced and cooling is more rapid, in the young (whose skin surface is greater relative to their body mass).
  2. Attempt resuscitation on any pulseless, nonbreathing patient who has been submerged in cold water.
  3. Seek medical direction and follow local protocol.
C. Assessment and care: water-related emergencies (pp. 657–660) (**Figs. 23-4, p. 659, 23-5, pp. 661–662, and 23-6, p. 663**)
  1. Scene size-up
    a. Study the scene to make sure that it is safe to enter.
    b. Wear a PFD anytime you are within 10 feet of water's edge.
    c. Do not enter water to rescue patient unless you are a capable swimmer, and you will not be putting yourself in danger.
    d. Take appropriate BSI precautions.
    e. Size up the scene to determine number of patients.
    f. Call for expert or extra assistance if required.
  2. Initial assessment
    a. Assess level of responsiveness and document it.
    b. Note reaction to painful stimuli in all four extremities.
    c. Assess airway, keeping in mind potential for spinal injury.
    d. Suction water, vomitus, and secretions from airway, inserting oral or nasal airway if the airway cannot be managed with manual maneuvers.
    e. Check breathing to be sure respirations are present and adequate.
    f. Assess for any open wounds to the chest that would impede breathing.
    g. If breathing is adequate, administer oxygen via nonrebreather mask.

On the Net
Statistics and information about drowning prevention. http://www.cdc.gov/ncipc/factsheets/drown.htm

Point to Emphasize
No one should be considered dead unless he or she is warm and dead. Don't give up. Resuscitation has been documented at a temperature as low as 18–20° C (66.2–68° F).

    h. If breathing is inadequate, provide positive-pressure ventilation with supplemental oxygen.

    i. Check circulation to make sure that patient has a pulse and that no life-threatening external bleeding needs to be controlled.

    j. Assess for signs or symptoms of internal bleeding or hypoperfusion (shock).

    k. Determine transport priority; give highest priority to
- **(1)** Patients with high spinal injuries affecting respirations
- **(2)** Patients with respiratory distress
- **(3)** Unresponsive patients

3. Focused history and physical exam

    a. Conduct rapid assessment.

    b. If patient is alert, conduct SAMPLE history and a focused physical exam.

    c. Look for signs or symptoms of any of the following injuries or medical problems
- **(1)** Airway obstruction
- **(2)** Absent or inadequate breathing
- **(3)** Pulselessness (cardiac arrest)
- **(4)** Spinal injury or head injury
- **(5)** Soft-tissue or musculoskeletal injuries
- **(6)** External or internal bleeding
- **(7)** Shock
- **(8)** Hypothermia
- **(9)** Alcohol or drug abuse
- **(10)** Drowning

4. Emergency medical care—drowning

    a. Responsive patient with suspected spinal injury
- **(1)** Apply manual in-line stabilization and remove patient from water on backboard.

    b. Patient with no suspected spinal injury
- **(1)** Place patient on left side to allow water, vomitus, and secretions to drain from upper airway.

    c. Suction as needed.

    d. Establish an airway, and begin positive pressure ventilations with supplemental oxygen.

    e. Once you have determined that there are no foreign objects in the airway, apply ventilations with more force until you see patient's chest rise and fall.

    f. If patient is pulseless and apneic and qualifies for AED, proceed with the AED protocol.
- **(1)** If patient is also hypothermic, deliver only three individual shocks.
- **(2)** If unsuccessful, continue with CPR and transport immediately.

    g. If gastric distention interferes with your ability to ventilate the patient, place patient on his left side and—if suction is immediately available—place your hand over the epigastric area of patient's abdomen and apply firm pressure to relieve the distention.

    h. Manage the resultant regurgitation by turning patient on his side (turning the patient and backboard as a unit if immobilized) and using suction.

i. Manage any other medical or trauma conditions associated with the drowning event.

   j. Transport patient as quickly as possible, continuing resuscitative measures during transport, keeping patient warm, and providing high-flow oxygen.

5. Detailed physical exam and ongoing assessment

   a. If time and patient's condition permit, perform a detailed physical exam.

   b. Be alert for signs that the patient is deteriorating into respiratory or cardiac arrest.

   c. Unstable patient

      (1) Perform the ongoing assessment (repeating initial assessment, focused history, physical exam and vital signs, and checking interventions) every 5 minutes.

   d. Stable patient

      (1) Perform the ongoing assessment every 15 minutes.

ENRICHMENT (OPTIONAL)

The following sections contain information that is valuable as background for the EMT, but that goes substantially beyond the U.S. Department of Transportation's EMT-Basic National Standard Curriculum.

II. Scuba or deep-water diving emergencies (pp. 660–666)

  A. Decompression sickness (bends) (pp. 662–665)

  B. Arterial gas embolism (p. 665)

  C. Barotrauma (p. 665)

  D. Emergency medical care (pp. 665–666)

    1. Keep patient in supine position if spine injury is suspected or if patient is alert. If no spine injury but patient has an altered mental status, place him in a lateral recumbent position.

    2. Administer oxygen at 15 liters per minute by nonrebreather mask or positive-pressure ventilation with supplemental oxygen as appropriate.

    3. Initiate CPR and apply AED, if needed.

    4. Transport patient immediately.

    5. Try to obtain the patient's diving log and transport it to the hospital with patient.

    6. Contact medical direction to consider transporting to a facility with a recompression chamber.

CASE STUDY FOLLOW-UP

Ask a student volunteer to read the Case Study that begins on page 652 of the textbook. You may wish to use the following questions to engage students in a discussion of the Case Study Follow-up that begins on page 666 of the textbook. Provide missing information and clarify ideas as needed.

Q1. According to the manager, what is the probable mechanism of injury?

A1. *According to the manager, the patient had been drinking and suddenly dived into the shallow end of the pool.*

On the Net
For more about the Diver Alert Network (DAN), go to: www. diversalertnetwork.org

On the Net
SCUBA Diving Emergencies. www.diversalertnetwork .org/medical/faq/index.asp

Reading/Reference
Margolis, G. et al., "The Pressure Is On: Hyperbaric Oxygen Treatment as an Adjunct to Prehospital Care," *JEMS,* May 2000.

Q2. How do you extricate Robby from the pool while protecting his spinal column?

A2. *A lifeguard's float board is maneuvered into position under Robby. Robby's torso is immobilized, a cervical spinal immobilization collar is applied, and Robby is immobilized to the board. Then the board is gently pushed to the side of the pool, where, with the assistance of the employee and two police officers, the board and Robby are removed as a unit from the water.*

Q3. Describe the results of your detailed physical exam in regard to Robby's lower extremities.

A3. *The extremities show good pulses. However, there is no voluntary motor function and Robby cannot feel anything in either hand or foot.*

Q4. How do you react when Robby vomits?

A4. *The nonrebreather mask is removed and the board is turned so that Robby is on his left side. Suction equipment is used to clear his mouth and airway as he vomits, after which he is returned to the normal position.*

Q5. What is Robby's prognosis according to the emergency department physician?

A5. *He is not optimistic about the possibility that Robby will walk again.*

IN REVIEW

Assess students' ability to apply what they have just learned by discussing the Review Questions on page 668 in the textbook.

Q1. List at least five common causes of drowning.

A1. *Common causes of drowning include: (1) getting exhausted in the water; (2) losing control and getting swept into water that is too deep; (3) losing a support (such as a sinking boat); (4) getting trapped or entangled while in the water; (5) suffering seizures while in the water; (6) using poor judgment in the water; (7) suffering hypothermia; (8) suffering trauma; and (9) having a diving accident. (pp. 653–656)*

Q2. Explain the conditions that must apply before an EMT enters the water to attempt a rescue.

A2. *The conditions that must apply before an EMT enters the water to attempt a rescue are that the body of water must be open, shallow, and have a stable, uniform bottom. If those conditions are not met, the EMT must never go into the water unless the following criteria are met: the EMT must be a good swimmer, must be specially trained in water rescue, must be wearing a PFD, and must be accompanied by other rescuers. (p. 655)*

Q3. Describe the four basic methods used in attempting to rescue a patient from the water.

A3. *The four basic methods used in attempting to rescue a patient from the water are "reach, throw, row, and go": (1) try to reach the patient with some object and pull him ashore; (2) throw the patient an object that will float attached to a rope and pull him to shore; (3) row out to the patient in a boat; (4) go into the water to reach the patient by wading or swimming. (p. 655)*

©2008 by Pearson Education, Inc.
Prehospital Emergency Care, 8th ed.

Q4. Explain why patients who have been submerged in cold water can often be resuscitated after 30 minutes or more.

A4. *Patients who have been submerged in cold water can often be resuscitated after 30 minutes or more because, in cold water, the body's mammalian diving reflex kicks in, restricting blood flow to the extremities, but maintaining it to the heart and brain, increasing the likelihood of resuscitating the patient, even after prolonged immersion. (pp. 656–657)*

Q5. List the injuries and medical problems whose signs and symptoms the EMT should be alert for when assessing the water-related emergency patient.

A5. *Injuries and medical problems whose signs and symptoms the EMT should be alert for when assessing the water-related emergency patient include airway obstruction, absent or inadequate breathing, pulselessness (cardiac arrest), spinal injury or head injury, soft-tissue injuries, musculoskeletal injuries, external or internal bleeding, shock, hypothermia, alcohol or drug abuse, and drowning. (pp. 657–658)*

Q6. List the steps for removing a drowning patient with a possible spine injury from the water.

A6. *The steps for removing a drowning patient with a possible spine injury from the water are as follows: (1) Apply manual in-line stabilization and if patient is not breathing, begin rescue breathing using a pocket mask; (2) slide a backboard under the patient and secure the torso and legs to it; (3) apply a cervical spinal immobilization collar and head immobilization device; (4) float the board to the water's edge and remove the patient on the board from the water. (p. 658)*

Q7. List the steps of emergency medical care for a drowning patient that should take place after the patient is removed from the water and, if necessary, immobilized to a spine board.

A7. *The steps of emergency medical care for a drowning patient that should take place after the patient is removed from the water and, if necessary, immobilized to a spine board are (1) place patient on side and suction as needed; (2) establish an airway, begin positive-pressure ventilation with supplemental oxygen; (3) apply an AED, if needed and if patient qualifies for its use (follow local protocols); (4) relieve gastric distention, if necessary; (5) transport rapidly. (pp. 658–660)*

CRITICAL THINKING

Assess students' ability to respond to real-life emergency situations by discussing the Critical Thinking questions on page 668 in the textbook.

Q1. How would you proceed with the emergency care of the patient?

A1. *After immediately removing the patient from the cold environment and removing his wet clothes, place him on his left side so that any water, vomitus, or secretions can drain from his upper airway, place him back into a supine position, and suction as necessary. Next, establish an airway using a head-tilt chin-lift maneuver or a jaw thrust maneuver if there is any suspicion of a spine injury, insert an oropharyngeal airway, and begin positive pressure ventilation with supplemental oxygen connected to the ventilation device. The EMTs should then immediately begin CPR. After 5 cycles of CPR, apply the AED and follow the AED protocol for hypothermic patients. Watch for* *(and treat) severe gastric distention and transport without delay while continuing resuscitative efforts.*

Q2. Would you apply the AED and proceed with defibrillation?

A2. *The AED must be applied; however, because the cardiac arrest was not witnessed or it may have been greater than 4 to 5 minutes since the cardiac arrest, perform 5 cycles of CPR prior to activating the AED. Even though the patient is only 4 years of age, an adult AED and pads can be used if a pediatric attenuating system is not available. Because of the probability of hypothermia, only one shock should be delivered. If it is not successful, CPR should be continued and the patient should be transported immediately.*

Q3. What are some other special considerations when managing this patient?

A3. *There are numerous special considerations related to managing this patient, but the following should all be included: the ambient temperature, the patient's core temperature, the patient's age, the temperature of the water (and its affect on resuscitation), and the AED protocol for hypothermic patients.*

GUEST PRESENTATION AND DIALOGUE

Arrange to have a guest speaker who has experienced a drowning. Explain that you are now going to turn the class over to a person who has actually experienced a drowning emergency. Ask students to write down any questions that come to mind while the guest is sharing his or her experience. Tell students that they will have an opportunity to ask their questions after the presentation.

Introduce the guest by name. Allow the guest to share his or her drowning experience.

After the presentation, invite students to ask questions. Deflect questions that are too personal. Provide clarification of any questions beyond the medical knowledge of the guest.

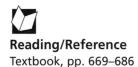

Reading/Reference
Textbook, pp. 669–686

Workbook
Chapter 23 Activities

Chapter Quiz
Handout 23-2

TestGen
Chapter 23 Test

Online Test Preparation
Send your students to
http://www.prenhall.com/
EMTAchieve

ASSIGNMENTS

Assign Chapter 24, "Behavioral Emergencies," to be read before the next class. Also ask students to complete Chapter 23 of the Workbook.

EVALUATION

Chapter Quiz Distribute copies of the Chapter Quiz provided in Handout 23-2 to evaluate student understanding of this chapter. Remind students not to refer to their textbooks or notes while taking the quiz.

Test Manager You may wish to create a custom-tailored test using Prentice Hall *TestGen for Prehospital Emergency Care, Eighth Edition* to evaluate student understanding of this chapter.

Online Test Preparation (for students and instructors) Additional test preparation is available through *EMT Achieve: Basic Test Preparation* at http://www.prenhall.com/EMTAchieve. Instructors can also monitor student mastery online.

©2008 by Pearson Education, Inc.
Prehospital Emergency Care, 8th ed.

REINFORCEMENT

Handouts If classroom discussions or performance on the quiz indicates that some students have not fully mastered the chapter content, you may wish to assign some or all of the Reinforcement Handouts for this chapter.

TECH EXTRAS

Brady Skills Series EMT-B Videos/CD Have your students watch the skills come to life on either VHS or CD-ROM.

PowerPoint Presentation (for instructors) The PowerPoint material developed for this chapter offers useful reinforcement of chapter content.

Student CD A wide variety of material on this CD-ROM will reinforce and also expand student knowledge and skills.

Companion Website (for students) Additional review quizzes and links to EMS resources will contribute to further reinforcement of this chapter. Please visit http://www.prenhall.com/mistovich.

Handouts 23-3 to 23-5
Reinforcement Activities

Brady Skills Series EMT-B Videos/CD
Visual Reinforcement

PowerPoint Presentation
Chapter 23

Student CD
Chapter 23

Companion Website
http://www.prenhall.com/mistovich

OBJECTIVES CHECKLIST

OBJECTIVES

Cognitive	Date Mastered
4-7.6 Recognize the signs and symptoms of water-related emergencies.	
4-7.7 Describe the complications of drowning.	

Psychomotor	Date Mastered
4.7.11 Demonstrate the assessment and emergency medical care of a drowning patient.	
4.7.12 Demonstrate completing a prehospital care report for patients with environmental emergencies.	

CHAPTER 23 QUIZ

Write the letter of the best answer in the space provided.

_____ 1. The term _____ describes a drowning event where a patient is pronounced dead within 24 hours of the event.
   A. drowning   C. water rescue
   B. submersion   D. drowning-related death

_____ 2. Death that occurs 24 hours after a drowning is called a
   A. drowning.   C. water rescue.
   B. submersion.   D. drowning-related death.

_____ 3. If a swimmer may have been involved in a diving accident or may have been struck by a boat, water skier, surfboard, or another object, the EMT should suspect
   A. spinal injury.   C. ARDS.
   B. air embolism.   D. hypothermia.

_____ 4. A condition in which the stomach fills with water, enlarging the abdomen to the point that it interferes with the ability to inflate the lungs, is called
   A. hydrothorax.   C. distended pleura.
   B. water in the lungs.   D. gastric distention.

_____ 5. As a guideline, the EMT should attempt resuscitation on any pulseless, nonbreathing patient who has been submerged in _____ water, even if the drowning has been longer than 30 minutes.
   A. warm   C. fresh
   B. cold   D. salt

_____ 6. All of the following are signs and symptoms of arterial gas embolism *except*
   A. dizziness.   C. chest pain.
   B. delayed onset.   D. difficulty breathing.

_____ 7. If you suspect that a patient has a spine injury, maintain in-line stabilization and then secure the patient to a backboard before
   A. evaluating breathing.   C. starting rescue breathing.
   B. starting CPR.   D. removing from water.

_____ 8. Signs and symptoms of barotrauma include all of the following *except*
   A. extreme dizziness.   C. nausea.
   B. palpitations.   D. disorientation.

_____ 9. Decompression sickness may occur up to _____ following a dive.
   A. 2 days   C. one week
   B. 72 hours   D. two weeks

_____ 10. The most important factor in determining whether EMTs enter the water to rescue a patient is
   A. the quality of their equipment.
   B. their training.
   C. the depth of the water.
   D. their ability to use a rowboat.

IN THE FIELD

Read the following real-life situation. Then answer the question that follows.

It is 1400 in the afternoon and you and your partner are dispatched to a local neighborhood for a possible drowned child. As you arrive, you note that the police are already on the scene. One officer leads you to the backyard where another officer is performing CPR on a small child. A young woman is standing nearby. The officer explains that the 2-year-old had apparently snuck out of the house and had fallen in the pool. It is estimated that the child had been in the water for about 20 minutes before being discovered by the babysitter. Your partner instructs the officer to stop CPR, verifies that the child is apneic and pulseless, and then resumes CPR.

1. What additional actions should you and your partner take?

©2008 by Pearson Education, Inc.
Prehospital Emergency Care, 8th ed.

CHAPTER 23 REVIEW

Write the word or words that best complete each sentence in the space provided.

1. The term _____ describes a drowning where a patient is pronounced dead within 24 hours of the event.

2. Drownings can be additionally complicated in cases where _____ is involved, which can produce additional trauma.

3. The EMT should always assume that a diver has sustained _____ injuries.

4. If a patient is responsive and close to shore, use the _____, _____, _____, and _____ strategy.

5. In the case of a drowning involving a possible spine injury, the goal is to support the back and stabilize the _____ and _____ as other care is provided.

6. When a person dives into cold water, the _____ diving reflex can prevent death, even after prolonged submersion.

7. Some experts advise _____ _____ for every drowning patient, regardless of water temperature, even those who have been in the water for a prolonged period.

8. A(n) _____ _____ _____ is a blocking of blood vessels by an air bubble or clusters of air bubbles.

9. The signs and symptoms of an arterial gas embolism have a(n) _____ _____.

10. _____ sickness usually occurs when a diver ascends too quickly from a deep, prolonged dive.

REINFORCEMENT

DROWNING AND DIVING EMERGENCIES: TRUE OR FALSE

Indicate if the following statements are true or false by writing T or F in the space provided.

_____ **1.** Drowning is the leading cause of accidental death in children under age 5.

_____ **2.** Drownings always occur in large bodies of water.

_____ **3.** The best prognosis for drowning patients occurs among those who are submerged in warm, dirty, or brackish (salty) water.

_____ **4.** During resuscitation of a drowning patient, gastric distention should be relieved whether or not it interferes with ventilations.

_____ **5.** Drowning patients may be unresponsive, not breathing, or pulseless, or they may be responsive and possibly gasping or coughing up water.

_____ **6.** In a water-related emergency, the EMT must reach the patient as soon as possible without regard for personal safety to initiate life-saving measures.

_____ **7.** Injuries to the cervical spine are seen with many water-related accidents.

_____ **8.** The onset of decompression sickness may occur up to 72 hours after a dive.

_____ **9.** Divers with upper respiratory infections or allergies are at increased risk of barotrauma.

_____ **10.** Provision of oxygen is critical in cases of decompression sickness because it reduces the size of nitrogen bubbles and improves circulation.

LECTURE MASTER 23

Drowning and Diving Emergencies

Water-Related Emergencies
Incidence of Drowning

Overview of Disease Process

Diving Emergencies

Safety Measures

Spine Injury

Resuscitation

Assessment and Care

Scuba or Deep-Water Diving Emergencies
Decompression Sickness

Arterial Gas Embolism

Barotrauma

HANDOUT 23-2: Chapter 23 Quiz

1. A	**4.** D	**7.** D	**9.** B
2. D	**5.** B	**8.** B	**10.** B
3. A	**6.** B		

HANDOUT 23-3: In the Field

1. It is not known how the child fell into the water, and spinal injuries have to be suspected. The head and neck must be stabilized and the child secured to a backboard. As rapidly as possible, an airway should be established (suction as needed) and positive-pressure ventilations initiated. If gastric distention interferes with ventilations, it must be relieved. Manage any other trauma conditions and transport the patient as quickly as possible, continuing resuscitative measures during transport.

HANDOUT 23-4: Chapter 23 Review

1. Drowning
2. diving
3. spine
4. reach, throw, row, go
5. head, neck
6. mammalian
7. artificial ventilation (or positive-pressure ventilation)
8. arterial gas embolism
9. rapid onset
10. Decompression sickness

HANDOUT 23-5: Drowning and Diving Emergencies: True of False

1. F	**4.** F	**7.** T	**9.** T
2. F	**5.** T	**8.** T	**10.** T
3. F	**6.** F		

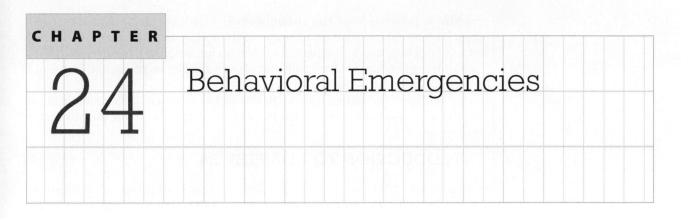

24 Behavioral Emergencies

This chapter covers Lesson 4-8 and portions of Lesson 4-10 of the U.S. Department of Transportation's EMT-Basic National Standard Curriculum.

OBJECTIVES

Numbered objectives are from the U.S. Department of Transportation's EMT-Basic National Standard Curriculum. Asterisked objectives, if any, pertain to material that is supplemental to the DOT curriculum. Page numbers refer to pages in the textbook.

Cognitive

4-8.1   Define behavioral emergencies. (p. 671)

4-8.2   Discuss the general factors that may cause an alteration in a patient's behavior. (p. 671)

4-8.3   State the various reasons for psychological crises. (pp. 671–673)

4-8.4   Discuss the characteristics of an individual's behavior that suggest that the patient is at risk for suicide. (pp. 672–673)

4-8.5   Discuss special medical/legal considerations for managing behavioral emergencies. (pp. 683–684)

4-8.6   Discuss the special considerations for assessing a patient with behavioral problems. (pp. 675–678, 679)

4-8.7   Discuss the general principles of an individual's behavior that suggest that he or she is at risk for violence. (pp. 672–673)

4-8.8   Discuss methods to calm behavioral emergency patients. (pp. 673–674)

Affective

4-8.9   Explain the rationale for learning how to modify your behavior toward the patient with a behavioral emergency. (p. 673)

Psychomotor

4-8.10   Demonstrate the assessment and emergency medical care of the patient experiencing a behavioral emergency.

4-8.11   Demonstrate various techniques to safely restrain a patient with a behavioral problem.

REVIEW

In the last lesson, "Drowning and Diving Emergencies," students learned that water-related incidents make up a category of environmental emergencies posing special challenges for EMTs. Patients in such incidents often sustain life-threatening injuries. They need emergency medical care as

Total Teaching Time
180 minutes

Resources Needed
- Scored Chapter 23 Quizzes
- Set of restraining devices approved for use in your area
- Complete jump kit, including BSI equipment and refusal of treatment form
- Oxygen equipment
- Portable suction unit
- Stretcher

Additional Resources
Larmon/Davis, *Basic Life Support Skills*

Elling, *EMT Achieve: Basic Test Preparation*

Limmer/Mistovich/O'Keefe, *Audio Lecture & Study Guide: EMT*

Mistovich/Kuvlesky, *SUCCESS! for the EMT, Second Edition*

rapidly as possible. But the circumstances in which patients receive their injuries may expose medical personnel attempting to assist them to the risk of injury. Thus, caring for patients in such circumstances requires of EMTs not only emergency medical skills but also the ability to recognize and avoid or reduce potential hazards at the scene.

Distribute the scored quizzes from the last class. Go over each question on the quiz and handle any concerns students may have about the answers.

INTRODUCTION TO CHAPTER 24

Chapter 24, "Behavioral Emergencies," is the 13th lesson of Module 4. Emergency care for behavioral emergencies is different from emergency care for physical problems. You cannot readily see the comfort that your words or your mere presence provides to someone who is panicked or agitated. It is hard to gauge the immediate results of your care for someone who is depressed. But the care you give patients in behavioral emergencies can just as easily save lives as the care you give for physical problems.

Distribute the Chapter 24 Objectives Checklist and give students a few minutes to look it over. Then briefly paraphrase the objectives of this lesson in your own words.

LECTURE

The following suggested lecture outline is based on the Department of Transportation's EMT-Basic National Standard Curriculum. In some places, the DOT curriculum has been rearranged or expanded upon so that it is more complete or easier for the student to understand. The page numbers in parentheses refer to pages in the textbook. The parenthetical references in dark, heavy type are to figures, tables, and scans in the textbook.

BEHAVIORAL EMERGENCIES

I. Behavioral problems (p. 671)
  A. Behavior (p. 671)
    1. The way a person acts or performs
    2. Any or all of that person's activities and responses, especially those responses that can be observed
  B. Behavioral emergency (p. 671)
    1. Situation in which a person exhibits "abnormal" behavior that is unacceptable or intolerable to the patient, the family, or the community.
    2. The abnormal behavior that precipitates the emergency may be due to a psychological condition (such as a mental illness), to extremes of emotion, or even to a physical condition (such as lack of oxygen or low blood sugar)
II. Behavioral change (p. 671)
  A. A number of factors may cause a change in a person's behavior, among them situational stresses, medical illnesses, psychiatric problems, and alcohol or drugs. Below are some common reasons for behavioral change (p. 671)
    1. Low blood sugar in a person with diabetes
    2. Hypoxia (lack of oxygen)
    3. Inadequate blood flow to the brain
    4. Head trauma

Handout 24-1
Chapter 24 Objectives Checklist

● ➤
Lecture Master
You may wish to display Lecture Master 24 when presenting the lecture to the class.

Point to Emphasize
Always consider the possibility that the unusual behavior is caused by something other than a psychological problem.

5. Mind-altering substances
6. Psychogenic substances
7. Excessive cold or heat
8. Infections of the brain or its coverings

B. Be sure that problem is behavioral, not physical. Clues that the problem may be physical are: (p. 671)
1. Relatively sudden onset of symptoms
2. Visual but not auditory hallucinations
3. Memory loss or impairment
4. Dilated, constricted, or unequal pupils; or pupils that respond differently to light
5. Excessive salivation
6. Incontinence (loss of bladder or bowel control)
7. Unusual breath odor

C. Remember that behavioral changes and crises often follow (or are the result of) physical trauma or illness. (p. 671)

III. Psychiatric problems (pp. 671–672)
A. Anxiety (pp. 671–672)
1. State of painful uneasiness about impending problems
2. Agitation
3. Restlessness
4. Panic attack
    a. Intense fear, tension, or restlessness

B. Phobia (p. 672)
1. Irrational fear of specific thing, place, or situation
2. Is closely related to anxiety

C. Depression (p. 672)
1. Deep feelings of sadness, worthlessness, and discouragement
2. Is one of the most common psychiatric conditions
3. Is a factor in approximately 50 percent of all suicides

D. Bipolar disorder (manic-depressive disorder) (p. 672)
1. Patient swings to opposite sides of the mood spectrum, from inflated view of self to depressive state

E. Paranoia (p. 672)
1. Highly exaggerated or unwarranted mistrust or suspiciousness

F. Schizophrenia (p. 672)
1. Group of mental disorders
2. Rarely manifests as multiple-personality disorder as is commonly believed
3. Characterized distortions of speech and thought, bizarre delusions, hallucinations, social withdrawal, lack of emotional expressiveness

IV. Violence (pp. 672–673)
A. Suicide attempt (pp. 672–673)
1. Any willful act designed to end one's own life.
2. Men more successful but women make three times as many attempts.
3. More than half committed with firearms.
4. Drug ingestion and wrist slashing among most common unsuccessful attempts.
5. Tenth leading cause of death in the United States among all ages; second leading cause among college-age students.
6. At least half of successful suicides have attempted it previously.
7. Seventy-five percent give clear warning.

Teaching Tip
Ask students how many of them have experienced an anxiety attack. Ask them to describe what it felt like.

On the Net
For facts about depression and numerous links to other sites, go to: www.psych.helsinki.fi/~janne/asdfaq

On the Net
For the National Foundation for Depressive Illness, Inc., go to: www.depression.org

Point of Interest
Depression is the most common mental illness in the United States.

On the Net
For facts and resources about suicide and prevention, go to: www.spanusa.org

8. The four most common methods of suicide, in order:
   a. Self-inflicted gunshot wound
   b. Hanging
   c. Poisoning by ingestion
   d. Carbon monoxide poisoning
9. Too often dismissed as "just trying to get attention."
10. Take every suicidal act or gesture seriously and transport the patient for evaluation.
11. Statistical data about those most likely to take their own lives:
    a. Men over age 40 who are single, widowed, or divorced
    b. Men and women who are widowed or divorced
    c. Those with histories of alcoholism or drug abuse
    d. Those with severe depression
    e. Those who have formulated a highly lethal plan and who have told others about it (highest risk)
    f. Those who gather articles that could be used to commit suicide (purchasing a gun or stockpiling a large quantity of pills)
    g. Those with a previous history of self-destructive behavior
    h. Those recently diagnosed with a serious illness, particularly an illness that signals a loss of independence
    i. Those who have recently lost a loved one or who perceive that those to whom they are closely emotionally attached are in danger
    j. Those who have lost control or are unable to manage life (Arrest, imprisonment, and job loss are signs.)

B. Violence to others (p. 673)
   1. Sixty to 75 percent of all behavioral emergency patients will become assaultive or violent.
   2. Violence to others can be caused by the following:
      a. Patient mismanagement (real or perceived)
      b. Psychosis
      c. Alcohol or drug intoxication
      d. Fear
      e. Panic
      f. Head injury
   3. Early signs that a patient may become violent include:
      a. Nervous pacing
      b. Shouting
      c. Threatening
      d. Cursing
      e. Throwing objects
      f. Clenched teeth and/or fists

V. **Dealing with behavioral emergencies** (p. 673)
   A. Dealing with patients with behavioral emergencies requires extreme sensitivity. (p. 673)
   B. Basic principles (p. 673)
      1. Every person has limitations.
      2. Each person has a right to his or her feelings.
      3. Each person has more ability to cope with crisis than he or she might think.
      4. Everyone feels some emotional disturbance when involved in a disaster or when injured.
      5. Emotional injury is just as real as physical injury.

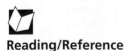

Reading/Reference
Tracy, S., "Emotional Medical Services," *JEMS,* Sept. 2000.

6. People who have been through a crisis do not just "get better."

7. Cultural differences have special meaning when you are called to intervene in behavioral emergencies.

VI. Techniques for treating behavioral emergency patients (pp. 673–674)

   A. Speak in a calm, reassuring voice directly to the patient. (p. 674)

   B. Maintain a comfortable distance between yourself and the patient. (p. 674) **(Fig. 24-1, p. 674)**

   C. Seek the patient's cooperation. (p. 674)

   D. Maintain good eye contact with the patient. (p. 674)

   E. Do not make any quick movements. (p. 674)

   F. Respond honestly to the patient's questions, but don't foster unrealistic expectations. (p. 674)

   G. Never threaten, challenge, belittle, or argue with disturbed patients. (p. 674)

   H. Always tell the truth; never lie to the patient. (p. 674)

   I. Do not "play along" with visual or auditory disturbances. (p. 674)

   J. When you can, involve trusted family members or friends. (p. 674)

   K. Be prepared to stay at the scene for a long time. (p. 674)

   L. Never leave the patient alone. (p. 674)

   M. Avoid the use of restraint. (p. 674)

   N. Do not force the patient to make decisions. (p. 674)

   O. Encourage the patient to participate in a motor activity that helps reduce anxiety. (p. 674)

   P. If the patient has attracted a crowd, do what you can to disperse it. (p. 674)

VII. Assessment and care: behavioral emergencies (pp. 674–682) **(Figs. 24-3 and 24-4, pp. 679–681)**

   A. Scene size-up (p. 675)

     1. Take steps to ensure your safety even before you arrive at the scene.

       a. Pay close attention to dispatch.

       b. Check with dispatch to see whether police are on the way.

       c. Begin scene size-up immediately upon arrival.

       d. Never enter a potentially violent situation without support.

     2. If you cannot guarantee your own safety, call the police and wait for them to arrive before you leave your vehicle.

     3. Be alert when responding to the scene of a suicide or potential suicide that you do not fall victim to the mechanism the patient planned to use to end his or her own life (carbon monoxide, gas, electrical devices, etc.)

     4. Locate the patient visually before you enter the scene. **(Fig. 24-2, p. 675)**

     5. Never let down your guard or turn your back on the patient.

     6. Scan quickly for instruments the patient may use to injure himself or others.

     7. If the patient displays a weapon, never ignore or disregard it.

     8. Stay outside the danger zone—for a knife, 22 feet; for a gun, much farther.

     9. Before physically approaching the patient, determine whether you and your partner can handle the situation alone.

On the Net
Behavioral emergencies.
www.psychguides.com/
Behavioral20Emergencies
.pdf

Point to Emphasize
Whenever called to care for a patient who has attempted or may be about to attempt suicide, the first concern must be personal safety.

©2008 by Pearson Education, Inc.
Prehospital Emergency Care, 8th ed.

10. Scan scene for signs of things that may have contributed to the crisis or that the patient might have used in a suicide attempt.
11. Study the scene for clues to the nature of the emergency, looking for a mechanism of injury or a sign of the nature of illness.
12. Always determine the number of patients, not automatically assuming there is just one.
13. Call for additional resources as needed.

B. Initial assessment (p. 676)
1. Gather a general impression of the patient.
2. Assess the patient's mental status by asking specific questions that will help you measure the patient's level of responsiveness and orientation.
3. Watch the patient's appearance, level of activity, and speech patterns.
4. Try to determine whether the patient is oriented to time, person, and place.
5. Pay particular attention to the patient's airway and breathing.
6. Be prepared to provide oxygen by nonrebreather mask at 15 liters per minute or positive-pressure ventilation with supplemental oxygen, if necessary.
7. If the patient has attempted suicide, make the medical problem rather than the behavioral problem your priority.

C. Focused history and physical exam (pp. 676–677)
1. Conduct the focused history and physical exam once any life threats have been managed.
2. Try to obtain a SAMPLE history if the patient is alert and has no significant injury.
3. Note carefully events leading to the emergency.
4. Inform the patient of what you are doing, and explain what is likely to be done to help.
5. Stay polite, use good manners, show respect, and make no unsupported assumptions.
6. Allow the patient to tell you what happened.
7. Avoid asking questions that can be answered with a simple "yes" or "no."
8. Show that you are listening by rephrasing or repeating part of what the patient says.
9. Determine the patient's chief complaint and then conduct a focused physical exam centered on those areas.
10. Take a set of baseline vital signs.
11. Follow the specific tips below for assessing suicidal patients:
    a. Make your primary concern injuries or medical conditions related to the suicide attempt.
    b. Listen carefully.
    c. Accept all the patient's complaints and feelings.
    d. Do not trust "rapid recoveries."
    e. Be specific in your actions.
    f. Never show disgust or horror when caring for the patient.
    g. Do not try to deny that the suicide attempt occurred.
    h. Never try to shock a patient out of a suicidal act.

12. Follow the guidelines below when assessing violent patients:
  a. Take a history from bystanders, family members, and friends at the scene.
  b. Look at the patient's posture.
  c. Listen to the patient.
  d. Monitor the patient's physical activity.
  e. Be firm and clear.
  f. Be prepared to use restraints, but only if necessary.

13. Signs and symptoms that may indicate a behavioral emergency:
  a. Fear
  b. Anxiety
  c. Confusion
  d. Behavioral changes
  e. Anger
  f. Mania
  g. Depression
  h. Withdrawal
  i. Loss of contact with reality
  j. Sleeplessness
  k. Loss of appetite
  l. Loss of sex drive
  m. Constipation
  n. Crying
  o. Tension
  p. Irritability

D. Emergency medical care (p. 677)
  1. Make your own safety your first priority.
  2. Assess the patient for trauma or a medical condition.
  3. Calm the patient and stay with the patient.
  4. If it is necessary to protect yourself and others, or the patient from harming herself, use restraints.
  5. Transport the patient to a facility where she can get physical and psychological treatment.

E. Detailed physical exam and ongoing assessment (p. 678)
  1. Perform a detailed physical exam en route to the hospital.
  2. Perform an ongoing assessment as warranted by the patient's condition.
  3. Monitor the patient's airway, breathing, circulation, and mental status.
  4. Repeat vital signs assessment and check any interventions.
  5. Continue to calm and reassure the patient.

F. Restraining a patient (pp. 678–682) **(Fig. 24-5, p. 682)**
  1. Restraints should be avoided unless the patient is a danger to himself and/or others.
  2. Use only padded, humane restraints that will not injure the patient who struggles.
  3. Plan how to restrain patient in advance.

VIII. Legal considerations (pp. 682–684)
  A. Consent (p. 683)
    1. Informed consent
      a. Forcing a person to have treatment against his or her will—without consent—is grounds for a charge of assault and battery.
      b. If the patient is under age 18 and is not an emancipated minor, consent to treat should come from a parent, guardian, or blood relative.

Slides/Videos
Brady Skill Series: EMT-B, "Soft Restraints"

Teaching Tip
Identify local laws regarding the use of restraints and forcibly moving patients.

c. If you cannot find a responsible adult to consent to the treatment of a minor or of a mentally incompetent patient, or if the patient is unresponsive, you may go ahead and treat, acting on the principle of implied consent.
2. Implied consent
   a. Belief that the person who could grant consent would if he or she were present and able to do so
B. Refusal of care (p. 683)
   1. Emotionally disturbed patients—especially those who are intoxicated or who have taken a drug overdose—commonly refuse treatment.
   2. If the person is alert and oriented, unless considered mentally incompetent, he must still legally consent before you can treat him.
   3. Depending on state and local law, a patient who is disoriented, in shock, mentally ill, or under the influence of drugs or alcohol may not be considered competent to refuse care.
   4. Your best protection against legal problems is to document carefully and thoroughly all aspects of the encounter.
   5. If the patient refuses care, complete a refusal of care form, and have it signed and witnessed by a police officer.
   6. If the patient threatens to hurt himself or others and you can demonstrate reason to believe the patient's threats are real, you can transport the patient without consent.
C. Using reasonable force (pp. 683–684)
   1. The amount of force deemed reasonable depends on the circumstances of the situation. As a general guide, consider the following:
      a. Size and strength of the patient
      b. Type of behavior exhibited by the patient
      c. Mental state of the patient
      d. Method of restraint
D. Police and medical direction (p. 684)
   1. Before you restrain any patient for any reason, seek medical direction.
   2. Involve law enforcement personnel when you need to restrain or transport a patient without consent or if there is any threat of violence.
E. False accusations (p. 684)
   1. The best way to protect yourself against false accusations by the patient is to carefully and completely document everything that happens during the encounter.
   2. Another source of protection against false accusations is to have witnesses, preferably throughout the entire course of treatment and transportation.

CASE STUDY FOLLOW-UP

Ask a student volunteer to read the Case Study that begins on page 670 of the textbook. You may wish to use the following questions to engage the students in a discussion of the Case Study Follow-up that begins on page 685 of the textbook. Provide missing information and clarify ideas as needed.

Q1. What hazards to yourself do you find at the scene?

A1. *Blood and a hunting knife.*

Q2. How do you deal with both hazards?

A2. *To deal with the blood, don appropriate body substance isolation gear. To deal with the knife, request that the patient put the knife on top of the sink and slide back from it a little. Only after she complies would it be safe to move into the bathroom, pick up the knife, and secure it.*

Q3. How does Maria describe the cause of her injury?

A3. *Maria says, "No one cares. I got so tired of it. I just wanted it all over. All of it. I thought I'd come here where nobody knows me and slit my wrists and that would be it. Over. I had a couple of drinks and I was going to do it, I really was. I thought I could go through with it. I did one wrist and then I saw the blood and I chickened out. I called 9-1-1. Now I'm sorry I did. No, I'm not. Oh, I don't know. I'm so confused. I don't know . . ." She trails off into sobs.*

Q4. How do you respond to Maria story?

A4. *By trying to show concern and by acknowledging the patient's feelings.*

Q5. How do you assess and treat Maria's injured wrist?

A5. *By inspecting and palpating the area around the wrist wound, noting that a radial pulse is present and the skin below the wound is slightly pale, cool, and dry to the touch. Maria is able to wiggle the fingers of her left hand, and she can identify which of her fingers is being touched. The wound is then dressed and bandaged.*

IN REVIEW

Assess students' ability to apply what they have just learned by discussing the Review Questions on page 686 of the textbook.

Q1. List some of the clues that a behavioral problem may be due to physical rather than psychological causes.

A1. *Clues that a behavioral problem may be due to physical rather than psychological causes include sudden onset of symptoms; visual but not auditory hallucinations; memory loss or impairment; dilated, constricted, or unequal pupils with different responses to light; excessive salivation; incontinence; and unusual odors on the breath. (p. 671)*

Q2. Explain some of the causes that can lead to violence in the behavioral patient.

A2. *Some of the causes that can lead to violence in the behavioral patient include real or perceived patient mismanagement, psychosis, alcohol or drug intoxication, fear, panic, and head injury. (p. 671)*

Q3. Explain basic steps to follow during the assessment of a potentially suicidal patient.

A3. *Basic steps to follow during the assessment of a potentially suicidal patient are as follows: Make injuries or medical conditions related to the suicide attempt your primary concern; listen carefully; accept all the patient's complaints and feelings; do not trust "rapid recoveries"— transport the patient even if he seems to be better; be specific in your actions—do something tangible for the patient; never show disgust or* *horror when caring for the patient; do not deny that a suicide attempt occurred; never try to shock a patient out of a suicidal act. (p. 674)*

Q4. Explain basic steps to follow during assessment of a violent patient.

A4. *Basic steps to follow during assessment of a violent patient are as follows: get a history from bystanders or family; study the patient's posture; listen to the patient; monitor the patient's physical activity; be firm and clear in your directions to the patient; and be prepared to use restraints, if necessary. (pp. 675–677)*

Q5. List some of the basic signs and symptoms of a behavioral emergency.

A5. *Basic signs and symptoms of a behavioral emergency include fear, anxiety, confusion, behavioral changes, anger, mania, depression, withdrawal, loss of contact with reality, sleeplessness, loss of appetite, loss of sex drive, constipation, crying, tension, and irritability. (p. 677)*

Q6. Explain the basic steps of emergency medical care in a behavioral emergency.

A6. *Ensure EMT safety; assess the patient for trauma or a medical condition; calm the patient and stay with the patient; use restraints if it's necessary to prevent the patient from harming himself or others; transport the patient for further medical and psychological treatment; and bring pills and/or medications if they were involved in a suicide attempt. (pp. 677–678)*

Q7. Explain the proper way to restrain a violent patient.

A7. *Restrain a patient in a supine position with humane restraints— padded soft leather or cloth restraints rather than metal handcuffs. (p. 678)*

Q8. List factors that would be considered in determining if the force used with a patient was reasonable.

A8. *Factors that would be considered in determining whether the force used with a patient was reasonable are size and strength of patient, type of behavior patient exhibits, patient's mental state, and method of restraint. (p. 678)*

Q9. Explain the circumstances in which you can transport a patient without his consent.

A9. *You can transport a patient without his consent if you can demonstrate that you believe the patient's threats to hurt himself or others are real. (pp. 683–684)*

Q10. Explain basic steps to protect yourself against false accusations by a patient.

A10. *Basic steps to protect yourself against false accusations by a patient are as follows: Thoroughly document the encounter; involve the medical chain of command and law enforcement; have witnesses, and, if possible, have witnesses sign the written report of the event. (p. 684)*

CRITICAL THINKING

Assess students' ability to respond to real-life emergency situations by discussing the Critical Thinking questions on page 686 in the textbook.

Q1. What scene safety issues are involved?

A1. *The patient's aggressive and violent behavior and the knife that he is holding are definite scene safety issues and both may present a personal hazard to you and your partner.*

Q2. How would you proceed in providing care for this patient?

A2. *The very first step would be to stay clear of the patient, ensure your safety at all times, and call for law enforcement to disarm him. If at any time the scene becomes unstable or hazardous, retreat and wait for the law enforcement officers to instruct you to enter once it has been made safe. Once the patient has been taken into law enforcement custody and restrained, the EMTs can then proceed with the assessment, emergency care, and transport.*

Q3. What is your primary responsibility in managing the patient?

A3. *The EMT's primary responsibility when managing this patient is their own safety. An injured EMT is no good to any patient. Once the scene has been deemed safe, the next priority shifts to assessing and providing emergency care to the patient. Even though this patient may be experiencing a behavioral emergency, it is not your responsibility to determine the specific behavioral emergency or attempt to manage it; however, it is your primary responsibility to provide emergency care to the patient for his wounds.*

Q4. Would you consider restraining this patient?

A4. *Based on the patient's actions and aggressive behavior, it would be necessary to restrain him to adequately assess and provide emergency care. The restraint should be done with law enforcement assistance.*

Q5. What criteria would you use to make the decision to restrain the patient?

A5. *Since this patient is obviously a danger to himself and others, he should be restrained for care and transport. It is not possible to assess or provide emergency care without the patient being restrained.*

Q6. How would you proceed in restraining the patient?

A6. *Once the patient is disarmed by law enforcement, make sure there are enough responders for each person to control one of the patient's limbs. Then, all responders should approach the patient at the same time, take him down in a controlled manner, and bring him under control. Once under control, the patient should then be immediately placed in a face-up (supine) position and then moved and restrained to the cot with soft or humane restraints.*

Q7. What are some hazards involving patient restraint?

A7. *Hazards of restraining patients may include injuries to rescuers, injuries to the patient, and positional asphyxia. Placing a patient in a supine position may lead to ineffective spontaneous ventilation and your inability to properly assess the patient. The patient who begins to struggle more aggressively while in a supine position may be a sign of worsening hypoxia. As the patient becomes more hypoxic, he becomes more agitated and aggressive. As the patient becomes more hypercarbic from poor ventilation and retention of carbon dioxide, the patient becomes more confused. The EMT may interpret this as the patient becoming more violent; however, it may be a clear indication that he is becoming more hypoxic and hypercarbic.*

*Q*8. What legal issues are of concern in this patient?

*A*8. *When dealing with this patient, the EMTs should be concerned with legal issues involving consent, refusal of care, reasonable force, and the potential for false accusations.*

SKILLS DEMONSTRATION AND PRACTICE

Ask for one student to be a patient and four students to assist with the application of restraint devices. Caution students to be extremely careful when applying restraints in order to avoid injury to themselves or the patient.

Step by step, describe the procedure for restraining a patient. Direct assistants to perform each step in the procedure as it is described. Show the correct way to apply restraining devices.

Select another group of students and repeat the process, this time allowing a student to apply the restraints. Repeat the process until all students have had the opportunity to participate in the practice activity.

ROLE PLAY

Provide students with the opportunity to apply what they have learned to a real-life situation encountered by EMS personnel. Ask two volunteers to play the role of EMTs who are responding to a 9-1-1 call, two volunteers to be bystanders, and one volunteer to be the patient. Take the two EMT players outside the classroom and provide them with a complete jump kit containing BSI equipment, oxygen equipment, a portable suction unit, and a stretcher. Also provide restraints and a patient refusal form. Describe the following situation to them: You are dispatched to a suburban home around 1:00 A.M. on a Saturday. The dispatcher said that the patient is an intoxicated adolescent male. You should act appropriately on what you find there. The emphasis of the scene is on dealing with behavioral emergencies. However, you should use all the skills you have learned to date. Tell the volunteers playing the EMTs that you will call them to the scene in just a minute.

Have the bystanders and the patient come to the front of the classroom. Describe the following situation to them and to the class:

Sixteen-year-old Todd Hoerchle came home at 12:30 A.M. on Saturday, an hour and a half past his curfew. His parents were waiting up for him. Todd was obviously drunk. A loud argument developed. Todd became angry and began breaking things. He injured his hand when he put his fist through the TV. His parents called 9-1-1. The police have not been called. Todd is still yelling and breaking things when the EMTs arrive. Todd threatens to kill himself. Mr. and Mrs. Hoerchle want Todd treated, but they do not want him transported.

Tell the patient and bystanders to take their places and to start acting. Call the EMTs back into the classroom. Allow the role play to progress naturally. Intervene only if the players seem to be at a loss for what to do.

End the play when the EMTs have prepared the patient for transport to the ambulance or obtained a signed refusal form.

With the entire class, discuss the following:

- What did the EMTs do well?

- What, if anything, could they have done differently? Discuss the laws for your state regarding the involuntary restraint and transport of a minor.

ASSIGNMENTS

Assign students to read Chapter 25, "Obstetric and Gynecological Emergencies," before the next class. Also ask them to complete Chapter 24 of the Workbook.

EVALUATION

Chapter Quiz Distribute copies of the Chapter Quiz provided in Handout 24-2 to evaluate student understanding of this chapter. Remind students not to refer to their textbooks or notes while taking the quiz.

Test Manager You may wish to create a custom-tailored test using Prentice Hall *TestGen for Prehospital Emergency Care, Eighth Edition* to evaluate student understanding of this chapter.

Online Test Preparation (for students and instructors) Additional test preparation is available through *EMT Achieve: Basic Test Preparation* at http://www.prenhall.com/EMTAchieve. Instructors can also monitor student mastery online.

REINFORCEMENT

Handouts If classroom discussions or performance on the quiz indicates that some students have not fully mastered the chapter content, you may wish to assign some or all of the Reinforcement Handouts for this chapter.

TECH EXTRAS

Brady Skills Series EMT-B Videos/CD Have your students watch the skills come to life on either VHS or CD-ROM.

PowerPoint Presentation (for instructors) The PowerPoint material developed for this chapter offers useful reinforcement of chapter content.

Student CD A wide variety of material on this CD-ROM will reinforce and also expand student knowledge and skills.

Companion Website (for students) Additional review quizzes and links to EMS resources will contribute to further reinforcement of this chapter. Please visit http://www.prenhall.com/mistovich.

Reading/Reference
Textbook, pp. 687–723

Workbook
Chapter 24 Activities

Chapter Quiz
Handout 24-2

TestGen
Chapter 24 Test

Online Test Preparation
Send your students to
http://www.prenhall.com/
EMTAchieve

Handouts 24-3 to 24-6
Reinforcement Activities

**Brady Skills Series
EMT-B Videos/CD**
Visual Reinforcement

**PowerPoint
Presentation**
Chapter 24

Student CD
Chapter 24

Companion Website
http://www.prenhall.com/
mistovich

OBJECTIVES CHECKLIST

Cognitive	Date Mastered
4-8.1 Define behavioral emergencies.	
4-8.2 Discuss the general factors that may cause an alteration in a patient's behavior.	
4-8.3 State the various reasons for psychological crises.	
4-8.4 Discuss the characteristics of an individual's behavior that suggest that the patient is at risk for suicide.	
4-8.5 Discuss special medical/legal considerations for managing behavioral emergencies.	
4-8.6 Discuss the special considerations for assessing a patient with behavioral problems.	
4-8.7 Discuss the general principles of an individual's behavior that suggest that he or she is at risk for violence.	
4-8.8 Discuss methods to calm behavioral emergency patients.	

Affective	Date Mastered
4-8.9 Explain the rationale for learning how to modify your behavior toward the patient with a behavioral emergency.	

Psychomotor	Date Mastered
4-8.10 Demonstrate the assessment and emergency medical care of the patient experiencing a behavioral emergency.	
4-8.11 Demonstrate various techniques to safely restrain a patient with a behavioral problem.	

CHAPTER 24 QUIZ

Write the letter of the best answer in the space provided.

_____ **1.** A situation in which a person exhibits actions that are unacceptable to the patient, family, or community is known as

   A. a panic attack.   **C.** a behavioral emergency.

   B. depression.   **D.** psychosis.

_____ **2.** Which one of the following is *not* a factor in determining whether the use of force with an emotionally disturbed patient is reasonable or not?

   A. size and strength of patient   **C.** mental state of patient

   B. dispatch information   **D.** method of restraint

_____ **3.** The medical condition most likely to cause restlessness and confusion, cyanosis, and altered mental status is

   A. excessive heat.   **C.** excessive cold.

   B. inadequate blood to the brain.   **D.** lack of oxygen.

_____ **4.** One method of protecting against false accusations by a behavioral emergency patient is

   A. using medical responders of a different gender than the patient.

   B. involving third-party witnesses.

   C. limiting the involvement of other medical responders.

   D. sharply limiting documentation.

_____ **5.** The first step that an EMT takes in a behavioral emergency is to

   A. gather a thorough patient history.

   B. complete an initial assessment.

   C. identify him- or herself.

   D. perform a careful scene size-up.

_____ **6.** A state of painful uneasiness about impending problems is called

   A. anxiety.   **C.** psychosis.

   B. depression.   **D.** mania.

_____ **7.** In talking with a behavioral patient, an EMT should take all of the following actions *except*

   A. identifying him- or herself.

   B. avoiding direct eye contact.

   C. being as honest as possible.

   D. standing at least 3 feet from the patient.

_____ **8.** Of the groups listed, the highest suicide rates have been found in the following age group

   A. women under age 25   **C.** men ages 15 to 25

   B. men over age 40   **D.** women over age 50

_____ **9.** A patient who has attempted suicide in the past is
   A. looking for attention.
   B. less likely to commit suicide than one who has not.
   C. a candidate for forceful restraint.
   D. more likely to commit suicide than one who has not.

_____ **10.** In most localities, an EMT cannot legally restrain a patient without orders from
   A. dispatch.   **C.** the police.
   B. the patient's physician.   **D.** the patient's family.

IN THE FIELD

Read the following real-life situation. Then answer the questions that follow.

The emergency medical dispatcher reports a 14-year-old girl who is "acting in a bizarre manner." Her father is currently trying to keep her from leaving the house.

Upon the EMS unit's arrival at the scene, the father guides the team into the house. He states that his daughter has been depressed for the past few weeks. Today the daughter's behavior changed dramatically. Instead of appearing to be lethargic, the daughter has become hyperactive. The father indicates that the family has a history of manic depression. "The doctor has a new word for it," laughs the father nervously. "They call it bipolar disorder." The father indicates that his daughter is on medication for the condition, but feels that she has stopped using it. The girl's psychiatrist recommended that the father call 9-1-1.

The father takes you to meet his daughter, Stephanie. You see a clean, well-dressed young woman who appears to be happy. She speaks very fast and occasionally exhibits muscle twitches of the face and hands. Although Stephanie indicates no physical complaints, her vital signs are on the high side of normal. She doesn't want to talk about her medical condition. She also doesn't want to be transported to the hospital. With her eyes averted, Stephanie says a little too lightly, "My father worries much too much. I'm just fine."

1. How should you proceed with patient care?

2. What information might you use to persuade the patient to accompany you to the hospital?

CHAPTER 24 REVIEW

Write the word or words that best complete each sentence in the space provided.

1. _____ is defined as the manner in which a person acts or performs.

2. A(n) _____ _____ exists when a person exhibits abnormal behavior.

3. There are many _____ conditions as well as psychological conditions that are likely to alter a patient's behavior.

4. _____ is a condition characterized by deep feelings of sadness, worthlessness, and discouragement—feelings that often do not seem connected to the actual circumstances of the patient's life.

5. In providing patient care during a behavioral emergency, an EMT should treat any life-threatening conditions during the _____ _____.

6. In talking with a patient experiencing a behavioral emergency, maintain good _____ _____ and avoid any quick _____.

7. Whenever you are called to care for a patient who has attempted suicide, your first concern must be for _____ _____ _____.

8. Suicide is more common among people with a history of _____ or _____ _____.

9. Before you restrain any patient for any reason, contact _____ _____.

10. The best way to protect yourself against false accusations by a patient is to carefully and completely _____ everything that happens during the encounter, including detailed aspects of the patient's abnormal behavior.

©2008 by Pearson Education, Inc.
Prehospital Emergency Care, 8th ed.

BEHAVIORAL EMERGENCIES: LISTING

1. List seven physical conditions that are likely to alter a person's behavior.

2. List seven basic principles to keep in mind whenever you encounter a behavioral emergency.

BEHAVIORAL EMERGENCIES: TRUE OR FALSE

Indicate if the following statements are true or false by writing T or F in the space provided.

_____ **1.** During a behavioral emergency, an EMT should only call the police as a last resort.

_____ **2.** When dealing with a patient with a behavior problem always consider that the problem may be caused by a physical condition.

_____ **3.** Whenever an EMT is called to the scene of a suicide attempt, his or her first concern should be for the patient's safety.

_____ **4.** Every suicidal act or gesture should be taken seriously, and the patient should be transported for evaluation.

_____ **5.** If a patient's fear or aggression increases, an EMT should not push the issue of transport.

_____ **6.** In treating a behavioral emergency, an EMT should not leave the patient alone.

_____ **7.** Once a patient is acting rationally, an EMT may remove soft restraints.

_____ **8.** Under most state laws, any adult of sound mind has the right to determine whether he or she will be treated or, more specifically, touched by another person in the course of treatment.

_____ **9.** The patient who has become calm following a period of combativeness will most likely not revert to the earlier behavior.

_____ **10.** Depending on state and local law, a patient who is disoriented, in shock, mentally ill, or under the influence of drugs or alcohol may *not* be considered competent to refuse care.

Behavioral Emergencies

Behavioral Problems

Behavioral Change
- Behavioral emergencies versus physical emergencies

Psychiatric Problems
- Anxiety
- Phobias
- Depression
- Bipolar disorder
- Paranoia
- Schizophrenia

Violence
- Suicide
- Violence to others

Dealing with Behavioral Emergencies

Basic Principles

Techniques for Treating Behavioral Emergency Patients

Assessment and Care

Restraining a Patient

Legal Considerations
- Consent
- Refusal of care
- Reasonable force
- Police and medical direction
- False accusations

HANDOUT 24-2: Chapter 24 Quiz

1. C	**4.** B	**7.** B	**9.** D
2. B	**5.** D	**8.** B	**10.** C
3. D	**6.** A		

HANDOUT 24-3: In the Field

1. Sample response: Several factors indicate that the girl should be convinced to accept treatment: she's a minor; her psychiatrist directed the father to call 9-1-1; she has a potentially hazardous condition. Medical direction should be contacted. Depending on local protocols, paperwork may have to be filled out if the girl refuses transport. The police may also need to intervene. The patient should be made aware of all possible options, but she should also understand that the outcome will be the same—a trip to the hospital.

2. Sample response: The girl might be told: "You are experiencing muscle twitches, which need to be checked out. Your father is worried about you, and we can set his mind at ease. Your doctor requested that you be checked out at the hospital."

HANDOUT 24-4: Chapter 24 Review

1. Behavior
2. behavioral emergency
3. physical
4. Depression
5. initial assessment
6. eye contact, movements
7. your own safety
8. alcoholism, drug abuse
9. medical direction
10. document

HANDOUT 24-5: Behavioral Emergencies: Listing

1. Any seven of the following: low blood sugar, lack of oxygen, inadequate blood to the brain, head trauma, mind-altering substances, excessive cold, excessive heat, psychogenic substances, infections of the brain or its coverings

2. Every person has limitations. Each person has a right to his or her feelings. Each person has more ability to cope with crisis than he or she might think. Everyone feels some emotional disturbance when involved in a disaster or when injured. Emotional injury is just as real as physical injury. People who have been through a crisis do not just "get better." Cultural differences have special meaning when you are called to intervene in behavioral emergencies.

HANDOUT 24-6: Behavioral Emergencies: True or False

1. F	**4.** T	**7.** F	**9.** F
2. T	**5.** T	**8.** T	**10.** T
3. F	**6.** T		

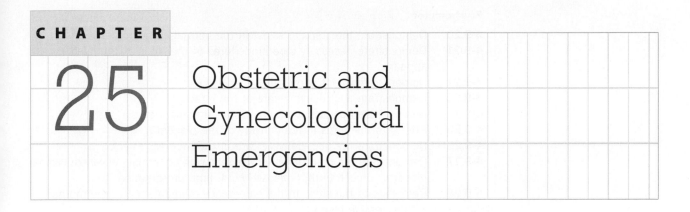

CHAPTER

25 Obstetric and Gynecological Emergencies

This chapter covers Lesson 4-9 and portions of Lesson 4-10 of the U.S. Department of Transportation's EMT-Basic National Standard Curriculum.

OBJECTIVES

Numbered objectives are from the U.S. Department of Transportation's EMT-Basic National Standard Curriculum. Asterisked objectives, if any, pertain to material that is supplemental to the DOT curriculum. Page numbers refer to pages in the textbook.

Cognitive

4-9.1   Identify the following structures: uterus, vagina, fetus, placenta, umbilical cord, amniotic sac, perineum. (pp. 689–691)

4-9.2   Identify and explain the use of the contents of an obstetrics kit. (p. 698)

4-9.3   Identify predelivery emergencies. (pp. 693–696)

4-9.4   State indications of an imminent delivery. (pp. 696, 698)

4-9.5   Differentiate the emergency medical care provided to a patient with predelivery emergencies from a normal delivery. (pp. 694–695, 698–703, 708)

4-9.6   State the steps in the predelivery preparation of the mother. (pp. 700–701)

4-9.7   Establish the relationship between body substance isolation and childbirth. (pp. 698, 700)

4-9.8   State the steps to assist in the delivery. (pp. 698–703, 708)

4-9.9   Describe care of the infant as the head appears. (pp. 701, 708)

4-9.10   Describe how and when to cut the umbilical cord. (pp. 702, 708)

4-9.11   Discuss the steps in the delivery of the placenta. (pp. 702–703, 708)

4-9.12   List the steps in the emergency medical care of the mother post-delivery. (pp. 703, 708)

4-9.13   Summarize neonatal resuscitation procedures. (pp. 711–713)

4-9.14   Describe the procedures for the following abnormal deliveries: breech birth, prolapsed cord, limb presentation. (pp. 703–705)

4-9.15   Differentiate the special considerations for multiple births. (p. 705–706)

4-9.16   Describe special considerations of meconium. (p. 706)

4-9.17   Describe special considerations of a premature baby. (p. 706)

4-9.18   Discuss the emergency medical care of a patient with a gynecological emergency. (pp. 713–715)

Affective

4-9.19   Explain the rationale for understanding the implications of treating two patients (mother and baby). (pp. 696, 703)

Total Teaching Time
180 minutes

Resources Needed
- Scored Chapter 24 Quizzes
- Obstetrics kit, one for every three students
- Birthing model
- Infant CPR models or toy dolls, one for every three students

Additional Resources
Larmon/Davis, *Basic Life Support Skills*

Elling, *EMT Achieve: Basic Test Preparation*

Limmer/Mistovich/O'Keefe, *Audio Lecture & Study Guide: EMT*

Mistovich/Kuvlesky, *SUCCESS! for the EMT, Second Edition*

4-9.20   Demonstrate the steps to assist in the normal cephalic delivery.
4-9.21   Demonstrate necessary care procedures of the fetus as the head appears.
4-9.22   Demonstrate infant neonatal procedures.
4-9.23   Demonstrate post-delivery care of the infant.
4-9.24   Demonstrate how and when to cut the umbilical cord.
4-9.25   Attend to the steps in the delivery of the placenta.
4-9.26   Demonstrate the post-delivery care of the mother.
4-9.27   Demonstrate the procedures for the following abnormal deliveries: vaginal bleeding, breech birth, prolapsed cord, limb presentation.
4-9.28   Demonstrate the steps in the emergency medical care of the mother with excessive bleeding.
4-9.29   Demonstrate completing a prehospital care report for patients with obstetric/gynecological emergencies.

REVIEW

In the last lesson, "Behavioral Emergencies," students learned that, as EMTs, they will respond to many emergencies in which the patient is behaving in unexpected and sometimes dangerous ways. The unusual behavior may be the result of stress, physical trauma, illness, drug and alcohol abuse, or mental illness. Whatever the cause, students learned not to hesitate to request police assistance whenever they feel it is necessary or when local protocol requires it. Appropriate emergency care may be provided only after the scene is secure.

Distribute the scored quizzes from the last class. Go over each question on the quiz and handle any concerns students may have about the answers.

INTRODUCTION TO CHAPTER 25

Chapter 25, "Obstetric and Gynecological Emergencies," is the 14th and last lesson of Module 4. A pregnant woman is too often rushed to a hospital, usually because the EMT is afraid that the infant will be born before the mother can get there. In most cases, there is no need for such haste. Childbirth is a normal, natural process. Only in a few situations involving complications is there a need to see that the mother reaches the hospital quickly. Care of patients in an emergency involving reproductive organs is not a common event. However, students must be prepared to deal with these emergencies in an absolutely professional, effective, and compassionate way. They should be sure to review assessment and emergency medical care procedures for these kinds of emergencies as often as possible.

Distribute the Chapter 25 Objectives Checklist and give students a few minutes to look it over. Then briefly paraphrase the objectives for this lesson in your own words.

LECTURE

The following suggested lecture outline is based on the Department of Transportation's EMT-Basic National Standard Curriculum. In some places, the DOT curriculum has been rearranged or expanded upon so that it is more complete or easier for the student to understand. The page numbers in parentheses refer to pages in the textbook. The parenthetical references in dark, heavy type are to figures, tables, and scans in the textbook.

Handout 25-1
Chapter 25 Objectives
Checklist

● ➤

Lecture Master
You may wish to display
Lecture Master 25 when
presenting the lecture to
the class.

I. Childbirth and obstetric emergencies (pp. 689–693)

    A. Anatomy of pregnancy (pp. 689–690) **(Fig. 25-1, p. 689)**

        1. Uterus

        2. Fetus

        3. Cervix

        4. Bloody show

            a. Blood-tinged mucus plug that may be expelled from the vagina signaling the first stage of labor

        5. Placenta

            a. Fetal organ through which fetus receives oxygen and nourishment from the mother and discharges carbon dioxide and waste products during pregnancy

        6. Afterbirth

            a. Delivery of the placenta after the birth of the infant

        7. Umbilical cord

            a. Placental cord containing one vein and two arteries; the vein carries blood and nutrients to the fetus, and the arteries carry deoxygenated blood and waste products back to the placenta

        8. Wharton's jelly

            a. Protective substance on the umbilical cord

        9. Amniotic sac (bag of waters)

            a. Sac containing insulating and protecting amniotic fluid in which the fetus floats within the uterus

       10. Vagina (birth canal)

            a. Lower part of the birth canal

       11. Perineum

            a. Skin area between vagina and anus, commonly torn during delivery

       12. Crowning

            a. The infant's presenting part (usually the head) appearing at the opening of the birth canal

    B. Labor (pp. 690–693)

        1. Process of birth; divided into three stages **(Fig. 25-2, p. 691)**

            a. First stage: dilation

            b. Second stage: expulsion **(Fig. 25-3, p. 692)**

            c. Third stage: placental

II. Assessment and care—Predelivery emergency (pp. 693–696) **(Figs. 25-4 and 25-5, pp. 697–699)**

    A. Scene size-up (p. 693)

        1. Obstetric emergency

            a. Emergency having to do with pregnancy and childbirth

        2. First indication usually from dispatcher, but any woman of child-bearing age (12–50) could potentially be experiencing an obstetric emergency

    B. Initial assessment (p. 693)

        1. Perform after taking BSI precautions and ensuring that scene is safe

        2. Same as for patient who is not pregnant (mental status, airway, breathing)

    C. Focused history and physical exam (pp. 693–694)

        1. Use SAMPLE questions, including OPQRST.

            a. Are you experiencing any pain or discomfort?

On the Net

For more on childbirth, go to: www.childbirth.org

On the Net

For more on obstetric and gynecological emergencies, go to: www.obgyn.net

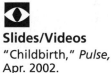

Slides/Videos

"Childbirth," *Pulse,* Apr. 2002.

    b. When was your last menstrual period?

    c. Have you missed a menstrual period?

    d. Have you had any unusual vaginal discharge?

    e. When (if the patient knows she is pregnant) is your due date?

    f. Have you ever been pregnant before?

2. If patient is experiencing abdominal pain, perform focused medical assessment.

3. Obtain baseline vitals.

D. Signs and symptoms of predelivery emergency (p. 694)

  1. Abdominal pain, nausea, vomiting

  2. Vaginal bleeding, passing of tissue

  3. Weakness, dizziness

  4. Altered mental status

  5. Seizures

  6. Excessive swelling of face and/or extremities

  7. Abdominal trauma

  8. Shock (hypoperfusion) (Pregnancy may mask early signs of shock.)

E. Emergency medical care (pp. 694–695)

  1. If close to full term, take precautions against supine hypotensive syndrome by placing patient in a sitting position or lying on either side.

  2. Ensure adequate airway, breathing, and circulation.

    a. Administer oxygen at 15 liters per minute by nonrebreather mask to any pregnant patient.

    b. Provide positive-pressure ventilation with supplemental oxygen if breathing is inadequate.

  3. Care for bleeding from the vagina.

    a. Place sanitary napkin over vaginal opening.

    b. Never touch vaginal area.

    c. Never pack vagina in attempt to control bleeding.

    d. Replace soaked pads.

    e. Save and transport with patient any passed tissue or evidence of blood loss.

  4. Treat for shock (hypoperfusion) if indicated.

  5. Provide emergency medical care as you would for the nonpregnant patient based on any other signs and symptoms.

  6. Transport patient on left side.

F. Ongoing assessment (p. 695)

G. Specific predelivery emergencies (pp. 695–696)

  1. Spontaneous abortion (miscarriage)

    a. Delivery of fetus and placenta before fetus is viable (usually 20th week)

    b. Signs and symptoms

      (1) Cramp-like lower abdominal pain similar to labor

      (2) Moderate to severe vaginal bleeding, which may be bright red or dark red

      (3) Passage of tissue or blood clots

    c. Emergency care in addition to general guidelines

      (1) Ask when last menstrual period began.

      (2) Provide emotional support.

  2. Seizures during pregnancy

    a. Provide emergency care same as for any seizure patient.

    b. Take extra care to protect patient from injuring herself.

    c. Be sure to transport patient on her left side.

    d. Transport in as calm and as quiet a manner as possible.

3. Vaginal bleeding

    a. Follow general guidelines for emergency care.

    b. Place sanitary napkins over vaginal opening.

    c. Transport patient as soon as possible.

    d. Be alert for signs and symptoms of shock (hypoperfusion).

4. Trauma to a pregnant woman

    a. Severe blunt trauma to the abdomen can damage uterus and injure fetus, as well as rupture the mother's spleen, liver, and diaphragm.

    b. Treat same as you would any other trauma patient.

    c. Remember that early signs of shock may be minimal or absent.

    d. Patient's breathing adequate—administer oxygen at 15 liters per minute by nonrebreather mask.

    e. Patient's breathing inadequate—administer positive-pressure ventilation with supplemental oxygen.

    f. If you suspect neck or back injury, immobilize patient using normal immobilization, but then place pillows on right side to tilt patient left and relieve pressure on the inferior vena cava.

    g. Transport as soon as possible.

III. Assessment and care: active labor and normal delivery (pp. 696–703) **(Figs. 25-12 and 25-13, pp. 707–709)**

  A. Predelivery considerations (pp. 696–698)

    1. Delivery not imminent

      a. Transport

    2. Patient in active labor

      a. Focus on assisting the mother with delivery and providing initial care to the neonate (newborn infant).

    3. Questions to ask to determine whether to transport or commit to delivery

      a. Is this the patient's first delivery? If not, how many times has she been pregnant? How many deliveries?

      b. How long has the patient been pregnant?

      c. Has there been any bleeding or discharge (bloody show or amniotic fluid)?

      d. Are there any contractions or pain?

      e. What is the frequency and duration of contractions?

      f. Is crowning occurring with contractions?

      g. Does the patient feel the need to push?

      h. Does the patient feel as if she is having a bowel movement with increasing pressure in the vaginal area?

      i. Is the abdomen (uterus) hard upon palpation?

    4. Situations when you must assist in the delivery

      a. When you have no suitable transportation

      b. When the hospital or physician cannot be reached due to bad weather, a natural disaster, or some other catastrophe

      c. If delivery is imminent

    5. Signs and symptoms of imminent delivery

      a. Crowning has occurred.

      b. Contractions are closer than 2 minutes apart, they are intense, and they last from 60 to 90 seconds.

On the Net

Labor basics plus handling emergency labor. http://pregnancy.about.com/library/weekly/aa071199.htm

Point to Emphasize

All third-trimester patients should be transported on their left side. A pillow or rolled blanket should be placed behind the back to maintain proper position.

    c. Patient feels the infant's head moving down the birth canal (sensation of bowel movement).

    d. Patient has a strong urge to push.

    e. Patient's abdomen is very hard.

6. What to do if birth is imminent

    a. Contact medical direction for a decision to commit to delivery.

    b. If delivery does not occur in 10 minutes, contact medical direction for permission to transport.

    c. If you must assist in the delivery

        (1) Take all appropriate BSI precautions, including gloves, gown, and eye protection.

        (2) Do not touch the patient's vaginal area except during delivery and in the presence of your partner.

        (3) Do not allow patient to use the bathroom.

        (4) If patient urinates or moves her bowels, replace the linens with clean ones.

        (5) Do not hold patient's legs together or attempt to delay delivery.

        (6) Use a sterile obstetrics (OB) kit.

7. Contents of an OB kit **(Fig. 25-6, p. 700)**

    a. Surgical scissors or scalpel (for cutting umbilical cord)

    b. Cord clamps or cord ties

    c. Umbilical tape or sterilized cord

    d. Bulb syringe

    e. Towels, five or more

    f. Gauze sponges, 2×10

    g. Sterile gloves

    h. One infant blanket

    i. Individually wrapped sanitary napkins, three or more

    j. Large plastic bag, at least one

    k. Germicidal wipes

B. Emergency medical care: patient in active labor for normal delivery (pp. 698–703) **(Fig. 25-7, pp. 700–701)**

1. Position the patient on firm surface with knees drawn up and spread apart, buttocks elevated, feet flat on surface, and head, neck, and shoulders supported with pillows or folded blankets.

2. Create a sterile field around the vaginal opening.

3. Monitor patient for vomiting

4. Continually assess for crowning.

5. Place your gloved fingers on the bony part of the infant's skull when it crowns, and exert very gentle pressure to prevent explosive delivery.

6. Rupture amniotic sac with your fingers if it is not already broken, and push it away from infant's head and face as they appear.

7. Determine position of umbilical cord.

    a. If around neck, use two fingers to slip it over infant's shoulder.

    b. If you cannot move the cord, place two clamps 3 inches apart and cut between them.

8. Remove fluids from infant's airway.

    a. Suction two or three times with a bulb syringe—mouth first and then nostrils.

      b. Be sure to compress syringe before bringing it to infant's face.

      c. Insert syringe tip 1 to 1.5 inches into infant's mouth and slowly release bulb.

      d. Avoid touching the back of the mouth.

      e. Remove syringe, discharge contents into a towel, and repeat.

      f. Use same procedure to suction each nostril.

  9. Support newborn with both hands as torso and full body are expelled.

      a. Never pull infant from vagina.

      b. Do not put your fingers in infant's armpits. (Pressure there can damage nerve centers.)

      c. Receive newborn in clean or sterile towel.

10. Grasp feet as they are born.

11. Clean newborn's mouth and nose.

      a. Wiping with sterile gauze

      b. Suctioning mouth and nose again

12. Dry, wrap, warm, and position the infant.

      a. Placing on side or back with neck in neutral position

      b. Keeping level with mother's vagina until umbilical cord is cut

13. Assign your partner to monitor and complete initial care of newborn while you attend to mother.

14. Clamp, tie, and cut umbilical cord as pulsations cease. **(Fig. 25-8, p. 702)**

      a. Using two clamps or ties on cord about 3 inches apart

      b. Placing first clamp approximately four finger widths (6 inches) from infant

      c. Cutting between two clamps with sterile surgical scissors or scalpel

      d. Controlling any cord bleeding by placing another clamp or tie proximal to one already placed on cord

15. Observe for delivery of placenta.

      a. Expecting delivery within 10 to 20 minutes of delivery of infant

      b. Guiding placenta from vagina when it appears by grasping and rotating it—never pulling

      c. Not delaying transport to wait for delivery of placenta

16. Wrap delivered placenta in a towel and place it in a plastic bag for transport.

17. Place one or two sanitary napkins over vaginal opening.

18. Record the time of delivery

19. Transport mother, infant, and placenta to hospital.

C. Emergency medical care: excessive post-delivery blood loss (p. 703)

  1. Place medial edge of one hand (fingers extended) horizontally across abdomen, just above symphysis pubis.

  2. Cup your other hand around the uterus.

  3. Use a kneading or circular motion to massage the area.

  4. Allow infant to suckle on the mother's breast to help uterus contract.

  5. If bleeding continues to be excessive, check your massage technique, continue massage, and transport immediately.

D. Ongoing assessment (p. 703)

◎

Point to Emphasize
Note the exact time of birth.

IV. Assessment and care: active labor with abnormal delivery
(pp. 703–706)

 A. Signs and symptoms of abnormal delivery emergency (p. 703)

  1. Any fetal presentation other than normal crowning of the fetal head

  2. Abnormal color or smell of amniotic fluid

  3. Labor before 38 weeks of pregnancy

  4. Recurrence of contractions after first infant is born (indicating multiple births)

 B. Emergency medical care and ongoing assessment (p. 703)

  1. In general, similar to that of normal delivery

  2. Exceptions include an emphasis on immediate transport, administration of high-flow oxygen, and continuous monitoring of vital signs.

 C. Specific abnormal delivery emergencies (pp. 703–706)

  1. Prolapsed cord (**Fig. 25-9, p. 704**)

   a. Cord presents through birth canal before delivery of head, a serious emergency that endangers life of unborn infant.

   b. Position patient head down in "knee–chest" position (kneeling and bent forward, face down, chest to knees), or raise buttocks with pillows to reduce pressure of fetal head on cord.

   c. Insert sterile gloved hand into vagina, pushing presenting part of fetus away from the pulsating cord.

   d. Cover cord with sterile towel moistened with saline solution.

   e. Transport patient rapidly, continuing pressure on infant's head or buttocks to keep pressure off cord.

   f. Monitor cord pulsations—should be present.

  2. Breech birth presentation (**Fig. 25-10, p. 705**)

   a. Buttocks or lower extremities are low in uterus and are first to be delivered

   b. Immediate rapid transportation upon recognition.

   c. Place mother on oxygen.

   d. Place mother in head-down position with pelvis elevated.

  3. Limb presentation (**Fig. 25-11, p. 705**)

   a. Infant's limb protrudes from birth canal

   b. Transport immediately. (Surgery is likely to be required.)

   c. Administer oxygen.

   d. Keep mother in head-down position with pelvis elevated.

   e. Never pull infant by its limb.

   f. Never attempt delivery in this situation.

   g. Instruct mother to pant if she has the urge to push with contractions.

  4. Multiple births

   a. Signs and symptoms

    (1) Abdomen is still very large after one infant is delivered.

    (2) Uterine contractions continue to be extremely strong after delivering first infant.

Reading/Reference

Mattera, C., "Obstetrical Complications," *JEMS,* Mar. 1999.

Point of Interest

The highest number of children ever produced from a multiple birth is reported to be 10.

©2008 by Pearson Education, Inc.
Prehospital Emergency Care, 8th ed.

      (3) Uterine contractions begin again about 10 minutes after one infant has been delivered.

      (4) Infant's size is small in proportion to size of mother's abdomen.

  b. Follow general guidelines for normal delivery.

  c. Call for assistance.

  d. If second infant is not breech, handle delivery as you would for single infant.

  e. Expect and manage hemorrhage following second birth.

  f. Be prepared for infants to each have own placenta or to share placenta.

  g. If second infant has not delivered within 10 minutes of first, transport mother and infant to hospital.

5. Meconium staining

  a. Fetal bowel movement in amniotic fluid, turning it greenish or brownish-yellow rather than clear; an indication of possible fetal distress.

  b. Suction infant's mouth and nose as soon as head emerges from birth canal.

  c. Do not stimulate before suctioning

      (1) Goal is to clear mouth and nose before infant takes first breath.

  d. Transport infant as soon as possible, maintaining airway and supporting ventilation as necessary throughout transport.

6. Premature birth

  a. Infant weighing less than 5 pounds or one born before 38 weeks of development

  b. At risk for hypothermia and respiratory distress

  c. May require more vigorous resuscitation than full-term infant

  d. Additional care for premature infant

      (1) Dry thoroughly and keep warm with warmed blankets or plastic bubble-bag swaddle, making sure head is covered.

      (2) Use gentle suction with bulb syringe.

      (3) Prevent bleeding from umbilical cord.

      (4) Administer supplemental oxygen by blowing oxygen across infant's face with end of oxygen tube approximately an inch above infant's mouth and nose.

      (5) Support ventilation if breathing is inadequate.

      (6) Prevent contamination and do not let anyone breathe into infant's face.

      (7) Wrap infant securely to keep it warm, and heat vehicle during transport.

V. Assessment and care: the newborn infant (pp. 706–713) **(Figs. 25-18 and 25-19, pp. 713–714)**

  A. Initial care of the newborn (p. 706)

    1. Keep warm by drying, wrapping in blanket, and drying and covering head.

    2. Repeat suctioning.

  B. Assessment using APGAR memory aid (pp. 706–710)

    1. Appearance

Point to Emphasize
The most important step after establishing the infant's airway is to dry and cover the head to prevent heat loss.

Point to Emphasize

If assessment of the infant's breathing reveals shallow, slow, or absent respirations, provide artificial ventilations at a rate of 40–60 per minute. Reassess respiratory effort after 30 seconds.

2. Pulse
3. Grimace
4. Activity
5. Respiration

C. Interpreting your assessment findings (p. 710)
   1. 7–10 points
     a. Newborn active and vigorous; provide routine care
   2. 4–6 points
     a. Newborn moderately depressed; provide stimulation and oxygen
   3. 0–3 points
     a. Newborn severely depressed; provide extensive care including oxygen with bag-valve mask ventilations and CPR
   4. Stimulation methods **(Fig. 25-14, p. 710)**
     a. Flick soles of feet.
     b. Rub infant's back.

D. Signs and symptoms of severely depressed infant needing aggressive care (p. 710)
   1. Respiratory rate over 60/min.
   2. Diminished breath sounds
   3. Heart rate over 180/min. or under 100/min.
   4. Obvious signs of delivery trauma
   5. Poor or absent skeletal muscle tone
   6. Respiratory arrest or severe distress
   7. Heavy meconium staining of amniotic fluid
   8. Weak pulses
   9. Cyanotic body (core and extremities)
   10. Poor peripheral perfusion
   11. Lack of or poor response to stimulation
   12. Apgar score under 4

E. Emergency medical care (resuscitation) of severely depressed infant (pp. 710–713)
   1. Majority of newborn infants respond to routine care; only a few require aggressive resuscitation. **(Fig. 25-15, p. 711)**
   2. Provide free-flow oxygen with tube an inch from nose and mouth if **(Fig. 25-16, p. 711)**:
     a. Bluish discoloration of skin
     b. Spontaneous breathing
     c. Adequate heart rate
   3. Provide ventilations by bag-valve mask at 40–60/min. and reassess after 30 seconds if: **(Fig. 25-17, p. 712)**
     a. Breathing is shallow, slow, gasping, or absent following brief stimulation
     b. Heart rate is less than 100/min.
     c. Trunk remains cyanotic despite provision of blow-by oxygen
   4. If heart rate drops to less than 60/min., continue ventilations and begin chest compressions at 120/min.

VI. **Gynecological emergencies** (pp. 713–715)
A. Scene size-up and initial assessment (p. 713)
   1. Note any mechanism of injury that may have caused abdominal or pelvic trauma.
   2. If crime scene (e.g., sexual assault), do not approach patient until police ensure that scene is secure.

      3. Have female EMT conduct assessment on sexual assault victim whenever possible.

      4. After taking all BSI precautions, perform initial assessment.

  B. Focused history and physical exam (pp. 713–714)

      1. Get sample history using OPQRST and remain nonjudgmental.

      2. If sexual assault, make treatment of injuries priority.

      3. Question discreetly about potential injuries.

      4. Do your best to protect patient's privacy.

      5. Do not examine the genitalia of a sexual assault victim unless profuse or life-threatening bleeding.

      6. Obtain set of baseline vital signs.

      7. Help preserve evidence in cases of sexual assault.

         a. Discourage victim from taking a bath, douching, urinating, washing hands, or cleaning wounds.

         b. Handle patient's clothing as little as possible.

         c. Bag all items of clothing and other items separately.

         d. Follow local protocol for crime scene protection.

      8. Signs and symptoms of injury to female genitalia

         a. Abdominal pain

         b. Vaginal bleeding

         c. Soft tissue injuries

         d. Shock (hypoperfusion) if blood loss is great

  C. Emergency medical care (p. 715)

      1. Ensure adequate airway, breathing, and circulation.

      2. Care for vaginal bleeding

         a. Place sanitary napkin over vaginal opening

         b. Never pack vagina in an attempt to control bleeding.

         c. Replace pad if it becomes soaked with blood.

      3. Provide emergency medical care as for any patient, based on any other signs and symptoms.

  D. Transport with detailed physical exam, if appropriate, and ongoing assessment. (p. 715)

ENRICHMENT (OPTIONAL)

The following sections contain information that is valuable as background for the EMT, but that goes substantially beyond the U.S. Department of Transportation's EMT-Basic National Standard Curriculum.

VII. More about predelivery emergencies (pp. 715–719)

  A. Placenta previa (pp. 715–716) **(Fig. 25-20, p. 715)**

      1. Tearing or separation of abnormally low placenta resulting in hemorrhaging that is painless

      2. Overview of disease process

      3. Assessment

      4. Emergency medical care

         a. Follow general guidelines for predelivery emergency.

         b. Administer oxygen at 15 liters per minute by nonrebreather mask.

         c. Provide immediate transport.

  B. Abruptio placenta (pp. 716–717) **(Fig. 25-21, p. 716)**

      1. Placenta separates from uterine wall prior to birth of baby

      2. Overview of disease process

      3. Assessment

      4. Emergency medical care

          a. Follow general guidelines for predelivery emergency.

          b. Administer oxygen at 15 liters per minute by nonrebreather mask.

          c. Provide immediate transport.

C. Preeclampsia/eclampsia (p. 717)

    1. Once known as toxemia or "poisoning of blood"

    2. Overview of disease process

    3. Assessment

    4. Emergency medical care

        a. Follow general guidelines for predelivery emergency.

        b. Administer oxygen at 15 liters per minute by nonrebreather mask.

        c. Keep suction close at hand.

        d. If seizure begins, provide positive-pressure ventilation during seizure.

        e. Transport patient in as quiet and as calm a manner as possible.

D. Ruptured uterus (pp. 717–718) **(Fig. 25-22, p. 718)**

    1. Spontaneous or traumatic rupture of the uterine wall, thereby releasing fetus into abdominal cavity

    2. Overview of disease process

    3. Assessment

    4. Emergency medical care

        a. Follow general guidelines for predelivery emergency.

        b. Administer oxygen at 15 liters per minute by nonrebreather mask.

        c. Provide immediate transport.

E. Ectopic pregnancy (pp. 718–719) **(Fig. 25-23, p. 718)**

    1. Egg is implanted in the fallopian tube, on the abdominal peritoneal covering, on the outside wall of the uterus, on an ovary, or on the cervix

    2. Overview of disease process

    3. Assessment

    4. Emergency medical care

        a. Follow general guidelines for predelivery emergency.

        b. Treat patient for shock (hypoperfusion)

        c. Administer oxygen at 15 liters per minute by nonrebreather mask.

        d. Constantly reassess vital signs.

        e. Provide immediate transport.

F. Braxton-Hicks contractions (p. 719)

G. Precipitous delivery (p. 719)

H. Shoulder dystocia (p. 719)

CASE STUDY FOLLOW-UP

Ask a student volunteer to read the Case Study that begins on page 688 of the textbook. You may wish to use the following questions to engage the students in discussion of the Case Study Follow-up that begins on page 720 of the textbook. Provide missing information and clarify ideas as needed.

Q1. In your initial assessment, what does the condition of Mrs. Baker's slacks indicate?

A1. *That her water has already broken.*

Q2. In your focused history and physical exam, what do you discover about Mrs. Baker's contractions?

A2. *They are occurring every 2 minutes, with a 50-second duration.*

Q3. How does your visual examination of Mrs. Baker's perineum help you decide to deliver the baby in the laundromat?

A3. *There is crowning, with the head bulging out further with each contraction, and the amniotic fluid appears to be clear.*

Q4. What is the baby's initial and second Apgar score?

A4. *7 and 10*

Q5. What does Joe do with the placenta after it is delivered by Mrs. Baker?

A5. *He places it in a container for the emergency department staff to examine.*

IN REVIEW

Assess students' ability to apply what they have just learned by discussing the Review Questions on page 722 of the textbook.

Q1. List the signs and symptoms that would indicate a predelivery emergency, and describe the general guidelines for emergency medical care.

A1. *Signs and symptoms of predelivery emergency include abdominal pain, nausea, vomiting; vaginal bleeding, passage of tissue; weakness, dizziness; altered mental status; seizures; excessive swelling of the face and/or extremities; abdominal trauma; and shock (hypoperfusion). General guidelines for emergency medical care of predelivery emergencies are as follows: Ensure adequate airway, breathing, and circulation. Care for bleeding from the vagina. Treat for shock (hypoperfusion) if indicated. Provide emergency medical care as for the nonpregnant patient based on any other signs and symptoms. Transport the patient on her left side. (pp. 694)*

Q2. Describe signs that would indicate an imminent delivery.

A2. *Delivery is imminent if crowning has occurred; contractions are 2 minutes apart or closer, are intense, and last from 60 to 90 seconds; patient feels infant's head moving down birth canal (sensation of bowel movement); patient has a strong urge to push; patient's abdomen is very hard. (pp. 696–698)*

Q3. Describe how to properly position a mother in active labor and how to create a sterile field around the vaginal opening.

A3. *To position a mother in active labor, position the patient on a firm surface with knees drawn up and spread apart, with patient's feet flat on surface beneath her. Elevate patient's buttocks several inches with a folded blanket, sheet, towels, or other clean objects, buttocks several feet in from the edge of the surface. Support mother's head, neck, and shoulders with pillows or folded blankets. To create a sterile field* *around the vaginal opening, use sheets from the OB kit, sterile towels, or paper barriers. Remove patient's clothing or push it up above her waist. Place one sheet under the woman's hips, unfolding it toward her feet, and another sheet over her abdomen and legs. Place the OB kit or equipment close enough to reach but away from the birth canal so it will not be contaminated. (pp. 700–701)*

Q4. Describe the emergency medical care for a patient in active labor for a normal delivery.

A4. *The emergency medical care for a patient in active labor for a normal delivery is as follows: (1) Position the patient supine. (2) Create a sterile field around the vaginal opening. (3) Monitor the patient for vomiting. Be ready to suction. (4) Continually assess for crowning. (5) When crowning occurs, exert very gentle pressure to the infant's head to prevent explosive delivery. Also exert gentle pressure horizontally across the perineum to reduce the risk of traumatic tears. (6) Tear the amniotic sac if it is not already broken and move it away from infant's head and face. (7) Remove umbilical cord from around the infant's neck, if necessary. (8) As soon as the head is delivered, suction infant's mouth and nostrils. (9) As the torso and full body are born, support the newborn with both hands. Receive the newborn in a clean or sterile towel. (10). Grasp the feet as they are born. (11) Wipe blood and mucus from the infant's mouth and nose with sterile gauze. Then suction the mouth and nose again. (12) Dry the infant with towels and place it in a blanket on its back or side with the neck in a neutral position. Keep the infant level with the mother's vagina until the umbilical cord is cut. (13) Assign one partner to care for the mother, the other to monitor and care for the newborn. (14) Clamp, tie, and cut the umbilical cord when pulsations cease. Periodically check the end of the cord for bleeding, and control any that may occur. (15) Expect the placenta to be delivered within 10 to 20 minutes of the infant. (16) Wrap the delivered placenta in a towel and place it in a plastic bag for transport to the hospital. (17) Place one or two sanitary napkins over the vaginal opening. Then lower the patient's legs and help her hold them together. Elevate her feet, if necessary. (18) Record the time of delivery and transport the mother, infant, and placenta to the hospital. Keep both the mother and the infant warm. Transport gently. (pp. 698–703)*

Q5. Describe how you would recognize an abnormal delivery.

A5. *An abnormal delivery can be recognized by observing one or more of the following: any fetal presentation other than the normal crowning of the fetal head; abnormal color or smell of the amniotic fluid; labor before 38 weeks of pregnancy; recurrence of contractions after the first infant is born. (p. 703)*

Q6. Describe the specific steps you would take to provide emergency medical care for (a) a prolapsed cord, (b) a breech birth or limb presentation, (c) a multiple birth, (d) meconium staining, and (e) a premature birth.

A6. *(a) For a prolapsed cord, position the patient with her head down to allow gravity to reduce the pressure on the cord. Insert a sterile, gloved hand into the vagina, and push the presenting part of the fetus away from the pulsating cord. Follow local protocol and seek medical direction. Cover the umbilical cord with a sterile towel moistened with saline solution. Transport the patient rapidly, maintaining pressure on the presenting part and monitoring pulsations in the cord. (pp. 703–704)*

©2008 by Pearson Education, Inc.
Prehospital Emergency Care, 8th ed.

(b) For a breech birth or a limb presentation, transport immediately upon recognition. Administer oxygen to the mother, and keep the mother in a head-down position so gravity will discourage the progress of the fetus. (pp. 704–705)

(c) For a multiple birth, call for assistance. Be prepared for one or more placentas and more than one resuscitation. If the second infant is not breech, handle the delivery as you would for a single infant. Expect and manage hemorrhage following the second birth. If the second infant has not delivered within 10 minutes of the first, transport to the hospital for delivery of the second infant. (pp. 705–706)

(d) For meconium staining, suction the infant's mouth and nose as soon as the head emerges from the birth canal. Do not stimulate the infant to breathe before suctioning. Transport as soon as possible, maintaining the airway throughout. (p. 706)

(e) For a premature birth, dry the infant and keep it warm. Prevent bleeding from the umbilical cord. Blow oxygen across the infant's face. Prevent contamination and do not let anyone breathe into the infant's face. (p. 706)

Q7. Describe the initial care that is required for the majority (80 percent) of newborns that do not require aggressive resuscitation.

A7. *Approximately 80 percent of newborns require no resuscitation beyond keeping them warm and suctioning the airway. If their responses are slightly depressed, most will respond to oxygen blown by the face or to bag-valve-mask ventilations with supplemental oxygen. (p. 711)*

Q8. Describe the indications and procedures for neonatal resuscitation.

A8. *The indications and procedures for neonatal resuscitation are as follows: (1) If the infant has bluish discoloration but has spontaneous breathing and adequate heart rate, direct a flow of oxygen across the face. (2) Provide ventilations by bag-valve mask with supplemental oxygen at the rate of 40–60 per minute if the infant's breathing is shallow, slow, gasping, or absent following brief stimulation; the heart rate is less than 100/minute; the core body remains cyanotic (blue) despite provision of blow-by oxygen. Reassess after 30 seconds. If the breathing and/or heart rate has not improved, continue ventilations and reassess every 30 seconds. (3) If, despite adequate ventilations, the infant's heart rate drops to less than 60 beats per minute, continue ventilations and begin chest compressions at a rate of 120/minute. (pp. 711–712)*

Q9. List the most common signs and symptoms of a gynecological emergency.

A9. *The most commons signs and symptoms of a gynecological emergency are abdominal pain, vaginal bleeding, and soft tissue injuries. If blood loss is significant, the patient also will display the characteristic signs and symptoms of shock (hypoperfusion). (p. 715)*

Q10. Describe the general guidelines for emergency medical care of a gynecological emergency, including special consideration of the sexual assault victim.

A10. *The general guidelines for emergency medical care of a gynecological emergency are as follows: Take BSI precautions; ensure adequate airway, breathing, and circulation; administer high-flow oxygen and treat for shock (hypoperfusion) if indicated; provide emergency medical care based on the patient's signs and symptoms; care for bleeding from* *the vagina; monitor and record vital signs; and transport. If the emergency is the result of sexual assault, be sure the scene is safe before you enter, examine genitalia only if there is profuse bleeding, use a female EMT for care when possible, discourage the patient from cleaning to help preserve evidence, and follow local protocol on reporting requirements. (p. 715)*

CRITICAL THINKING

Assess students' ability to respond to real-life emergency situations by discussing the Critical Thinking questions on page 723 in the textbook.

Q1. What signs would lead you to believe the labor is true labor and not Braxton-Hicks?

A1. *True labor is distinguished from Braxton-Hicks primarily by three characteristics of the contractions: intensity, duration, and frequency. Contractions of true labor will progressively become more intense (more painful), longer in duration, and more frequent. Braxton-Hicks contractions typically present with a very irregular pattern. The contraction intensity, duration, and frequency vary from contraction to contraction. Braxton-Hicks, also commonly known as false labor, were once thought to have no physiologic purpose; however, more recently it has been found that Braxton-Hicks contractions are involved with the preparation of the pregnant patient for true labor.*

Q2. Why is the patient experiencing lightheadedness?

A2. *This patient is most likely experiencing supine hypotensive syndrome. This condition typically presents in the pregnant patient who is in her third trimester. It is due to the large heavy fetus and uterus falling backward and compressing the inferior vena cava while the patient is in a supine position. The compressed vena cava reduces venous blood flow to the right atrium, which in turn decreases the amount of blood filling the left ventricle prior to its contraction. The reduced blood volume being ejected from the left ventricle results in a decreased blood pressure. The reduced blood pressure decreases perfusion to the brain resulting in lightheadedness or fainting (syncope). To reverse the condition, move the patient into a lateral recumbent or seated position, or simply elevate the hip to one side with pillows or blankets. If the patient is severely lightheaded, do not attempt to place her in a seated position. Also, it was once thought that a left lateral recumbent position or lifting the left hip was preferable since the inferior vena cava is located to the right of the midline. However, it has been found that lifting either hip or placing the patient in either a left or right lateral recumbent position would remove the pressure of the fetus off of the vena cava and reverse the condition.*

Q3. How would you proceed with the emergency care of the patient?

A3. *Since it is obvious that delivery is imminent, the EMTs should prepare the mother and immediate area for a normal delivery. First, the EMTs must be sure to take the necessary standard precautions to include gloves and eye protection. Also, move the mother to an acceptable location for delivery, preferably on the floor or on a bed with her hips and buttocks near the edge. Place the mother on a nonrebreather at 15 lpm. Then open the obstetrical kit and prepare the items inside. If time permits, place an absorbent pad under the mother's buttocks, and drape her legs with the enclosed sheets. Be cautious of an explosive delivery. Time the* *contractions and coach the mother to push during the contractions and to relax and breathe deep between contractions. Only instruct her to push if she is crowning. If she is not crowning, do not have her push during contractions. Instead, have her pant. Coach her strongly not to push. Consider transport.*

Q4. What signs are indicative of imminent delivery?

A4. *The most conclusive sign of imminent delivery is crowning. Other signs include contractions that are regularly occurring 2 minutes or less apart, are intense, and are lasting approximately 60 seconds.*

Q5. What is the significance of the green substance in the fluid on the sheets?

A5. *The green substance found in the amniotic fluid is meconium. Meconium is a substance resulting from a fetal bowel movement, which typically indicates fetal distress. The most important consideration is to keep the newborn from aspirating any of the meconium. Frequent and aggressive suctioning of the nasopharynx and oropharynx with a bulb syringe must be done to prevent aspiration of the meconium as soon as the head is delivered. Suctioning should continue throughout and after the delivery. Aspiration of the meconium could lead to respiratory distress and possible infection in the lungs.*

ROLE PLAY

Provide students with the opportunity to apply what they have learned to a real-life situation encountered by EMS personnel. Ask for one female student to play the role of a pregnant patient in labor and a second student to be your partner. Step-by-step, describe the procedure for assessing and preparing the mother and delivering the infant. After your demonstration, divide the class into groups of three. Provide each group with an obstetrics kit and a birthing model or simulated infant. In each group, one member should be the mother, one the EMT who is assisting with the delivery, and the third an EMT assistant. Tell the students to role-play the steps in the assessment, preparation, and delivery process. Tell them to rotate positions and repeat the role play until every member of the team, regardless of gender, plays all three roles.

Observe each group as it performs the role play. Provide corrective feedback and answer questions as needed.

ASSIGNMENTS

Assign students to read Chapter 26, "Mechanisms of Injury: Kinetics of Trauma," before the next class. Also ask them to complete Chapter 25 of the Workbook.

EVALUATION

Chapter Quiz Distribute copies of the Chapter Quiz provided in Handout 25-2 to evaluate student understanding of this chapter. Remind students not to refer to their textbooks or notes while taking the quiz.

Reading/Reference
Textbook, pp. 724–745

Workbook
Chapter 25 Activities

Chapter Quiz
Handout 25-2

TestGen
Chapter 25 Test

Online Test Preparation
Send your students to
http://www.prenhall.com/
EMTAchieve

Handouts 25-3 to 25-6
Reinforcement Activities

**Brady Skills Series
EMT-B Videos/CD**
Visual Reinforcement

**PowerPoint
Presentation**
Chapter 25

Student CD
Chapter 25

Companion Website
http://www.prenhall.com/
mistovich

Test Manager You may wish to create a custom-tailored test using Prentice Hall *TestGen for Prehospital Emergency Care, Eighth Edition* to evaluate student understanding of this chapter.

Online Test Preparation (for students and instructors) Additional test preparation is available through *EMT Achieve: Basic Test Preparation* at http://www.prenhall.com/EMTAchieve. Instructors can also monitor student mastery online.

REINFORCEMENT

Handouts If classroom discussions or performance on the quiz indicates that some students have not fully mastered the chapter content, you may wish to assign some or all of the Reinforcement Handouts for this chapter.

TECH EXTRAS

Brady Skills Series EMT-B Videos/CD Have your students watch the skills come to life on either VHS or CD-ROM.

PowerPoint Presentation (for instructors) The PowerPoint material developed for this chapter offers useful reinforcement of chapter content.

Student CD A wide variety of material on this CD-ROM will reinforce and also expand student knowledge and skills.

Companion Website (for students) Additional review quizzes and links to EMS resources will contribute to further reinforcement of this chapter. Please visit http://www.prenhall.com/mistovich.

OBJECTIVES CHECKLIST

Cognitive		Date Mastered
4-9.1	Identify the following structures: uterus, vagina, fetus, placenta, umbilical cord, amniotic sac, perineum.	
4-9.2	Identify and explain the use of the contents of an obstetrics kit.	
4-9.3	Identify predelivery emergencies.	
4-9.4	State indications of an imminent delivery.	
4-9.5	Differentiate the emergency medical care provided to a patient with predelivery emergencies from a normal delivery.	
4-9.6	State the steps in the predelivery preparation of the mother.	
4-9.7	Establish the relationship between body substance isolation and childbirth.	
4-9.8	State the steps to assist in the delivery.	
4-9.9	Describe care of the infant as the head appears.	
4-9.10	Describe how and when to cut the umbilical cord.	
4-9.11	Discuss the steps in the delivery of the placenta.	
4-9.12	List the steps in the emergency medical care of the mother post-delivery.	
4-9.13	Summarize neonatal resuscitation procedures.	
4-9.14	Describe the procedures for the following abnormal deliveries: breech birth, prolapsed cord, limb presentation.	
4-9.15	Differentiate the special considerations for multiple births.	
4-9.16	Describe special considerations of meconium.	
4-9.17	Describe special considerations of a premature baby.	
4-9.18	Discuss the emergency medical care of a patient with a gynecological emergency.	

Affective		Date Mastered
4-9.19	Explain the rationale for understanding the implications of treating two patients (mother and baby).	

Psychomotor		Date Mastered
4-9.20	Demonstrate the steps to assist in the normal cephalic delivery.	
4-9.21	Demonstrate necessary care procedures of the fetus as the head appears.	
4-9.22	Demonstrate infant neonatal procedures.	
4-9.23	Demonstrate post-delivery care of the infant.	
4-9.24	Demonstrate how and when to cut the umbilical cord.	
4-9.25	Attend to the steps in the delivery of the placenta.	
4-9.26	Demonstrate the post-delivery care of the mother.	
4-9.27	Demonstrate the procedures for the following abnormal deliveries: vaginal bleeding, breech birth, prolapsed cord, limb presentation.	
4-9.28	Demonstrate the steps in the emergency medical care of the mother with excessive bleeding.	
4-9.29	Demonstrate completing a prehospital care report for patients with obstetric/gynecological emergencies.	

EVALUATION

CHAPTER 25 QUIZ

Write the letter of the best answer in the space provided.

_____ 1. The organ that contains the developing fetus is called the
   A. cervix.
   B. vagina.
   C. uterus.
   D. placenta.

_____ 2. The disk-shaped inner lining of the uterus that begins to develop after the ovum attaches itself to the uterine wall is the
   A. cervix.
   B. vagina.
   C. uterus.
   D. placenta.

_____ 3. The fetus floats in a bag of waters containing _____ fluid.
   A. placental
   B. amniotic
   C. umbilical
   D. CSF

_____ 4. The 9-month period of pregnancy is divided into
   A. quarters.
   B. months.
   C. trimesters.
   D. halves.

_____ 5. A delivery in which the baby's buttocks present first at the vaginal opening is called a _____ presentation.
   A. breech
   B. cephalic
   C. normal
   D. prolapsed

_____ 6. All of the following are examples of abnormal deliveries *except*
   A. breech presentation.
   B. cephalic presentation.
   C. prolapsed presentation.
   D. abruptio placenta.

_____ 7. The term used to describe the point at which the presenting part of the baby first bulges from the vaginal opening is
   A. staining.
   B. a bloody show.
   C. placentae preview.
   D. crowning.

_____ 8. The third stage of labor ends with the
   A. birth of the baby.
   B. full dilation of the cervix.
   C. expulsion of the placenta.
   D. entry of the baby into the birth canal.

_____ 9. The second stage of labor begins when
   A. regular contractions start.
   B. dilation of the cervix occurs.
   C. birth of the baby is complete.
   D. the baby enters the birth canal.

_____ 10. Meconium staining may be an indication of
   A. breech birth.
   B. a premature birth.
   C. fetal distress.
   D. bleeding in the uterus.

_____ 11. The placenta is usually delivered after the baby and is called the
   A. afterbirth.
   B. womb.
   C. bloody show.
   D. postpartum.

_____12. Delivery of the baby may be imminent if contractions last _____ and are _____ apart.
  A. 1–2 minutes; 6–8 minutes
  B. 2–3 minutes; 5–6 minutes
  C. 60–90 seconds; 2–3 minutes
  D. 45 seconds–1 minute; 3–4 minutes

_____13. The EMT should clamp, tie, and cut the umbilical cord after
  A. it appears.
  B. the baby is delivered.
  C. the placenta is delivered.
  D. its pulsations have ceased.

_____14. If this is the woman's first delivery, she is not straining, and there is no crowning, then
  A. birth will probably occur too soon for transport.
  B. you will probably have time to transport to a medical facility for delivery.
  C. birth will probably occur during transport in the ambulance.
  D. a surgical delivery will probably be necessary.

_____15. The EMT must assist in the delivery of the infant in all of the following cases *except* when
  A. you have no suitable transportation.
  B. the hospital or physician cannot be reached due to bad weather.
  C. the mother requests your assistance.
  D. delivery is imminent.

_____16. If the pregnant mother gets dizzy and has a drop in blood pressure when she is in a supine position, the condition is called
  A. supine hypotensive syndrome.
  B. supine hypertensive crisis.
  C. eclampsia.
  D. abruptio placentae.

_____17. The Apgar score of a newborn who can be expected to need only routine care would be
  A. –3 to 0.
  B. 0 to 3.
  C. 4 to 6.
  D. 7 to 10.

_____18. Which one of the following statements is *true* about the afterbirth?
  A. Pull on the umbilical cord to encourage its delivery.
  B. It usually delivers in about 20 minutes.
  C. It may be discarded as soon as it is delivered.
  D. It can remain in the uterus and pose no serious problem.

_____19. To control vaginal bleeding after birth
  A. massage the uterus.
  B. have the mother squeeze her legs together.
  C. pack the vagina with gauze dressings.
  D. don't allow the mother to nurse the baby.

_____20. If the umbilical cord presents first during delivery
  A. provide the mother with oxygen and transport immediately because the problem can be handled only at the hospital.
  B. keep pressure off the cord by placing your gloved hand in the vagina and transport immediately.
  C. immediately clamp and cut the cord.
  D. place a mask with high-concentration oxygen at the vaginal opening.

IN THE FIELD

Read the following real-life situation. Then answer the questions that follow.

Patty O'Hara is pregnant, and her delivery date was several days ago. She was experiencing back pain all evening before going to bed. About 1:30 A.M., she is awakened with abdominal cramps and realizes her clothes and bed sheets are wet. She wakes her husband, Brian, telling him it's time to go to the hospital. Her labor quickly develops, and soon her contractions are about 1 minute long and coming every 2 minutes. Before Brian can get dressed and start the car, Patty tells him she doesn't think she can make it to the hospital before the baby is born. She lies back on the bed, and Brian calls 9-1-1.

An anxious Brian meets the ambulance in front of their house about 7 minutes later. Upon entering the bedroom, George and Edwin, both EMTs, are greeted by Patty, who is still lying supine on the bed. George introduces himself and Edwin as they don BSI equipment. George notes that Patty is having a contraction and that her bag of waters has ruptured. Patty informs George that her contractions are coming about every 2 minutes and that she feels the need to move her bowels. Edwin times her next contraction and it lasts about 1 minute.

Patty tells the EMTs that this is her fourth child, it is about a week overdue, and that the pregnancy has been normal up to now. George explains that he needs to look for crowning, and Brian assists Patty in removing clothing. George notes crowning of the baby's head, so he and Edwin prepare to deliver the baby. They open their OB kit and place the drapes under Patty's buttocks, on her abdomen, and on her legs. Edwin places a pillow under Patty's buttocks to elevate her hips. George instructs Brian to stay with Patty at the head of the bed. George positions himself at the foot of the bed, while Edwin takes Patty's vitals.

As the baby's head begins to appear, George positions his hands at the vaginal opening. He places his hand on the baby's head, gently, to prevent an explosive delivery. As the head delivers, George notes meconium staining of the amniotic fluid. As soon as the head delivers, George uses a bulb syringe to quickly suction the mouth and nose. As the baby's body is delivered, George supports the head, the shoulders, and the rest of the body as it appears. The baby begins crying as George repeats the suctioning. George keeps the baby at about the same level as Patty's vagina, clamps and cuts the umbilical cord, and wraps the infant in a warm blanket. Edwin writes the exact time of birth in his notepad. With the baby and mother doing well, George and Edwin prepare for a calm, careful transport to the hospital.

1. What signs led to George's decision to deliver the baby at the house instead of transporting?

2. What BSI equipment would be appropriate for a delivery at home?

3. Bob noted meconium staining during the delivery. What is the cause of this, and what complications might this cause? What can the EMT do at the time of delivery to help prevent complications?

4. Why did George suction the mouth of the baby first?

5. Why did George keep the baby at the same level as the mother's vagina?

6. What signs did George look for that told him it was appropriate to cut the umbilical cord?

CHAPTER 25 REVIEW

Write the word or words that best complete each sentence in the space provided.

1. The _____ is a muscular organ in which the fetus grows.

2. Blood from the fetus is sent through blood vessels in the _____

   _____ to the placenta where the blood picks up nourishment from the

   mother.

3. The lower part of the birth canal is called the _____.

4. During the first stage of labor, the cervix becomes _____

   _____.

5. During the third stage of labor, the _____ separates from the uterine wall

   and is _____ from the uterus.

6. Greenish or brownish-yellow coloring in the amniotic fluid is called _____

   _____.

7. When suctioning a newborn with a bulb syringe, suction the _____ first,

   then the _____, remembering to compress the bulb syringe

   _____ placing it in the baby.

8. If a newborn's heart rate is less than _____ beats per minute, provide

   _____ _____ _____ at a

   rate of 40–60 per minute.

9. When clamping the umbilical cord, place two clamps or ties on the cord about

   _____ inches apart; the first clamp should be approximately

   _____ inches from the infant.

10. It is critical to keep a newborn baby _____.

11. The placenta, umbilical cord, membranes of the amniotic sac, and some of the tissues lining the

    uterus are called the _____ and may take up to

    _____ _____ to deliver.

12. To control vaginal bleeding after delivery of the baby and placenta, you should

    _____ the mother's abdomen, just above the uterus.

13. To care for a breech presentation, place the mother in a(n) _____

_____ position with the _____ elevated.

14. With a limb presentation, _____ _____ is essential

for the baby's survival.

15. An infant who weighs less than 5 pounds at birth or is born before the 38th week of pregnancy is

called a(n) _____ _____.

16. A life-threatening condition in which the placenta separates from the uterine wall is called

_____ _____.

17. _____ _____ is a condition in which the placenta

has formed in an abnormally low position that can lead to tearing or separation of the uterus.

18. Implantation of the fertilized egg in an oviduct, the cervix, or in the abdominopelvic cavity is called

a(n) _____ _____.

19. A common condition called _____ is usually associated with high blood

pressure and swelling of the extremities.

©2008 by Pearson Education, Inc.
Prehospital Emergency Care, 8th ed.

OBSTETRIC AND GYNECOLOGICAL EMERGENCIES: LISTING

1. List at least five recommended items found in the standard obstetric kit.

2. List at least five things to consider when evaluating a mother in labor in order to make a transport decision.

3. List the steps in the general procedure for umbilical cord care.

4. List the two methods of controlling vaginal bleeding after birth.

Student's Name _____

OBSTETRIC AND GYNECOLOGICAL EMERGENCIES: MATCHING

Write the letter of the term in the space next to the appropriate description.

_____ 1. Spontaneous abortion

_____ 2. When the baby appears buttocks first during birth

_____ 3. When an infant's extremity protrudes first from the vagina

_____ 4. Amniotic fluid that is greenish or brownish-yellow rather than clear

_____ 5. "Poisoning" of the blood during pregnancy characterized by high blood pressure and swollen extremities

_____ 6. A condition in which the placenta is positioned too close to the cervix and will not allow a normal delivery of the fetus

_____ 7. Any newborn weighing less than 5 pounds or born before the 38th week

_____ 8. When the umbilical cord presents first and is squeezed between the vaginal wall and the baby's head

_____ 9. Dizziness and a drop in blood pressure caused by the baby compressing the inferior vena cava when the woman is supine

_____ 10. A condition in which the placenta separates from the uterine wall, causing extreme prebirth bleeding

A. abruptio placenta

B. breech presentation

C. limb presentation

D. meconium

E. miscarriage

F. placenta previa

G. preeclampsia/eclampsia

H. premature birth

I. prolapsed cord

J. supine hypotensive syndrome

Obstetric and Gynecological Emergencies

Anatomy of Pregnancy

Stages of Labor

- Dilation
- Expulsion
- Placental

Assessment and Care: Predelivery Emergency

Supine Hypotensive Syndrome

Spontaneous Abortion

Seizures

Vaginal Bleeding

Trauma

Assessment and Care: Normal Delivery

Assessment and Care: Abnormal Delivery

Prolapsed Cord

Breech Birth

Limb Presentation

Multiple Births

Meconium

Premature Birth

Assessment and Care: The Newborn Infant

Apgar Score

Resuscitation

Assessment and Care: Gynecological Emergencies

Additional Predelivery Emergencies

Placenta Previa

Abruptio Placenta

Preeclampsia/Eclampsia

Ruptured Uterus

Ectopic Pregnancy

HANDOUT 25-2: Chapter 25 Quiz

1. C	**6.** B	**11.** A	**16.** A
2. D	**7.** D	**12.** C	**17.** D
3. B	**8.** C	**13.** D	**18.** B
4. C	**9.** D	**14.** B	**19.** A
5. A	**10.** C	**15.** C	**20.** B

HANDOUT 25-3: In the Field

1. This is Patty's fourth child, her bag of waters broke, and her contractions were lasting 1 minute and coming every 2 minutes. She felt a need to move her bowels.

2. BSI equipment for a delivery should include gloves, mask, protective eyewear, and a gown to protect clothing.

3. Meconium is the material expelled from the bowels of a fetus before delivery. It usually indicates either fetal or maternal distress. When meconium staining is seen, it is important for the EMT to suction the mouth and nose of the baby as soon as the head is delivered to prevent the baby from aspirating the material into the lungs, which can lead to pneumonia or other infections.

4. The mouth of a newborn should be suctioned first. Infants are obligate nose breathers. If the nose is suctioned first, the baby may attempt to take a breath. Any material in the baby's mouth would then be aspirated into the lungs.

5. It is important to keep the baby at the level of the mother's vagina before the umbilical cord is cut so that blood from the baby will not return into the placenta. For this reason, do not place the baby on the mother's abdomen until the cord is clamped and cut.

6. The umbilical cord can be clamped and cut when the baby begins breathing on his or her own, and after the cord has stopped pulsating.

HANDOUT 25-4: Chapter 25 Review

1. uterus
2. umbilical cord
3. vagina
4. fully dilated
5. placenta, expelled
6. meconium staining

7. mouth, nose, before
8. 100, positive-pressure ventilations
9. 3, 6
10. warm
11. afterbirth, 20 minutes
12. massage
13. knee–chest, pelvis
14. rapid transport
15. premature infant
16. abruptio placenta
17. Placenta previa
18. ectopic pregnancy
19. Preeclampsia/eclampsia

HANDOUT 25-5: Obstetric and Gynecological Emergencies: Listing

1. Any five of the following: surgical scissors or scalpel; cord clamps or cord ties; umbilical tape or sterilized cord; bulb syringe; towels, five or more; gauze sponges, 2 10; sterile gloves; one infant blanket; individually wrapped sanitary napkins; large plastic bag; germicidal wipes

2. Any five of the following: Is this the patient's first delivery? If not, how many has she experienced? How long has the patient been pregnant? Has there been any bleeding or discharge? Are there any contractions or pain present? What is the frequency and duration of contractions? Is crowning occurring with contractions? Does the patient feel the need to push? Does the patient feel as if she is having a bowel movement? Is the abdomen hard upon palpation?

3. (1) Place two clamps or ties on the cord about 3 inches apart. The first clamp should be approximately 6 inches from the infant. (2) Use sterile surgical scissors or a scalpel to cut the cord between the two clamps. (3) Periodically check the end of the cord for bleeding.

4. Massage the uterus. Allow the infant to suckle on the mother's breast.

HANDOUT 25-6: Obstetric and Gynecological Emergencies: Matching

1. E	**4.** D	**7.** H	**9.** J
2. B	**5.** G	**8.** I	**10.** A
3. C	**6.** F		

26 Mechanisms of Injury: Kinetics of Trauma

This chapter covers portions of Lesson 3-1 of the U.S. Department of Transportation's EMT-Basic National Standard Curriculum.

OBJECTIVES

Numbered objectives are from the U.S. Department of Transportation's EMT-Basic National Standard Curriculum. Asterisked objectives, if any, pertain to material that is supplemental to the DOT curriculum. Page numbers refer to pages in the textbook.

Cognitive

3-1.4 Discuss common mechanisms of injury/nature of illness. (pp. 730–742)

* Explain how the following affect the force of impact: mass and velocity, acceleration and deceleration, energy changing form and direction. (pp. 727–728)

* Describe the three main impacts that occur in a vehicle collision. (pp. 729–730)

* Discuss the following mechanisms of injury and their effects on the human body: motor-vehicle collisions, vehicle–pedestrian collisions, motorcycle collisions, falls, penetrating injuries, and blast injuries. (pp. 730–742)

* Discuss the steps of patient assessment, including the priority decision, as they relate to and are guided by the mechanism of injury. (p. 743)

REVIEW

In Chapter 25, "Obstetric and Gynecological Emergencies," students learned that only in a few situations involving complications does the EMT need to see that the mother reaches a hospital quickly. EMTs must be prepared to deal with these emergencies in an absolutely professional, effective, and compassionate way. In addition, they need to be sure to review assessment and emergency medical care procedures as often as they can.

Distribute the scored quizzes from the last class. Go over each question on the quiz, and handle any concerns students may have about the answers.

Explain that Module 4, "Medical, Behavioral, and Obstetric/Gynecological Emergencies," is now complete. In Module 4, students learned about some of the medications EMTs can help patients administer. They also learned how to handle breathing problems, cardiac emergencies, and crises related to diabetes, allergies, poisoning, overdose, behavioral emergencies, and problems during pregnancy and birth.

Total Teaching Time
120 minutes

Resources Needed
• Scored Chapter 25 Quizzes

• Newspaper articles with accounts of incidents involving trauma

Additional Resources
Larmon/Davis, *Basic Life Support Skills*

Elling, *EMT Achieve: Basic Test Preparation*

Limmer/Mistovich/O'Keefe, *Audio Lecture & Study Guide: EMT*

Mistovich/Kuvlesky, *SUCCESS! for the EMT, Second Edition*

INTRODUCTION TO MODULE 5

In Module 5, students will learn how to care for patients who have been injured. In this module, students will learn about mechanisms of injury; how to control bleeding and shock; how to treat soft tissue injuries; how to care for burns; and how to handle injuries to the muscles, bones, head, spine, and other parts of the body.

INTRODUCTION TO CHAPTER 26

Chapter 26, "Mechanisms of Injury: Kinetics of Trauma," is the first lesson of Module 5. Since the early 1970s, trauma (injury) has been recognized as the leading cause of death for those between the ages of 14 and 40 (now exceeded only by AIDS among young adults) and is the third leading cause of death for all age groups, after cardiovascular disease and cancer. Trauma makes up a significant percent of the calls to which prehospital personnel respond. With any trauma patient, determining the possible extent of injury is critical to making good priority decisions regarding on-scene assessment and care versus rapid transport with assessment and care continuing en route. To make these judgments, the EMR must not only recognize obvious injuries but also must maintain a high index of suspicion for hidden injuries. An understanding of mechanisms of injury is the chief component of this crucial assessment skill.

Distribute the Chapter 26 Objectives Checklist, and give students a few minutes to look it over. Then briefly paraphrase the objectives for this lesson in your own words.

LECTURE

The following suggested lecture outline is based on the Department of Transportation's EMT-Basic National Standard Curriculum. In some places, the DOT curriculum has been rearranged or expanded upon so that it is more complete or easier for the student to understand. The page numbers in parentheses refer to pages in the textbook. The parenthetical references in dark, heavy type are to figures, tables, and scans in the textbook.

MECHANISMS OF INJURY: KINETICS OF TRAUMA

I. The kinetics of trauma (pp. 727–730) **(Fig. 26-1, p. 728)**
    A. Mass and velocity (pp. 727–728)
        1. The amount of kinetic energy a moving body contains.
    B. Acceleration and deceleration (p. 728)
        1. The faster a change in speed, the greater the force exerted.
        2. Law of inertia
            a. A body at rest will remain at rest, and a body in motion will remain in motion, unless acted upon by an outside force.
        3. Acceleration
            a. Rate at which a body in motion increases its speed
        4. Deceleration
            a. Rate at which a body in motion decreases its speed
    C. Energy changes form and direction (p. 728)
        1. Interruption of kinetic energy traveling through the body can cause injury
    D. Impacts (pp. 729–730) **(Fig. 26-2, p. 729)**

Handout 26-1
Chapter 26 Objectives Checklist

●➤

Lecture Master
You may wish to display Lecture Master 26 when presenting the lecture to the class.

1. Vehicle collision
    a. Vehicle is suddenly stopped
2. Body collision
    a. Patient comes to quick stop against part(s) inside vehicle
3. Organ collision
    a. Patient's internal organs come to quick stop against other body parts (skull, chest, or abdomen)
II. **Mechanisms of injury** (pp. 730–742)
    A. Vehicle collisions (pp. 730–739)
        1. The greater the speed at collision, the greater the chance for life-threatening injury (**Fig. 26-3, p. 731**)
        2. High index of suspicion for trauma
            a. Death of another occupant of vehicle
            b. Unresponsive patient
            c. Patient with an altered mental status
        3. Frontal impact collision (**Fig. 26-4, p. 731**)
            a. Driver continues to move forward at same speed vehicle is traveling (**Fig. 26-5, p. 731**)
            b. May proceed up and over steering wheel, causing injuries to head, neck, chest, and abdomen, and possible ejection (**Figs. 26-6 and 26-7, p. 732**)
                (1) Abdominal injury
                (2) Chest injury (**Figs. 26-8 and 26-9, p. 733**)
                (3) Face, head, and neck injury (**Fig. 26-10, p. 733**)
            c. May proceed down and under steering wheel, causing injuries to knees, femurs, hips, acetabulum, and spine.
        4. Rear-end impact (**Fig. 26-11, p. 734**)
            a. Initial movement is backward, causing potential neck injury. (**Fig. 26-12, p. 734**)
            b. Initial neck injury followed by either frontal up-and-over or down-and-under injuries
        5. Lateral (side) impact (**Figs. 26-13 and 26-14, p. 735**)
            a. Head and neck
            b. Chest and abdomen
            c. Pelvis
        6. Rotational or rollover impact
            a. Rotational impact (**Fig. 26-15, p. 735**)
            b. Rollover impact (**Figs. 26-16 and 26-17, p. 736**)
        7. Vehicle–pedestrian collision
            a. Extent of injury depends on (**Fig. 26-18, p. 737**)
                (1) How fast vehicle is traveling
                (2) Part of pedestrian's body hit
                (3) How far pedestrian thrown
                (4) Surface pedestrian lands on
                (5) Body part that first strikes ground
            b. Common child injuries: combination of injuries to femur, chest, abdomen, and head
            c. Common adult injuries: fractures of tibia and fibula; injuries to back, chest, shoulders, arms, abdomen; and head and neck injuries
        8. Restraints: a cause of hidden injuries (**Fig. 26-19, p. 737**)
        9. Considerations for infants and children
            a. Seat restraints should restrain at one or two points on mid-pelvis, one point on each shoulder.
            b. Seat should face backward in upright position.

Point to Emphasize

EMTs are the eyes and ears of the receiving facility. They must be alert, while on the scene, for any clues that might warn doctors and nurses of potential problems. They might consider photographing the emergency scene, if possible.

On the Net

National statistics on mechanisms of injury. http://www.facs.org/ntdbreport2001/resourceutil.html

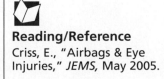

Reading/Reference

Criss, E., "Airbags & Eye Injuries," *JEMS,* May 2005.

c. Children should always be restrained in backseat of vehicle.

10. Motorcycle collisions **(Fig. 26-20, p. 738)**
    a. Head-on impact **(Figs. 26-21 and 26-22, p. 738)**
       (1) Most often associated with ejection
    b. Angular impact
       (1) Rider and motorcycle strike an object, usually a protruding object, at an angle
    c. Ejection
       (1) Occurs if the rider clears the motorcycle's handlebars
    d. "Laying the bike down"
       (1) Bike turned sideways and "laid down" with driver's inside leg dragging on pavement or ground

11. All-terrain vehicles **(Fig. 26-23, p. 739)**

B. Falls (pp. 739–740)
   1. Most common mechanism of injury; damage varies according to distance, surface, and body part that impacts first.
   2. Feet-first falls **(Fig. 26-24, p. 739)**
   3. Head-first falls

C. Penetrating injuries (pp. 740–741) **(Fig. 26-25, p. 740)**
   1. Damage results from amount of kinetic energy transferred to tissue and the area of the body it penetrates
   2. Low-velocity injuries
      a. Usually due to a knife or other impaling objects
   3. Medium- and high-velocity injuries
      a. Usually due to bullets or pellets; amount of damage depends on:
      b. Trajectory
         (1) Path or motion of projectile during travel
      c. Dissipation of body energy
         (1) Drag
            (a) Factors that slow bullet down
         (2) Profile
            (a) Impact point of bullet
         (3) Cavitation
            (a) Pathway or cavity in the body tissues formed by entering bullet
      d. Shotgun pellets increase impact surface area. **(Fig. 26-26, p. 741)**
   4. Gunshot wounds
      a. Head
      b. Chest
      c. Abdomen
      d. Extremities

D. Blast injuries (pp. 741–742) **(Fig. 26-27, p. 741 and Fig. 26-28, p. 742)**
   1. Primary phase injuries
      a. Due to pressure wave of blast
      b. Primarily affect gas-containing organs (lungs, stomach, intestines, inner ears, sinuses)
      c. Patient may suffer severe damage and death with no external signs of injury.
   2. Secondary phase injuries
      a. Due to flying debris from blast

On the Net

Fall statistics. http://www. tf.org/tf/injuries/fall.html

On the Net

Wound ballistics. www.firearmstactical.com/ wound.htm

Reading/Reference

Criss, E., "Ballistic Basics," *JEMS,* May 1999.

            3. Tertiary phase injuries
                a. Due to patient being thrown away from blast
III. The "golden hour" (p. 743)
   A. "Golden hour" (p. 743)
      1. Severely injured patient has best chance for survival if
         surgical intervention takes place within 1 hour from time of
         injury
   B. "Platinum 10 minutes" (p. 743)
      1. Maximum time out of the golden hour that EMT teams
         should devote to on-scene activities for severely injured
         patient
      2. Standard parameter for emergency care
   C. "High index of suspicion" (p. 743)
      1. Presumption by EMTs that patient has severe injuries if there
         is any indication that this is possible **(Table 26-1, p. 743)**

CASE STUDY FOLLOW-UP

Ask a student volunteer to read the Case Study that begins on page 727 of the
textbook. You may wish to use the following questions to engage the students
in a discussion of the Case Study Follow-up that begins on page 744 of the
textbook. Provide missing information and clarify ideas as needed.

Q1. From what direction was the patient's vehicle struck?

A1. *From the rear.*

Q2. Because Mike was not wearing his seatbelt, what pathway did his
body take during the impact?

A2. *He went down and under the dashboard during the impact.*

Q3. As a precaution, what does your partner do to Mike during the
initial assessment?

A3. *Gets into the back seat and reaches from behind to hold Mike's head
still.*

Q4. How do you extricate Mike from his vehicle?

A4. *A cervical spine immobilization collar and a KED immobilization
vest are applied; then Mike is transferred to a long spine board,
immobilized, and finally extricated.*

Q5. In addition to his painful knees, what new complaint does Mike
make during your focused history?

A5. *That he now also has an ache in his lumbar spine.*

IN REVIEW

Assess students' ability to apply what they have just learned by discussing the
Review Questions on page 745 of the textbook.

Q1. Based on the formulas for kinetic energy and force, explain how the
following are likely to affect the severity of an injury: (a) mass and
velocity; (b) acceleration and deceleration.

A1. *Mass, velocity, acceleration, and deceleration affect the kinetic energy
and force of impact. (a) Velocity is a more significant factor than mass.
When mass is doubled, kinetic energy is doubled; when velocity is doubled,*

kinetic energy is squared. (b) When the rate of either acceleration or deceleration increases, so does the force that is exerted. (pp. 727–728)

Q2. Name and describe, in sequence, the three impacts that take place in a vehicular collision.

A2. *First the vehicle strikes an object (vehicle collision). Next, the patient comes to a quick stop on parts of the inside of the vehicle (body collision). Finally, the patient's internal organs strike the internal body and the tissues that support them (organ collision). (p. 729)*

Q3. Name and describe four types of motorcycle collisions.

A3. *Four types of motorcycle collisions are the following: (a) head-on impact, when the cycle tends to tip forward and the rider to strike the handlebars; (b) angular impact, when the rider strikes an object at an angle; (c) ejection, when the rider clears the handlebars and strikes the object of the collision, the ground, or both; and (d) "laying the bike down," when the bike is laid on its side with the rider's inside leg dragging on the pavement or ground. (p. 738)*

Q4. Describe the path of energy and possible patterns of injury for each of the following kinds of falls: (a) feet first; (b) landing on outstretched hands; (c) head first.

A4. *(a) In a feet-first fall, energy travels up the skeletal system, possibly causing fracture of the heels, ankles, knees, hips, pelvis, and/or spine. (b) In a landing on outstretched hands, energy travels up the arms with possible fracture to the wrist, elbow, and/or shoulder. (c) In a head-first fall, energy may travel through the arms to the shoulder; the head and spine may be hyperextended, flexed, or compressed; and there may be injuries to the torso and legs as the body is thrown forward or backward. (pp. 739–740)*

Q5. Define cavitation and tell which of the following kinds of weapons would be likely to produce it: knife, handgun, M-16 rifle.

A5. *Sometimes called pathway expansion, cavitation is the cavity in the body tissues formed by a pressure wave resulting from the kinetic energy of a bullet. The cavity formed is larger than the diameter of the projectile itself. A knife does not produce cavitation because it is a low-velocity weapon. A bullet fired from a handgun (medium velocity) or M-16 rifle (high velocity) would produce cavitation. (pp. 740–741)*

Q6. Explain the cause of each of the following phases of blast injury: primary, secondary, and tertiary.

A6. *In a blast, the cause of primary-phase injuries is the pressure wave from the blast; the cause of secondary-phase injuries is flying debris propelled by the blast; and the cause of tertiary-phase injuries is the impact of the patient being thrown by the blast. (pp. 741–742)*

Q7. Name mechanisms of injury that should cause the EMT to have a high index of suspicion of significant injury.

A7. *Mechanisms that should cause the EMT to have a high index of suspicion of significant injury are the following: ejection from an automobile; death or a patient with an altered mental status in the same passenger compartment; extrication time greater than 20 minutes; falls greater than 20 feet; rollover; high-speed auto crash (initial speed greater than 40 mph, major auto deformation greater than 20 inches, intrusion into passenger compartment greater than*

12 inches); auto–pedestrian/auto–bicycle injury with greater than 5 mph impact; pedestrian thrown or run over; motorcycle crash greater than 20 mph or separation of rider from bike. (Table 26-1, p. 743)

CRITICAL THINKING

Assess students' ability to respond to real-life emergency situations by discussing the Critical Thinking questions on page 745 in the textbook.

Q1. Based on the mechanism of injury, what injuries do you suspect the patient possibly has suffered?

A1. *In a frontal collision, the injury patterns typically involve the head, neck, anterior chest, abdomen, pelvis, and lower extremities. The upper extremities may also be involved depending on their position during impact. Based on the pattern of injury typical in a frontal collision, many organs or structures may be injured including the brain, spinal cord, vertebral column, chest wall, lungs, heart, aorta, vena cava, spleen, liver, intestines, bladder, pelvis, femur, tibia, fibula, humerus, radius, or ulna.*

Q2. What type of impact was involved in the collision?

A2. *A head-on collision produces a frontal impact mechanism of injury. Based on the laws of motion, once the car impacts the cement barrier at 65 mph, the body continues moving forward until it impacts the inside of the car at 65 mph. Once the body impact occurs, the organs will continue moving forward at 65 mph until they strike the inside of the body. This will typically produce the tearing and shearing injuries to the organs and internal structures.*

Q3. What two different pathway patterns of injury may be involved in this collision?

A3. *This frontal impact may have caused either an up-and-over injury pattern or a down-and-under injury pattern. The up-and-over pattern occurs when the patient's body moves up out of the seat and over the steering wheel with the head moving toward the windshield. This will typically cause injury to the head, neck, chest, and abdomen. The down-and-under movement causes the patient to slide under the steering wheel. This movement typically causes injury to the feet, tibia, fibula, femurs, pelvis, and abdomen.*

IDENTIFYING MECHANISM OF INJURY

Bring in several copies of local newspapers that contain articles describing incidents involving trauma in the community. Read the accounts to students, and ask them to suggest possible mechanisms of injury for each of the incidents you have chosen. You might also ask students to describe what precautions they would have taken at each scene if their EMS unit had been assigned to it.

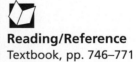

Reading/Reference
Textbook, pp. 746–771

ASSIGNMENTS

Assign students to read Chapter 27, "Bleeding and Shock," before the next class. Also ask them to complete Chapter 26 of the Workbook.

Workbook
Chapter 26 Activities

Chapter Quiz
Handout 26-2

TestGen
Chapter 26 Test

Online Test Preparation
Send your students to
http://www.prenhall.com/
EMTAchieve

Handouts 26-3 to 26-7
Reinforcement Activities

**Brady Skills Series
EMT-B Videos/CD**
Visual Reinforcement

**PowerPoint
Presentation**
Chapter 26

Student CD
Chapter 26

Companion Website
http://www.prenhall.com/
mistovich

EVALUATION

Chapter Quiz Distribute copies of the Chapter Quiz provided in Handout 26-2 to evaluate student understanding of this chapter. Remind students not to refer to their textbooks or notes while taking the quiz.

Test Manager You may wish to create a custom-tailored test using Prentice Hall *TestGen for Prehospital Emergency Care, Eighth Edition* to evaluate student understanding of this chapter.

Online Test Preparation (for students and instructors) Additional test preparation is available through *EMT Achieve: Basic Test Preparation* at http://www.prenhall.com/EMTAchieve. Instructors can also monitor student mastery online.

REINFORCEMENT

Handouts If classroom discussions or performance on the quiz indicates that some students have not fully mastered the chapter content, you may wish to assign some or all of the Reinforcement Handouts for this chapter.

TECH EXTRAS

Brady Skills Series EMT-B Videos/CD Have your students watch the skills come to life on either VHS or CD-ROM.

PowerPoint Presentation (for instructors) The PowerPoint material developed for this chapter offers useful reinforcement of chapter content.

Student CD A wide variety of material on this CD-ROM will reinforce and also expand student knowledge and skills.

Companion Website (for students) Additional review quizzes and links to EMS resources will contribute to further reinforcement of this chapter. Please visit http://www.prenhall.com/mistovich.

©2008 by Pearson Education, Inc.
Prehospital Emergency Care, 8th ed.

OBJECTIVES CHECKLIST

Cognitive		Date Mastered
3-1.4	Discuss common mechanisms of injury/nature of illness.	
*	Explain how the following affect the force of impact: mass and velocity, acceleration and deceleration, energy changing form and direction.	
*	Describe the three main impacts that occur in a vehicle collision.	
*	Discuss the following mechanisms of injury and their effects on the human body: motor-vehicle collisions, vehicle–pedestrian collisions, motorcycle collisions, falls, penetrating injuries, and blast injuries.	
*	Discuss the steps of patient assessment, including the priority decision, as they relate to and are guided by the mechanism of injury.	

OBJECTIVES

CHAPTER 26 QUIZ

Write the letter of the best answer in the space provided.

_____ 1. Newton's first law of motion states that a body at rest will remain at rest and a body in motion will remain in motion unless acted upon by
   A. inertia.
   B. condensation.
   C. an outside force.
   D. convection.

_____ 2. The term for the energy that is contained in a moving body is
   A. kinetic.
   B. thermal.
   C. potential.
   D. chemical.

_____ 3. An increase in which one of the following causes the greatest increase in kinetic energy?
   A. mass
   B. velocity
   C. size
   D. width

_____ 4. Shearing or tearing forces are placed on the organs and their supportive tissues in the mechanism of injury called
   A. acceleration/deceleration.
   B. machine/body collision.
   C. rollover collisions.
   D. penetrating injuries.

_____ 5. A bullet traveling through a body part produces a temporary indentation around the bullet's actual path. This process is known as
   A. penetration.
   B. compression.
   C. cavitation.
   D. levitation.

_____ 6. The chance of sustaining a fatal injury in a vehicle collision is increased by 300% when the occupant is
   A. unrestrained.
   B. ejected.
   C. an infant or a child.
   D. improperly restrained.

_____ 7. In every motor-vehicle collision there are at least how many impacts?
   A. two
   B. three
   C. four
   D. five

_____ 8. A fall should be considered severe any time an adult patient has fallen _____ feet.
   A. 2
   B. 5
   C. 10
   D. 15

_____ 9. On what does the extent of injury depend when a vehicle hits a pedestrian?
   A. how fast the vehicle was going
   B. what part of the pedestrian's body was hit
   C. how far the pedestrian was thrown
   D. all of the above

_____ 10. Which one of the following may be useful in determining nature of illness/mechanism of injury?
   A. the patient
   B. bystanders
   C. family members
   D. all of the above

©2008 by Pearson Education, Inc.
Prehospital Emergency Care, 8th ed.

EVALUATION

IN THE FIELD

Review the following real-life situation. Then answer the questions that follow.

Your EMS unit is dispatched to a one-vehicle automobile collision. You arrive and find a 22-year-old female who reportedly dodged an animal that was in the roadway. She ran off the road and hit a large cedar tree. After repeated questioning, she admits that she had just taken her seatbelt off. You assess the car to find that the steering column is bent and that there is a starburst pattern on the windshield in front of the driver's seat. The driver, meanwhile, is very anxious and restless. You note a large bruise over her sternum.

1. What injuries would you expect to find, considering the mechanism of injury?

2. How would you expect the injuries to be different if the patient had been wearing a seatbelt? If the airbag had deployed?

REINFORCEMENT

CHAPTER 26 REVIEW

Write the word or words that best complete each sentence in the space provided.

1. Since the early 1970s, _____ has been recognized as the leading cause of death for those between the ages of 14 and 40.

2. The science of analyzing the mechanism of injury is sometimes called the

   _____ _____ _____.

3. The factors and forces that may have caused injury to a patient are the

   _____ _____ _____.

4. The amount of kinetic energy an object contains depends on two factors: the body's

   _____ and the body's _____.

5. During the assessment of a patient who was involved in an MVC, the EMT must maintain a high

   _____ _____ _____

   based on the mechanism of injury.

6. Understanding the factor of _____ is important in evaluating the mechanism of injury in vehicle collisions.

7. _____ travels in a straight line unless it meets and is deflected by some type of interference.

8. The rate at which a body in motion increases its speed is known as _____.

9. Over one-third of all deaths due to trauma occur from _____

   _____.

10. The up-and-over pathway causes impact to the _____,

    _____, _____, and

    _____.

©2008 by Pearson Education, Inc.
Prehospital Emergency Care, 8th ed.

KINETICS OF TRAUMA: LISTING

1. List four major factors in determining the force of an impact.

2. In the typical vehicular collision, there are actually three impacts. List these.

3. List five common mechanisms of injury.

4. List five types of motor-vehicle collisions.

REINFORCEMENT

RECOGNIZING INJURY PATTERNS

For each of the three types of collisions pictured below, identify the type of collision and the type of injuries commonly associated with it.

1. _____ collision

Type of injuries:

2. _____ collision

Type of injuries:

3. _____ collision

Type of injuries:

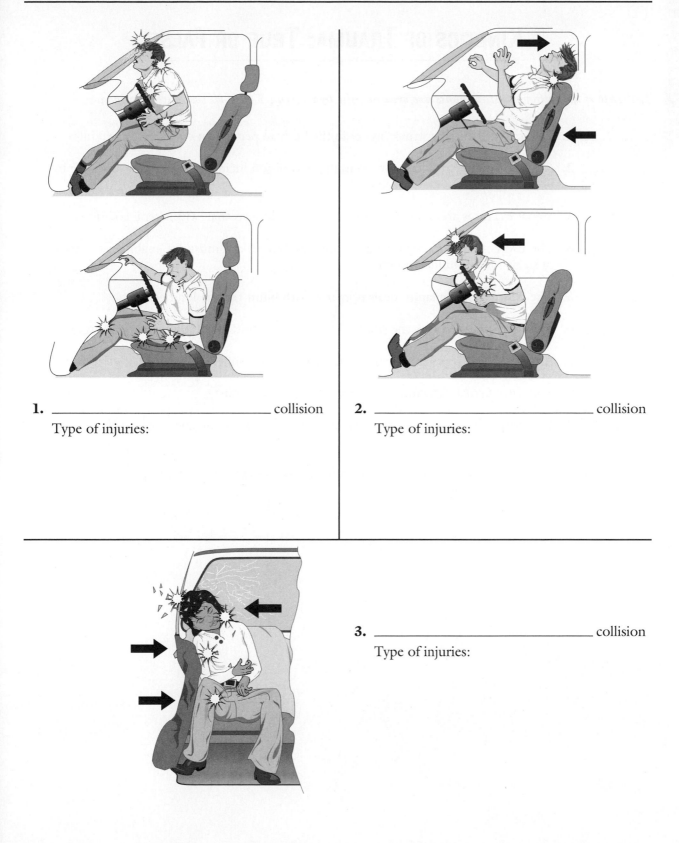

1. _____ collision

Type of injuries:

2. _____ collision

Type of injuries:

3. _____ collision

Type of injuries:

REINFORCEMENT

KINETICS OF TRAUMA: TRUE OR FALSE

Indicate if the following statements are true or false by writing T or F in the space provided.

_____ **1.** Children are initially struck higher in the body in pedestrian collisions than adults.

_____ **2.** Airbags are extremely effective in multiple collision incidents but are not effective in initial impact head-on collisions.

_____ **3.** Spinal fractures are more common with rear collisions than with lateral collisions.

_____ **4.** The EMT must not only recognize obvious injuries but must also maintain a high index of suspicion for hidden injuries.

_____ **5.** The concept of cavitation deals primarily with blunt trauma injuries.

_____ **6.** Trauma is nearly always the result of two or more bodies colliding with each other.

_____ **7.** A knife wound is potentially more traumatic than a bullet wound.

_____ **8.** The fall is actually the most common mechanism of injury.

_____ **9.** The "paper bag syndrome" results from compression of the chest against the steering column.

_____ **10.** Injuries from rotational crashes or rollover crashes are not as easy to predict as injuries from other crashes.

©2008 by Pearson Education, Inc.
Prehospital Emergency Care, 8th ed.

Mechanisms of Injury: Kinetics of Trauma

Kinetics of Trauma

Mass and Velocity

Acceleration and Deceleration

Energy Changes Form and Direction

Impacts

Mechanisms of Injury

Vehicle Collisions

- Frontal impact
- Rear-end impact
- Lateral impact
- Rotational or rollover crash
- Vehicle–pedestrian crash
- Restraints and hidden injuries
- Infant/child considerations
- Motorcycle collisions

Falls

- Feet-first
- Head-first

Penetrating Injuries

- Low-velocity
- Medium- and high-velocity

Blast Injuries

The "Golden Hour"

HANDOUT 26-2: Chapter 26 Quiz

1. C	**4.** A	**7.** B	**9.** D
2. A	**5.** C	**8.** D	**10.** D
3. B	**6.** B		

HANDOUT 26-3: In the Field

1. Closed and/or open head injuries, soft tissue and blunt force injuries to the chest, abdominal injuries
2. *Seatbelt:* Head and neck injuries are still likely, as the seatbelt does not hold them immobile. Deceleration injuries may be present without any outward signs of trauma. *Airbag:* Deceleration injuries are still likely. The airbag immediately deflates, allowing secondary impact with the steering wheel and/or windshield. Abrasions are likely on the arms and face from contact with the rapidly deploying airbag.

HANDOUT 26-4: Chapter 26 Review

1. trauma
2. kinetics of trauma
3. mechanisms of injury
4. mass, velocity
5. index of suspicion
6. velocity
7. Energy
8. acceleration
9. vehicle collisions
10. head, neck, chest, abdomen

HANDOUT 26-5: Kinetics of Trauma: Listing

1. Mass, velocity, acceleration, deceleration
2. Vehicle, body, organs
3. Falls, vehicular collisions, penetrating gunshots or stabbings, explosions, blast injuries
4. Head-on, rear-end, side impact, rollover, rotational

HANDOUT 26-6: Recognizing Injury Patterns

1. Head-on collision. Types of injuries: up-and-over-head, neck, chest, abdominal injuries; down-and-under-knee, hip, and leg injuries
2. Rear-end collision. Types of injuries: neck (most common), head, chest
3. Lateral-impact collision. Types of injuries: head and neck, chest abdomen, pelvis, thighs.

HANDOUT 26-7: Kinetics of Trauma: True or False

1. T	**4.** T	**7.** F	**9.** T
2. F	**5.** F	**8.** T	**10.** T
3. F	**6.** T		

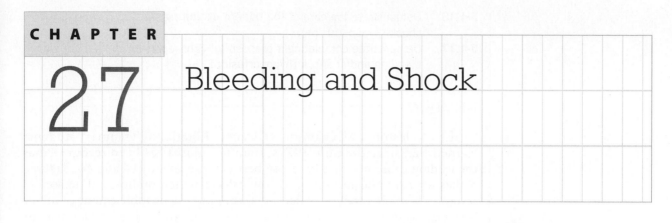

CHAPTER

27 Bleeding and Shock

This chapter covers Lesson 5-1 and portions of Lesson 5-5 of the U.S. Department of Transportation's EMT-Basic National Standard Curriculum.

OBJECTIVES

Numbered objectives are from the U.S. Department of Transportation EMT-Basic National Standard Curriculum. Asterisked objectives, if any, pertain to material that is supplemental to the DOT curriculum. Page numbers in parentheses refer to pages in the textbook.

Cognitive

5-1.1 List the structure and function of the circulatory system. (p. 748)

5-1.2 Differentiate between arterial, venous, and capillary bleeding. (p. 749)

5-1.3 State methods of emergency medical care of external bleeding. (pp. 749, 751–757)

5-1.4 Establish the relationship between body substance isolation and bleeding. (pp. 748, 751, 759, 760, 761)

5-1.5 Establish the relationship between airway management and the trauma patient. (pp. 746, 751, 758, 759, 761)

5-1.6 Establish the relationship between mechanism of injury and internal bleeding. (pp. 757–759)

5-1.7 List the signs of internal bleeding. (p. 759)

5-1.8 List the steps in emergency medical care of the patient with signs and symptoms of internal bleeding. (p. 759)

5-1.9 List signs and symptoms of shock (hypoperfusion). (p. 761)

5-1.10 State the steps in the emergency medical care of the patient with signs and symptoms of shock (hypoperfusion). (pp. 761–763)

Affective

5-1.11 Explain the sense of urgency to transport patients that are bleeding and show signs of shock (hypoperfusion). (pp. 746, 763)

Psychomotor

5-1.12 Demonstrate direct pressure as a method of emergency medical care of external bleeding.

5-1.13 Demonstrate the use of diffuse pressure as a method of emergency medical care of external bleeding.

5-1.14 Demonstrate the use of pressure points and tourniquets as a method of emergency medical care for external bleeding.

5-1.15 Demonstrate the care of the patient exhibiting signs and symptoms of internal bleeding.

Total Teaching Time
180 minutes

Resources Needed
- Scored Chapter 28 Quizzes
- Ample supplies of dressings, bandages, and tourniquet rods

Additional Resources
Larmon/Davis, *Basic Life Support Skills*

Elling, *EMT Achieve: Basic Test Preparation*

Limmer/Mistovich/ O'Keefe, *Audio Lecture & Study Guide: EMT*

Mistovich/Kuvlesky, *SUCCESS! for the EMT, Second Edition*

5-1.16   Demonstrate the care of the patient exhibiting signs and symptoms of shock (hypoperfusion).

5-1.17   Demonstrate completing a prehospital care report for the patient with bleeding and/or shock (hypoperfusion).

REVIEW

In the last lesson, "Mechanisms of Injury: Kinetics of Trauma," students learned that since the early 1970s, trauma (injury) has been recognized as the leading cause of death for those between the ages of 14 and 40. Trauma makes up a significant percent of the calls to which prehospital personnel respond. With any trauma patient, determining the possible extent of injury is critical to making good priority decisions regarding on-scene assessment and care versus rapid transport with assessment and care continuing en route. To make these judgments, the EMT must not only recognize obvious injuries but also must maintain a high index of suspicion for hidden injuries. An understanding of mechanisms of injury is the chief component of this crucial assessment skill.

Distribute the quizzes from the last class. Go over each question on the quiz and handle any concerns students may have about the answers.

INTRODUCTION TO CHAPTER 27

Chapter 27, "Bleeding and Shock," is the second lesson of Module 5. Bleeding can be a significant, life-threatening emergency. As EMTs, students must be able to recognize obvious or external bleeding problems, as well as not-so-obvious internal bleeding problems. If either type of bleeding is left untreated, it has the potential to lead to rapid patient deterioration, shock (hypoperfusion), and death. Control of severe external bleeding is performed during the initial assessment. Only airway and breathing have a higher priority. Internal bleeding and shock (hypoperfusion) are treated immediately following the initial assessment. Note that an important element of the emergency care of bleeding and shock (hypoperfusion) is to transport the patient to a medical facility as rapidly as possible.

Distribute the Chapter 27 Objectives Checklist, and give students a few minutes to look it over. Then briefly paraphrase the objectives for this lesson in your own words.

LECTURE

The following suggested lecture outline is based on the Department of Transportation's EMT-Basic National Standard Curriculum. In some places, the DOT curriculum has been rearranged or expanded upon so that it is more complete or easier for the student to understand. The page numbers in parentheses refer to pages in the textbook. The parenthetical references in dark, heavy type are to figures, tables, and scans in the textbook.

BLEEDING AND SHOCK

I. The circulatory system (p. 748)
    A. Heart, blood vessels, and blood (p. 748)
        1. Heart
            a. Left side pumps oxygen-rich blood to body.
            b. Right side pumps oxygen-depleted blood to lungs.

Handout 27-1
Chapter 27 Objectives Checklist

Lecture Master
You may wish to display Lecture Master 27 when presenting the lecture to the class.

Slides/Videos
Brady Skill Series: EMT-B,
"Bleeding and Shock"
"Dressing and Bandaging"

2. Blood vessels
   a. Arteries
   b. Capillaries
   c. Veins
3. Blood
   a. Red blood cells
   b. White blood cells
   c. Plasma
   d. Platelets
   e. Blood pressure
      (1) Pressure exerted against arterial walls during circulation
B. Perfusion (p. 748)
   1. Delivery of oxygen and other nutrients to the cells of all organ systems and the removal of carbon dioxide and other waste products.
   2. Shock (hypoperfusion)
      a. Insufficient supply of oxygen and other nutrients to some of the body's cells, which results in inadequate circulation of blood through an organ
   3. Organ systems especially sensitive to perfusion changes
      a. Heart
      b. Brain
      c. Spinal cord
      d. Kidneys

II. **External bleeding** (pp. 748–757)
   A. BSI precautions must be routinely taken to avoid skin and mucous membrane exposure to body fluids. (p. 748)
   B. Severity (pp. 748–749) **(Fig. 27-1, p. 748)**
      1. Based on patient's signs and symptoms **(Fig. 27-2, p. 750)**
      2. Serious injury may prevent effective clotting from occurring.
      3. Uncontrolled bleeding or significant blood loss leads to shock (hypoperfusion) and possibly death.
   C. Types of bleeding (p. 749) **(Fig. 27-3, p. 751)**
      1. Arterial bleeding
         a. Blood spurts from wound
         b. Blood bright, red, oxygen-rich
         c. Most difficult to control because of pressure at which arteries bleed
      2. Venous bleeding
         a. Flows slowly and steadily
         b. Blood dark red, oxygen-depleted
         c. Easier to control than arterial because of lower venous pressure
      3. Capillary bleeding **(Fig. 27-4, p. 751)**
         a. Blood oozes from wound
         b. Blood dark red
         c. Often clots spontaneously
   D. Assessment and care: external bleeding (pp. 749–752)
      1. Scene size-up, initial assessment, and rapid trauma assessment
         a. Begin preparing while en route by donning all necessary personal protective equipment.
         b. If responding to accident or scene of violence, notify appropriate support agencies.
         c. Make sure the scene is safe before you enter.

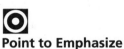

Point of Interest
About 2.5 million red blood cells die every second, but they are replaced just as quickly.

Point to Emphasize
Whenever bleeding is anticipated or discovered, the use of BSI precautions is essential to avoid exposure to skin and mucous membranes.

Point to Emphasize
No matter how small the blood loss appears to be, if the patient shows any signs or symptoms of shock (hypoperfusion), the bleeding is considered serious.

    d. Note number of patients at scene and any potential mechanism of injury.

    e. Get general impression of patient and patient's mental status as you approach.

    f. Ensure the ABCs and perform basic life support procedures, placing serious bleeding above all other emergency care except airway and breathing.

    g. Perform rapid trauma assessment, if patient condition permits.

       (1) With serious bleeding, should take not more than 90 seconds.

       (2) Obtain set of baseline vitals.

  2. Emergency medical care

    a. Maintain body substance isolation.

    b. Apply direct pressure to site of bleeding.

    c. Elevate the injured extremity, and apply ice or cold pack.

    d. If bleeding doesn't stop, use pressure points.

    e. Immobilize injured extremities.

    f. As a last resort, use a tourniquet.

    g. Provide care for signs and symptoms of shock.

  3. Remainder of assessment

    a. Continue to be alert for renewed bleeding.

    b. Focused history and physical exam

    c. Detailed physical exam

    d. Ongoing assessment

E. Methods of controlling external bleeding (pp. 752–756)

  1. Direct pressure

    a. Applying fingertip pressure and/or hand pressure directly to the point of bleeding. **(Fig. 27-5, p. 752)**

  2. Elevation

    a. Elevating injured extremity in conjunction with applying direct pressure

    b. Elevate arm or leg above the level of the heart.

    c. Elevate painful, swollen, deformed, or joint-injured extremity only after splinting.

  3. Pressure points (pulse points) **(Figs. 27-6, p. 753 and 27-7, p. 754)**

    a. Applying pressure to point where artery that lies close to surface of skin over a bony prominence creates a pulse point

    b. Use brachial pressure point for bleeding in upper extremity.

    c. Use femoral pressure point for bleeding in lower extremity.

  4. Pressure splints **(Fig. 27-8, p. 755)**

    a. Purpose

       (1) Splint open wounds to extremities having possible bone or joint injuries so that bone ends or fragments don't continue to damage surrounding tissue.

    b. Use of air-pressure splints can also help control bleeding.

    c. Pneumatic antishock garment can also be used as pressure splint.

  5. Cold application

a. Apply ice or cold pack to facilitate clotting, promote vasoconstriction, and reduce swelling.
6. Tourniquet
   a. Use only as last resort to control bleeding of an amputated extremity when all other methods of bleeding control have failed.
   b. Tourniquet use can cause permanent damage to nerves, muscles, and blood vessels, resulting in loss of an extremity.
   c. Procedures for application (**Fig. 27-9 and 27-10, p. 756**)
     (1) Use a bandage 4 inches wide and four to six layers thick.
     (2) Wrap bandage around extremity twice at point proximal to bleeding but as distal to extremity and as close to injury as possible.
     (3) Tie knot in bandage material and place stick-type object on top of it.
     (4) Tie ends of bandage in a square knot over the stick-type object.
     (5) Twist stick-type object until bleeding stops.
     (6) After bleeding has stopped, secure stick-type object in place.
     (7) Notify other emergency personnel that tourniquet has been applied.
     (8) Document the use of the tourniquet and the time that it was applied in the prehospital care report.
   d. Precautions with the use of a tourniquet
     (1) Use a wide bandage and secure tightly.
     (2) Never use wire, rope, a belt, or any other material that may cut into the skin and underlying tissue.
     (3) Do not remove or loosen the tourniquet once it is applied, unless directed to do so by medical direction.
     (4) Leave tourniquet in open view.
     (5) Do not apply a tourniquet directly over any joint, but as close to the injury as possible.

F. Bleeding from the nose, ears, or mouth (pp. 756–757) (**Fig. 27-11, p. 757**)
  1. Possible causes
    a. Skull injury
    b. Facial trauma
    c. Digital trauma (nose picking)
    d. Sinusitis and other upper respiratory tract infections
    e. Hypertension (high blood pressure)
    f. Clotting disorders
    g. Esophageal disease
  2. Suspect possible skull fracture if patient is bleeding from ears or nose.
  3. If patient has head injury, do not attempt to stop the flow of blood; instead, place loose dressing around area to limit exposure to infectious agents.
  4. Emergency medical care for epistaxis (nosebleed) (**Fig. 27-12, p. 757**)
    a. Place patient in a sitting position leaning forward.
    b. Apply direct pressure by pinching fleshy portion of nostrils together.

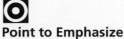

Point to Emphasize
Stress that a tourniquet should be used only as a last resort. It should be made of material wide enough as to not cut into the patient's skin, should be used only on extremities and not directly over joints, and once applied should never be loosened or removed.

      c. Keep the patient calm and quiet.

III. Internal bleeding (pp. 757–759)

  A. Severity (pp. 757–758)

    1. Depends on

      a. Patient's overall condition

      b. Patient's age

      c. Other medical conditions

      d. Source: two most common sources

        (1) Damaged internal organs

        (2) Fractured extremities, especially femur, pelvis, and hip

      e. Suspect internal bleeding if penetrating wounds to skull, chest, or abdomen.

  B. Assessment and care (pp. 758–759)

    1. Scene size-up and initial assessment

      a. Look for and evaluate potential mechanisms of injury.

      b. When you are certain scene is safe, approach patient.

      c. Evaluate mental status and ensure an open airway, adequate breathing, and adequate circulation.

      d. Provide basic life support as needed.

      e. Care for serious external bleeding.

    2. Focused history and physical exam

      a. If you suspect internal bleeding, conduct focused history and physical exam.

      b. Treat patient for internal bleeding if there is evidence of contusions, abrasions, deformity, impact marks, or swelling.

    3. Signs and symptoms of internal bleeding

      a. Pain, tenderness, swelling, or discoloration of suspected site of injury

      b. Bleeding from the mouth, rectum, vagina, or other orifice

      c. Vomiting bright red blood or blood the color of dark coffee grounds

      d. Dark, tarry stools or stools with bright red blood

      e. Tender, rigid, and/or distended abdomen

    4. Late signs and symptoms of internal bleeding that indicate shock (hypoperfusion)

      a. Anxiety, restlessness, combativeness, or altered mental status

      b. Weakness, faintness, or dizziness

      c. Thirst

      d. Shallow, rapid breathing

      e. Rapid pulse

      f. Pale, cool, clammy skin

      g. Delayed capillary refill

      h. Dropping blood pressure

      i. Narrow pulse pressure

      j. Dilated pupils that are sluggish to respond

      k. Nausea and vomiting

  C. Emergency medical care (p. 759)

    1. Take BSI precautions.

    2. Maintain an open airway and adequate breathing/artificial ventilation as necessary.

    3. Administer oxygen if not already done in initial assessment.

    4. Control external bleeding, applying splint, if necessary.

5. Provide immediate transport.
6. Care for symptoms of shock.
   D. Detailed physical exam and ongoing assessment (p. 759)
      1. Remain alert for renewed bleeding.
      2. Conduct detailed physical exam.
      3. Perform ongoing assessment every 5 minutes throughout transport.
IV. **Factors that may increase bleeding** (p. 759)
   A. Movement (p. 759)
   B. Low body temperature (p. 759)
   C. Medication (p. 759)
   D. Intravenous fluids (p. 759)
V. **Shock (hypoperfusion)** (pp. 760–763) **(Fig. 27-13, p. 760; Figs. 27-18 and 27-19, pp. 765–767)**
   A. Severity (p. 760)
      1. Shock (hypoperfusion) is direct result of inadequate perfusion of cells; when cells do not receive the oxygen and nutrients they require, they begin to fail and die.
      2. Prompt recognition and treatment is vital to patient survival; cell and organ malfunction and death can result from shock.
      3. Peripheral perfusion is drastically reduced due to reduction in circulating blood volume.
      4. Suspect shock in any patient who has suffered trauma.
   B. Scene size-up and initial assessment (pp. 760–761)
      1. Note any potential mechanism of injury.
      2. Seek law enforcement resources, if necessary.
      3. Approach the patient when it is safe and assess patient's mental status and ABCs.
      4. Pay particular attention to airway maintenance and, if needed, provide positive-pressure ventilation and high-flow oxygen.
   C. Focused history and physical exam (p. 761)
      1. Perform rapid trauma assessment
         a. If multiple injuries
         b. If internal bleeding is suspected
         c. If altered mental status
         d. If shock is suspected
      2. Monitor for signs and symptoms of shock throughout focused history and physical exam.
      3. Assess for internal or external bleeding if patient exhibits signs of shock.
      4. Monitor for peripheral perfusion and skin color, temperature, and condition.
   D. Signs and symptoms of shock (hypoperfusion) (p. 761) **(Fig. 27-14, p. 761)**
      1. Mental status
         a. Restlessness
         b. Anxiety
         c. Altered mental status
      2. Peripheral perfusion and perfusion of the skin
         a. Pale, cool, clammy skin
         b. Weak, thready peripheral pulses
         c. Delayed capillary refill
      3. Vital signs
         a. Increased pulse rate (early sign)
            (1) Weak and thready

Teaching Tip
Use the plumbing analogy of pipes, pumps, and fluid to describe the pathophysiology of shock.

Slides/Videos
"Shock," *Pulse,* Jan. 2000.

Reading/Reference
Stene, D., and Smith, M., "Shock: Inside and Out," *EMS Magazine,* Nov. 2001.

b. Increased breathing rate (early sign)
  - **(1)** Deep or shallow
  - **(2)** Labored
  - **(3)** Irregular
  - **c.** Decreased blood pressure (late sign)
  - **d.** Narrow pulse pressure
4. Other signs and symptoms
  - **a.** Dilated pupils (sluggish reaction)
  - **b.** Marked thirst
  - **c.** Nausea and vomiting
  - **d.** Pallor with cyanosis to the lips
5. Infants and children can maintain their blood pressure until their blood volume is depleted by almost one-third, then their condition suddenly deteriorates. If a child's blood pressure is dropping, it is an ominous sign.

E. Emergency medical care (pp. 761–763) **(Fig. 27-15, p. 762)**
1. Maintain BSI precautions.
2. Maintain an open airway.
3. Administer oxygen.
  - **a.** Breathing adequate
    - **(1)** Administer oxygen via nonrebreather mask at 15 liters per minute.
  - **b.** Breathing inadequate
    - **(1)** Begin positive-pressure ventilation with supplemental oxygen.
4. Control any external bleeding.
5. If signs of shock (hypoperfusion) are present and lower abdomen is tender and pelvic injury is suspected, with no evidence of chest injury, apply and inflate the pneumatic antishock garment **(Fig. 27-16, p. 763)** if approved by medical direction. **(Fig. 27-17, p. 764)**
6. Elevate the lower extremities approximately 8–12 inches. If the patient has serious injuries to the pelvis, lower extremities, head, chest, abdomen, neck, or spine, or if shock may be due to cardiac compromise, keep patient supine.
7. Splint suspected bone or joint injuries.
8. Prevent loss of body heat by covering patient with a blanket.
9. Transport the patient immediately.

F. Summary: assessment and care **(Figs. 27-18 and 27-19, pp. 765–767)**

G. Remainder of the assessment (p. 763)
1. Continue to assess for changes in mental status and vital signs throughout focused history, physical exam, detailed physical exam, and ongoing assessment.
2. Assessment can be conducted en route.

ENRICHMENT (OPTIONAL)

The following sections contain information that is valuable as background for the EMT, but that goes substantially beyond the U.S. Department of Transportation's EMT-Basic National Standard Curriculum.

VI. Hemophilia (p. 763)
  - **A.** Congenital disease that prevents normal clotting (p. 763)
  - **B.** Transport to medical facility for special medication (p. 763)

VII. More about shock (pp. 763–769)

A. Causes of shock (pp. 763–766)
　　1. Fluid loss
　　2. Pump failure
　　3. Vasodilation
　　4. Hypoxia (inadequate oxygen)
B. Types of shock (pp. 766–768)
　　1. Hypovolemic shock
　　　　a. Decrease in volume of blood available for perfusion of body's organs
　　2. Obstructive shock
　　　　a. Mechanical obstruction or compression that prevents blood flow to the heart
　　3. Distributive shock
　　　　a. Abnormal distribution of blood in the vessels or throughout the body that causes an insufficient amount of blood returning to the heart
　　　　b. Vasogenic or neurogenic shock
　　　　　　(1) Spinal cord or head injury that causes the nervous system to lose control over the vascular system
　　　　c. Anaphylactic shock
　　　　　　(1) Reaction to a foreign protein from a source such as bee venom, food, or certain medications
　　　　d. Septic shock
　　　　　　(1) Result of toxins produced by a severe (usually bacterial) infection
　　4. Cardiogenic shock
　　　　a. Result of inadequate pumping of heart
C. Stages of shock (pp. 768–769) **(Fig. 27-20, p. 768)**
　　1. Compensatory shock
　　　　a. First stage
　　　　b. Normal body defense mechanisms maintain perfusion and function
　　2. Decompensated (progressive) shock
　　　　a. Second stage
　　　　b. Blood shunted from less to more vital organs
　　3. Irreversible shock
　　　　a. Third and final stage
　　　　b. Multisystem organ damage
　　　　c. Even with treatment, death is the result

On the Net
Explanation of all types of shock. http://www.hhp.ufl.edu/ess/at/AbdomenWeb/Web%20page%20info/Types_of_Shock.htm

On the Net
Hypovolemic shock management. http://www.nlm.nih.gov/medlineplus/ency/article/000167.htm

CASE STUDY FOLLOW-UP

Ask a student volunteer to read the Case Study that begins on page 747 of the textbook. You may wish to use the following questions to engage the students in a discussion of the Case Study Follow-up that begins on page 770 of the textbook. Provide missing information and clarify ideas as needed.

Q1. Describe the patient's injury.

A1. *A large penetrating wound to the left upper quadrant of the abdomen with profuse bleeding*

Q2. What do you decide should be this patient's transport priority?

A2. *High priority—rapid transport*

Q3. Describe your initial assessment of the patient.

A3. *He is unconscious, unresponsive to verbal stimuli but will grimace to painful stimuli. His airway is patent with rapid and shallow breathing at a rate of 34 per minute. A radial pulse cannot be detected, but the carotid pulse is weak and rapid with a rate of 120. Dark red blood is flowing profusely from the abdominal wound.*

Q4. How do you treat the patient?

A4. *By packing the wound with sterile dressings and taping the dressings in place. Since there are no other signs of external trauma, spinal precautions are omitted. Once the patient is on the stretcher and in the ambulance, the patient's breathing is assisted with a bag-valve mask and supplemental oxygen.*

Q5. What was found in surgery?

A5. *The patient had a severely lacerated spleen and an abdomen filled with blood.*

IN REVIEW

Assess students' ability to apply what they have just learned by discussing the Review Questions on page 771 of the textbook.

Q1. Describe arterial, venous, and capillary bleeding.

A1. *Arterial bleeding is bright red, spurting blood. Venous bleeding is dark red, steadily flowing blood. Capillary bleeding is dark red, slowly oozing blood. (p. 749)*

Q2. List five ways to control external bleeding.

A2. *Five ways to control external bleeding are as follows: (1) direct pressure, (2) elevation and cold application, (3) splinting, (4) pressure splints, and (5) tourniquet. (pp. 752–756)*

Q3. Explain (a) when and (b) how to use a tourniquet to control bleeding.

A3. *(a) Tourniquets are used only as a last resort to control bleeding of an amputated extremity when all other methods have failed. (b) To apply a tourniquet to an extremity, use a bandage 4 inches wide and four to six layers thick. Wrap it around the extremity twice at a point proximal to the bleeding but as distal on the extremity as possible. Tie a knot in the bandage material, and place a stick on top of it. Tie the ends of the bandage in a square knot over the stick. Twist the stick until the bleeding stops, and then secure it in place. Notify other emergency personnel who will care for the patient that a tourniquet has been applied. Document the use of the tourniquet and the time it was applied in the prehospital care report. Do not loosen or remove the tourniquet unless you are directed to do so by medical direction. Never apply a tourniquet directly over any joint. Always make sure the tourniquet is in open view. (pp. 755–756)*

Q4. Name the two most common sources of internal bleeding.

A4. *The two most common sources of internal bleeding are injured or damaged organs and fractured extremities, especially the femur, hip, or pelvis. (p. 757)*

Q5. List the signs and symptoms of internal bleeding, including late signs.

A5. *The signs and symptoms of internal bleeding are pain, tenderness, swelling, or discoloration of suspected site of injury; bleeding from the mouth, rectum, vagina, or other orifice; vomiting bright red blood or blood the color of dark coffee grounds; dark, tarry stools, or stools with bright red blood; tender, rigid, and/or distended abdomen. Late signs, which also indicate shock, are anxiety, restlessness, combativeness, or altered mental status; weakness, faintness, or dizziness; thirst; shallow rapid breathing; rapid pulse; pale, cool, clammy skin; delayed capillary refill; dropping blood pressure; narrow pulse pressure; dilated pupils that are sluggish to respond to light; nausea and vomiting. (p. 759)*

Q6. Describe emergency medical care of internal bleeding.

A6. *The emergency medical care of internal bleeding is as follows: Maintain an open airway and adequate breathing. Provide artificial ventilations as necessary. Administer oxygen. Control external bleeding. Splint any painful, swollen, deformed extremity. Provide immediate transport to critical patients with signs and symptoms of shock (hypoperfusion). Provide emergency care for shock. (p. 759)*

Q7. List the signs and symptoms of shock (hypoperfusion).

A7. *The signs and symptoms of shock (hypoperfusion) are restlessness, anxiety, altered mental status; pale, cool, clammy skin; weak, thready, or absent peripheral pulses; delayed capillary refill; increased pulse rate (early sign), with weak and thready pulse; increased breathing rate, with shallow, labored, irregular breathing; decreased blood pressure (late sign); narrow pulse pressure; dilated pupils; marked thirst; nausea and vomiting; pallor with cyanosis to the lips. (p. 761)*

Q8. Describe emergency medical care of shock (hypoperfusion).

A8. *The emergency medical care of shock (hypoperfusion) is as follows: Maintain an open airway. If breathing is adequate, administer oxygen via nonrebreather mask at 15 liters per minute. If breathing is inadequate, begin positive-pressure ventilation with supplemental oxygen. Control external bleeding. If signs and symptoms of shock (hypoperfusion) are present, the lower abdomen is tender with a suspected pelvic injury, and there is no evidence of chest injury, apply and inflate the PASG if approved by medical direction. Elevate the lower extremities approximately 8 to 12 inches. If the patient has injuries to the pelvis, lower extremities, head, chest, abdomen, neck, or spine, or if the shock may be due to cardiac compromise, keep the patient supine, without elevating the feet. (Follow local protocol.) Splint suspected bone or joint injuries. Cover the patient to prevent loss of body heat. Transport immediately. (pp. 761–763)*

CRITICAL THINKING

Assess students' ability to respond to real-life emergency situations by discussing the Critical Thinking questions on page 771 in the textbook.

Q1. What emergency care would you provide in the initial assessment?

A1. *The EMTs should immediately provide manual in-line spinal stabilization, open the airway by performing a jaw-thrust, and apply a* *nonrebreather mask at 15 lpm (the respiratory rate and tidal volume are adequate).*

Q2. What signs and symptoms in this patient indicate shock?

A2. *The patient's decreased mental status; heart rate of 124 bpm; weak radial pulses; absent pedal pulses; pale, cool, and clammy skin; hypotension (low blood pressure); narrow pulse pressure; and tachypnea (rapid respiratory rate) are all indicators of shock.*

Q3. How severe a shock state do you suspect?

A3. *Based on the blood pressure, it is evident that this patient is in a decompensated (progressive) stage of shock. When the systolic blood pressure falls, typically below 90 mmHg, it is an indication that the patient's body is no longer able to compensate for the blood loss. If the bleeding is not stopped, and the perfusion to cells are not restored, the shock stage will continue to progress.*

Q4. What overall emergency care would you provide?

A4. *With the oxygen continuously flowing at 15 lpm, a rapid trauma assessment will be conducted. A cervical spinal immobilization collar will be applied while manual in-line spine stabilization is maintained. Following the rapid trauma assessment, a rapid extrication should be done to remove the patient from the vehicle. The patient will be completely immobilized to a backboard following extrication. Cover the patient to keep them warm. Continue with the oxygen therapy and rapidly transport to the most appropriate medical facility, preferably a trauma center.*

ROLE PLAY

Ask for a student to be a patient. You may wish to use moulage on the patient to simulate active bleeding.

Step by step, describe and demonstrate the procedures for external bleeding control. Begin with direct pressure, then proceed to elevation, pressure points, and tourniquet application.

Pair students and provide each team with dressings, bandages, and tourniquet rods. Tell students that you want each team to take turns going through all the steps in bleeding control that you have just demonstrated. Tell them that when practicing tourniquet application, they must be very careful not to make the tourniquet tight enough to stop blood flow.

Observe each group as it practices. Provide corrective feedback and answer questions as needed. Monitor tourniquet practice to ensure the safety of students.

ASSIGNMENTS

Assign students to read Chapter 28, "Soft Tissue Injuries," before the next class. Also ask them to complete Chapter 27 of the Workbook.

EVALUATION

Chapter Quiz Distribute copies of the Chapter Quiz provided in Handout 27-2 to evaluate student understanding of this chapter. Remind students not to refer to their textbooks or notes while taking the quiz.

Reading/Reference
Textbook, pp. 772–796

Workbook
Chapter 27 Activities

Chapter Quiz
Handout 27-2

©2008 by Pearson Education, Inc.
Prehospital Emergency Care, 8th ed.

Test Manager You may wish to create a custom-tailored test using Prentice Hall *TestGen for Prehospital Emergency Care, Eighth Edition* to evaluate student understanding of this chapter.

Online Test Preparation (for students and instructors) Additional test preparation is available through *EMT Achieve: Basic Test Preparation* at http://www.prenhall.com/EMTAchieve. Instructors can also monitor student mastery online.

REINFORCEMENT

Handouts If classroom discussions or performance on the quiz indicates that some students have not fully mastered the chapter content, you may wish to assign some or all of the Reinforcement Handouts for this chapter.

TECH EXTRAS

Brady Skills Series EMT-B Videos/CD Have your students watch the skills come to life on either VHS or CD-ROM.

PowerPoint Presentation (for instructors) The PowerPoint material developed for this chapter offers useful reinforcement of chapter content.

Student CD A wide variety of material on this CD-ROM will reinforce and also expand student knowledge and skills.

Companion Website (for students) Additional review quizzes and links to EMS resources will contribute to further reinforcement of this chapter. Please visit http://www.prenhall.com/mistovich.

TestGen
Chapter 27 Test

Online Test Preparation
Send your students to
http://www.prenhall.com/
EMTAchieve

Handouts 27-3 to 27-6
Reinforcement Activities

**Brady Skills Series
EMT-B Videos/CD**
Visual Reinforcement

**PowerPoint
Presentation**
Chapter 27

Student CD
Chapter 27

Companion Website
http://www.prenhall.com/
mistovich

OBJECTIVES (vertical, left margin)

OBJECTIVES CHECKLIST

Cognitive		Date Mastered
5-1.1	List the structure and function of the circulatory system.	
5-1.2	Differentiate between arterial, venous, and capillary bleeding.	
5-1.3	State methods of emergency medical care of external bleeding.	
5-1.4	Establish the relationship between body substance isolation and bleeding.	
5-1.5	Establish the relationship between airway management and the trauma patient.	
5-1.6	Establish the relationship between mechanism of injury and internal bleeding.	
5-1.7	List the signs of internal bleeding.	
5-1.8	List the steps in emergency medical care of the patient with signs and symptoms of internal bleeding.	
5-1.9	List signs and symptoms of shock (hypoperfusion).	
5-1.10	State the steps in the emergency medical care of the patient with signs and symptoms of shock (hypoperfusion).	

Affective		Date Mastered
5-1.11	Explain the sense of urgency to transport patients that are bleeding and show signs of shock (hypoperfusion).	

Psychomotor		Date Mastered
5-1.12	Demonstrate direct pressure as a method of emergency medical care of external bleeding.	
5-1.13	Demonstrate the use of diffuse pressure as a method of emergency medical care of external bleeding.	
5-1.14	Demonstrate the use of pressure points and tourniquets as a method of emergency medical care for external bleeding.	
5-1.15	Demonstrate the care of the patient exhibiting signs and symptoms of internal bleeding.	
5-1.16	Demonstrate the care of the patient exhibiting signs and symptoms of shock (hypoperfusion).	
5-1.17	Demonstrate completing a prehospital care report for the patient with bleeding and/or shock (hypoperfusion).	

CHAPTER 27 QUIZ

Write the letter of the best answer in the space provided.

_____ 1. A blood vessel that carries oxygen-depleted blood back to the heart is called a(n)
     A. capillary.   **C.** vein.
     B. aorta.   **D.** artery.

_____ 2. The insufficient supply of oxygen and other nutrients to the body's cells is known as
     A. perfusion.   **C.** hypoperfusion.
     B. avulsion.   **D.** apnea.

_____ 3. The first step that an EMT should take when encountering a patient with severe bleeding is to
     A. apply pressure to the wound.
     B. utilize appropriate BSI precautions.
     C. check the patient's blood pressure.
     D. apply a tourniquet.

_____ 4. The type of bleeding that is often the most difficult to control is _____ bleeding.
     A. arterial   **C.** capillary
     B. venous   **D.** "oozing"

_____ 5. All of the following are signs of shock *except*
     A. altered mental status.   **C.** warm, dry skin.
     B. nausea and vomiting.   **D.** vital sign changes.

_____ 6. After taking BSI precautions, the next step an EMT should take in treating cases of profuse bleeding is to
     A. elevate the extremity.   **C.** apply bandaging.
     B. apply a dressing.   **D.** apply direct pressure.

_____ 7. The last resort in controlling external bleeding is
     A. direct pressure.   **C.** cold applications.
     B. use of pressure points.   **D.** use of a tourniquet.

_____ 8. Based on local protocol and approval from medical direction, a useful method for controlling internal bleeding may be the use of a
     A. splint.   **C.** cold pack.
     B. tourniquet.   **D.** PASG.

_____ 9. An average adult weighing 154 pounds will have _____ liters of total blood volume.
     A. 8–10   **C.** 6.8
     B. 4.9   **D.** 12–14

_____ 10. Vomiting of blood the color of dark coffee grounds is a sign of
     A. external bleeding.   **C.** internal bleeding.
     B. epistaxis.   **D.** cardiogenic shock.

_____ 11. The type of shock most commonly caused by profound blood or fluid loss is _____ shock.
     A. hypovolemic   **C.** vasogenic
     B. cardiogenic   **D.** irreversible

_____ 12. A condition in which nerve paralysis causes uncontrolled dilation of blood vessels is called _____ shock.
- **A.** compensated
- **B.** hemorrhagic
- **C.** cardiogenic
- **D.** vasogenic

_____ 13. Signs of arterial bleeding include _____ blood.
- **A.** oozing dark
- **B.** oozing bright red
- **C.** spurting dark
- **D.** spurting bright red

_____ 14. In the average adult patient who weighs 154 pounds, a blood volume loss of _____ % or more is considered significant and can lead to shock.
- **A.** 5
- **B.** 15
- **C.** 1
- **D.** 7.5

_____ 15. Which one of the following patient variables is *not* among the factors to consider when determining the severity of blood loss?
- **A.** country of origin
- **B.** medical conditions
- **C.** age
- **D.** injuries

_____ 16. Applying a cold pack to an injured extremity that is painful, swollen, or deformed is meant to do all of the following *except*
- **A.** facilitate clotting.
- **B.** promote vasoconstriction.
- **C.** normalize blood pressure.
- **D.** reduce pain and swelling.

_____ 17. Arteries that lie over bony prominences near the skin create pulse points. These sites are also called _____ points.
- **A.** venous
- **B.** distal
- **C.** arterial
- **D.** pressure

_____ 18. Any patient who exhibits signs and symptoms of shock
- **A.** should be immediately transported.
- **B.** should be given fluid replacement by mouth.
- **C.** should be treated on-scene.
- **D.** will always be hypotensive.

_____ 19. Bleeding from the nose, which can result from injury, disease, or environmental causes, is called
- **A.** hypovolemia.
- **B.** epistaxis.
- **C.** anaphylaxis.
- **D.** hemataxis.

_____ 20. The stage of shock in which the body is able to maintain perfusion and function is called
- **A.** uncompensated.
- **B.** hypovolemic.
- **C.** irreversible.
- **D.** compensatory.

IN THE FIELD

Read the following real-life situation. Then answer the questions that follow.

The emergency medical dispatcher sends you and your partner to an accident at a local baseball field. She informs you that a 9-year-old boy fell and has sustained a cut on his leg caused by broken glass.

Upon assessment of the scene, you note that the boy's mother is applying pressure to the wound with a handkerchief. Both the handkerchief and the ground directly underneath the boy are blood soaked.

During your initial assessment, you observe that the patient's skin color is pale and that he is cool and clammy to the touch. His heart and respiratory rates are rapid. The mother wants you to bandage the wound quickly so that she can take the boy to the family doctor. As you talk to the mother, the boy lies down on the ground and complains of dizziness and weakness. You note that the patient becomes slow to respond and begins to shiver.

1. What safety precautions should you have taken at this scene?

2. Does the boy have blunt or penetrating trauma?

3. List the emergency medical care steps that you will use to control bleeding. State the rationale for each step.

4. In your opinion, should the patient be transported to the hospital? Why or why not?

5. How will you handle the parent's request to take the child to the family doctor?

REINFORCEMENT

CHAPTER 27 REVIEW

Write the word or words that best complete each sentence in the space provided.

1. Trauma accompanied by _____, whether internal or external, can be a significant life-threatening emergency.

2. The circulatory system has three main components: the _____, the _____ _____, and the _____.

3. The three major types of blood vessels include _____, _____, and _____.

4. The adequate circulation of blood and oxygen throughout the body is known as _____.

5. An insufficient circulation of blood and oxygen to the body's cells and tissues is known as _____.

6. Severe external bleeding should be controlled during the _____ _____ phase of the patient assessment process.

7. Whenever bleeding is anticipated or discovered, the use of _____ _____ _____ precautions is essential for the EMT to avoid exposure of the skin and mucous membranes.

8. _____ bleeding is often rapid and profuse, spurting with each heartbeat.

9. A(n) _____ _____ is a site where a large artery lies close to the surface of the body and directly over a bone.

10. The pressure points used to control bleeding in the extremities usually involve the _____ artery or _____ artery.

11. The use of a(n) _____ is a last resort limited to situations in which other methods of controlling life-threatening bleeding have failed.

12. Care for the patient with internal bleeding centers around the prevention and treatment of _____.

13. The final stage of shock, or _____ shock, exists when the body has lost the battle to maintain perfusion to the organ systems.

14. An important point to remember is that prompt _____ is an important

intervention in trauma care.

15. Always suspect internal bleeding if there are penetrating wounds to the

_____, _____, or _____.

BLEEDING AND SHOCK: LISTING

1. List four causes of shock.

2. List three types of external bleeding.

3. List five methods of controlling external bleeding.

4. List eight signs of possible internal bleeding.

5. List three major types of shock.

REINFORCEMENT

BLEEDING AND SHOCK: MATCHING

Write the letter of the term next to the appropriate description.

_____ **1.** Device of last resort for bleeding control on an extremity

_____ **2.** Inability of the body to adequately circulate blood to the cells and tissues

_____ **3.** Medical term for severe bleeding

_____ **4.** Adequate circulation of blood and oxygen to the body

_____ **5.** Blood vessel that carries blood back to the heart

_____ **6.** Slow and oozing dark blood

_____ **7.** Distributes blood to all parts of the body

_____ **8.** First stage of shock in which the body is still able to maintain perfusion

_____ **9.** Shock, or lack of perfusion, brought on by inadequate pumping action of the heart

_____ **10.** The major artery of the upper arm; a pressure point

_____ **11.** Microscopic blood vessel where exchanges of oxygen and carbon dioxide occur

_____ **12.** Steady flow of dark red or maroon-colored blood

_____ **13.** Blood vessel with thick muscular walls that carries blood away from the heart

_____ **14.** Stage of shock in which the body is no longer able to maintain perfusion adequately

_____ **15.** High-pressure, rapid, spurting of bright red blood

A. arterial bleeding

B. artery

C. brachial artery

D. capillary

E. capillary bleeding

F. cardiogenic shock

G. circulatory system

H. compensated shock

I. decompensated shock

J. hemorrhage

K. hypoperfusion

L. perfusion

M. tourniquet

N. vein

O. venous bleeding

Bleeding and Shock

The Circulatory System
Heart

Blood Vessels

Blood

Perfusion

External Bleeding
Severity

Types of Bleeding

- Arterial

- Venous

- Capillary

Assessment and Care

Methods of Controlling External Bleeding

- Direct pressure

- Elevation and cold application

- Pressure points

- Splints

- Tourniquet

Bleeding from the Nose, Ears, or Mouth

Internal Bleeding
Severity

Assessment and Care

Shock (Hypoperfusion)
Assessment and Care

Types of Shock

Stages of Shock

HANDOUT 27-2: Chapter 27 Quiz

1. C	**6.** D	**11.** A	**16.** C
2. C	**7.** D	**12.** D	**17.** D
3. B	**8.** D	**13.** D	**18.** A
4. A	**9.** B	**14.** B	**19.** B
5. C	**10.** C	**15.** A	**20.** D

HANDOUT 27-3: In the Field

1. In this situation, there are no obvious hazards. There appears to be a possibility that the mother will become overaggressive. Scene safety should always be foremost in your mind. Use of gloves is a minimum for BSI.

2. Penetrating trauma (caused by glass that penetrated and lacerated the skin)

3. To control bleeding, apply dressings over the blood-soaked handkerchief and secure with a bandage to make a pressure dressing. Then elevate the limb. Add more dressings if the first ones become soaked. Use a pressure point if the pressure dressing does not control bleeding. Prepare to transport. A tourniquet should not be necessary, but one can be applied if all other bleeding control steps have failed and if a life-threatening condition is detected. (Once applied, a tourniquet should not be removed.)

4. The boy should be transported as quickly as possible. He has apparently lost a large quantity of blood, which can be serious if calculated against his size, age, and build. He is also showing early signs of shock. Children compensate very efficiently but can decline rapidly once decompensated shock begins.

5. The mother should be taken aside. The boy's condition should then be explained to her in nontechnical terms. The EMT might offer to have medical direction call the family doctor to meet the ambulance at the hospital. If the mother refuses transport, the EMT should explain the possible consequences and have her sign appropriate documents. Witnesses should also sign.

HANDOUT 27-4: Chapter 27 Review

1. Bleeding
2. heart, blood vessels, blood
3. arteries, capillaries, veins
4. perfusion
5. hypoperfusion
6. initial assessment
7. body substance isolation
8. Arterial
9. pressure point (or arterial pulse point)
10. brachial, femoral
11. tourniquet
12. shock
13. Irreversible
14. transport
15. skull, chest, abdomen

HANDOUT 27-5: Bleeding and Shock: Listing

1. Fluid loss, pump failure, vasodilation, hypoxia
2. Arterial, venous, capillary
3. Direct pressure, elevation and cold application, pressure points, splinting, tourniquet
4. Signs of possible internal bleeding include (any eight): pain, tenderness, swelling, or discoloration of suspected injury site; bleeding from mouth, rectum, vagina, or other orifice; vomiting bright red blood or blood the color of dark coffee grounds; dark, tarry stools, or stools with bright red blood; tender, rigid, and/or distended abdomen. Answers might also include signs and symptoms of internal bleeding and shock: anxiety, restlessness, combativeness, altered mental status; weakness, faintness, dizziness; thirst; shallow, rapid breathing; rapid pulse; pale, cool, clammy skin; delayed capillary refill; dropping blood pressure; narrow pulse pressure; dilated, sluggish pupils; nausea and vomiting
5. Any three: hypovolemic, vasogenic, anaphylactic, cardiogenic, septic

HANDOUT 27-6: Bleeding and Shock: Matching

1. M	**5.** N	**9.** F	**13.** B
2. K	**6.** E	**10.** C	**14.** I
3. J	**7.** G	**11.** D	**15.** A
4. L	**8.** H	**12.** O	

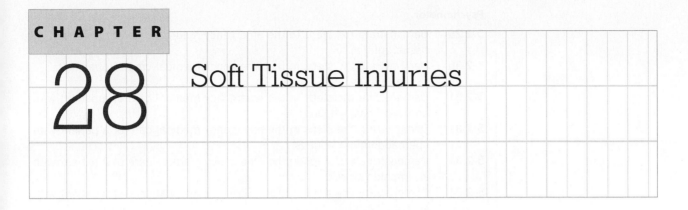

CHAPTER 28 — Soft Tissue Injuries

This chapter covers portions of Lesson 5-2 and Lesson 5-5 of the U.S. Department of Transportation's EMT-Basic National Standard Curriculum.

OBJECTIVES

Numbered objectives are from the U.S. Department of Transportation's EMT-Basic National Standard Curriculum. Asterisked objectives, if any, pertain to material that is supplemental to the DOT curriculum. Page numbers refer to pages in the textbook.

Cognitive

5-2.1 State the major functions of the skin. (p. 774)

5-2.2 List the layers of the skin. (p. 774)

5-2.3 Establish the relationship between body substance isolation (BSI) and soft tissue injuries. (p. 774)

5-2.4 List the types of closed soft tissue injuries. (p. 774)

5-2.5 Describe the emergency medical care of the patient with a closed soft tissue injury. (p. 776)

5-2.6 State the types of open soft tissue injuries. (pp. 777–781)

5-2.7 Describe the emergency medical care of the patient with an open soft tissue injury. (p. 782)

5-2.8 Discuss the emergency medical care considerations for a patient with a penetrating chest injury. (pp. 782–783)

5-2.9 State the emergency medical care considerations for a patient with an open wound to the abdomen. (p. 783)

5-2.10 Differentiate the care of an open wound to the chest from an open wound to the abdomen. (pp. 782–783)

5-2.21 List the functions of dressing and bandaging. (pp. 785–787)

5-2.22 Describe the purpose of a bandage. (p. 787)

5-2.23 Describe the steps in applying a pressure dressing. (p. 787)

5-2.24 Establish the relationship between airway management and the patient with chest injury, burns, and blunt and penetrating injuries. (pp. 774, 781)

5-2.25 Describe the effects of improperly applied dressings, splints, and tourniquets. (pp. 787, 789)

5-2.26 Describe the emergency medical care of a patient with an impaled object. (p. 783)

5-2.27 Describe the emergency medical care of a patient with an amputation. (pp. 783–785)

Total Teaching Time
270 minutes

Resources Needed

- Scored Chapter 27 Quizzes

- Large supply of sterile and nonsterile dressings, including Universal 4 × 4 Adhesive Occlusive

- Large supply of bandages, including self-adherent, gauze rolls, triangular adhesive tape, air splint

Additional Resources

Larmon/Davis, *Basic Life Support Skills*

Elling, *EMT Achieve: Basic Test Preparation*

Limmer/Mistovich/O'Keefe, *Audio Lecture & Study Guide: EMT*

Mistovich/Kuvlesky, *SUCCESS! for the EMT, Second Edition*

Psychomotor

5-2.29   Demonstrate the steps in the emergency medical care of closed soft tissue injuries.

5-2.30   Demonstrate the steps in the emergency medical care of open soft tissue injuries.

5-2.31   Demonstrate the steps in the emergency medical care of a patient with an open chest wound.

5-2.32   Demonstrate the steps in the emergency medical care of a patient with open abdominal wounds.

5-2.33   Demonstrate the steps in the emergency medical care of a patient with an impaled object.

5-2.34   Demonstrate the steps in the emergency medical care of a patient with an amputation.

5-2.35   Demonstrate the steps in the emergency medical care of an amputated part.

5-2.40   Demonstrate completing a prehospital care report for patients with soft tissue injuries.

Additional objectives from DOT Lesson 5-2 are addressed in Chapter 31, "Burn Emergencies." Some of the objectives from DOT Lesson 5-2 are also addressed in Chapter 36, "Chest, Abdomen, and Genitalia Injuries."

REVIEW

In the last chapter, "Bleeding and Shock," students learned that bleeding can be a significant, life-threatening emergency. EMTs must be able to recognize obvious or external bleeding problems, as well as not-so-obvious internal bleeding problems because if either type of bleeding is left untreated, it has the potential to lead to rapid patient deterioration, shock (hypoperfusion), and death. Control of severe external bleeding is performed during the initial assessment. Only airway and breathing have a higher priority. Internal bleeding and shock (hypoperfusion) are treated immediately following the initial assessment. An important element of the emergency care of bleeding and shock (hypoperfusion) is to transport the patient to a medical facility as rapidly as possible.

Distribute the quizzes from the last class. Go over each question on the quiz and handle any concerns students may have about the answers.

INTRODUCTION TO CHAPTER 28

Chapter 28, "Soft Tissue Injuries," is the third chapter in Module 5. Injuries to the soft tissues—the skin, muscles, nerves, blood vessels, and organs—are often dramatic but rarely life-threatening. However, they are serious if they lead to airway or breathing compromise, uncontrolled bleeding, or shock. In general, emergency medical care emphasizes the control of bleeding, prevention of further injury, and reduction of the risk of infection. Unless injuries are life-threatening, care is usually accomplished after the initial assessment and prior to lifting and moving. Failure to recognize and provide care for soft tissue injuries may lead to severe, uncontrolled bleeding, possible additional injury including shock (hypoperfusion), or further contamination of the wound leading to an increased risk of infection.

Distribute the Chapter 28 Objectives Checklist, and give students a few minutes to look it over. Then briefly paraphrase the objectives for this lesson in your own words.

Handout 28-1
Chapter 28 Objectives
Checklist

The following suggested lecture outline is based on the Department of Transportation's EMT-Basic National Standard Curriculum. In some places, the DOT curriculum has been rearranged or expanded upon so that it is more complete or easier for the student to understand. The page numbers in parentheses refer to pages in the textbook. The parenthetical references in dark, heavy type are to figures, tables, and scans in the textbook.

SOFT TISSUE INJURIES

I. **The skin** (p. 774) (Students may also review material on the skin in Chapter 4, "The Human Body.")

    A. Review description and function (p. 774)

        1. Protects body from environment, bacteria, and other organisms

        2. Helps to regulate the body's temperature

        3. Serves as a receptor organ that senses heat, cold, touch, pressure, and pain

        4. Aids in the elimination of water and various salts

    B. Layers (p. 774)

        1. Epidermis

        2. Dermis

        3. Subcutaneous

    C. Wound (pp. 774) **(Fig. 28-1, p. 775)**

        1. Injury to the skin and underlying tissues

II. **Closed soft tissue injuries** (pp. 774–776)

    A. Contusion (bruise) (p. 774)

        1. Intact epidermis with injury to the cells and blood vessels contained within the dermis **(Fig. 28-2, p. 776)**

        2. Will cause localized swelling and pain

        3. May cause some discoloration at injury site (ecchymosis)

    B. Hematoma (p. 774) **(Fig. 28-3, p. 776)**

        1. Similar to contusion but usually involves bigger blood vessel and larger amount of tissue

        2. Collection of blood beneath the skin

        3. Larger amount of tissue damage than contusion

        4. Larger vessels damaged than contusion

        5. Hematoma the size of a fist can equal a 10 percent blood loss.

    C. Crush injuries (p. 774)

        1. Caused by crushing force applied to body

        2. Can cause internal organ rupture

        3. May have severe internal bleeding resulting in shock (hypoperfusion)

        4. May be open or closed

    D. Assessment and care: closed soft tissue injuries (pp. 774–776)

        1. Scene size-up and initial assessment

            a. Scan for mechanism of injury.

            b. Take all body substance isolation (BSI) precautions.

            c. When safe, approach patient and conduct initial assessment.

            d. Provide in-line stabilization of cervical spine if you suspect possible spine injury.

            e. Assess mental status and ensure adequate airway and breathing; then check for and treat bleeding and shock.

Lecture Master

You may wish to display Lecture Master 28 when presenting the lecture to the class.

Point of Interest

The skin is the largest organ of the human body. It has a total surface area of over 20 square feet.

Slides/Videos

Trauma images. http://www.trauma.org/imagebank/imagebank.html

On the Net

Skin anatomy and the process of wound healing. http://www.angio.org/providers/woundcare/understandingWounds.html

Point to Emphasize

Always consider the possibility of closed soft tissue injuries when there is swelling, pain, or deformity and a mechanism of blunt trauma. Patients with a significant MOI should be considered to have internal bleeding and shock until ruled out in the Emergency Department.

    f. Administer oxygen by nonrebreather mask at 15 liters per minute if indicated.

    g. Administer positive-pressure ventilation with supplemental oxygen if breathing is inadequate.

  2. Focused history and physical exam

    a. Reconsider the mechanism of injury to estimate potential number and sites of impact.

    b. Perform rapid trauma assessment, including check for DCAP-BTLS.

    c. Assess baseline vitals and take SAMPLE history.

    d. Look for signs and symptoms of soft tissue injury.

      (1) Swelling, pain, discoloration at injury site

      (2) Signs and symptoms of internal bleeding and shock (hypoperfusion) with severe injuries

  3. Emergency medical care

    a. Take BSI precautions.

      (1) Wear protective gloves and personal protective equipment.

      (2) Wash hands thoroughly after a call, even if gloves were worn.

    b. Ensure an open airway and adequate breathing.

    c. Treat for shock (hypoperfusion), if necessary.

    d. Splint painful, swollen, deformed extremities.

  4. Detailed physical exam and ongoing assessment

III. Open soft tissue injuries (pp. 776–785)

  A. Classification (pp. 776–781) **(Fig. 28-4, p. 777)**

    1. Abrasion **(Fig. 28-5, p. 777)**

      a. Outermost layer of skin damaged by scraping, rubbing, or shearing forces.

      b. Painful injury, even though superficial, because of exposure of nerve endings

      c. No or very little oozing of blood controlled easily by direct pressure

    2. Laceration **(Figs. 28-6 and 28-7, p. 778)**

      a. Break in skin of varying depth

      b. May occur in isolation or together with other types of soft tissue injury

      c. May bleed more than other types of soft tissue injury

      d. May be linear (regular) injury

      e. May be stellate (irregular) injury

    3. Avulsion **(Fig. 28-8, p. 779)**

      a. Flaps of skin or tissue are torn loose or pulled completely off

      b. May be severe bleeding, although some blood vessels may tamponade (compress) themselves by retracting into soft tissue

      c. Prolonged healing

      d. May be extensive scarring

      e. Mechanism of injury: most commonly result of industrial accidents or home machinery and motor vehicle accidents

    4. Amputation **(Fig. 28-9, p. 779)**

      a. Disruption in continuity of extremity and other body parts

      b. Mechanism of injury: ripping or tearing forces associated with industrial or motor vehicle accidents

---

On the Net

Dealing with lacerations.
http://www.emedicine.com/
aaem/topic141.htm

Point to Emphasize

Do not underestimate the effects of a laceration. The patient may need stitches, plastic surgery, or a tetanus shot at the hospital, so don't put on butterfly bandages and leave the patient at the scene. Serious infection or scarring could result.

☑

Teaching Tip

Distribute local protocols regarding the care of avulsed tissue.

◎

Point to Emphasize

Never complete a partial amputation. Do not immerse the amputated part directly in saline or water. Do not let the part come in direct contact with ice or it may freeze.

  c. Most have very little bleeding (due to elasticity of blood vessels), but bleeding can be massive.

  d. Always consider shock (hypoperfusion) in cases of amputation.

 5. Penetration/puncture (**Figs. 28-10, p. 780 and 28-11, pp. 780–781**)

  a. Sharp, pointed object pushed or driven into soft tissues

  b. May be deep, damaging, and cause severe internal bleeding, even with small entry wound and no external bleeding

  c. Factors affecting wound severity

   (1) Wound location

   (2) Size of penetrating object

   (3) Depth of penetration

   (4) Forces involved in creating injury

  d. Gunshot wound

   (1) May have both entrance and exit wound

   (2) Exit wound may bleed more profusely than entrance wound.

   (3) Assess for multiple gunshot wounds, particularly in areas covered by hair.

  e. Stab wound

   (1) May be easily detected or small and hidden by clothing or extremity

   (2) Expose patient and carefully inspect all areas of body.

   (3) Always assess patient for underlying internal injuries and shock (hypoperfusion).

 6. Crush injuries (**Fig. 28-12, p. 781**)

  a. Blunt trauma or crushing force injures soft tissue and/or internal organs

  b. May cause painful, swollen, deformed extremities

  c. External bleeding may be minimal or absent.

  d. Internal bleeding may be severe.

  e. Patient may at first appear unaffected but can deteriorate rapidly into shock (hypoperfusion) when object causing injury is lifted from patient.

B. Assessment and care: open soft tissue injuries (pp. 781–785) (**Figs. 28-24 and 28-25, pp. 791–793**)

 1. Scene size-up and initial assessment

  a. Ensure that scene is safe before entering.

  b. Note potential mechanism of injury.

  c. Stabilize cervical spine if indicated.

  d. Get general impression of patient and patient's mental status as approaching patient.

  e. Ensure an open airway.

  f. Provide oxygen by nonrebreather mask at 15 liters per minute if severe injuries and breathing is inadequate.

  g. Initiate positive-pressure ventilation with supplemental oxygen if indicated.

  h. Bring severe bleeding under control.

 2. Focused history and physical exam

  a. Begin with rapid trauma assessment.

  b. Assess baseline and vital signs.

  c. Take a SAMPLE history.

Slides/Videos
"Penetrating Trauma," *Pulse,* Oct. 1999.

d. Perform focused trauma assessment for patients without a significant mechanism of injury.

e. Signs and symptoms of open soft tissue injuries

   (1) Break in skin and external bleeding

   (2) Localized swelling, pain, and discoloration at injury site

   (3) Possible signs and symptoms of internal bleeding and shock (hypoperfusion)

3. Emergency medical care

  a. Take BSI precautions.

  b. Ensure an open airway and adequate breathing.

  c. Expose the wound and assess for additional wounds.

  d. Control bleeding.

  e. Prevent further contamination.

  f. Dress and bandage the wound.

  g. Keep the patient calm and quiet.

  h. Treat for shock (hypoperfusion).

  i. Transport.

4. Detailed physical exam and ongoing assessment

  a. If rapid trauma assessment was performed, consider performing a detailed physical exam en route.

  b. Repeat initial assessment, rapid or focused assessment.

  c. Monitor vital signs.

  d. Recheck interventions.

5. Special considerations

  a. Chest injuries

   (1) Use an occlusive dressing (one that can form an air-tight seal) to prevent air entering chest cavity through wound (open pneumothorax). (**Fig. 28-13, p. 782**)

   (2) Secure dressing on only three sides to prevent a buildup of air in chest cavity that compresses lungs and heart toward uninjured side (tension pneumothorax).

   (3) Place patient in position of comfort if no spinal injury is suspected.

  b. Abdominal injuries with evisceration (organs protruding through the wound)

   (1) Do not touch or try to replace the exposed organs.

   (2) Cover exposed organs with sterile dressing moistened with sterile water or saline. Then cover with occlusive dressing taped on all four sides. (**Fig. 28-14, p. 783**)

   (3) Flex patient's hips and knees if uninjured and spinal injury is not suspected.

  c. Impaled objects still embedded in wound (**Fig. 28-15, p. 783**)

   (1) Do not remove the impaled object, unless it is through the cheek, it would interfere with chest compressions, or it interferes with transport.

   (2) Manually secure the object.

   (3) Expose the wound area by cutting away clothing.

   (4) Control bleeding.

   (5) Use a bulky dressing to help stabilize the object. (**Figs. 28-16, p. 784 and 28-17, p. 785**)

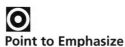

Point to Emphasize

An open chest wound is a *true emergency* that requires rapid initial care and immediate transport to a medical facility.

Point to Emphasize

The only impaled object that should be removed is one in the cheek. The danger of airway compromise is too great to leave it there. It should be removed in the direction that it entered the cheek. If it is in a deeper structure, such as the palate, do not try to remove it; stabilize the object and transport.

d. Amputations—concerns for reattachment

    (1) Wrap amputated part in a dry, sterile gauze dressing.

    (2) Wrap or bag the amputated part in plastic and keep cool.

        (a) Follow local protocol.

        (b) Label the bag with patient's name, date, body part, and time part was wrapped and bagged.

    (3) Keep amputated part cool.

        (a) Place in cooler or other suitable container with ice pack or ice on bottom.

        (b) Do not place directly on ice or ice pack.

        (c) Label container with patient's name, date, and body part.

    (4) Transport the amputated part with the patient if at all possible.

    (5) Do not complete partial amputations.

    (6) Immobilize injured area to prevent further injury.

e. Large, open neck injury (**Fig. 28-18, p. 785**)

    (1) Place a gloved hand over wound to control bleeding.

    (2) Apply an occlusive dressing.

    (3) Cover occlusive dressing with a regular dressing.

    (4) Apply only enough pressure to control the bleeding, compressing carotid artery only if it is severed and it is necessary to control bleeding.

    (5) Once bleeding is controlled, apply a pressure dressing.

    (6) Provide appropriate immobilization if spinal injury is suspected.

IV. Dressings and bandages (pp. 785–789)

  A. Dressings (pp. 785–787)

    1. Purpose

      a. Stop bleeding.

      b. Protect the wound from further damage.

      c. Prevent further contamination and infection.

    2. Common types of dressings (**Fig. 28-19, p. 786**)

      a. Sterile gauze pad

      b. Self-adhering dressing

      c. Universal or multitrauma dressing

      d. Occlusive dressing

  B. Bandages (p. 787) (**Fig. 28-19, p. 786**)

    1. Purpose

      a. To hold dressing in place

    2. Common types of bandages

      a. Self-adhering bandages

      b. Gauze rolls

      c. Triangular bandages (**Fig. 28-22, p. 790**)

      d. Air splint (**Fig. 28-23, p. 790**)

  C. Application of pressure dressings (p. 787) (**Figs. 28-20, p. 788 and 28-21, p. 789**)

    1. Cover the wound with several sterile gauze dressings or a sterile bulky dressing.

    2. Apply hand pressure over wound until bleeding is controlled.

◉

Point to Emphasize
Treatment of neck vein wounds is aimed at stopping bleeding and preventing an air embolus from entering circulation.

3. Bandage firmly to create enough pressure to maintain control of bleeding.
4. If blood soaks through the original dressing and bandage, indicating continued severe bleeding, remove them and apply direct fingertip pressure. Once the bleeding is controlled, apply dressings and bandage over the wound again.

D. General principles of dressing and bandaging (pp. 787–789)
1. Dressing materials should be as clean as possible.
2. Do not bandage a dressing in place until bleeding has stopped.
3. Make sure that the dressing adequately covers the entire wound.
4. If possible, remove all of the patient's jewelry from the injured body part.
5. Do not bandage a wound too loosely.
6. Bandage wounds snugly but not too tightly.
7. If you bandage a small wound on an extremity, cover a larger area with the bandage.
8. Always place the body part to be bandaged in the position in which it is to remain.
9. Apply a tourniquet only as a last resort .

E. Summary: assessment and care (p. 789) **(Figs. 28-24 and 28-25, pp. 791–793)**

ENRICHMENT (OPTIONAL)

The following sections contain information that is valuable as background for the EMT, but that goes substantially beyond the U.S. Department of Transportation's EMT-Basic National Standard Curriculum.

V. Other soft tissue injuries (pp. 789–794)
A. Bites (pp. 789–790) **(Fig. 28-26, p. 794)**
1. Generally combination of penetration/puncture and crush injuries
2. Complications of bites
3. Emergency medical care
   a. Essentially same as other soft tissue injuries
   b. Should always be evaluated at medical facility no matter how minor
   c. Always ensure scene safety before providing patient care.
B. Clamping injuries—body part caught or strangled by piece of machinery (pp. 790–794) **(Fig. 28-27, p. 794)**
1. Freeing body part
   a. Apply lubricant
   b. Slowly attempt to wiggle part loose, elevating body part above patient's head, if possible, as you work.
   c. If there is severe bleeding or shock and patient cannot be rapidly disentangled, immediately transport both patient and object.
   d. If object is too large to transport, specialized personnel may be required to cut away parts of machine or clamping object.

©2008 by Pearson Education, Inc.
Prehospital Emergency Care, 8th ed.

Ask a student volunteer to read the Case Study that begins on page 773 of the textbook. You may wish to use the following questions to engage the students in a discussion of the Case Study Follow-up that begins on page 795 of the textbook. Provide missing information and clarify ideas as needed.

Q1. Describe the nature of this call and how the scene was made safe.

A1. *This call is for a dog bite. The owner locked the dog in a garage across the street.*

Q2. From your initial assessment, describe the injury to Mr. Young's leg.

A2. *There are two 3-inch lacerations on the calf of the lower leg. Bleeding is dark red and moderate in rate. The puncture is through all layers of the skin and appears to extend into the muscle.*

Q3. How do you treat the wound?

A3. *By placing a sterile gauze dressing over the wounds and applying direct pressure. When bleeding has almost stopped, a pressure bandage is applied and secured with tape.*

Q4. What reason do you give Mr. Young for transporting him to the hospital?

A4. *There is a risk of infection from the dog's saliva. Also, because the wound is deep, it may need to be sutured.*

Q5. What essential pieces of information about the dog do you make sure have been collected?

A5. *The owner's name and address, and the dog's rabies vaccination status.*

IN REVIEW ◼

Assess students' ability to apply what they have just learned by discussing the Review Questions on page 796 of the textbook.

Q1. Describe each of three types of closed soft tissue injuries.

A1. *Three types of closed injuries include: (1) a contusion, or bruise; (2) a hematoma, similar to a contusion except it usually involves damage to a larger blood vessel and a larger amount of tissue; and (3) a crush injury, which may be closed or open. (p. 774)*

Q2. Identify the general signs and symptoms of closed soft tissue injuries.

A2. *The general signs and symptoms of closed soft tissue injuries include swelling, pain, and discoloration at the injury site, with the potential of internal bleeding and shock (hypoperfusion) if the underlying organs are injured. (pp. 774–776)*

Q3. Outline the general emergency medical care for closed soft tissue injuries.

A3. *The general emergency medical care for closed soft tissue injuries includes taking BSI precautions; ensuring an open airway and adequate breathing; treating for shock (hypoperfusion), if necessary; splinting painful, swollen, deformed extremities. (p. 776)*

Q4. Describe each of six types of open soft tissue injuries.

A4. *Six types of open soft tissue injuries are abrasions, lacerations, avulsions, penetrations/punctures, amputations, and crush injuries. Abrasions are generally caused by scraping, rubbing, or shearing away the outermost layer of the skin (epidermis). Lacerations are breaks in the skin caused by forceful impact with a sharp object. An avulsion is a loose flap of skin and soft tissue that has been torn loose or pulled completely off. A penetration or puncture wound generally is the result of a sharp, pointed object being pushed or driven into the soft tissue. Amputations involve a disruption in the continuity of an extremity or other body part as the result of ripping or tearing forces. Crush injuries are usually the result of blunt trauma or crushing forces. (pp. 776–781)*

Q5. Identify the general signs and symptoms of open soft tissue injuries.

A5. *The general signs and symptoms of open soft tissue injuries include a break in the skin and external bleeding; swelling, pain, and discoloration at the injury site; possible signs and symptoms of internal bleeding and shock (hypoperfusion). (p. 782)*

Q6. Outline the general emergency medical care for open soft tissue injuries.

A6. *The general emergency medical care for open soft tissue injuries includes taking BSI precautions; ensuring an open airway and adequate breathing; exposing the wound; controlling bleeding; preventing further contamination; dressing and bandaging the wound; keeping the patient calm and quiet; treating for shock (hypoperfusion); and transporting. (p. 782)*

Q7. Describe the special considerations that must be taken when providing emergency medical care to patients with the following injuries: penetrating chest wounds, abdominal evisceration, impaled object, amputated part, and large open injury to the neck.

A7. *Special considerations that must be taken when providing emergency medical care to patients with the following injuries are: Penetrating chest wounds—use an occlusive dressing to prevent air from entering the chest cavity through the wound; leave one side untaped to allow air to escape as the patient exhales. Patient may assume a position of comfort if there is no suspected spinal injury; however, spinal injury should be suspected with any significant mechanism of injury to the chest. Abdominal evisceration—avoid touching or trying to replace the abdominal organs; cover the exposed organs with a moistened sterile dressing, an occlusive dressing, additional layers of bulky dressings, and a bandage; flex the patient's hips and knees if they are uninjured and if spinal injury is not suspected. However, suspect spinal injury with any significant mechanism of injury to the abdomen. Do not use the abdominal portion of the PASG if it is used in your system. Impaled object—manually secure the object, expose the wound area, control bleeding, use a bulky dressing to help stabilize the object during transport. Amputated part—wrap the part in a dry, sterile gauze dressing, wrap or bag the amputated part in plastic, keep it cool, and transport the part with the patient. Large open injury to the neck— cover the wound with a gloved hand, apply an occlusive dressing covered by a regular dressing, apply pressure to control bleeding, apply a pressure bandage, and provide care for suspected spinal injury. (pp. 782–785)*

Q8. Describe the purpose of a dressing and name several available types.

A8. *A dressing covers an open wound to aid in the control of bleeding and to prevent further damage or contamination. In most cases, the dressing should be sterile. Common types of dressings include universal or multitrauma dressings, gauze pads, adhesive-type dressings, and occlusive dressings. (p. 785)*

Q9. Describe the purpose of a bandage and name several available types.

A9. *A bandage is used to hold or secure a dressing in place. Common types of bandages include self-adhering bandages, gauze rolls, triangular bandages, and air splints.(p. 787)*

Q10. Describe the purpose of a pressure dressing and outline the steps for applying a pressure dressing.

A10. *A pressure dressing is used to maintain control of bleeding. Apply a pressure dressing as follows: Cover the wound with several sterile gauze dressings or a bulky dressing. Apply hand pressure over the wound until the bleeding is controlled. Bandage firmly to create enough pressure to maintain control of the bleeding. (Check distal pulses to be sure the bandage is not too tight.) If blood soaks through the original dressing and bandage, remove them and apply fingertip pressure. When bleeding is under control, apply dressings and bandage over the wound again. (pp. 787–789)*

CRITICAL THINKING

Assess students' ability to respond to real-life emergency situations by discussing the Critical Thinking questions on page 796 in the textbook.

Q1. What immediate emergency care would you provide for the patient?

A1. *The EMT should immediately place a gloved hand over the gaping neck laceration and apply direct pressure to control the bleeding. The same EMT will establish and maintain manual in-line spinal stabilization as best as possible. Next, open the airway using a jaw-thrust maneuver, insert an oropharyngeal airway, and begin bag-valve-mask ventilation. Connect oxygen to the BVM reservoir and set the liter flow at 12 to 15 lpm.*

Q2. How would you manage the wound to the neck?

A2. *An occlusive dressing should be placed directly on the wound (replacing the gloved hand that would have been placed there initially) and then covered by a regular dressing. Pressure should be applied just until the bleeding is controlled and once it is, a pressure dressing should be applied. The occlusive dressing is used to prevent air from being sucked into a large lacerated vein, potentially creating an air embolism.*

Q3. What complications may be associated with the neck wound?

A3. *With this type of large open neck wound there is a risk of air being sucked into the lacerated vein that is draining blood toward the right atrium. An air bubble acts just like a blood clot and can obstruct blood flow through a vessel. If the air bubble was to enter the right atrium, it would then flow into the right ventricle and then into the pulmonary artery. The air bubble would then enter the pulmonary circulation and would likely cause an obstruction in a pulmonary vessel blocking forward blood flow and causing a disturbance in gas exchange in the lungs.*

Q4. How would you manage the knife impaled in the chest?

A4. *First, the knife should be manually stabilized, then the clothing should be cut away, exposing the wound area, and bleeding should be controlled with direct pressure to the wound edges. The knife should then be stabilized and bandaged in place with a bulky dressing.*

ROLE PLAY

Ask for a student volunteer to be a patient. Step-by-step, describe and demonstrate the procedures for bandaging the following parts of the body: forehead, elbow or knee, forearm or leg, hand, shoulder, and hip. Pair students and provide each team with dressings and bandages. Tell students that you want each team member to take turns practicing all the bandages that you have just demonstrated.

Observe each team as it practices. Provide corrective feedback and answer questions as needed.

ASSIGNMENTS

Assign students to read Chapter 29, "Burn Emergencies," before the next class. Also ask them to complete Chapter 28 of the Workbook.

EVALUATION

Chapter Quiz Distribute copies of the Chapter Quiz provided in Handout 28-2 to evaluate student understanding of this chapter. Remind students not to refer to their textbooks or notes while taking the quiz.

Test Manager You may wish to create a custom-tailored test using Prentice Hall *TestGen for Prehospital Emergency Care, Eighth Edition* to evaluate student understanding of this chapter.

Online Test Preparation (for students and instructors) Additional test preparation is available through *EMT Achieve: Basic Test Preparation* at http://www.prenhall.com/EMTAchieve. Instructors can also monitor student mastery online.

REINFORCEMENT

Handouts If classroom discussions or performance on the quiz indicates that some students have not fully mastered the chapter content, you may wish to assign some or all of the Reinforcement Handouts for this chapter.

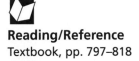

Reading/Reference
Textbook, pp. 797–818

Workbook
Chapter 28 Activities

Chapter Quiz
Handout 28-2

TestGen
Chapter 28 Test

Online Test Preparation
Send your students to http://www.prenhall.com/EMTAchieve

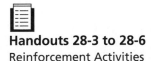

Handouts 28-3 to 28-6
Reinforcement Activities

TECH EXTRAS

Brady Skills Series EMT-B Videos/CD Have your students watch the skills come to life on either VHS or CD-ROM.

PowerPoint Presentation (for instructors) The PowerPoint material developed for this chapter offers useful reinforcement of chapter content.

Student CD A wide variety of material on this CD-ROM will reinforce and also expand student knowledge and skills.

Companion Website (for students) Additional review quizzes and links to EMS resources will contribute to further reinforcement of this chapter. Please visit http://www.prenhall.com/mistovich.

**Brady Skills Series
EMT-B Videos/CD**
Visual Reinforcement

**PowerPoint
Presentation**
Chapter 28

Student CD
Chapter 28

Companion Website
http://www.prenhall.com/
mistovich

OBJECTIVES (sidebar)

OBJECTIVES CHECKLIST

Cognitive		Date Mastered
5-2.1	State the major functions of the skin.	
5-2.2	List the layers of the skin.	
5-2.3	Establish the relationship between body substance isolation (BSI) and soft tissue injuries.	
5-2.4	List the types of closed soft tissue injuries.	
5-2.5	Describe the emergency medical care of the patient with a closed soft tissue injury.	
5-2.6	State the types of open soft tissue injuries.	
5-2.7	Describe the emergency medical care of the patient with an open soft tissue injury.	
5-2.8	Discuss the emergency medical care considerations for a patient with a penetrating chest injury.	
5-2.9	State the emergency medical care considerations for a patient with an open wound to the abdomen.	
5-2.10	Differentiate the care of an open wound to the chest from an open wound to the abdomen.	
5-2.21	List the functions of dressing and bandaging.	
5-2.22	Describe the purpose of a bandage.	
5-2.23	Describe the steps in applying a pressure dressing.	
5-2.24	Establish the relationship between airway management and the patient with chest injury, burns and blunt and penetrating injuries.	
5-2.25	Describe the effects of improperly applied dressings, splints, and tourniquets.	
5-2.26	Describe the emergency medical care of a patient with an impaled object.	
5-2.27	Describe the emergency medical care of a patient with an amputation.	

Psychomotor		Date Mastered
5-2.29	Demonstrate the steps in the emergency medical care of closed soft tissue injuries.	
5-2.30	Demonstrate the steps in the emergency medical care of open soft tissue injuries.	
5-2.31	Demonstrate the steps in the emergency medical care of a patient with an open chest wound.	
5-2.32	Demonstrate the steps in the emergency medical care of a patient with open abdominal wounds.	
5-2.33	Demonstrate the steps in the emergency medical care of a patient with an impaled object.	
5-2.34	Demonstrate the steps in the emergency medical care of a patient with an amputation.	
5-2.35	Demonstrate the steps in the emergency medical care of an amputated part.	
5-2.40	Demonstrate completing a prehospital care report for patients with soft tissue injuries.	

CHAPTER 28 QUIZ

Write the letter of the best answer in the space provided.

_____ 1. The injury that is similar to a contusion except that it usually involves damage to a larger blood vessel and a larger amount of tissue is a(n)

    A. abrasion.   **C.** wound.

    B. evisceration.   **D.** hematoma.

_____ 2. The outer layer of the skin is called the

    A. subcutaneous layer.   **C.** dermis.

    B. cutaneous layer.   **D.** epidermis.

_____ 3. A break in the skin of varying depth—either linear or stellate—is known as a(n)

    A. avulsion.   **C.** laceration.

    B. amputation.   **D.** abrasion.

_____ 4. All of the following are examples of closed wounds *except* a(n)

    A. contusion.   **C.** crush injury.

    B. hematoma.   **D.** abrasion.

_____ 5. Open wounds in which flaps of skin and tissue are torn loose or pulled off completely are called

    A. avulsions.   **C.** amputations.

    B. lacerations.   **D.** punctures.

_____ 6. Care for an abrasion is important because of the

    A. amount of blood and fluid lost.

    B. emotional trauma of the patient.

    C. underlying soft tissue damage.

    D. risk of contamination and infection.

_____ 7. In treating a patient with a puncture wound involving an impaled object, the usual emergency care includes all of the following steps *except*

    A. removing the impaled object.   **C.** controlling profuse bleeding.

    B. exposing the wound area.   **D.** keeping the patient at rest.

_____ 8. A major concern in caring for a patient with an impaled object in the cheek is

    A. dressing the wound.

    B. maintaining an open airway.

    C. checking to see if the tongue is cut.

    D. positioning the head for drainage.

_____ 9. The condition that is characterized by air entering the chest cavity through an open wound is called

    A. open flail chest.   **C.** open pneumothorax.

    B. paradoxical wound.   **D.** air embolism.

_____ 10. A severe buildup of air in the chest cavity that compresses the heart and the lungs toward the uninjured side is known as

    A. pneumothorax.   **C.** traumatic asphyxia.

    B. tension pneumothorax.   **D.** hemothorax.

_____11. Open wounds of the abdomen that are so large that organs protrude from them are known as
    A. avulsions.
    B. sucking abdominal wounds.
    C. eviscerations.
    D. hematomas.

_____12. The largest organ of the body is the
    A. heart.
    B. skin.
    C. liver.
    D. kidney.

_____13. The major layers of the skin are
    A. mid-dermis, dermis, and muscular tissue.
    B. subcutaneous tissue, mid-dermis, and dermis.
    C. epidermis, dermis, and subcutaneous layer.
    D. interdermis, dermis, and subcutaneous tissue.

_____14. When a part of the body is caught between two compressing surfaces, a _____ injury results.
    A. shear
    B. crush
    C. penetrating
    D. stretching

_____15. The medical term for any dressing that forms an airtight seal is a(n) _____ dressing.
    A. occlusive
    C. universal
    B. flutter-valve
    D. self-adherent

_____16. When attempting to control bleeding from an open wound, the first method to attempt is
    A. elevation.
    B. direct pressure.
    C. use of pressure points.
    D. a tourniquet.

_____17. In cases of amputation, save the amputated part by
    A. wrapping it in dry, sterile dressings.
    B. putting it in a plastic bag.
    C. putting it on a cool surface.
    D. all of the above.

_____18. The preferred position in which to place patients with abdominal injuries is
    A. on the back with legs flexed at the knees.
    B. the Trendelenburg position.
    C. the recovery position.
    D. on the stomach with arms tucked in.

_____19. Bleeding control and prevention of a(n) _____ are the major goals of emergency medical care of a large, open neck injury.
    A. air clot
    B. thrombus
    C. air embolism
    D. blood clot

_____20. Which one of the following is *not* a closed soft tissue injury?
    A. contusion
    B. crush injury
    C. hematoma
    D. avulsion

IN THE FIELD

Read the following real-life situation. Then answer the questions that follow.

A call comes into your station from the emergency medical dispatcher, who reports: "Head-on collision on Market Street. Four people involved."

Your unit reaches the scene in 2 minutes. Police have already closed off the one-way street. "Out-of-town driver," says the police officer. "He completely missed the one-way sign."

You quickly assess the scene and notice skid marks near one of the vehicles. "I tried to hit my brakes when I saw him coming," says the driver of the other car. "I wasn't going all that fast when we collided, but it was still quite a jolt."

The occupants of both cars were wearing seatbelts. Airbags deployed when the vehicles collided. One front-seat passenger, a 19-year-old male, is complaining of abdominal and chest pain. Upon initial assessment, you find marks across his body where the seatbelt confined him. As you palpate these areas, the patient complains of tenderness. You note that his abdomen is rigid and that he winces as you attempt to palpate it. There appear to be no other injuries to his body, so you place him on a stretcher with his knees flexed.

1. What type of injury do you suspect the patient has suffered?

2. What was the mechanism of injury?

3. Describe and explain the additional emergency medical care steps you would provide for this patient.

4. While assessing the patient, he becomes pale and less talkative. His pulse and respiratory rates have increased since you took the set of baseline vital signs. What do you think is happening to the patient? What actions should you take?

CHAPTER 28 REVIEW

Write the word or words that best complete each sentence in the space provided.

1. The largest organ in the human body is the _____.

2. The three layers of the skin are the _____, _____,
   and _____ _____.

3. A wound in which there is no open pathway from the outside to the injured site is called a(n)
   _____ _____.

4. An injury to the soft tissues characterized by swelling and discoloration caused by a mass of blood
   beneath the epidermis is called a(n) _____.

5. A(n) _____ is an injury to the cells and blood vessels contained within the
   dermis.

6. When the skin is interrupted, or broken, exposing the tissues underneath, the result is a(n)
   _____ _____.

7. Simple scrapes or scratches in the outer layer of the skin are known as
   _____.

8. A(n) _____ / _____ is generally caused by a
   sharp, pointed object being pushed into the soft tissues.

9. _____ are wounds in which flaps of skin and tissues are torn loose or pulled
   off completely.

10. In wounds to the neck, there is a possibility for a(n) _____
    _____ being sucked in through a vein.

11. The term _____ _____ is used when the chest
    cavity is open to the atmosphere.

12. A(n) _____ _____ occurs when the lung collapses
    as a result of air that has entered the chest cavity and organs are displaced.

13. Open abdominal wounds from which organs protrude are known as
    _____.

14. A(n) _____ _____ should never be removed in
    the field, unless it is in the cheek or neck and obstructing air flow through the trachea.

15. A dressing that can form an airtight seal over a wound is called a(n) _____

dressing.

16. A(n) _____ covers an open wound to aid in the control of bleeding and to

prevent further damage or contamination.

17. A(n) _____ _____ is usually a 40-inch square

piece of cloth and may be used as a bandage to secure a dressing in place.

18. A material used to secure a dressing in place is known as a(n) _____.

19. The term _____ indicates that the object is free from living

microorganisms such as bacteria, virus, or spores that may cause infection.

20. Plastic is preferred over _____ _____ as an

occlusive dressing.

SOFT TISSUE INJURIES: LISTING

1. List the steps in applying a pressure dressing.

2. List four functions of the skin.

3. List the basic emergency care steps in treating closed wounds.

4. List the basic emergency care steps in treating open wounds.

SOFT TISSUE INJURIES: TRUE OR FALSE

Indicate if the following statements are true or false by writing T or F in the space provided.

_____ 1. When treating a closed soft tissue injury, hyperventilate the patient at 24 liters per minute via nonrebreather mask.

_____ 2. A wound that is beneath unbroken skin is called a closed injury.

_____ 3. Signs and symptoms of a closed soft tissue injury include swelling, pain, and discoloration at the injury site.

_____ 4. An open injury may be the indicator of a deeper, more serious injury.

_____ 5. The healing of an avulsion may be prolonged and scarring may be extensive.

_____ 6. The most common sites of avulsions are the upper arms and buttocks.

_____ 7. With gunshot wounds, the entry wound usually appears larger than the exit wound.

_____ 8. An amputated part should be placed directly on ice and transported with the patient.

_____ 9. In the field, eviscerated abdominal organs should be replaced inside the body cavity, if at all possible.

_____ 10. A chest injury may prevent adequate breathing.

_____ 11. Dog bites are a common type of animal bite.

_____ 12. A common complication associated with bites is cellulitis.

_____ 13. Human bites most commonly involve the lower extremities.

_____ 14. Jewelry should be left in place for security's sake when splinting an injured hand.

_____ 15. If the injured part involves the hands or feet, leave the tips of the fingers or toes exposed to allow for assessment of distal circulation.

Soft Tissue Injuries

Review of Anatomy and Physiology of the Skin

Closed Soft Tissue Injuries

Types of Injuries

- Contusions
- Hematomas
- Crush injuries

Assessment and Care

Open Soft Tissue Injuries

Types of Injuries

- Abrasions
- Lacerations
- Avulsions
- Amputations
- Penetrations/punctures
- Crush injuries

Assessment and Care

Special Considerations

- Chest injuries
- Abdominal injuries
- Impaled objects
- Amputations
- Large open neck injuries

Dressings and Bandages
Dressings

Bandages

Pressure Dressings

General Principles of Dressing
and Bandaging

Other Soft Tissue Injuries
Bites

Clamping Injuries

HANDOUT 28-2: Chapter 28 Quiz

1. D	**6.** D	**11.** C	**16.** B
2. D	**7.** A	**12.** B	**17.** D
3. C	**8.** B	**13.** C	**18.** A
4. D	**9.** C	**14.** B	**19.** C
5. A	**10.** B	**15.** A	**20.** D

HANDOUT 28-3: In the Field

1. The injury is a closed, blunt trauma, crush injury.
2. The mechanism of injury is most likely the force of the restraining seatbelt against the patient's abdomen and chest. The force can be transmitted from the exterior body surface to interior structures even though the only visible injury may be a simple bruise.
3. Manage the patient as if there is internal bleeding and provide treatment to care for and prevent shock. Provide oxygen. Be alert for vomiting, and transport as quickly as possible.
4. The patient is apparently developing shock, probably due to internal bleeding. Transport rapidly.

HANDOUT 28-4: Chapter 28 Review

1. skin
2. epidermis, dermis, subcutaneous layers
3. closed wound
4. hematoma
5. contusion
6. open wound
7. abrasions
8. penetration/puncture
9. Avulsions
10. air embolus
11. open pneumothorax
12. tension pneumothorax
13. eviscerations
14. impaled object
15. occlusive
16. dressing
17. triangular bandage
18. bandage
19. sterile
20. aluminum foil

HANDOUT 28-5: Soft Tissue Injury: Listing

1. Cover the wound with several sterile gauze dressings or a sterile bulky dressing. Apply direct pressure over the wound until the bleeding is controlled. Bandage firmly to create enough pressure to maintain control of the bleeding. If blood soaks through the original dressing, remove it and apply fingertip pressure. Once bleeding is controlled, apply dressings and bandage over the wound.
2. Protection, temperature regulation, receptor organ for sensation, water regulation
3. Take appropriate BSI precautions. Manage the patient's airway, breathing, and circulation. Treat for shock. Splint extremities that are painful, swollen, or deformed.
4. Take BSI precautions; ensure an open airway and adequate breathing; expose the wound; control bleeding; prevent further contamination; dress and bandage the wound; keep the patient calm and quiet; treat for shock (hypoperfusion); transport.

HANDOUT 28-6: Soft Tissue Injury: True or False

1. F	**5.** T	**9.** F	**13.** F
2. T	**6.** F	**10.** T	**14.** F
3. T	**7.** F	**11.** T	**15.** T
4. T	**8.** F	**12.** T	

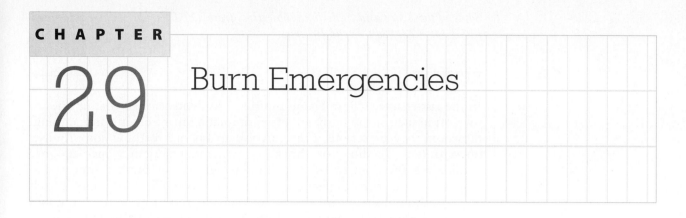

This chapter covers portions of Lesson 5-2 and Lesson 5-5 of the U.S. Department of Transportation's EMT-Basic National Standard Curriculum.

OBJECTIVES

Numbered objectives are from the U.S. Department of Transportation's EMT-Basic National Standard Curriculum. Asterisked objectives, if any, pertain to material that is supplemental to the DOT curriculum. Page numbers refer to pages in the textbook.

Cognitive

5-2.1 State the major functions of the skin. (pp. 798–799)
5-2.2 List the layers of the skin. (p. 798)
5-2.11 List the classifications of burns. (pp. 799–800)
5-2.12 Define superficial burn. (p. 799)
5-2.13 List the characteristics of a superficial burn. (pp. 799–800)
5-2.14 Define partial-thickness burn. (p. 800)
5-2.15 List the characteristics of a partial-thickness burn. (p. 800)
5-2.16 Define full-thickness burn. (p. 800)
5-2.17 List the characteristics of a full-thickness burn. (p. 800)
5-2.18 Describe the emergency medical care of a patient with a superficial burn. (pp. 808–809)
5-2.19 Describe the emergency medical care of a patient with a partial-thickness burn. (pp. 808–809)
5-2.20 Describe the emergency medical care of a patient with a full-thickness burn. (pp. 808–809)
5-2.24 Establish the relationship between airway management and the patient with chest injury, burns, and blunt and penetrating injuries. (pp. 799, 806–807, 808, 813, 814, 816)
5-2.28 Describe the emergency care for a chemical burn. (pp. 809–810)
5-2.29 Describe the emergency care for an electrical burn. (pp. 810–812)

Psychomotor

5-2.36 Demonstrate the steps in the emergency medical care of a patient with superficial burns.
5-2.37 Demonstrate the steps in the emergency medical care of a patient with partial-thickness burns.
5-2.38 Demonstrate the steps in the emergency medical care of a patient with full-thickness burns.
5-2.39 Demonstrate the steps in the emergency medical care of a patient with a chemical burn.

Total Teaching Time
180 minutes

Resources Needed
- Scored Chapter 28 Quizzes
- Adult, child, and infant mannequins

Additional Resources
Larmon/Davis, *Basic Life Support Skills*

Elling, *EMT Achieve: Basic Test Preparation*

Limmer/Mistovich/O'Keefe, *Audio Lecture & Study Guide: EMT*

Mistovich/Kuvlesky, *SUCCESS! for the EMT, Second Edition*

Some of the above and additional objectives from DOT Lesson 5-2 are addressed in Chapter 28, "Soft Tissue Injuries."

REVIEW

In the last chapter, "Soft Tissue Injuries," students learned that injuries to the soft tissues of the body are often dramatic but rarely life-threatening. However, they are serious if they involve airway or breathing compromise, uncontrolled bleeding, or shock. In general, emergency medical care emphasizes the control of bleeding, prevention of further injury, and reduction of the risk of infection. Unless injuries are life-threatening, care is usually accomplished after the initial assessment and prior to lifting and moving. Failure to recognize and provide care for soft tissue injuries may lead to severe, uncontrolled bleeding, possible additional injury including shock (hypoperfusion), or further contamination of the wound leading to infection.

Distribute the quizzes from the last class. Go over each question on the quiz and handle any concerns students may have about the answers.

INTRODUCTION TO CHAPTER 29

Chapter 29, "Burn Emergencies," is the fourth chapter in Module 5. Each year over 2 million people suffer burn injuries. Burn injuries are complicated because, contrary to what most people think, they are not just "skin deep." In addition to damaging the structure of the skin and compromising its functions, burn injuries impact most of the body's other systems in some way. For instance, burn injuries can impair the body's fluid and chemical balance and body temperature regulation, as well as its musculoskeletal, circulatory, and respiratory functions. Burn injuries may also affect a person's emotional well-being because of possible disfigurement and the need to cope with long healing processes. In order to properly assess and provide emergency care for burn patients, EMTs need to have a fundamental understanding of the kinds of burns, how burn injuries are classified, and how they affect adult, child, and infant patients.

Distribute the Chapter 29 Objectives Checklist, and give students a few minutes to look it over. Then briefly paraphrase the objectives for this lesson in your own words.

LECTURE

The following suggested lecture outline is based on the Department of Transportation's EMT-Basic National Standard Curriculum. In some places, the DOT curriculum has been rearranged or expanded upon so that it is more complete or easier for the student to understand. The page numbers in parentheses refer to pages in the textbook. The parenthetical references in dark, heavy type are to figures, tables, and scans in the textbook.

BURN EMERGENCIES

I. **The skin: Structure and function review** (pp. 798–799) (Also review information on skin in Chapter 4, "The Human Body," and Chapter 28, "Soft Tissue Injuries.")
    A. Structure (p. 798)
        1. Epidermis

Handout 29-1
Chapter 29 Objectives Checklist

●➤
Lecture Master
You may wish to display Lecture Master 29 as you present the lecture to the class.

✓
Teaching Tip
Have someone from a regional burn center visit the class and answer questions or present the burn lecture.

Slides/Videos
"Burns," *Pulse,* Jan. 2000.

           a. Outermost layer
     2. Dermis
           a. Second layer
     3. Subcutaneous
           a. Innermost layer composed of fatty connective tissue
  B. Functions (pp. 798–799)
     1. Provides barrier against infection
     2. Provides protection from bacteria or other harmful agents found in the environment
     3. Insulates and protects underlying structures and body organs from injury
     4. Aids in the regulation of body temperature
     5. Provides for transmission of sensory information
     6. Aids in elimination of some of the body's wastes
     7. Contains fluids necessary to functioning of other organs and systems

II. Airway, breathing, and circulation (p. 799)
  A. Most burn patients who die in the prehospital setting will die of an occluded airway, toxic inhalation, or other trauma and not from the burn itself. (p. 799)
  B. Control airway, breathing, and life-threatening bleeding first; then classify the burn. (p. 799)

III. Classifying burns by depth (pp. 799–800) **(Fig. 29-1, p. 799)**
  A. Superficial (first-degree burn) (pp. 799–800)
     1. Involves only the epidermis
     2. Red skin
     3. Pain at site
     4. Tenderness
  B. Partial thickness (second-degree burn) (p. 800)
     1. Involves both the epidermis and portions of the dermis **(Fig. 29-2, p. 801)**
     2. Causes intense pain as a result of nerve-end damage
     3. Further classified as:
           a. Superficial partial thickness
                (1) Thin-walled blisters
                (2) Skin is pink and moist
                (3) Skin is soft and tender to touch
           b. Deep partial thickness
                (1) Thick-walled blisters that often rupture
                (2) Skin is red and blanched white
                (3) Patient can still feel pressure at site
                (4) Poor capillary refill to burn site
  C. Full thickness (third-degree burn) (p. 800)
     1. Extends through all dermal layers and may involve subcutaneous layers, muscle, bone, or organs **(Fig. 29-3, p. 802)**
     2. Dark brown or white charring
     3. Skin dry, leathery, and may be hard to the touch
     4. Little or no pain because nerve endings have been destroyed
     5. Pain at periphery of burn
  D. Full-thickness (fourth-degree burn) (p. 800)
     1. Extends very deep and typically associated with electrical burns

IV. Determining the severity of burn injuries (pp. 800–809) **(Table 29-1, p. 804)**
  A. Classification of severity (p. 800) **(Fig. 29-4, p. 803)**

     1. Critical

     2. Moderate

     3. Minor

  B. Body surface area (BSA) percentage (pp. 803–805)

     1. Rule of nines **(Fig. 29-6, p. 805)**

       a. Adult

         (1) Head and neck—9%

         (2) Each upper extremity—9%

         (3) Chest—9%

         (4) Abdomen—9%

         (5) Upper back—9%

         (6) Lower back—9%

         (7) Anterior of each lower extremity—9%

         (8) Posterior of each lower extremity—9%

         (9) Genitalia—1%

       b. Infant (1 year of age or less)

         (1) Head and neck—18%

         (2) Chest and abdomen—18%

         (3) Entire back—18%

         (4) Each upper extremity—9%

         (5) Each lower extremity—14%

       c. Children over age 1 year—for each year beyond 1:

         (1) Add 0.5% to each leg

         (2) Subtract 1% for head

     2. Palm estimation method

       a. Compares burn area to patient's palm

       b. Palm equals approximately 1% of BSA

       c. Can be used to estimate burn area of patient at any age

  C. Burn injury location (p. 801)

     1. Face and upper airway **(Fig. 29-5, p. 804)**

       a. Potential for respiratory compromise or eye injuries

     2. Hands and feet

       a. Potential for loss of function

     3. Genitalia and groin region

       a. Potential for loss of genitourinary function and increased chances of infection

     4. Circumferential (those that encircle a body area) burns to arm or leg

       a. Potential for circulatory compromise and nerve damage caused by constriction or swelling tissues

     5. Regions with major joint function

       a. Potential loss of joint function

       b. Circumferential burns to chest; potential for respiratory compromise caused by limiting expansion of chest

  D. Age and preexisting medical conditions (pp. 801–803)

     1. Age of patient as it affects severity of burn injury

       a. Under 5 years old

       b. Over 55 years old

     2. Preexisting medical conditions that affect severity of burn injury

       a. Respiratory illness

         (1) Adversely affects severity if further respiratory compromise

       b. Cardiovascular problem

         (1) May increase complications

©2008 by Pearson Education, Inc.
Prehospital Emergency Care, 8th ed.

    c. Diabetes

       (1) May compromise patient's ability to heal

    d. Other injury in addition to burn injury

       (1) Increases life threat or potential for shock (hypoperfusion)

  3. Special considerations for infants and children (**Table 29-1, p. 804**)

    a. Large body surface in relation to mass

    b. Fluid and heat loss greater than in adults

    c. At higher risk for

       (1) Shock (hypoperfusion)

       (2) Airway difficulties

       (3) Hypothermia

    d. Consider possibility of abuse. (See assessing and reporting child abuse, Chapter 36, "Infants and Children.")

E. Causes of burns (pp. 805–806) (**Fig. 29-7, p. 806**)

  1. Flame burn—contact with an open flame

  2. Contact burn—contact with hot object

  3. Scald—contact with hot liquid

  4. Steam burn—contact with hot steam

  5. Gas burn—contact with hot gases

  6. Electrical burn—contact with electrical energy

  7. Flash burn—contact with a flaming gas or liquid

F. Assessment and care: burn injuries (pp. 806–809)

  1. Scene size-up

    a. Determine whether scene is safe to enter.

    b. Take appropriate BSI precautions.

    c. Begin assessing mechanism of injury and number of patients.

  2. Initial assessment

    a. Stop the burning process.

       (1) Within first 10 minutes of injury, if possible, use water or saline to cool burn injury for 60–120 seconds.

       (2) Remove jewelry and any smoldering clothing.

       (3) Cut around areas of clothing that adhere to patient; do not attempt to remove adhered fabric.

       (4) Do not keep the burn immersed as this may cause hypothermia.

    b. Continue the initial assessment once you have stopped the burning process.

       (1) Evaluate patient's airway, breathing, and mental status.

       (2) Look for any indications that the airway may be injured.

          (a) Sooty deposits in mouth or nose

          (b) Singed facial or nose hairs

          (c) Signs of smoke inhalation

          (d) Any facial burns

    c. Provide oxygen by nonrebreather mask at a rate of 15 liters per minute.

    d. If breathing is inadequate, provide positive-pressure ventilations with supplemental oxygen.

    e. Determine the patient's priority for transport.

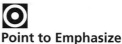

Point to Emphasize

Do not attempt to rescue persons trapped by fire unless you are trained to do so and you have the equipment and personnel required. The simple act of opening a door might cost a life.

Point to Emphasize

Body heat loss through evaporation is 70 times greater in a burn wound area.

3. Focused history and physical exam
   a. Reassess mechanism of injury and chief complaint.
   b. Alert patient with no significant mechanism of injury
      (1) Conduct focused trauma assessment.
   c. Patient has altered mental status or evidence of additional injuries
      (1) Perform rapid trauma assessment.
   d. Take and record baseline vital signs.
   e. Obtain a SAMPLE history from patient, patient's family, or bystanders.
   f. Look for signs and symptoms of burn depth and possible inhalation injuries.
      (1) Superficial burns
         (a) Pink or red, dry skin
         (b) Slight swelling
         (c) Pain and tenderness to touch
      (2) Partial-thickness burns
         (a) White to cherry red skin
         (b) Moist and mottled skin
         (c) Blistering and intense pain
         (d) Pain on peripheral edges of burns
      (3) Full-thickness burns
         (a) Dry, hard, tough, leathery skin
         (b) White waxy to dark brown or black charred (eschar) skin color
         (c) Inability to feel pain because of damaged nerve endings
      (4) Inhalation injuries
         (a) Singed nasal hairs
         (b) Facial burns
         (c) Burned flecks of carbon in sputum
         (d) Sooty or smoky smell on breath
         (e) Respiratory distress accompanied by
            (i) Restriction of chest wall movement
            (ii) Restlessness
            (iii) Chest tightness
            (iv) Stridor
            (v) Wheezing
            (vi) Difficulty swallowing
            (vii) Hoarseness
            (viii) Coughing
            (ix) Cyanosis
         (f) Presence of actual burns of the oral mucosa
4. Emergency medical care (**Fig. 29-8, p. 808**)
   a. Remove patient from source of burn and stop the burning process.
      (1) Use water or saline but do not keep burn immersed.
      (2) If burn source is semisolid or liquid, cool with water or saline but do not attempt to remove the substance.
      (3) Brush away dry chemicals before flushing with water.
   b. Remove any smoldering clothing and any jewelry.
   c. Establish and maintain an airway and breathing.
   d. Classify the severity of the burn and transport immediately if critical. (**Table 29-1, p. 804**)

On the Net
Burns and burn treatment.
www.survivingburns.org/

On the Net
Ways to help burn victims and their families.
http://theburncenter.org/services.htm

On the Net
Treatment methods for burns. http://gaga.essortment.com/burntreatmentp_relj.htm

  e. Cover the burned area with a dry, sterile dressing.

  f. Keep the patient warm, and treat other injuries as needed.

  g. Transport patient to appropriate facility.

 5. Special considerations for dressing burns

  a. Avoid using any material that sheds or leaves particles.

  b. Never apply any type of ointments, lotions, or antiseptics to burn injury.

  c. Never attempt to break or drain blisters.

  d. Burns of hands and toes

   (1) Remove all rings and jewelry that may constrict with swelling.

   (2) Separate all digits with dry, sterile dressing material. **(Fig. 29-9, p. 809)**

  e. Burns of eyes **(Fig. 29-10, p. 810)**

   (1) Do not attempt to open eyelids.

   (2) Determine if burn is thermal or chemical.

   (3) If thermal burn, apply sterile dressing to both eyes.

   (4) If chemical burn, flush with water for at least 20 minutes while en route to hospital.

   (5) Flush from medial to lateral side to avoid washing chemical into opposite eye.

 6. Detailed physical exam and ongoing assessment

  a. Perform detailed physical exam en route to burn center or hospital, if warranted and patient's condition permits, and perform ongoing assessment(s).

  b. Because swelling and closure of airway can be rapid, always consider advanced life support (ALS) response when dealing with airway complications in burn patients.

V. Chemical burns (pp. 809–810) **(Figs. 29-11 through 29-14, pp. 810–811)**

 A. Protect yourself before entering the burn scene. (p. 810)

  1. Wear gloves and eye protection.

  2. Wear impervious (fluid-proof) gown or suit in cases of large exposure.

 B. Brush off dry chemicals before flushing with water. (p. 810)

 C. Flush most chemical burns with large amounts of water. (p. 810)

 D. Continue flushing contaminated area while en route to receiving facility. (p. 810)

VI. Electrical burns (pp. 810–812) **(Fig. 29-16, p. 812)**

 A. Scene safety (pp. 810–811)

  1. Do not attempt to remove patient from the electrical source unless trained and equipped to do so.

  2. Never touch a patient still in contact with electrical source.

 B. Emergency medical care (pp. 811–812)

  1. Administer oxygen by nonrebreather mask at 15 liters per minute or positive-pressure ventilations with supplemental oxygen, if necessary.

  2. Monitor the patient closely for respiratory and cardiac arrest. (Consider need for AED.)

  3. Assess for muscle tenderness with or without twitching and any seizure activity.

  4. Always assess for an entrance and exit burn injury.

Point to Emphasize

The major problem caused by electrical shock is usually not the burn. Respiratory and cardiac arrest are real possibilities. Be prepared to provide basic cardiac life support measures with automated defibrillation.

5. Transport as soon as possible (often more severe than external indications).

VII. Summary: Assessment and care (p. 812) **(Figs. 29-17 and 29-18, pp. 813–815)**

ENRICHMENT (OPTIONAL)

The following sections contain information that is valuable as background for the EMT, but that goes substantially beyond the U.S. Department of Transportation's EMT-Basic National Standard Curriculum.

VIII. Circulatory system (pp. 814–816)
  A. Extreme fluid loss and increased stress on heart (pp. 814–816)
  B. Increased capillary permeability, decreasing fluid volume in vessels (pp. 814–816)
  C. Edema (24 hours after injury, edema may double in size from normal) (pp. 814–816)
  D. Burn shock (pp. 814–816)
    1. Extensive vascular bed damage allowing both fluid and protein in the plasma to leak into surrounding tissues
  E. Shock (hypoperfusion) caused by fluid loss (p. 816)

IX. Respiratory system (p. 816)
  A. Airway closure from swelling of face or throat (p. 816)
  B. Fluid accumulation in lungs from inhalation of superheated air (p. 816)
  C. Respiratory arrest, poisoning, or compromise from inhaling noxious fumes (p. 816)
  D. Restricted chest expansion if chest is circumferentially burned (p. 816)

 X. Renal system (kidneys) (p. 816)
  A. Decreased urinary output because of decreased blood flow (p. 816)
  B. Waste formation in blood because of cell destruction (p. 816)
  C. Blockage in kidneys possibly leading to loss of kidney function (p. 816)

XI. Nervous and musculoskeletal systems (p. 816)
  A. Loss of function to extremities or other body parts due to nerve damage (p. 816)
  B. Long-term muscle wasting and joint dysfunction due to scarring (p. 816)
  C. Fear and anxiety due to extreme pain and scarring (p. 816)

XII. Gastrointestinal system (p. 816)
  A. Normal chemical balances upset because of nausea or vomiting (p. 816)
  B. Ulcers due to long-term stress (p. 816)

CASE STUDY FOLLOW-UP

Ask a student volunteer to read the Case Study that begins on page 798 of the textbook. You may wish to use the following questions to engage the students in a discussion of the Case Study Follow-up that begins on page 817 of the textbook. Provide missing information and clarify ideas as needed.

  Q1. What is this patient's transport priority?
  A1. *High priority.*

©2008 by Pearson Education, Inc.
Prehospital Emergency Care, 8th ed.

Q2. What do you do to help stop the burning?

A2. *Pour sterile saline over the patient's burned areas and remove clothing and jewelry.*

Q3. What percentage of the patient's body surface area has experienced a full-thickness burn and how do you classify the severity of the patient's burns?

A3. *It is a full-thickness burn over 50% BSA; the patient's burns are critical.*

Q4. How does your partner protect the airway and breathing?

A4. *Through insertion of an airway adjunct and use of the bag-valve unit for positive-pressure ventilation with supplemental oxygen.*

Q5. How do you dress the burns?

A5. *By covering the patient with a sterile burn sheet and placing sterile dressings between his fingers and toes.*

IN REVIEW

Assess students' ability to apply what they have just learned by discussing the Review Questions on page 818 in the textbook.

Q1. Define and list the characteristics of superficial, partial-thickness, and full-thickness burns.

A1. *Superficial burns involve the epidermis and are characterized by pink or red, dry skin and slight swelling.*

Partial-thickness burns will cause intense pain. Superficial partial-thickness burns are characterized by thin-walled blisters and pink and moist, soft and tender skin. Deep partial-thickness burns are characterized by thick-walled blisters that often rupture, red and blanched white skin, poor capillary refill at burn site, and patient can still feel pressure at site.

Full-thickness burns are characterized by dry, hard, tough, and leathery skin that may appear white-waxy to dark brown or black and charred (eschar). These are usually painless due to nerve-end damage. (pp. 799–800)

Q2. Define the rule of nines and describe how it is used on both adult and infant or child burn injury patients.

A2. *The rule of nines is a standardized way to identify the amount of skin surface that is burned. In an adult, the head and neck, each upper extremity, the chest, the abdomen, the upper back, the lower back, the anterior of each lower extremity, and the posterior of each lower extremity each represent 9%. The genital region represents a 1% BSA. In infants the head and neck are counted as 18%, the chest and abdomen as 18%, the entire back as 18%, each upper extremity as 9%, each lower extremity as 14%. For children over the age of 1 year, add 0.5% to each leg and subtract 1% for the head for each year beyond 1. (p. 803–805)*

Q3. Using the rule of nines, name the percentage of body surface area (BSA) burned if (A) a 4-year-old child has superficial burn injuries to the front and back of both legs as well as the chest, abdomen, and back; (B) an adult has partial-thickness burn injuries to the front of one lower extremity and to the front and back of the other lower extremity.

A3. *Using the rule of nines, (A) a 4-year-old child with superficial burn injuries to the front and back of both legs as well as the chest, abdomen, and back has a BSA of 67%; (B) an adult with partial-thickness burn injuries to the front of one lower extremity and the front and back of the other has a BSA of 27%. (p. 805)*

Q4. Determine the burn severity classification for patients A and B in Question 3.

A4. *The burn severity classification for patient A is critical, for patient B is moderate. (Table 29-1, p. 804)*

Q5. Describe the basic emergency care steps for burn injuries.

A5. *Basic emergency medical care steps for a burn injury are as follows: (1) stop the burning process with water or saline; (2) remove smoldering clothing and jewelry; (3) assess the patient's airway, breathing, and mental status, administering oxygen by nonrebreather mask at 15 liters per minute or positive-pressure ventilation with supplemental oxygen as necessary; (4) classify severity of burns and transport immediately if critical; (5) cover the burned area with a dry, sterile dressing or burn sheet; (6) keep the patient warm and treat other injuries as needed; and (7) transport to a facility in accord with local protocol. (pp. 808–809)*

Q6. List the three things an EMT should not do when applying dry, sterile dressings to a burn injury patient.

A6. *The three things an EMT should not do when applying dry, sterile dressings to a burn injury patient are as follows: (1) Use material that shreds or leaves particles; (2) apply any type of ointments, lotions, or antiseptics; (3) attempt to break or drain blisters. (p. 809)*

Q7. List the emergency medical care guidelines for chemical burns.

A7. *The emergency medical care guidelines for chemical burns are as follows: Protect yourself from exposure to hazardous materials. Wear gloves and eye protection at a minimum. Brush off dry powders prior to flushing with water. Immediately begin to flush with large amounts of water. Continue flushing the contaminated area for at least 20 minutes while en route to the receiving facility, taking care not to contaminate uninjured areas when flushing. (p. 810)*

Q8. List the emergency medical care guidelines for electrical burns.

A8. *The emergency medical care guidelines for electrical burns are as follows: Do not attempt to remove the patient from the electrical source unless properly trained to do so. If the patient is still in contact with the electrical source (or you are unsure), do not touch the patient. Administer oxygen at 15 liters per minute by nonrebreather mask or positive-pressure ventilation with supplemental oxygen if indicated. Monitor the patient for cardiac arrest, be prepared to provide CPR, and have AED available, if possible. Assess the patient for muscle tenderness with or without twitching or seizure activity. Treat all soft tissue injuries associated with the burn and look for both entrance and exit injuries. Transport as soon as possible. (pp. 810–812)*

©2008 by Pearson Education, Inc.
Prehospital Emergency Care, 8th ed.

CRITICAL THINKING

Assess students' ability to respond to real-life emergency situations by discussing the Critical Thinking questions on page 818 in the textbook.

Q1. Would these burns be considered mild, moderate, or severe?

A1. *The burns to the patient's eyes should be considered severe. Any chemical burn to the eyes could lead to loss of sight.*

Q2. What is your rationalization for the above answer?

A2. *Due to the potential for serious and continued damage to the patient's eyes, which could result in a total loss of function, these should be treated as severe burns.*

Q3. How is the eye injuries best managed while en route to the hospital?

A3. *Chemical burns to the eyes should be treated by continued flushing with water during transport.*

Q4. What is the recommended process for flushing chemical eye injuries before arriving at the hospital?

A4. *The affected eye(s) should be flushed with water in a medial to lateral direction for at least 20 minutes during transport to the hospital. Remove any contacts and lift the eyelids to ensure that the chemical is flushed from under the lids.*

Q5. If there was a community hospital within 2 minutes of the university, and a regional burn/trauma center within 15 minutes of the university, which facility should the EMT elect to transport the patient to?

A5. *Local protocols or on-line medical direction should be consulted to determine the appropriate facility for this situation.*

SKILLS PRACTICE

Before class, prepare as many adult, infant, and child mannequins as you can obtain with makeup to simulate different types of burns over different amounts of body surface area.

Divide the class into small groups. Have half the groups estimate BSA burned on each mannequin, using the rule of nines and the other half using the palmar method. Have the groups record their results. When all groups are done, have them compare the results and discuss their findings.

Alternatively, project a drawing of the human body using an overhead projector. Use a marker to color body areas to represent different degrees of burns. Have students use the rule of nines to calculate the total BSA burned.

ASSIGNMENTS

Assign students to read Chapter 30, "Musculoskeletal Injuries," before the next class. Also ask them to complete Chapter 29 of the Workbook.

Reading/Reference
Textbook, pp. 819–846

Workbook
Chapter 29 Activities

Chapter Quiz
Handout 29-2

TestGen
Chapter 29 Test

Online Test Preparation
Send your students to
http://www.prenhall.com/
EMTAchieve

Handouts 29-3 to 29-6
Reinforcement Activities

**Brady Skills Series
EMT-B Videos/CD**
Visual Reinforcement

**PowerPoint
Presentation**
Chapter 29

Student CD
Chapter 29

Companion Website
http://www.prenhall.com/
mistovich

EVALUATION

Chapter Quiz Distribute copies of the Chapter Quiz provided in Handout 29-2 to evaluate student understanding of this chapter. Remind students not to refer to their textbooks or notes while taking the quiz.

Test Manager You may wish to create a custom-tailored test using Prentice Hall *TestGen for Prehospital Emergency Care, Eighth Edition* to evaluate student understanding of this chapter.

Online Test Preparation (for students and instructors) Additional test preparation is available through *EMT Achieve: Basic Test Preparation* at http://www.prenhall.com/EMTAchieve. Instructors can also monitor student mastery online.

REINFORCEMENT

Handouts If classroom discussions or performance on the quiz indicates that some students have not fully mastered the chapter content, you may wish to assign some or all of the Reinforcement Handouts for this chapter.

TECH EXTRAS

Brady Skills Series EMT-B Videos/CD Have your students watch the skills come to life on either VHS or CD-ROM.

PowerPoint Presentation (for instructors) The PowerPoint material developed for this chapter offers useful reinforcement of chapter content.

Student CD A wide variety of material on this CD-ROM will reinforce and also expand student knowledge and skills.

Companion Website (for students) Additional review quizzes and links to EMS resources will contribute to further reinforcement of this chapter. Please visit http://www.prenhall.com/mistovich.

Objectives Checklist

Cognitive		Date Mastered
5-2.1	State the major functions of the skin.	
5-2.2	List the layers of the skin.	
5-2.11	List the classifications of burns.	
5-2.12	Define superficial burn.	
5-2.13	List the characteristics of a superficial burn.	
5-2.14	Define partial-thickness burn.	
5-2.15	List the characteristics of a partial-thickness burn.	
5-2.16	Define full-thickness burn.	
5-2.17	List the characteristics of a full-thickness burn.	
5-2.18	Describe the emergency medical care of a patient with a superficial burn.	
5-2.19	Describe the emergency medical care of a patient with a partial-thickness burn.	
5-2.20	Describe the emergency medical care of a patient with a full-thickness burn.	
5-2.24	Establish the relationship between airway management and the patient with chest injury, burns, and blunt and penetrating injuries.	
5-2.28	Describe the emergency care for a chemical burn.	
5-2.29	Describe the emergency care for an electrical burn.	

Psychomotor		Date Mastered
5-2.36	Demonstrate the steps in the emergency medical care of a patient with superficial burns.	
5-2.37	Demonstrate the steps in the emergency medical care of a patient with partial-thickness burns.	
5-2.38	Demonstrate the steps in the emergency medical care of a patient with full-thickness burns.	
5-2.39	Demonstrate the steps in the emergency medical care of a patient with a chemical burn.	

OBJECTIVES

EVALUATION

CHAPTER 29 QUIZ

Write the letter of the best answer in the space provided.

_____ 1. In estimating BSA of a burn, each upper extremity in an adult represents what percentage of the total body area?
   A. 7%   **C.** 18%
   B. 27%   **D.** 9%

_____ 2. The three layers of the skin include the
   A. outer dermis, dermis, and subcutaneous tissue.
   B. endodermis, dermis, and muscle tissue.
   C. mid-dermis, dermis, and subcutaneous tissue.
   D. epidermis, dermis, and subcutaneous tissue.

_____ 3. The innermost layer of the skin is the
   A. endodermis.   **C.** epidermis.
   B. subcutaneous layer.   **D.** dermis.

_____ 4. An example of a superficial burn would be a(n)
   A. severe scalding.   **C.** thermal flame burn.
   B. eschar.   **D.** sunburn.

_____ 5. One method that the EMT can use to estimate the body surface area damaged by a burn is the
   A. rule of nines.   **C.** rule of sixes.
   B. BSC rule.   **D.** plantar system.

_____ 6. In a child under age 5, any partial-thickness burn involving between 10 and 20% of BSA should be considered
   A. minor.   **C.** critical.
   B. moderate.   **D.** superficial.

_____ 7. All of the following are important factors to consider in determining burn severity *except*
   A. percentage of body surface area involved.
   B. location of the burn.
   C. patient age and preexisting medical conditions.
   D. ambient environmental temperature.

_____ 8. A burn that encircles a body area such as the chest, an arm, or a leg is called
   A. full thickness.   **C.** immersional.
   B. circumferential.   **D.** severe.

_____ 9. When determining the BSA involved in a burn, the EMT should remember that the palm of the patient's hand is equal to about what percentage of total body area?
   A. 2%   **C.** 1%
   B. 3%   **D.** ½%

©2008 by Pearson Education, Inc.
Prehospital Emergency Care, 8th ed.

_____ **10.** Burns are classified according to
    A. location of the injury.   **C.** type of heat involved.
    B. depth of the injury.   **D.** amount of heat involved.

_____ **11.** The most important treatment for a patient who has sustained a chemical burn to the eyes is
    A. rapid application of dry, sterile dressings to both eyes.
    B. application of gauze pads soaked with saline.
    C. copious irrigation with water.
    D. provision of oxygen via nonrebreather mask.

_____ **12.** A burn in which the epidermis is burned through and the dermis is damaged is known as a _____ burn.
    A. superficial   **C.** full-thickness
    B. partial-thickness   **D.** third-degree

_____ **13.** Absence of pain in a patient with a severe burn is most commonly associated with a _____ burn.
    A. first-degree   **C.** third-degree
    B. second-degree   **D.** superficial

_____ **14.** In managing a burn correctly, an EMT may take all of the following steps *except*
    A. apply dry, sterile dressings.
    B. apply ointments or sprays.
    C. keep the patient warm.
    D. keep the burn site clean.

_____ **15.** A partial-thickness (second-degree) burn will appear
    A. white to cherry red.   **C.** charred.
    B. dark brown or black.   **D.** pink.

_____ **16.** When the EMT is dealing with the victim of an electrical burn, the primary concern should be
    A. patient care.   **C.** rapid AED use.
    B. personal safety.   **D.** bystander history.

_____ **17.** When administering emergency medical care to a burn patient, clothing that has adhered to a burned area should be
    A. covered with an antiseptic ointment.
    B. covered with a dry, sterile dressing.
    C. carefully removed from the burned skin.
    D. left in place after cutting around the adhered area.

_____ **18.** When dealing with chemical burns, the EMT should remember that dry chemicals should be
    A. brushed away before irrigating.
    B. irrigated without delay.
    C. removed with a damp sterile gauze pad.
    D. irrigated with neutralizing vinegar.

_____**19.** In cases of chemical burns to the eyes, the EMT should flood the eyes with

   A. vinegar.

   B. baking soda and water.

   C. water.

   D. hydrogen peroxide solution.

_____**20.** The most serious problem usually associated with electrical shocks is

   A. internal bleeding.

   B. hypertension.

   C. hypothermia.

   D. respiratory and/or cardiac arrest.

IN THE FIELD

Read the following real-life situation. Then answer the questions that follow.

You receive a call to the side of a county highway where it is reported that a utility worker is "on fire and still up in his bucket." While responding, you ask your dispatcher to arrange for aerial rescue apparatus to assist you.

    Upon arrival at the scene, you notice a charred utility bucket still in the air near several electrical lines. The utility worker, while still on fire, has jumped from the bucket and landed on the roadside.

1. What are your immediate considerations at this scene?

2. Utility officials are on the scene and assure you that the power is off. The fire has been extinguished, and you approach the patient. He is a male in his early 30s, conscious, and oriented to person, place, and time. He is complaining of severe pain all over his body. His facial hair has been singed off and his face is cherry red. He is able to control his own airway. You apply high-flow oxygen via nonrebreather mask. What types of injuries do you suspect that the patient has suffered? What was the mechanism of injury?

3. What other emergency care steps would you provide for this patient?

CHAPTER 29 REVIEW

Write the word or words that best complete each sentence in the space provided.

1. Burns are classified according to the _____ of the injury.

2. The three layers of the skin are the _____, _____, and _____ _____.

3. Most burn patients who die in the prehospital setting will die from a(n)

   _____ _____, _____

   _____, or other _____.

4. Examples of superficial burns include _____ or a minor

   _____ injury.

5. The tough and leathery dead soft tissue formed in a full-thickness burn injury is called

   _____.

6. A superficial burn is an injury that involves only the _____.

7. A partial-thickness burn is also called a(n) _____-degree burn.

8. When calculating BSA, the EMT should remember that the genital region represents

   _____ % of the total BSA.

9. Burn injuries need to be _____ _____ within

   approximately the first 10 minutes of injury.

10. Once the EMT has determined that the scene of a burn emergency is safe to enter, he or she should

    immediately take _____ _____.

11. _____ burns can cause severe damage not only to soft tissues, but to the

    body as a whole.

12. A(n) _____ _____ burn, or third-degree burn, is

    a burn in which all layers of the skin are damaged.

13. An alternative to the rule of nines for estimating the BSA of a burn involves using a comparison of

    the burned area to the patient's _____.

14. All burns normally classified as moderate should be reclassified as _____ in

    a person younger than 5 or older than 55 years of age.

15. If dry lime is the burn agent, do not irrigate the burn with _____ until it

    has been _____ _____ the patient.

BURN EMERGENCIES: LISTING

1. List the signs and symptoms of partial-thickness burns.

2. List the signs and symptoms of full-thickness burns.

3. List the four most important factors in determining burn severity.

4. List three considerations when treating burns of the eye.

REINFORCEMENT

THE RULE OF NINES

The rule of nines is used to estimate the extent of the burn area on a patient's body. On the figures below, write in the percentage that each body area represents on the lines provided.

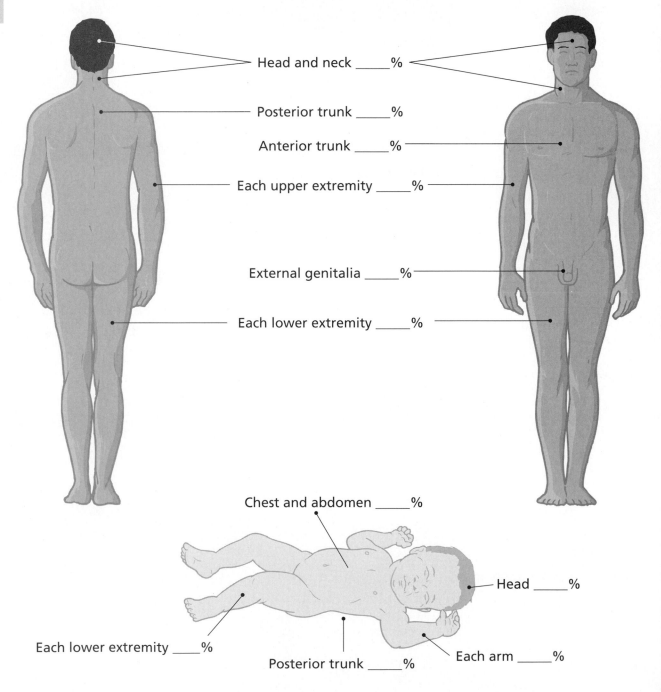

Head and neck _____%

Posterior trunk _____%

Anterior trunk _____%

Each upper extremity _____%

External genitalia _____%

Each lower extremity _____%

Chest and abdomen _____%

Head _____%

Each lower extremity _____%

Posterior trunk _____%

Each arm _____%

LECTURE MASTER 29

Burn Emergencies

Review of the Skin's Structure and Function

Burns and the ABCs

Classifying Burns by Depth

Superficial

Partial Thickness

Full Thickness

Determining Severity of Burn Injuries

Body Surface Area

Burn Location

Patient's Age

Preexisting Medical Conditions

Assessment and Care

Special Considerations

Hands and Toes

Eyes

Chemical Burns

Electrical Burns

Burns and Body Systems

Circulatory

Respiratory

Renal (Kidneys)

Nervous and Musculoskeletal

Gastrointestinal

HANDOUT 29-2: Chapter 29 Quiz

1. D	**6.** B	**11.** C	**16.** B
2. D	**7.** D	**12.** B	**17.** D
3. B	**8.** B	**13.** C	**18.** A
4. D	**9.** C	**14.** B	**19.** C
5. A	**10.** B	**15.** A	**20.** D

HANDOUT 29-3: In the Field

1. Personal/EMS crew safety, scene safety, patient safety

2. Thermal and electrical burns should be considered as well as multiple injuries related to the trauma of the fall. The mechanism of injuries to consider are primarily burns and then injuries associated with a fall from over 20 feet.

3. Remove any smoldering clothing and any jewelry. Establish and maintain cervical spine immobilization. Continue to monitor the airway and provide adequate ventilation with oxygen. Classify the severity of the burn. Arrange for rapid advanced life support transport to a burn center. Cover the burned areas with dry, sterile dressings. Maintain the patient's body temperature and treat any other injuries.

HANDOUT 29-4: Chapter 29 Review

1. depth
2. epidermis, dermis, subcutaneous layers
3. occluded airway, toxic inhalation, trauma
4. sunburn, scald
5. eschar
6. epidermis
7. second
8. 1
9. cooled down
10. BSI precautions
11. Electrical
12. full-thickness
13. palm
14. critical
15. water, brushed off

HANDOUT 29-5: Burn Emergencies: Listing

1. Blisters, intense pain, white to cherry red skin, moist and mottled skin, pain on peripheral edges of burn

2. Dry, hard, tough, leathery skin that appears white-waxy to dark brown or black and charred; little or no pain

3. Percentage of BSA involved; location of burn; patient's age; preexisting medical conditions

4. Do not attempt to open eyelids if they are burned. If dealing with a thermal burn, apply a dry, sterile dressing to both eyes in order to prevent simultaneous movement of both eyes. Chemical burns should be flushed with water for at least 20 minutes while en route to the hospital. Flush the eye from medial to lateral to avoid washing the chemical into the other eye.

HANDOUT 29-6: The Rule of Nines

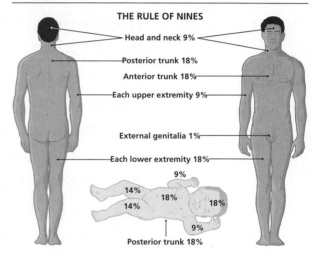

THE RULE OF NINES

Head and neck 9%
Posterior trunk 18%
Anterior trunk 18%
Each upper extremity 9%
External genitalia 1%
Each lower extremity 18%

9%
14%
18%
14%
18%
9%
Posterior trunk 18%

This chapter covers Lesson 5-3 and portions of Lesson 5-5 of the U.S. Department of Transportation's EMT-Basic National Standard Curriculum.

OBJECTIVES

Numbered objectives are from the U.S. Department of Transportation EMT-Basic National Standard Curriculum. Asterisked objectives, if any, pertain to material that is supplemental to the DOT curriculum. Page numbers in parentheses refer to pages in the textbook.

Cognitive

5-3.1 Describe the function of the muscular system. (pp. 820–821)
5-3.2 Describe the function of the skeletal system. (p. 821)
5-3.3 List the major bones or bone groupings of the spinal column; the thorax; the upper extremities; the lower extremities. (p. 821)
5-3.4 Differentiate between an open and a closed painful, swollen, deformed extremity. (p. 824)
5-3.5 State the reasons for splinting. (pp. 823, 825, 828)
5-3.6 List the general rules of splinting. (pp. 830–831)
5-3.7 List the complications of splinting. (pp. 833–834)
5-3.8 List the emergency medical care for a patient with a painful, swollen, deformed extremity. (pp. 825, 826, 834–844)

Affective

5-3.9 Explain the rationale for splinting at the scene versus load and go. (pp. 824, 825, 828)
5-3.10 Explain the rationale for immobilization of the painful, swollen, deformed extremity. (p. 828)

Psychomotor

5-3.11 Demonstrate the emergency medical care of a patient with a painful, swollen, deformed extremity.
5-3.12 Demonstrate completing a prehospital care report for patients with musculoskeletal injuries.

REVIEW

In the last chapter, "Burn Emergencies," students learned that burn injuries are complicated because, contrary to what most people think, they are not just "skin deep." In addition to damaging the structure of the skin and compromising its functions, burn injuries impact most of the body's other

Total Teaching Time

240 minutes (Note: Due to the time needed to teach this lesson, you may wish to teach it in two different class periods. The first class period can conclude with the lecture section, and the second class period can begin with the skills demonstration and practice section.)

Resources Needed

- Scored Chapter 29 Quizzes

- EMTs to serve as teaching assistants, one per practice station.

- Volunteers to serve as "patients"

- Ample supplies of the following for practice stations:
  - Triangular bandages
  - Padding materials
  - Soft splints
  - Padded splints
  - Roller bandages
  - Bandaging tape
  - Tongue depressors
  - Pillows
  - Air splints
  - Traction splints used in your area

- Pneumatic antishock garment used in your area (may be omitted if not used in your area)

Additional Resources

Larmon/Davis, *Basic Life Support Skills*

Elling, *EMT Achieve: Basic Test Preparation*

Limmer/Mistovich/O'Keefe, *Audio Lecture & Study Guide: EMT*

Mistovich/Kuvlesky, *SUCCESS! for the EMT, Second Edition*

Handout 30-1
Chapter 30 Objectives Checklist

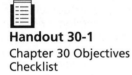

Lecture Master
You may wish to display Lecture Master 30 when presenting the lecture to the class.

On the Net
Musculoskeletal Atlas. http://eduserv.hscer.washington.edu/hubio553/atlas/content.html

Slides/Videos
Brady Skill Series: EMT-B, "Long Bone Splinting" "Joint Splinting" "Hare Traction Splint" "Sager Traction Splint" "Sling and Swathe"

systems in some way. For instance, burn injuries can impair the body's fluid, chemical balance, and body temperature regulation, as well as its musculoskeletal, circulatory, and respiratory functions. Burn injuries may also affect a person's emotional well-being because of possible disfigurement and the need to cope with long healing processes. In order to properly assess and provide emergency care for burn patients, EMTs need to have a fundamental understanding of the kinds of burns, how burn injuries are classified, and how they affect adult, child, and infant patients.

Distribute the quizzes from the last class. Go over each question on the quiz and handle any concerns students may have about the answers.

INTRODUCTION TO CHAPTER 30

Chapter 30, "Musculoskeletal Injuries," is the fifth chapter in Module 5. Injuries to muscles, joints, and bones are some of the most common emergencies you will encounter in the field. These injuries can range from the simple and non-life-threatening (such as a broken finger or sprained ankle) to the critical and life-threatening (such as a fracture of the femur or spine). Regardless of whether the injury is mild or severe, your ability to provide emergency care efficiently and quickly may prevent further painful and damaging injury and may even keep the patient from suffering permanent disability or death.

Distribute the Chapter 30 Objectives Checklist, and give students a few minutes to look it over. Then briefly paraphrase the objectives for this lesson in your own words.

LECTURE

The following suggested lecture outline is based on the Department of Transportation's EMT-Basic National Standard Curriculum. In some places, the DOT curriculum has been rearranged or expanded upon so that it is more complete or easier for the student to understand. The page numbers in parentheses refer to pages in the textbook. The parenthetical references in dark, heavy type are to figures, tables, and scans in the textbook.

  I. Musculoskeletal system review (pp. 820–821) (Students may also review material on the musculoskeletal system in Chapter 4, "The Human Body.")

    A. Functions of the musculoskeletal system (p. 820)

      1. To give the body shape

      2. To protect the internal organs

      3. To provide for movement

    B. Muscles (pp. 820–821)

      1. Voluntary (skeletal)

      2. Involuntary (smooth)

      3. Cardiac

      4. Muscle injury

        a. Overexertion can cause broken fibers.

        b. Trauma can cause bruises, crushing, cuts, tearing, or other injuries, even though skin not broken.

        c. All injured muscles tend to swell and become tender, painful, or weak.

    C. Tendons and ligaments (p. 821) (**Fig. 30-1, p. 821**)

    D. Skeletal system (p. 821) (**Fig. 30-2, p. 821**)

      1. Basic components

a. Skull
b. Spinal column
c. Thorax
d. Pelvis
e. Lower extremities
f. Upper extremities
2. Joints
a. Places where bones meet

II. Injuries to bones and joints (pp. 821–828)
  A. Kinds of musculoskeletal injuries (pp. 821–822)
    1. Fracture **(Fig. 30-3, p. 822)**
      a. Broken bone
    2. Strain
      a. Injury to muscle or muscle tendon possibly by being overextended or stretched
    3. Sprain
      a. Injury to a joint or possible damage to or tearing of ligaments
    4. Dislocation
      a. Displacement of a bone from its normal position in a joint **(Fig. 30-4, p. 822)**
  B. Mechanism of injury (pp. 822–823) **(Fig. 30-5, p. 823)**
    1. Direct force
      a. Occurs at point of impact
    2. Indirect force
      a. Force impacts on one end of limb, causing injury some distance away from point of impact
    3. Twisting force
      a. One part of extremity remains stationary while rest twists
  C. Assessment and care: bone or joint injuries (pp. 823–826)
    1. Scene size-up and initial assessment
      a. Take appropriate BSI precautions.
      b. Consider the mechanism of injury.
      c. Ask questions of bystanders, family, and patient.
      d. Form general impression of patient's injury and determine priority of care.
      e. Check for obvious signs of severe hemorrhage.
      f. Look for signs and symptoms of shock; treat for shock as appropriate.
      g. Look for pulselessness and cyanosis distal to injured extremity; if found, transport immediately following focused history and physical exam.
      h. If patient has life-threatening injury not directly related to extremity injury, transport immediately and immobilize extremity en route.
    2. Focused history and physical exam
      a. Unresponsive patient or multiple injuries or significant mechanism of injury
        (1) Begin focused history and physical exam with a rapid trauma assessment.
      b. Responsive patient and insignificant mechanism of injury
        (1) Conduct focused physical exam.
      c. Check for DCAP-BTLS at injury site. **(Fig. 30-6, p. 824)**
      d. Check for capillary refill time.

Teaching Tip
Use a skeleton to review the major bones that are often injured from various traumatic MOIs.

On the Net
Radiology of fractures. http://www.gentili.net/fracturemain.asp

Point of Interest
While most fractures are not life-threatening, bones are living tissue and bleed. A simple closed tibia–fibula fracture typically causes 1 pint (500 cc) of blood loss. Femur fractures typically cause a 2-pint (1,000 cc) blood loss, and pelvic fractures cause a 3- to 4-pint (1,500–2,000 cc) blood loss.

Teaching Tip
To assess compromise to an extremity when musculoskeletal injury is suspected, use the five p's: *pain* (of the distal extremity), *pallor* (pale skin or poor capillary refill), *paresthesia* (sensation of "pins and needles"), *pulses* (diminished or absent in injured extremity), and *paralysis* (inability to move).

  e. Assess baseline vitals.

  f. Obtain SAMPLE history from patient.

3. Types of bone and joint injuries (**Figs. 30-7, 30-8, and 30-9, pp. 825–826**)

 a. Open

  (1) An open wound is associated with the fracture; bone may or may not protrude through wound

 b. Closed

  (1) Overlying skin is intact

4. Signs and symptoms of bone and joint injuries (**Fig. 30-10, p. 826**)

 a. Deformity or angulation

 b. Pain and tenderness

 c. Grating, or crepitus (sound or feeling of broken bone fragments grinding against each other)

 d. Swelling

 e. Disfigurement

 f. Severe weakness and loss of function

 g. Bruising (discoloration)

 h. Exposed bone ends

 i. Joint locked into position

5. Emergency medical care

 a. Take proper BSI precautions before approaching patient.

 b. Administer oxygen if needed.

 c. Maintain in-line spinal stabilization if spinal injury is suspected.

 d. Splint bone and joint injuries, checking distal pulses, motor function, and sensation both before and after splinting.

 e. Apply cold packs to the painful, swollen, or deformed extremity.

 f. Elevate the extremity (if spinal injury is not suspected) and keep it elevated during transport.

 g. Transport.

6. Detailed physical exam and ongoing assessment

 a. Conduct detailed physical exam during transport.

 b. Perform ongoing assessment, including recheck of patient's vital signs and interventions.

D. Summary: assessment and care (pp. 826–828) (**Figs. 30-11 and 30-12, pp. 827–829**)

III. Basics of splinting (pp. 828–844)

A. Splint (p. 828)

 1. Any device used to immobilize a body part

B. Reasons for splinting (p. 828)

 1. To reduce chance for further injury by preventing movement of bone fragments, bone ends, or dislocated joints.

 2. To reduce pain and minimize the following complications:

  a. Damage to muscles, nerves, or blood vessels caused by movement of bone fragments or bone ends

  b. Conversion of a closed fracture to an open fracture

  c. Restriction of blood flow due to bone ends or dislocations compressing blood vessels

  d. Excessive bleeding due to tissue damage caused by bone ends

Point to Emphasize

Stress to students that they should not allow the blood and gore associated with open fractures to distract them from the ABCs. Manage the patient based on vital signs and assessment. Musculoskeletal injuries are rarely life-threatening.

On the Net

Causes of and treatments for fractures. http://orthopedics.about.com/blfracture.htm

  e. Increased pain associated with movement of bone ends or dislocated bones

  f. Paralysis of extremities due to a damaged spine

C. General rules of splinting (pp. 830–831) **(Fig. 30-13, pp. 830–831)**

  1. Both before and after applying splint, assess pulse, motor, and sensation distal to injury.

  2. Immobilize joints both above and below an injury to a long bone.

  3. Immobilize the bones above and below an injury to a joint.

  4. Remove or cut away clothing and remove all jewelry around injury site.

  5. Cover open wounds with sterile dressings.

  6. Align extremity with gentle manual traction before splinting if there is a severe deformity, absence of distal pulses, or cyanosis.

  7. Never intentionally replace protruding bones or push them back beneath the skin.

  8. Pad each splint to prevent discomfort and unnecessary pressure.

  9. Apply the splint before moving the patient; do not release manual traction until after splint is applied.

  10. When in doubt, splint the injury.

  11. If patient shows signs of shock (hypoperfusion), align patient in normal anatomical position, treat for shock, and transport immediately (unless femur or pelvis fracture is suspected, then splint as a bleeding control measure).

D. Splinting equipment (pp. 831–833) **(Fig. 30-14, p. 832)**

  1. Rigid splints

  2. Traction splints **(Fig. 30-15, p. 832)**

  3. Vacuum splints **(Fig. 30-16, p. 833)**

  4. Pressure splints

    a. Air splint

    b. Pneumatic antishock garment (PASG)

  5. Improvised splints **(Fig. 30-17, p. 834)**

  6. Sling and swathe

E. Hazards of improper splinting (pp. 833–834)

  1. Compression of nerves, tissues, and blood vessels under splint aggravating existing injury or causing new injury

  2. Delay in transport of a patient with life-threatening injury

  3. Reduction of distal circulation, compromising the viability of extremity

  4. Aggravation of bone or joint injury

  5. Causing or aggravating tissue, nerve, vessel, or muscle damage from excessive bone or joint movement

F. Splinting long bone injuries (p. 834) **(Fig. 30-18, p. 835)**

  1. Look for signs and symptoms of long bone injury.

    a. Exposed bone ends

    b. Joints locked into position

    c. Paresthesia (prickling or tingling sensation) indicating some loss of sensation

    d. Paralysis

    e. Pallor of injury site

  2. Apply manual stabilization to injured extremity

  3. Assess the distal pulse and monitor for pulse, motor, and sensory function below the injury site.

Point to Emphasize

Whether immobilizing a finger or an entire body, the principles are the same—perform distal PMS checks on all extremities before and after splinting.

4. Align with gentle manual traction if deformity is severe, distal pulses are absent, or distal extremity is cyanotic.
5. Measure splint for proper length.
6. Secure the entire injured extremity, mobilizing a hand or foot in the position of function.
7. Reassess pulse, motor, and sensory function.

G. Splinting joint injuries (p. 834) **(Fig. 30-19, p. 836)**
  1. Manually stabilize joint in position found.
  2. Assess pulse, motor, and sensory function below the injury site.
  3. Look for paresthesia or paralysis.
  4. Align joint with gentle traction if distal extremity is cyanotic or lacks pulses.
  5. Apply the splint to immobilize the bone above and below the joint.
  6. Reassess distal pulses and motor and sensory function after splint is applied.
  7. Transport.

H. Traction splinting (pp. 834–836)
  1. Indicated for femur fracture and some fractures below the knee
  2. Contraindicated (do not use) if
    a. Injury is within 1 or 2 inches of knee or ankle
    b. Knee itself has been injured
    c. Hip has been injured
    d. Pelvis has been injured
    e. There is partial amputation or avulsion with bone separation; distal limb is connected only by marginal tissue. (Traction would risk separation.)
  3. Applying a bipolar traction splint **(Fig. 30-20, pp. 838–839)**
  4. Applying a unipolar traction splint **(Fig. 30-21, p. 840)**

I. Splinting specific injuries (pp. 836–837) **(Fig. 30-22 and 30-23, pp. 841–844)**
  1. Pelvic fracture
    a. PASG
    b. Pelvic wrap

J. Compartment syndrome (p. 837)
  1. Overview of condition
  2. Signs and symptoms
  3. Emergency care

CASE STUDY FOLLOW-UP

Ask a student volunteer to read the Case Study that begins on page 820 in the textbook. You may wish to use the following questions to engage the students in a discussion of the Case Study Follow-up that begins on page 845 in the textbook. Provide missing information and clarify ideas as needed.

Q1. Describe the mechanism of injury.

A1. *The patient was "tackled pretty hard" by two or three other football players.*

Q2. Where does Tom complain of pain?

A2. *His right leg and right arm.*

Q3. Describe the appearance of Tom's arm and leg.

A3. *Tom's right arm is tender and swollen. Approximately 6 inches below Tom's right knee, bone ends are protruding through a fracture site.*

Q4. How do you splint Tom's arm and leg?

A4. *By applying a vacuum splint to Tom's right arm; by covering the protruding bone ends below the knee with a trauma pad and applying padded board splints to Tom's right leg.*

Q5. Why do you take spinal precautions?

A5. *Because of the mechanism of injury.*

IN REVIEW

Assess students' ability to apply what they have just learned by discussing the Review Questions on page 846 in the textbook.

Q1. List three functions of the musculoskeletal system.

A1. *Three functions of the musculoskeletal system are the following: to give the body shape, to protect the internal organs, and to provide for movement. (p. 820)*

Q2. Explain the difference between an open and a closed bone injury.

A2. *In a closed bone injury the skin over the fracture site is intact. In an open bone injury an open wound is associated with the fracture. (p. 824)*

Q3. List the indications that would lead you to suspect a bone or joint injury.

A3. *A mechanism of injury consistent with a bone or joint injury; deformity or angulation, pain and tenderness, crepitus, swelling, disfigurement, severe weakness and loss of function, bruising, exposed bone ends, joint locked in position. (pp. 824–825)*

Q4. Explain the reasons for splinting a bone or joint injury.

A4. *The reasons for splinting a bone or joint injury are the following: First, splinting prevents movement of any bone fragments, bone ends, or dislocated joints, reducing the chance for further injury. Second, splints usually reduce pain and minimize complications from bone and joint injuries. (p. 828)*

Q5. List the emergency medical care steps for treating a bone or joint injury.

A5. *The emergency medical care steps for treating a bone or joint injury are the following: Practice body substance isolation, administer oxygen if needed, maintain spinal stabilization if spine injury is suspected, splint bone and joint injuries, apply cold packs, elevate the extremity if spinal injury is not suspected, and transport. Assess pulse, motor, and sensory function distal to the injury site both before and after splinting. (pp. 825–826)*

Q6. Outline the general rules for splinting a bone or joint injury.

A6. *The general rules for splinting a bone or joint injury are the following: Assess distal pulse, motor function, and sensation both before and after splinting. Immobilize the joints both above and below a long bone injury or the bones above and below a joint injury. Remove or cut away clothing and jewelry. Cover all wounds, including open fractures, with* *a sterile dressing. If there is a severe deformity or the distal extremity is cyanotic or lacks pulses, align with gentle traction before splinting. Do not align if pain, resistance, or crepitus increase. Generally do not align a wrist, an elbow, a knee, or a shoulder. Never try to push bone ends back underneath the skin. Pad splints. Maintain manual traction until after the splint is applied. When in doubt, splint the injury. If the patient shows signs of shock, transport at once without splinting, unless you suspect a femur or pelvis fracture; in those cases, splinting should be conducted as a bleeding control measure. (pp. 830–831)*

Q7. Describe the complications that can arise from improper splinting of a bone or joint.

A7. *Complications that can arise from improper splinting of a bone or joint are as follows: nerve tissue and blood vessel compression under the splint; transport delay in patients with life-threatening conditions; reduction of distal circulation; possible aggravation of bone or joint injuries; damage to tissues, nerves, blood vessels, or muscles due to excessive movement. (pp. 833–834)*

Q8. List contraindications for (reasons for not using) a traction splint on a suspected femur fracture.

A8. *Contraindications for using a traction splint are as follows: an injury within 2 inches of the knee or ankle, an injury of the knee itself, hip or pelvic injury, and partial amputation or avulsion with bone separation. (p. 836)*

CRITICAL THINKING

Assess students' ability to respond to real-life emergency situations by discussing the Critical Thinking questions on page 846 in the textbook.

Q1. What initial emergency care would you provide to the patient?

A1. *An EMT should immediately establish and maintain manual in-line spinal stabilization. The patient's airway is open and the respirations are adequate; thus, apply a nonrebreather mask at 15 lpm.*

Q2. What specific injuries do you suspect?

A2. *Based on the assessment finding and the patient complaints, it is likely this patient has a fractured pelvis due to the instability and pain, and a possible fractured right tibia and fibula evident by the deformity.*

Q3. How would you manage the possible fractures?

A3. *The possible pelvic fracture should be quickly stabilized with a pelvic wrap or the pneumatic antishock garment (PASG). Due to the apparent onset of shock and the need for rapid transport, the lower leg injury should be initially immobilized with the long spine board. If there is an opportunity during transport, the lower leg should be splinted with a vacuum, board, pneumatic, or other acceptable rigid splint.*

Q4. What complications would occur with the suspected fractures?

A4. *Pelvic fractures are often associated with severe bleeding. The pelvis will often fracture in more than one place. The pelvic bone itself may bleed profusely along with lacerated or disrupted vessels in close proximity to the fractured pelvic bone. The lower leg fracture could result in either* *reduced distal circulation, and muscle, vessel, nerve, and other tissue damage from the fractured bone ends.*

ROLE PLAY

Before class, set up the practice stations listed below. Be sure each station has adequate supplies available to manage the injury it is demonstrating. If space is limited, you may wish to combine some of the stations. Arrange to have EMTs on hand to serve as teaching assistants at the stations as well as volunteers who will serve as "patients." Write the following on a chalkboard, flipchart, or overhead transparency:

1. Sling and swath
2. Humerus—soft splinting
3. Arm and elbow fractures and dislocations
4. Injuries to forearm, wrist, and hand
5. Air-inflated splints
6. Traction splints
7. Knee injuries, knee-bent, two-splint method
8. Ankle hitch
9. Knee injuries, knee-straight, single-splint method
10. Knee injuries, knee-straight, two-splint method
11. Leg injuries, two-splint method
12. Leg injuries, single-splint method
13. Antishock garment

Have students pair up. If there are an odd number of students, create a team of three.

Tell students that each team is to visit the 13 listed demonstration and practice stations. At each station they will find a "patient" and an EMT who will demonstrate and help each of them practice the station's splinting skill.

Tell students the location of each demonstration and practice station. Direct each pair to its first practice station. Visit each station to monitor progress of practice. Provide help to the teaching assistants, if necessary. Make sure that each team visits each practice station. When pairs have completed all stations, make sure that they return to the main classroom.

ASSIGNMENTS

Assign students to read Chapter 31, "Injuries to the Head," before the next class. Also ask them to complete Chapter 30 of the Workbook.

EVALUATION

Chapter Quiz Distribute copies of the Chapter Quiz provided in Handout 30-2 to evaluate student understanding of this chapter. Remind students not to refer to their textbooks or notes while taking the quiz.

Test Manager You may wish to create a custom-tailored test using Prentice Hall *TestGen for Prehospital Emergency Care, Eighth Edition* to evaluate student understanding of this chapter.

Reading/Reference
Textbook, pp. 847–866

Workbook
Chapter 30 Activities

Chapter Quiz
Handout 30-2

TestGen
Chapter 30 Test

Online Test Preparation
Send your students to
http://www.prenhall.com/
EMTAchieve

Handouts 30-3 to 30-7
Reinforcement Activities

**Brady Skills Series
EMT-B Videos/CD**
Visual Reinforcement

**PowerPoint
Presentation**
Chapter 30

Student CD
Chapter 30

Companion Website
http://www.prenhall.com/
mistovich

Online Test Preparation (for students and instructors) Additional test preparation is available through *EMT Achieve: Basic Test Preparation* at http://www.prenhall.com/EMTAchieve. Instructors can also monitor student mastery online.

REINFORCEMENT

Handouts If classroom discussions or performance on the quiz indicates that some students have not fully mastered the chapter content, you may wish to assign some or all of the Reinforcement Handouts for this chapter.

TECH EXTRAS

Brady Skills Series EMT-B Videos/CD Have your students watch the skills come to life on either VHS or CD-ROM.

PowerPoint Presentation (for instructors) The PowerPoint material developed for this chapter offers useful reinforcement of chapter content.

Student CD A wide variety of material on this CD-ROM will reinforce and also expand student knowledge and skills.

Companion Website (for students) Additional review quizzes and links to EMS resources will contribute to further reinforcement of this chapter. Please visit http://www.prenhall.com/mistovich.

OBJECTIVES CHECKLIST

Cognitive		Date Mastered
5-3.1	Describe the function of the muscular system.	
5-3.2	Describe the function of the skeletal system.	
5-3.3	List the major bones or bone groupings of the spinal column; the thorax; the upper extremities; the lower extremities.	
5-3.4	Differentiate between an open and a closed painful, swollen, deformed extremity.	
5-3.5	State the reasons for splinting.	
5-3.6	List the general rules of splinting.	
5-3.7	List the complications of splinting.	
5-3.8	List the emergency medical care for a patient with a painful, swollen, deformed extremity.	

Affective		Date Mastered
5-3.9	Explain the rationale for splinting at the scene versus load and go.	
5-3.10	Explain the rationale for immobilization of the painful, swollen, deformed extremity.	

Psychomotor		Date Mastered
5-3.11	Demonstrate the emergency medical care of a patient with a painful, swollen, deformed extremity.	
5-3.12	Demonstrate completing a prehospital care report for patients with musculoskeletal injuries.	

EVALUATION

CHAPTER 30 QUIZ

Write the letter of the best answer in the space provided.

_____ 1. All of the following are part of the musculoskeletal system *except*
  A. bones.   **C.** cartilage.
  B. joints.   **D.** skin.

_____ 2. The sound or feel of broken bone fragments grinding together is referred to as
  A. crepitus.   **C.** assonance.
  B. stridor.   **D.** dissonance.

_____ 3. There are three kinds of muscle: voluntary, involuntary, and
  A. periosteum.   **C.** cardiac.
  B. flexible.   **D.** skeletal.

_____ 4. The bones of the upper extremities include all of the following *except* the
  A. radius.   **C.** femur.
  B. humerus.   **D.** carpal.

_____ 5. Tissues or fibers that cause movement of the body parts or organs are called
  A. periosteum.   **C.** cartilage.
  B. muscles.   **D.** tendons.

_____ 6. The mechanism that causes the crushed tissues and fractures found in a patient struck by an auto is _____ force.
  A. direct   **C.** twisting
  B. indirect   **D.** rotational

_____ 7. An injury in which the skin over a fracture site is broken may be described as a(n)
  A. closed fracture.   **C.** vertical injury.
  B. open injury.   **D.** compromised injury.

_____ 8. An injury to a joint in which the bone ends become separated from each other is called a(n)
  A. dislocation.   **C.** sprain.
  B. angulation.   **D.** fracture.

_____ 9. The soft pliable splints that are easily shaped for use with deformed extremities are called _____ splints.
  A. box   **C.** vacuum
  B. long bone   **D.** traction

_____ 10. After taking BSI precautions, exposing the area, and controlling any external bleeding, the next step in immobilizing a long bone fracture is
  A. replacing protruding bones.
  B. assessing distal PMS.
  C. measuring the splint.
  D. applying the splint.

_____ **11.** If a patient's injured leg appears either internally or externally rotated, an EMT should suspect
    A. patella injury.
    B. ankle dislocation.
    C. fibula injury.
    D. hip dislocation.

_____ **12.** The term for a prickling or tingling feeling that indicates some loss of sensation is
    A. paresthesia.
    B. anesthesia.
    C. paraplegia.
    D. quadriplegia.

_____ **13.** The splint best suited for stabilization of a dislocated shoulder or a foot/ankle injury is a(n) _____ splint.
    A. air-inflatable
    B. soft or pillow
    C. formable
    D. rigid

_____ **14.** The splint best suited for easing pain of muscle spasm associated with fractures of the femur is a(n) _____ splint.
    A. air-inflatable
    B. traction
    C. vacuum
    D. PASG

_____ **15.** Muscle injuries resulting from overstretching or overexertion of the muscle are called
    A. sprains.
    B. strains.
    C. dislocations.
    D. sublocations.

_____ **16.** The mechanism that operates when one part of an extremity is held stationary while the rest rotates is _____ force.
    A. direct
    B. indirect
    C. twisting
    D. torsional

_____ **17.** Another term for the collar bone is the
    A. clavicle.
    B. humerus.
    C. scapula.
    D. patella.

_____ **18.** The displacement of a bone from its normal position in a joint is a
    A. fracture.
    B. sprain.
    C. dislocation.
    D. strain.

_____ **19.** The bones of the lower extremities include all of the following _except_ the
    A. pelvis.
    B. patella.
    C. femur.
    D. scapula.

_____ **20.** Use of a traction splint is indicated for a painful, swollen, deformed
    A. ankle.
    B. hip.
    C. elbow.
    D. femur.

REINFORCEMENT

IN THE FIELD

Read the following real-life situation. Then answer the questions that follow.

Your unit responds to a 9-1-1 call from a mother who reports that her 7-year-old son "has fallen from his tree house." When you arrive on the scene, the mother leads you into the backyard, where you see the boy grimacing in pain. He is holding his right leg. As you approach, he tells you that "it hurts all the way down to my toes."

You introduce yourself and learn that the patient's name is Roger. Roger tells you that he was climbing into the tree house and fell off of the ladder. You ask Roger if he remembers how he landed. "I think I landed on my feet first," he says. "It hurt so much that I couldn't stand up."

1. Explain the mechanism of injury associated with Roger's injuries.

2. What bones or joints do you suspect have been injured?

3. What type of splint will you use to immobilize Roger? Why?

4. What are four basic questions that should be asked of this patient?

CHAPTER 30 REVIEW

Write the word or words that best complete each sentence in the space provided.

1. The _____ system is composed of all the bones, joints, and muscles of the body.

2. As components of the skeleton, bones provide the body's _____.

3. _____ are the places where bones meet and are a critical element in the body's ability to move.

4. A common type of bone injury is a break, or _____.

5. With _____ _____, the force impacts on one end of the limb causing injury some distance away from the point of impact.

6. _____ are bands of connective tissue that bind the muscles to the bones.

7. Three types of mechanisms that cause musculoskeletal injuries include

   _____ force, _____ force, and

   _____ force.

8. The _____ splint applies constant pull along the length of the femur to stabilize fractures and reduce muscle spasms.

9. The EMT should splint suspected dislocations in position unless _____

   _____ are absent.

10. Proper _____ and prehospital care of musculoskeletal injuries help prevent

    closed injuries from becoming _____ injuries.

11. If the patient's thigh is painful, swollen, or deformed, the EMT should treat the patient as if the

    _____ is fractured.

12. To splint an injured extremity, an EMT must assess _____,

    _____ _____, and _____

    before and after splinting.

13. Dramatic-looking or painful extremity injuries can sometimes distract an untrained person from

    looking for other _____ - _____ conditions.

14. For any splint to be effective, it must immobilize the extremity or joint

    _____ and _____ the injury.

15. The point of realignment of deformed extremities is to assist in restoring effective

_____.

16. A traction splint is indicated if there is an isolated _____ fracture.

17. A patient with a hip fracture should be managed for _____.

18. Any device used to immobilize a body part is referred to as a(n) _____.

19. A(n) _____ is an injury to a joint with possible damage to or tearing of

ligaments.

20. A triangular bandage used to support the shoulder and arm is called a(n)

_____.

MUSCULOSKELETAL INJURIES: LISTING

1. List the six basic components of the skeletal system.

2. List four types of musculoskeletal injuries.

3. List three types of mechanisms that cause musculoskeletal injury.

4. List the signs and symptoms of musculoskeletal injuries.

REINFORCEMENT

IDENTIFYING MAJOR BONES

Write the name of the following bones in the correct location on the diagram below.

Carpals

Clavicle

Femur

Fibula

Humerus

Metacarpals

Metatarsals

Patella

Phalanges

Radius

Scapula

Sternum

Tarsals

Tibia

Ulna

Vertebrae

Xiphoid process

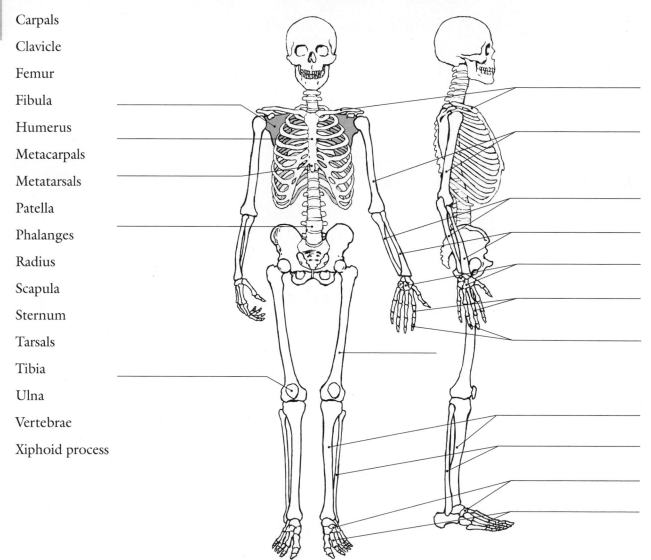

REINFORCEMENT

MUSCULOSKELETAL INJURIES: TRUE OR FALSE

Indicate if the following statements are true or false by writing T or F in the space provided.

_____ **1.** Proper splinting may serve to decrease the incidence of permanent injury.

_____ **2.** The three kinds of muscles include voluntary, skeletal, and cardiac.

_____ **3.** Voluntary muscles are those that are under the control of a person's will.

_____ **4.** Pulselessness and cyanosis distal to an injured extremity are signs of a very serious condition.

_____ **5.** Both before and after applying a splint, assess pulses, movement, and sensation distal to the injury.

_____ **6.** The most appropriate splint for a shoulder dislocation is the traction splint.

_____ **7.** The EMT should align an extremity with gentle traction if there is severe deformity or absence of distal pulses.

_____ **8.** Some types of rigid splints are often pliable enough to be molded to fit any appendage.

_____ **9.** The major type of pressure splint is a rigid splint.

_____ **10.** Improvised splints can be made from a cardboard box, an ironing board, a rolled-up magazine, a broom handle, or any similar object.

Musculoskeletal Injuries

Musculoskeletal System Review
Muscles
Tendons and Ligaments
Skeletal System

Injuries to Bones and Joints
Types
- Fracture
- Strain
- Sprain
- Dislocation

Mechanism of Injury
- Direct force
- Indirect force
- Twisting force

Fractures of Femur and Pelvis
Assessment and Care

Basics of Splinting
General Rules
Splinting Equipment
- Rigid splints
- Traction splints
- Vacuum splints
- Pressure splints
- Improvised splints
- Sling and swathe

Hazards of Improper Splinting

Specific Splinting Techniques

- Splinting long-bone injuries
- Splinting joint injuries
- Traction splinting
- Splinting specific injuries

HANDOUT 30-2: Chapter 30 Quiz

1. D	**6.** A	**11.** D	**16.** C
2. A	**7.** B	**12.** A	**17.** A
3. C	**8.** A	**13.** B	**18.** C
4. C	**9.** C	**14.** B	**19.** D
5. B	**10.** B	**15.** B	**20.** D

HANDOUT 30-3: In the Field

1. The mechanism of injury involves both direct force and indirect force. The impact of the fall is transmitted along the bone shafts and damages bones farther up the extremity.

2. The bones and joints that could be injured include bones and joints of the feet and ankle (by direct force) and the tibia, fibula, and femur and joints of the knee, hip, pelvis, and spinal column (by indirect force).

3. Because the injury could involve the entire leg from hip to toes (as well as a spinal injury), the injury can be treated as a pelvic fracture. The boy can be secured on a long spine board with his legs stabilized by a folded blanket between them and secured with cravats. This will splint him rapidly and take care of all injuries at one time.

4. When did the injury occur? What happened? Where does it hurt? What did you feel at the time of injury?

HANDOUT 30-4: Chapter 30 Review

1. musculoskeletal
2. framework
3. Joints
4. fracture
5. indirect force
6. Tendons
7. direct, indirect, twisting
8. traction
9. distal pulses
10. splinting, open
11. femur
12. pulse, motor function, sensation
13. life-threatening
14. above, below
15. circulation
16. femur
17. shock
18. splint
19. sprain
20. sling

HANDOUT 30-5: Musculoskeletal Injuries: Listing

1. Skull, spinal column, thorax, pelvis, upper extremities, lower extremities
2. Fracture, dislocation, sprain, strain
3. Direct force, indirect force, twisting force
4. Pain and tenderness; deformity or angulation; crepitus; swelling; bruising; exposed bone ends; joints locked into position; severe weakness and loss of function; disfigurement

HANDOUT 30-6: Identifying Major Bones

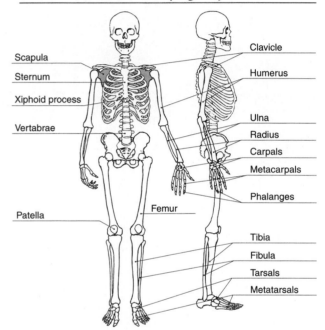

HANDOUT 30-7: Musculoskeletal Injuries: True or False

1. T	**4.** T	**7.** T	**9.** F
2. F	**5.** T	**8.** T	**10.** T
3. T	**6.** F		

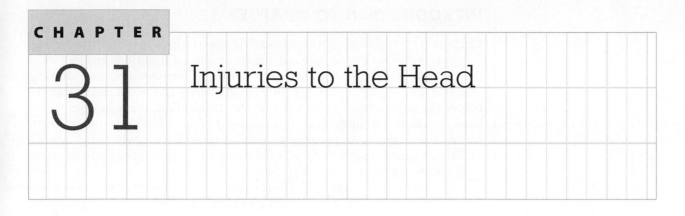
This chapter covers portions of Lesson 5-4 and Lesson 5-5 of the U.S. Department of Transportation's EMT-Basic National Standard Curriculum.

OBJECTIVES

Numbered objectives are from the U.S. Department of Transportation's EMT-Basic National Standard Curriculum. Asterisked objectives, if any, pertain to material that is supplemental to the DOT curriculum. Page numbers refer to pages in the textbook.

Cognitive

5-4.1 State the components of the nervous system. (pp. 848–850)

5-4.2 List the functions of the central nervous system. (pp. 848–850)

5-4.3 Define the structure of the skeletal system as it relates to the nervous system. (p. 848)

5-4.4 Relate mechanism of injury to potential injuries of the head and spine. (pp. 850–853)

5-4.11 Establish the relationship between airway management and the patient with head and spine injuries. (pp. 851, 858, 859, 860)

Psychomotor

5-4.44 Demonstrate completing a prehospital care report for patients with head and spinal injuries.

The above and additional objectives from DOT Lesson 5-4 are also addressed in Chapter 32, "Injuries to the Spine."

REVIEW

In the last chapter, "Musculoskeletal Injuries," students learned that injuries to muscles, joints, and bones are some of the most common emergencies they will encounter in the field. These injuries can range from the simple and non-life-threatening (such as a broken finger or sprained ankle) to the critical and life-threatening (such as a fracture of the femur or spine). Regardless of whether the injury is mild or severe, an EMT's ability to provide emergency care efficiently and quickly may prevent further painful and damaging injury and may even keep the patient from suffering permanent disability or death.

Distribute the scored quizzes from the last lesson. Go over each question on the quiz and handle any concerns students may have about the answers.

Total Teaching Time
165 minutes

Resources Needed
- Scored Chapter 30 quizzes
- Complete jump kit containing BSI equipment, oxygen equipment, a cervical collar, and a refusal-of-treatment form

Additional Resources
Larmon/Davis, *Basic Life Support Skills*

Elling, *EMT Achieve: Basic Test Preparation*

Limmer/Mistovich/O'Keefe, *Audio Lecture & Study Guide: EMT*

Mistovich/Kuvlesky, *SUCCESS! for the EMT, Second Edition*

INTRODUCTION TO CHAPTER 31

Chapter 31, "Injuries to the Head," is the sixth chapter in Module 5. Injuries to the head pose some of the most serious situations students will face as EMTs. The patient is often confused or unresponsive, making assessment of his condition difficult. Head injuries can occur days or weeks before the onset of any signs or symptoms. In addition, many injuries to the head are life-threatening. Such injuries are, in fact, a leading cause of death among this nation's young people. Many patients who survive head injuries suffer permanent disability. So it is clear that the cost of failing to recognize or properly treat such injuries can be very high.

Distribute the Chapter 31 Objectives Checklist and give students a few minutes to look it over. Then briefly paraphrase the objectives for this lesson in your own words.

Handout 31-1
Chapter 31 Objectives Checklist

●➤

Lecture Master
You may wish to display Lecture Master 31 when presenting the lecture to the class.

LECTURE

The following suggested lecture outline is based on the Department of Transportation's EMT-Basic National Standard Curriculum. In some places, the DOT curriculum has been rearranged or expanded upon so that it is more complete or easier for the student to understand. The page numbers in parentheses refer to pages in the textbook. The parenthetical references in dark, heavy type are to figures, tables, and scans in the textbook.

INJURIES TO THE HEAD

I. Anatomy of the skull and brain (pp. 848–850) (Students may also review material on the nervous system in Chapter 4, "The Human Body.")
   A. Skull (p. 848) **(Fig. 31-1, p. 849)**
      1. Cranial skull
         a. Helmet-like bony covering
      2. Basilar skull
         a. Floor of skull
   B. Brain (pp. 848–850) **(Fig 31-2, p. 849)**
      1. Cerebrospinal fluid
         a. Colorless fluid that circulates throughout skull and spinal column, protects brain and spinal cord against impact, and combats infection and cleanses brain and spinal cord
      2. Meninges
         a. Layers of tissue that enclose brain, brainstem, and spinal cord
         b. Dura mater ("hard mother")
            (1) Outermost meninges; composed of a double layer of tough, fibrous tissue
         c. Arachnoid
            (1) Middle meninges
         d. Pia mater ("soft mother")
            (1) Innermost meninges in contact with brain
         e. Subarachnoid space
            (1) Fibrous, spongy tissue filled with cerebrospinal fluid; separates arachnoid membrane and pia mater
         f. Bleeding in the meninges
            (1) Epidural bleeding

Point of Interest
The brain is a mass of over 10 billion cells that, once destroyed, cannot regenerate. On average, the adult brain weighs about 3 pounds and reaches 90 percent of its full adult size by the age of 5. Before birth, nerve cells in the fetal brain form at a rate of 250,000 a minute. After age 20, we lose about 10,000 brain cells each day.

Point of Interest
The term *arachnoid* means "resembling or related to arachnids (spiders)." The arachnoid membrane is so named because it is composed of hair-like fibers that resemble a fine spider web.

           (a) Bleeding that occurs between dura mater and
                 skull
       (2) Subdural bleeding
           (a) Bleeding that occurs beneath dura mater;
                 usually venous
       (3) Subarachnoid hemorrhage
           (a) Bleeding that occurs between arachnoid
                 membrane and surface of brain (can be fatal
                 in minutes)
   3. Parts of the brain
       a. Cerebrum
           (1) Largest part of brain (three-fourths of brain's
                 volume)
           (2) Made up of four lobes
           (3) Is responsible for most conscious and sensory
                 functions, the emotions, and the personality
       b. Cerebellum
           (1) Tucked under cerebellum
           (2) Controls equilibrium and coordinates muscle
                 activity
       c. Brainstem
           (1) Brain's funnel-shaped inferior part and the most
                 primitive and best protected part of brain
           (2) Controls most automatic functions, including
                 cardiac, respiratory, and vasomotor
           (3) Made up of pons, midbrain, and medulla
                 oblongata
II. Types of head injury (pp. 850–851)
   A. Scalp injuries (p. 850)
       1. Very vascular; tend to bleed very heavily
       2. Underlying fascia may be torn while skin stays intact.
       3. Bleeding under the skin can mimic skull deformity.
   B. Skull injuries (p. 850)
       1. Open skull deformity
           a. Break in the continuity of skin and bone
       2. Closed skull deformity
           a. Intact scalp
   C. Brain injuries (pp. 850–851) (**Fig. 31-5, p. 852**)
       1. Direct
           a. From penetrating trauma
       2. Indirect
           a. From a blow to the skull
       3. Secondary
           a. From lack of oxygen, buildup of carbon dioxide,
                 change in blood pressure
       4. Closed head injury
           a. No opening to brain yet brain damage can be extensive
                 (**Fig. 31-3, p. 851**)
       5. Open head injury
           a. Break in skull, providing an opening to the brain
                 (**Fig. 31-4, p. 851**)
           b. May be caused by an impaled object or impact with a
                 windshield
           c. Involves direct local damage to involved tissue

On the Net
Links to information,
illustrations, and resources
regarding head injuries.
http://www.nlm.nih.gov/
medlineplus/ency/article/
000028.htm

Point to Emphasize
With a blow of sufficient
force to the face, there
may also be brain injury.
Treat the patient as if a
skull or brain injury is
suspected.

      d. Can result in brain damage due to infection, brain tissue laceration, or punctures of brain by objects that invade cranium after penetrating skull

    6. Diffuse axonal injury (DAI)

    7. Specific types of brain injuries

      a. Concussion

        (1) Temporary loss of brain's ability to function

      b. Contusion

        (1) Bruising or swelling of the brain

      c. Hematoma

        (1) Pooling of blood within the brain

      d. Laceration

        (1) Tearing of brain tissue

III. Assessment and care: Head injuries (pp. 851–859) **(Figs. 31-18 and 31-19, pp. 860–862)**

  A. Scene size-up (p. 851)

    1. Always be alert for signs of head injury during trauma scene size-up.

      a. Unresponsiveness

      b. Altered mental status

      c. Bleeding from the scalp or face

      d. Apparent mechanism of injury (e.g., shattered windshield, deformed bicycle helmet) **(Fig. 31-6, p. 853)**

    2. Nontraumatic injuries to the brain can be caused by clots or hemorrhaging and can cause altered mental status and signs and symptoms similar to those of trauma cases.

  B. Initial assessment (pp. 851–854)

    1. Be alert for cervical-spine injury.

    2. Apply manual in-line stabilization of spine as the first step. **(Fig. 31-7, p. 853)**

    3. If patient is unresponsive or with altered mental status, establish an airway using jaw-thrust maneuver while holding in-line stabilization.

    4. Assess breathing. **(Fig. 31-8, p. 853)**

      a. If patient is breathing adequately, provide oxygen by nonrebreather mask at 15 liters per minute.

      b. If patient is not breathing adequately, provide positive-pressure ventilation with supplemental oxygen.

    5. Assess mental status.

      a. Assess initially using the AVPU memory aid (Alert, responds to Verbal stimulus, responds to Painful stimulus, or Unresponsive).

      b. Keep in mind that patient's mental status may change.

      c. Note patient's responses to pain.

        (1) Purposeful response

          (a) Patient tries to move away from or remove pain.

        (2) Nonpurposeful response

          (a) Patient may react to pain but not try to stop it.

          (b) Decorticate posturing (indicative of upper-level brainstem injury)

            (i) Patient postures by flexing arms across chest and extending legs.

          (c) Decerebrate posturing (indicative of lower-level brainstem injury)

　　　　(i) Patient postures by extending both arms down at sides, extending the legs, and sometimes arching the back.
　　　(3) Unresponsive
　　　　(a) Patient shows no response at all to verbal or painful stimuli.
　6. Record your observations of mental status accurately, noting the types of stimuli administered and the patient's responses.
　7. Determine a baseline for level of responsiveness.
　8. Use Glasgow Coma Scale to assess types of response to specific stimuli. **(Table 31-1, p. 854 and Table 31-2, p. 855)**
C. Focused history and physical exam (p. 854)
　1. First perform rapid trauma assessment.
　2. Next check vital signs and obtain a SAMPLE history.
　3. If patient's mental status worsens at any stage of the assessment or treatment, transport immediately and monitor during transport.
D. Rapid trauma assessment (pp. 854–857)
　1. Head
　　a. Palpate gently for deformities, depressions, lacerations, or impaled objects. **(Figs. 31-9, p. 855 and 31-10, p. 856)**
　2. Eyes **(Fig. 31-11, p. 856)**
　　a. Check patient's pupils with bright light (Equal size? React equally?)
　　b. Check eye movements (Do the eyes track?)
　　c. Note any discoloration ("Raccoon sign" may indicate intracranial injury or be late sign of skull fracture.)
　3. Ears and nose **(Fig. 31-12, p. 856)**
　　a. Check ears and nose for leakage of blood or clear fluid (may indicate skull fracture or intracranial bleeding).
　　b. Look for Battle's sign, a purplish discoloration of the mastoid area behind the ear (can be delayed sign of skull fracture).
　4. Motor/sensory assessment **(Fig. 31-13, p. 857)**
　　a. Alert patient
　　　(1) Check ability to move fingers and toes.
　　　(2) Have patient squeeze your fingers with both hands simultaneously to test for equal grip strength.
　　　(3) Ask patient to tell which finger or toe you are touching.
　　　(4) Pinch each extremity and ask patient to identify pain.
　　　(5) Ask if patient feels any weakness on one side of body.
　　b. Patient responsive only to verbal or painful stimuli
　　　(1) Watch for grimace response.
　　　(2) Watch for withdrawal from painful stimulus.
E. Baseline vital signs (p. 857)
　1. Check and record every 5 minutes, staying alert to any changes
　2. Blood pressure
　　a. If systolic is high or rising, suspect pressure inside skull.
　　b. If systolic is low or dropping, suspect blood loss that has led to shock, and check rest of body for bleeding.

Point to Emphasize
Bruising around the eyes or behind the ears may not be present for 12 to 24 hours following the trauma. It is not a good discriminator for head trauma in the field.

Point of Interest
Often patients with cerebrospinal fluid in the mouth complain of a "salty" taste.

    3. Pulse
        a. If high or rising, suspect hemorrhage elsewhere in body or early onset of hypoxia.
        b. If slow or dropping, suspect pressure inside the skull or severe hypoxia.
    4. Respiration
        a. Assess rate, depth, and pattern.
            (1) Look for respiratory patterns that indicate intercranial pressure:
                (a) Extremely fast and shallow
                (b) Completely irregular
                (c) Absent (apnea)
            (2) Look for Cushing's reflex (a sign of severe head injury)
        b. If definite signs of severe head injury, consider hyperventilation at a rate of 20 ventilations/minute with supplemental oxygen.
        c. If no definite signs of severe head injury and positive-pressure ventilation is needed, ventilate at a rate of 10–12 ventilations/minute with supplemental oxygen.
F. Take a SAMPLE history. (p. 857)
    1. When did the incident occur?
    2. What is the patient's chief complaint?
    3. Does the patient feel tingling, numbness, or paralysis? Where?
    4. How have the symptoms changed since the accident?
    5. How did the accident occur?
    6. Did the patient lose consciousness at any time? For how long?
    7. Did the patient suddenly lose consciousness and then gradually reawaken or did the patient pass out immediately, suddenly wake up, and then gradually lose consciousness again?
    8. Was the patient moved after the incident?
    9. Is there any history of a serious blow to the head?
G. Look for signs and symptoms of head injury. (pp. 857–858)
    1. Altered mental status; decreasing mental status
    2. Irregular breathing pattern (severe)
    3. Increasing blood pressure and decreasing pulse (a late finding) (severe)
    4. Obvious signs of injury
        a. Contusions, lacerations, scalp hematoma, skull deformity
    5. Blood or cerebrospinal fluid leaking from ears or nose **(Fig. 31-14, p. 858)**
    6. Discoloration (bruising) around eyes in absence of trauma to eyes (raccoon sign) (very late sign) **(Fig. 31-15, p. 858)**
    7. Discoloration (bruising) behind ears or at mastoid process (Battle's sign) (very late sign)
    8. Absent motor or sensory functions (severe or poor response)
    9. Nausea and/or vomiting, which may be forceful or repeated
    10. Unequal pupil size with altered mental status (severe)
    11. Diplopia (double vision)
    12. Possible seizures
    13. Visible damage to the skull (visible through laceration to the scalp)

14. Pain, tenderness, or swelling at the site of injury
15. Nonpurposeful response to painful stimuli (severe)
   (**Fig. 31-16, p. 858**)
16. Retrograde amnesia
   a. Unable to remember circumstances leading up to the incident.
17. Antegrade amnesia
   a. Unable to remember circumstances after the incident.
H. Emergency medical care (pp. 858–859)
   1. Take BSI precautions.
   2. Apply manual in-line stabilization, maintaining until patient is completely immobilized to a backboard. (**Fig. 31-17, p. 859**)
   3. Maintain patient airway and adequate oxygen.
      a. Use jaw-thrust maneuver to open airway.
      b. Remove foreign bodies from mouth and suction mucus.
      c. Protect against aspiration by keeping suction available at all times.
      d. Be prepared to roll secured patient to clear airway.
      e. Administer oxygen by nonrebreather mask at 15 liters per minute if breathing is adequate or positive-pressure ventilation with supplemental oxygen at 12 per minute if breathing is inadequate and signs of head injury are present.
      f. If signs of severe head injury present, consider hyperventilation at a rate of 20–24 breaths per minute.
   4. Monitor airway, breathing, pulse, and mental status for deterioration.
   5. Control bleeding.
      a. Do not apply pressure to an open or depressed skull injury.
      b. Dress and bandage open head wounds as indicated in treatment of soft tissue injuries.
      c. Do not attempt to stop the flow of blood or cerebrospinal fluid flowing from ears or nose; cover loosely and completely with a sterile gauze dressing.
      d. For other wounds, use gentle, continuous direct pressure with sterile gauze.
      e. Never try to remove a penetrating object; instead, immobilize object in place and dress wound.
   6. Be prepared for seizures.
   7. Transport immediately.
I. Detailed physical exam and ongoing assessment—repeat assessment every 5 minutes
IV. **Summary: Assessment and care** (p. 859) (**Figs. 31-18 and 31-19, pp. 860–862**)

ENRICHMENT (OPTIONAL)

The following sections contain information that is valuable as background for the EMT, but that goes substantially beyond the U.S. Department of Transportation's EMT-Basic National Standard Curriculum.

V. **More about brain injuries** (pp. 859–864)(**Fig. 31-20, p. 863**)
   A. Concussion (pp. 859–861)
      1. Effects appear soon after impact, then disappear

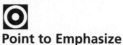

Point to Emphasize
Whenever you suspect skull or brain injury, also suspect spine injury.

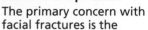

Point to Emphasize
The primary concern with facial fractures is the patient's airway. Be prepared to suction and remove debris and blood from the airway.

On the Net
Brain Trauma Foundation.
www.braintrauma.org

On the Net
Traumatic brain injuries and their treatment.
http://www.findarticles
.com/cf_0/m0984/2_122/
90868726/p1/article
.jhtml?term=%2Bbrain+
%2Binjury+%2B2002

B. Contusion (p. 861)
  1. Bruising or swelling of the brain
C. Subdural hematoma (pp. 861–864)
  1. Venous bleeding between brain and dura mater, causing pressure within skull
D. Epidural hematoma (p. 864)
  1. Arterial bleeding between skull and brain's protective cover; extreme emergency
E. Laceration of brain tissue (p. 864)

CASE STUDY FOLLOW-UP

Ask a student volunteer to read the Case Study that begins on page 848 of the textbook. You may wish to use the following questions to engage the students in a discussion of the Case Study Follow-up that begins on page 865 of the textbook. Provide missing information and clarify ideas as needed.

Q1. How do you secure Mike's airway?
A1. *By using a jaw-thrust maneuver and then inserting an oral airway.*

Q2. What is Mike's response to painful stimuli?
A2. *His arms flex across his chest and his legs stiffen.*

Q3. Describe the results of your examination of Mike's eyes.
A3. *Mike's left pupil is dilated and does not react to light.*

Q4. Describe Mike's pertinent past history as described by his family.
A4. *Mike was knocked unconscious for about 3 minutes 2 weeks ago after a rollerblading accident. He said he was fine and never sought medical care. This morning he was playing basketball and, according to his brother Sean, was hit in the head with an elbow. After that, the two brothers walked home. Sean states he noticed that Mike was walking oddly and complained of being tired. Once home, Mike went up to his room to lie down.*

Q5. How do you prepare Mike for transport?
A5. *A cervical collar is applied and he is then moved onto a backboard. When immobilization is complete, Mike is taken to the ambulance.*

IN REVIEW

Assess students' ability to apply what they have just learned by discussing the Review Questions on page 866 in the textbook.

Q1. Name the two parts of the central nervous system.
A1. *The two parts of the central nervous system are the brain and the spinal cord. (p. 848)*

Q2. Define the meninges and name the three layers of the meninges.
A2. *The meninges are layers of tissue that enclose and protect the brain. They are the dura mater, arachnoid, and pia mater. (pp. 849–850)*

Q3. Name the three anatomical components of the brain.
A3. *The three anatomical components of the brain are the cerebrum, cerebellum, and brain stem. (p. 850)*

©2008 by Pearson Education, Inc.
Prehospital Emergency Care, 8th ed.

Q4. Describe an open and a closed head injury.

A4. *In an open head injury, there is a break in the skull. In a closed head injury, the skull is not exposed and there is no opening to the brain. (pp. 850–851)*

Q5. Name other types of injury that may be present and related to a head injury.

A5. *Such injuries include cervical spine injury and bleeding, both internal and external, as well as airway problems. (p. 850–853)*

Q6. Name some of the major types of brain injury.

A6. *Major types of brain injury include concussion, contusion, hematoma, and laceration. (pp. 859–864)*

Q7. Explain why determining a baseline level of responsiveness is important in cases of head injury.

A7. *Determining a baseline level of responsiveness is important in cases of head injury because the level of responsiveness may deteriorate, a sign of a serious problem. (pp. 853–854)*

Q8. Explain why a SAMPLE history is important in cases of head injury.

A8. *A SAMPLE history is important in cases of head injury because the SAMPLE history can provide vital information about the mechanism, course, and seriousness of the injury. (p. 857)*

Q9. List the signs and symptoms of head injury.

A9. *The signs and symptoms of head injury include altered mental status; decreasing mental status; irregular breathing pattern; increasing blood pressure and decreasing pulse; obvious signs of injury—contusions, lacerations, scalp hematoma, skull deformity; blood or cerebrospinal fluid leaking from the ears or nose; discoloration around the eyes in the absence of eye trauma (raccoon sign); discoloration behind ears (Battle's sign); poor or absent motor or sensory function; nausea and/or vomiting; unequal pupil size with altered mental status; seizures; visible damage to the skull (through laceration in the scalp); pain, tenderness, or swelling at the site of injury; nonpurposeful response to painful stimuli. (pp. 857–858)*

Q10. Outline the steps of emergency medical treatment in cases of head injury.

A10. *The steps of emergency medical treatment in cases of head injury are: (1) Take BSI precautions before handling the patient. (2) Take manual, in-line spinal stabilization. (3) Maintain a patent airway with adequate breathing and adequate oxygenation (by nonrebreather mask at 15 liters per minute or positive-pressure ventilation with supplemental oxygen, as appropriate). (4) Monitor the airway, breathing, pulse, and mental status for deterioration. (5) Control bleeding. (6) Be prepared for seizures. (7) Transport immediately. (pp. 858–859)*

CRITICAL THINKING

Assess students' ability to respond to real-life emergency situations by discussing the Critical Thinking questions on page 866 in the textbook.

Q1. What immediate emergency care would you provide for the patient?

A1. *One EMT should immediately establish in-line manual spinal stabilization while performing a jaw-thrust maneuver to open the airway. Suction the blood until clear from the airway. Insert an oropharyngeal airway and immediately begin bag-valve-make ventilation. Connect oxygen to the BVM reservoir at a rate of 12 to 15 lpm.*

Q2. What do the vital signs indicate?

A2. *The slow heart rate (bradycardia), increasing systolic blood pressure (bounding radial pulses), and irregular respiratory pattern indicate a brain injury with increasing pressure inside the cranium (intracranial pressure). This is known as Cushing's Reflex. It is a protective reflex that is intended to keep the brain perfused with blood. The abnormal flexion (decorticate) posturing also is a strong indicator of a brain injury with compression of the brain.*

Q3. Would you hyperventilate the patient or not? And based on what criteria would you make the decision?

A3. *This patient should be hyperventilated with the BVM at a rate of 20 per minute. The decision to hyperventilate would be based on the patient's flexion posturing, irregular respirations, and slow heart rate – which all suggest an increased intracranial pressure. The criteria to hyperventilate include a fixed or dilated pupil(s), Cushing's Reflex, and abnormal posturing.*

Q4. How would you manage the impaled screwdriver?

A4. *Any bleeding from around the screwdriver wound should be controlled with gentle pressure on the wound edges followed by stabilization of the screwdriver with a bulky dressing. The wound and screwdriver should then be securely bandaged in place with all reasonable attempts being made to not disrupt fingerprints, which may be on the handle of the weapon.*

ROLE PLAY

Request the assistance of four volunteers, two to play the role of EMTs responding to a 9-1-1 call, one to be the patient, and one to be a coworker of the patient.

Take the two EMT players outside the classroom and provide them with a complete jump kit containing BSI equipment, oxygen equipment, a cervical collar, and a refusal-of-treatment form. Describe the following situation to them:

You have been dispatched to a convenience store on a Tuesday afternoon for a woman reported injured. You should act appropriately on what you find there. The emphasis of the scenario is dealing with head injuries. However, you should utilize all the skills you have learned to this point. We will call you to the scene in just a minute.

Have the patient and the coworker come to the front of the classroom. Describe the following situation to them and the class:

Lisa, a young woman, works at the local convenience store. She was stocking shelves in the back room when a heavy box fell from a top shelf and hit her on the right side of the head. Ted, a coworker, saw that Lisa was hit and that she dropped to the floor unconscious. The coworker moved the box away from Lisa and called 9-1-1. Lisa rapidly regained consciousness but she now has a headache. The spot where the box hit is swollen and tender to the touch but is not bleeding. Lisa denies neck or back pain. She has a slight weakness in her left hand. She is oriented to person/self and place, but is unsure of time, thinking it may be Saturday.

Decide who will play the patient and coworker. (Names may be changed according to the gender of the actors.) You may wish to use moulage on the volunteer playing the patient to simulate a swollen bruise on the side of the head.

Tell Lisa and Ted to take their places and start acting. Call the EMTs back into the classroom.

Allow the role play to progress naturally. Provide appropriate vital signs—pulse, strong and slightly rapid; breathing, adequate; skin, warm and pink and dry—and other objective information about the patient if the EMTs assess this information. Intervene only if the players seem to be at a loss for what to do.

End the play when the EMTs have made a final decision on transport or have obtained a signed refusal form.

With the entire class, discuss the following:

- What did the EMTs do well?
- What, if anything, should they have done differently?

ASSIGNMENTS

Assign students to read Chapter 32, "Injuries to the Spine" before the next class. Also ask them to complete Chapter 31 of the Workbook.

EVALUATION

Chapter Quiz Distribute copies of the Chapter Quiz provided in Handout 31-2 to evaluate student understanding of this chapter. Remind students not to refer to their textbooks or notes while taking the quiz.

Test Manager You may wish to create a custom-tailored test using Prentice Hall *TestGen for Prehospital Emergency Care, Eighth Edition* to evaluate student understanding of this chapter.

Online Test Preparation (for students and instructors) Additional test preparation is available through *EMT Achieve: Basic Test Preparation* at http://www.prenhall.com/EMTAchieve. Instructors can also monitor student mastery online.

REINFORCEMENT

Handouts If classroom discussions or performance on the quiz indicates that some students have not fully mastered the chapter content, you may wish to assign some or all of the Reinforcement Handouts for this chapter.

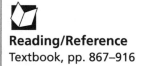

Reading/Reference
Textbook, pp. 867–916

Workbook
Chapter 31 Activities

Chapter Quiz
Handout 31-2

TestGen
Chapter 31 Test

Online Test Preparation
Send your students to
http://www.prenhall.com/
EMTAchieve

Handouts 31-3 to 31-6
Reinforcement Activities

©2008 by Pearson Education, Inc.
Prehospital Emergency Care, 8th ed.

TECH EXTRAS

Brady Skills Series EMT-B Videos/CD Have your students watch the skills come to life on either VHS or CD-ROM.

PowerPoint Presentation (for instructors) The PowerPoint material developed for this chapter offers useful reinforcement of chapter content.

Student CD A wide variety of material on this CD-ROM will reinforce and also expand student knowledge and skills.

Companion Website (for students) Additional review quizzes and links to EMS resources will contribute to further reinforcement of this chapter. Please visit http://www.prenhall.com/mistovich.

OBJECTIVES CHECKLIST

Cognitive		Date Mastered
5-4.1	State the components of the nervous system.	
5-4.2	List the functions of the central nervous system.	
5-4.3	Define the structure of the skeletal system as it relates to the nervous system.	
5-4.4	Relate mechanism of injury to potential injuries of the head and spine.	
5-4.11	Establish the relationship between airway management and the patient with head and spine injuries.	

Psychomotor		Date Mastered
5-4.44	Demonstrate completing a prehospital care report for patients with head and spinal injuries.	

OBJECTIVES

CHAPTER 31 QUIZ

Write the letter of the best answer in the space provided.

_____ 1. The major components of the central nervous system include the brain and the
   A. cranium.   **C.** spinal cord.
   B. spinous process.   **D.** dura mater.

_____ 2. If a patient tries to move away from or remove a painful stimulus, this response is termed _____ movement.
   A. purposeful   **C.** catatonic
   B. nonpurposeful   **D.** decorticate

_____ 3. The helmet-like structure that protects the brain is called the
   A. basilar skull.   **C.** dura mater.
   B. cranial skull.   **D.** meninges.

_____ 4. The weakest portion of the skull is made up of many separate bones. It is called the _____ skull.
   A. basilar   **C.** parietal
   B. temporal   **D.** occipital

_____ 5. Because of the scalp's rich blood supply, one likely result of a scalp injury is
   A. Battle's sign.
   B. bleeding from the ears.
   C. cerebrospinal fluid from the nose.
   D. profuse bleeding.

_____ 6. After taking BSI precautions, the first step in providing emergency care to a patient with skull fractures and brain injuries is to
   A. apply a cervical collar.
   B. control bleeding.
   C. provide manual stabilization of the head.
   D. transport the patient immediately.

_____ 7. A collection of blood within the skull or brain tissue is called a
   A. hematoma.   **C.** concussion.
   B. contusion.   **D.** laceration.

_____ 8. Within the skull, the brain is cushioned in a dense serous substance called _____ fluid.
   A. cerebrospinal   **C.** pericardial
   B. meningeal   **D.** peritoneal

_____ 9. All of the following structures are part of the brainstem *except* the
   A. pons.   **C.** medulla.
   B. midbrain.   **D.** arachnoid.

_____ 10. All of the following are highly vascular membranes separating the cranium and the brain *except* the
   A. subarachnoid space.   **C.** dura mater.
   B. pia mater.   **D.** arachnoid.

_____ **11.** All of the following are signs of Cushing's reflex *except* a(n)
    A. increase in blood pressure.   **C.** increase in heart rate.
    B. decrease in heart rate.   **D.** change in respiratory status.

_____ **12.** The bruising and swelling of brain tissue that may accompany concussion is called a(n)
    A. contusion.   **C.** epidural rupture.
    B. stroke.   **D.** subdural avulsion.

_____ **13.** The extreme emergency following a skull fracture in which arterial bleeding pools between the skull and the protective covering of the brain is called a(n)
    A. subdural hematoma.   **C.** contusion.
    B. laceration.   **D.** epidural hematoma.

_____ **14.** In documenting a possible head or spine injury, it is critical to note whether the patient, even briefly, lost
    A. his breath.   **C.** his balance.
    B. consciousness.   **D.** capillary refill.

_____ **15.** A head injury in which the scalp is lacerated but there is no opening in the skull is a(n)
    A. open head injury.   **C.** epidural hematoma.
    B. closed head injury.   **D.** subdural hematoma.

REINFORCEMENT

IN THE FIELD

Read the following real-life situation. Then answer the questions that follow.

At 1800 hours on a hot summer afternoon, you and your crew are called to a domestic dispute. Dispatch informs you that guns were involved. When you arrive, the police have secured the scene and it is safe. As you approach the scene, you find a 32-year-old male patient who is combative and responds only to painful stimuli. You note an entrance wound on the left parietal area. In addition, you note the presence of Battle's sign. Initial assessment reveals an increasing blood pressure, decreasing heart rate, and altered respirations.

1. What are your initial management considerations?

2. Explain your transport decision.

3. What five interventions should be carried out while en route to the definitive care facility?

CHAPTER 31 REVIEW

Write the word or words that best complete each sentence in the space provided.

1. The major components of the _____ _____
   _____ are the brain and the spinal cord.

2. The serous substance called _____ _____ protects
   the brain and spinal cord against impact.

3. Because head injuries can be so serious, the EMT must always be alert for signs of the mechanism of
   injury during the _____ _____
   _____.

4. The _____ skull is made up of plates of large, flat bones that are fused
   together to form a helmet-like covering.

5. Inside the skull, the brain is protected from injury by three _____.

6. The scalp has many _____ _____, so any scalp
   injury may bleed profusely.

7. _____ hematoma is the most common type of head injury.

8. Bruising and swelling of the brain tissue, or a(n) _____, occurs when the
   force of a blow is great enough to rupture blood vessels.

9. In addition to APVU, some EMS systems use the _____
   _____ _____ for determining a patient's level of
   responsiveness.

10. A late finding in a patient with isolated head trauma is that blood pressure
    _____ and heart rate _____.

11. Two nonpurposeful responses that a patient with a head injury might make include
    _____ and _____.

12. In a rapid trauma exam of a patient with a, head injury examine the head for
    _____, _____, _____, or
    _____ _____ around the head and face.

13. The lowest level on the AVPU scale is _____.

14. A purplish discoloration of the soft tissues around one or both eyes is called

_____ _____ and may be an indication of

intracranial injury.

15. In documenting injuries to the head and spine, carefully note any changes in the patient's

_____ _____ throughout assessment, treatment,

and transport.

HEAD INJURIES: LISTING

1. List four types of brain injuries.

2. List, in order from outer to inner, the meninges.

3. List the three anatomical components of the brain and give one function or characteristic of each.

4. List four mechanisms of injury that commonly produce head injuries.

5. List the three signs indicative of Cushing's reflex.

RECOGNIZING BRAIN STRUCTURE

Demonstrate your familiarity with the anatomy of the brain by writing the names of the following structures in the appropriate places on the diagram below.

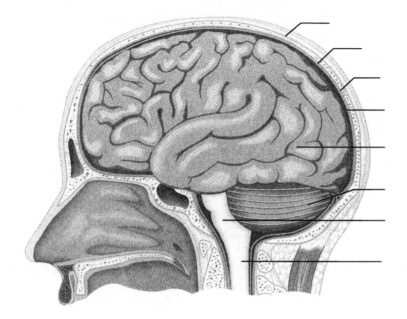

Arachnoid	Cerebral cortex	Dura mater	Pia mater
Cerebellum	Cranium	Medulla oblongata	Spinal cord

Injuries to the Head

Anatomy of the Skull and Brain
Skull

- Cranial skull
- Basilar skull

Brain

- Meninges
- Dura mater
- Arachnoid
- Pia mater
- Parts of the brain
- Cerebrum
- Cerebellum
- Brainstem

Types of Head Injury
Scalp Injuries

Skull Injuries

Brain Injuries

- Open and closed
- Concussion
- Hematoma
- Contusion
- Laceration

Assessment and Care

HANDOUT 31-2: Chapter 31 Quiz

1. C	**5.** D	**9.** D	**13.** D
2. A	**6.** C	**10.** A	**14.** B
3. B	**7.** A	**11.** C	**15.** B
4. A	**8.** A	**12.** A	

HANDOUT 31-3: In the Field

1. Cervical spine immobilization; ABCs (airway, breathing, circulation)
2. Based on the patient's condition, mechanism of injury, and mental status compromise, you should immediately package and rapidly transport this patient.
3. The interventions include continued airway management and oxygen administration; constant evaluation of the level of consciousness; frequent obtaining of vital signs and comparison to the baseline vital signs; wound management; frequent assessment of neurological status. If it is available, a request for advanced life support assistance would be appropriate.

HANDOUT 31-4: Chapter 31 Review

1. central nervous system
2. cerebrospinal fluid
3. scene size-up
4. cranial
5. meninges
6. blood vessels
7. Subdural
8. contusion
9. Glasgow Coma Scale
10. increases, decreases
11. flexion, extension
12. deformities, depressions, lacerations, impaled objects
13. unresponsive
14. raccoon sign
15. mental status

HANDOUT 31-5: Head Injuries: Listing

1. Concussion, contusion, hematoma, laceration
2. Dura mater, arachnoid, pia mater
3. Cerebrum—largest portion of the brain, responsible for most conscious and sensory functions, emotions, personality; cerebellum—controls equilibrium and coordinates muscle activity, controls muscle movement and coordination, coordinates reflexes; brainstem—most primitive and best protected part of brain, controls most automatic functions of the body.
4. Motor-vehicle crashes, assaults/violence, falls, sports injuries
5. Increase in systolic blood pressure, decrease in heart rate, change in respiratory pattern

HANDOUT 31-6: Recognizing Brain Structure

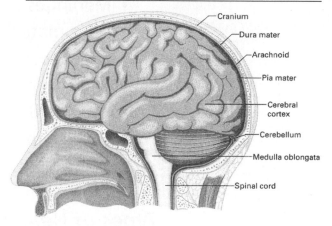

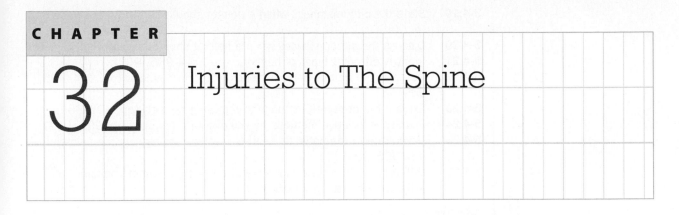

32 Injuries to The Spine

This chapter covers portions of Lesson 5-4 and Lesson 5-5 of the 1994 U.S. Department of Transportation's EMT-Basic National Standard Curriculum.

OBJECTIVES

Numbered objectives are from the U.S. Department of Transportation's EMT-Basic National Standard Curriculum. Asterisked objectives, if any, pertain to material that is supplemental to the DOT curriculum. Page numbers refer to pages in the textbook.

Cognitive

5-4.1 State the components of the nervous system. (p. 869)

5-4.2 List the functions of the central nervous system. (p. 869)

5-4.3 Define the structure of the skeletal system as it relates to the nervous system. (pp. 869–871)

5-4.4 Relate mechanism of injury to potential injuries of the head and spine. (pp. 871–873)

5-4.5 Describe the implications of not properly caring for potential spine injuries. (p. 867)

5-4.6 State the signs and symptoms of a potential spine injury. (pp. 878–879)

5-4.7 Describe the method of determining if a responsive patient may have a spine injury. (pp. 871–880)

5-4.8 Relate the airway emergency medical care techniques to the patient with a suspected spine injury. (pp. 873, 874, 881, 882, 883, 886, 904, 905, 907, 908, 909)

5-4.9 Describe how to stabilize the cervical spine. (pp. 880–904)

5-4.10 Discuss indications for sizing and using a cervical spine immobilization device. (pp. 885–890)

5-4.11 Establish the relationship between airway management and the patient with head and spine injuries. (pp. 873, 874, 881, 882, 883, 886, 904, 905, 907, 908, 909)

5-4.12 Describe a method for sizing a cervical spine immobilization device. (p. 886)

5-4.13 Describe how to log roll a patient with a suspected spine injury. (pp. 895, 897, 898)

5-4.14 Describe how to secure a patient to a long spine board. (pp. 893–901)

5-4.15 List instances when a short spine board should be used. (pp. 893–894)

5-4.16 Describe how to immobilize a patient using a short spine board. (pp. 894–895, 898, 901–904)

5-4.17 Describe the indications for the use of rapid extrication. (pp. 902–903)

5-4.18 List steps in performing rapid extrication. (pp. 903–904)

Total Teaching Time
225 minutes

Resources Needed

- Scored Chapter 31 Quizzes
- 5 EMTs to serve as teaching assistants
- 5 nonstudents to serve as patients
- 2 automobiles
- Cervical collars of various sizes
- Short spine boards or similar devices used in your area
- Long spine boards
- Straps
- Padding material
- Head immobilization device
- Football or bicycle helmet
- Child safety seat
- Towels
- Wide adhesive tape
- Knife

Additional Resources

Larmon/Davis, *Basic Life Support Skills*

Elling, *EMT Achieve: Basic Test Preparation*

Limmer/Mistovich/O'Keefe, *Audio Lecture & Study Guide: EMT*

Mistovich/Kuvlesky, *SUCCESS! for the EMT, Second Edition*

5-4.19	State the circumstances when a helmet should be left on the patient. (p. 904)
5-4.20	Discuss the circumstances when a helmet should be removed. (p. 904)
5-4.21	Identify different types of helmets. (pp. 904–905, 907)
5-4.22	Describe the unique characteristics of sports helmets. (pp. 904–905, 907)
5-4.23	Explain the preferred methods to remove a helmet. (pp. 905–906)
5-4.24	Discuss alternative methods for removal of a helmet. (pp. 905, 907)
5-4.25	Describe how the patient's head is stabilized to remove the helmet. (pp. 905–909)
5-4.26	Differentiate how the head is stabilized with a helmet compared to without a helmet. (pp. 905–909)

Affective

5-4.27	Explain the rationale for immobilization of the entire spine when a cervical spine injury is suspected. (pp. 867, 885)
5-4.28	Explain the rationale for utilizing immobilization methods apart from the straps on the cots. (pp. 885–904)
5-4.29	Explain the rationale for utilizing a short spine immobilization device when moving a patient from the sitting to the supine position. (pp. 893–894)
5-4.30	Explain the rationale for utilizing rapid extrication approaches only when they indeed will make the difference between life and death. (pp. 902–903)
5-4.31	Defend the reasons for leaving a helmet in place for transport of a patient. (p. 904)
5-4.32	Defend the reasons for removal of a helmet prior to transport of a patient. (pp. 904–905)

Psychomotor

5-4.33	Demonstrate opening the airway in a patient with suspected spinal cord injury.
5-4.34	Demonstrate evaluating a responsive patient with a suspected spinal cord injury.
5-4.35	Demonstrate stabilization of the cervical spine.
5-4.36	Demonstrate the four-person log roll for a patient with a suspected spinal cord injury.
5-4.37	Demonstrate how to log roll a patient with a suspected spinal cord injury using two people.
5-4.38	Demonstrate securing a patient to a long spine board.
5-4.39	Demonstrate using the short board immobilization technique.
5-4.40	Demonstrate procedure for rapid extrication.
5-4.41	Demonstrate preferred methods for stabilization of a helmet.
5-4.42	Demonstrate helmet removal techniques.
5-4.43	Demonstrate alternative methods for stabilization of a helmet.
5-4.44	Demonstrate completing a prehospital care report for patients with head and spinal injuries.

Some of the objectives from DOT Lesson 5-4 are also addressed in Chapter 31, "Injuries to the Head."

REVIEW

In the last chapter, "Injuries to the Head," students learned that injuries to the head pose some of the most serious situations they will face as EMTs. The patient is often confused or unresponsive, making assessment of his condition difficult. Head injuries to a patient can occur days or weeks before

©2008 by Pearson Education, Inc.
Prehospital Emergency Care, 8th ed.

the onset of any signs or symptoms. In addition, many injuries to the head are life-threatening. Such injuries are, in fact, a leading cause of death among this nation's young people. Many patients who survive head injuries suffer permanent disability. So it is clear that the cost of failing to recognize or properly treat such injuries can be very high.

Distribute the quizzes from the last class. Go over each question on the quiz and handle any concerns students may have about the answers.

INTRODUCTION TO CHAPTER 32

Chapter 32, "Injuries to the Spine," is the seventh chapter in Module 5. Spine injuries are among of the most formidable and traumatic EMTs manage. Yet they may face such injuries on almost a daily basis. Automobile crashes, shallow-water diving accidents, motorcycle crashes, and falls are all common causes of spine injury. Likewise, accidents during skiing, sledding, football, and gymnastics can result in spine injury. It is the job of the EMT to recognize injuries that could damage the spinal column or spinal cord and to provide appropriate emergency care. EMTs also must be aware that improper movement and handling of patients in such situations can easily lead to permanent disability or even death.

Distribute the Chapter 32 Objectives Checklist, and give students a few minutes to look it over. Then briefly paraphrase the objectives for this lesson in your own words.

Handout 32-1
Chapter 32 Objectives Checklist

LECTURE

The following suggested lecture outline is based on the Department of Transportation's EMT-Basic National Standard Curriculum. In some places, the DOT curriculum has been rearranged or expanded upon so that it is more complete or easier for the student to understand. The page numbers in parentheses refer to pages in the textbook. The parenthetical references in dark, heavy type are to figures, tables, and scans in the textbook.

● ➤
Lecture Master
You may wish to display Lecture Master 32 when presenting the lecture to the class.

INJURIES TO THE SPINE

I. Anatomy and physiology of spine injury (pp. 869–884)
  A. Nervous system (Students may also review material on the nervous system in Chapter 4, "The Human Body.")
  1. Functions
      a. Communication
      b. Control
  2. Structural divisions **(Fig. 32-1, p. 870)**
      a. Central nervous system
          (1) Brain
          (2) Spinal cord
      b. Peripheral nervous system—nerves located outside the brain and spinal cord
  3. Functional divisions
      a. Voluntary nervous system
          (1) Influences activity of voluntary (skeletal) muscles
      b. Automatic nervous system
          (1) Influences activities of involuntary muscles and glands

B. Skeletal system (pp. 869–871) (Students may also review material on the skeletal system in Chapter 4, "The Human Body.")
  1. Functions
  2. Components
    a. Skull
    b. Spinal column (**Fig. 32-2, p. 870**)
      (1) Body's principal support system
      (2) Vertebrae
        (a) 33 irregularly shaped bones that compose the spinal column
      (3) Disc
        (a) Fluid-filled pad of tough elastic cartilage between each two vertebrae
      (4) Surrounds and protects the spinal cord and divided into five parts
        (a) Cervical spine
          (i) First seven vertebrae that form the neck
        (b) Thoracic spine
          (i) Twelve vertebrae that form the upper back
        (c) Lumbar spine
          (i) Five vertebrae that form the lower back
        (d) Sacral spine (sacrum)
          (i) Five fused vertebrae that form rigid posterior portion of pelvis
        (e) Coccyx (tailbone)
          (i) Four fused vertebrae that form the lower end of the spine
    c. Spinal cord
      (1) Carries messages from brain to various parts of body through nerve bundles
      (2) Motor tract
      (3) Pain tract
      (4) Light touch tract
C. Common mechanisms of spine injury (p. 871) (**Fig. 32-3, p. 872**)
  1. Compression
    a. Weight of body driven against head
    b. Falls
    c. Diving accidents
    d. Motor-vehicle collisions in which person impacts an object head first
  2. Flexion
    a. Severe forward movement of head in which chin meets chest, or when torso is excessively curled forward
  3. Extension
    a. Severe backward movement of head in which neck is stretched, or when torso is severely arched backward
  4. Rotation
    a. Lateral movement of head or spine beyond its normal rotation
  5. Lateral bending
    a. Body bent severely from side
  6. Distraction
    a. Vertebrae and spinal cord stretched and pulled apart (hangings)

7. Penetration
  a. Injury from gunshots, stabbings, or other types of penetrating trauma
D. Assessment (pp. 871–874) (Fig. 32-9, pp. 875–876)
  1. Scene size-up
    a. Look for likely mechanism of spine injury at any of the following scenes:
      (1) Motorcycle crashes
      (2) Motor-vehicle crashes
      (3) Pedestrian–vehicle collisions
      (4) Falls
      (5) Blunt trauma
      (6) Penetrating trauma to the head, neck, or torso
      (7) Hangings
      (8) Diving accidents and submersions
      (9) Gunshot wounds to the head, neck, chest, abdomen, back, or pelvis
      (10) Unresponsive trauma patient
      (11) Electrical injuries
    b. Look for clues to the mechanism of injury.
    c. Maintain a high index of suspicion for spine injury.
    d. Do not rule out spine injury even if the patient is walking or sitting and there are no overt signs of trauma.
    e. Know that suspicion of spine injury sets standard for subsequent emergency care.
  2. Initial assessment
    a. Avoid excessive movement and manipulation of the body.
    b. Maintain in-line stabilization throughout entire patient contact.
    c. Open the airway, using the jaw-thrust maneuver.
    d. Suction fluids rather than turning patient's head to drain fluids.
    e. Assess chest and abdominal movement—if little or none, be prepared to provide positive-pressure ventilation with supplemental oxygen.
    f. Assess pulse, skin color, temperature, and condition
      (1) May appear normal despite injury to the vertebrae.
    g. Assess pulse
      (1) Weak or absent radial pulse may indicate spine injury due to reduced blood pressure.
    h. Assess skin temperature
      (1) May be warm and dry below a spinal cord injury site and cool, pale, and moist above the injury site.
    i. Assess patient's mental status
      (1) May range from completely alert and oriented to unresponsive in a patient with a spine injury.
    j. Categorize patient as either high or low priority for emergency care or transport. High-priority patients include:
      (1) Unresponsive patient
      (2) Responsive patient unable to obey commands
      (3) Patient with abnormal respiratory pattern
      (4) Patient with obvious signs of spine injury such as numbness or paralysis

Point of Interest
The greatest number of spinal cord injuries occurs among 16- to 20-year-olds.

Point to Emphasize
The EMT should overtreat a patient with potential spinal injury because a spinal injury cannot be ruled out in the field. The cost in terms of pain, suffering, disability, and money are very high when a spine-injured patient is unintentionally made worse by failure to immobilize the spine.

E. Focused history and physical exam (pp. 874–878)
   1. Conduct a focused history and physical exam.
   2. Continue manual in-line stabilization.
   3. Reassess patient's mental status.
   4. Conduct a rapid trauma assessment.
      a. Instruct patient to be still and not attempt to move.
      b. Cut clothing away to reduce unnecessary movement.
      c. Inspect and palpate head, neck, chest, abdomen, pelvis, extremities, and posterior body for DCAP-BTLS.
      d. Pay particular attention to the following when a spine injury is suspected:
         (1) Injuries associated with spine injury
         (2) Cervical spine immobilization collar (CSIC)
            (a) Apply after your assessment
         (3) Motor function assessment
         (4) Pain perception
         (5) Light touch perception
         (6) Posterior exam
      e. Obtain baseline vital signs.
         (1) Look for neurogenic shock
            (a) Low blood pressure
            (b) Slow heart rate associated with spine or brain injury
         (2) Look for spinal shock
            (a) Warm, dry skin
            (b) Motor and/or sensory deficit associated with spine injury
         (3) Closely reassess patient for deterioration, and report findings to emergency department.
      f. Obtain a SAMPLE history (responsive patient):
         (1) Does your neck or back hurt?
         (2) Where does it hurt?
         (3) Can you move your hands and feet?
         (4) Do you have any pain or muscle spasms along your back or to the back of your neck?
         (5) Do you have any numbness or tingling sensations in any of your arms or legs?
         (6) Was the onset of pain associated with a fall or other injury?
         (7) Did you move or did someone move you before our arrival?
         (8) Were you up and walking around before our arrival?
      g. Obtain a SAMPLE history (unresponsive patient):
         (1) Ask bystanders at scene.
         (2) Try to determine patient's mental status before your arrival.
F. Signs and symptoms (pp. 878–879) **(Figs. 32-5 and 32-6, pp. 879–880)**
   1. Ability to walk, move extremities, feel sensation, or lack of pain to spinal column does not rule out possibility of spinal column or cord damage.
   2. Tenderness in area of injury
   3. Pain associated with moving
      a. Do not ask patient to move to try to elicit a pain response.

On the Net
Spinal injuries. http://www.nlm.nih.gov/medlineplus/spinalcordinjuries.html

    b. Do not move patient to test for a pain response.

  4. Pain independent of movement or palpation

    a. Along spinal column

    b. Lower legs

    c. May be intermittent

  5. Obvious deformity of spine upon palpation

  6. Soft tissue injuries associated with trauma

    a. Head and neck

      (1) Cervical spine trauma

    b. Shoulders, back, or abdomen

      (1) Thoracic, lumbar trauma

    c. Lower extremities

      (1) Lumbar, sacral trauma

  7. Numbness, weakness, or tingling in extremities

  8. Loss of sensation or paralysis below suspected level of injury

  9. Loss of sensation or paralysis in upper or lower extremities

 10. Loss of bowel or bladder control (incontinence)

 11. Priapism (persistent erection of the penis)

 12. Impaired or diaphragmatic breathing

G. Complications of spine injury (p. 879)

  1. Inadequate breathing effort

  2. Paralysis

  3. Inadequate circulation

H. Incomplete spinal cord injury (pp. 879–880)

  1. Cord injury not involving all three tracts

I. Emergency medical care (pp. 880–883) **(Figs. 32-8 and 32-9, pp. 882–884)**

  1. When in doubt, immobilize patient.

  2. Take necessary BSI precautions.

  3. Immediately establish and maintain in-line stabilization. **(Fig. 32-7, p. 881)**

  4. Perform initial assessment.

    a. Open airway with jaw-thrust maneuver and maintain in-line stabilization.

    b. Suction secretions without turning patient's head.

    c. Provide positive-pressure ventilation while maintaining in-line stabilization.

  5. Assess pulse, motor function, and sensation in all extremities.

  6. Assess cervical region and neck.

  7. Apply a rigid cervical immobilization collar.

    a. Refer to manufacturer's instructions on proper sizing.

    b. If collar does not fit, loosely wrap a towel or blanket around the patient's neck, and tape to backboard while maintaining in-line stabilization.

  8. If found in a supine position, immobilize patient to a long backboard.

  9. Once patient is immobilized, reassess, record, and document pulses and motor and sensory function in all extremities.

 10. Transport to hospital.

 11. Perform detailed physical exam.

    a. Perform en route to the hospital if time and patient's condition permit.

    b. Inspect and palpate for further evidence of injury without unnecessarily moving patient.

    c. Assess and record any change in motor and sensory function in extremities.

Slides/Videos
"Spinal Injury," *Pulse,* May 1998.

On the Net
Spinal injury support. http://neurosurgery.mgh. harvard.edu/paral-r.htm

12. Perform ongoing assessment every 5 minutes en route to hospital.

    a. Be alert for the following:

        (1) Decreasing level of responsiveness is an early sign of head injury.

        (2) Rising systolic blood pressure and decreasing heart rate are late signs of head injury.

    b. Reevaluate the following interventions:

        (1) Airway adjuncts

        (2) Positive-pressure ventilation devices

        (3) Mask seal

        (4) Oxygen therapy

        (5) Splints

        (6) Immobilization devices

II. Summary: Assessment and care (p. 884) **(Figs. 32-8 and 32-9, pp. 882–884)**

III. Guidelines for immobilization (pp. 885–904)

    A. Tools (pp. 885–892)

        1. Cervical spine immobilization collars **(Fig. 32-10, p. 885)**

          a. Should be used any time you suspect injury to spine

          b. Should never use a soft collar, which permits too much lateral movement, flexion, and extension

          c. Should be used to

            (1) Prevent head from moving in relation to spine

            (2) Reduce compression of cervical spine during movement and transport

          d. Should never be used as sole means of immobilization

          e. Should be sized to patient based on design of device **(Fig. 32-11, p. 886)**

          f. Should be applied according to manufacturer's instructions or local protocols

            (1) To a sitting patient **(Fig. 32-12, p. 877 and 32-14, pp. 889–890)**

            (2) To a supine patient **(Fig. 32-13, p. 888 and 32-15, p. 891)**

        2. Full body spinal immobilization devices **(Fig. 32-16, p. 892)**

          a. Generally used to immobilize patients who are found in a lying or standing position

          b. May also be used in conjunction with short backboards

        3. Short spinal immobilization devices **(Fig. 32-16, p. 892)**

          a. Two types: vest and rigid

          b. Used to provide stabilization and immobilization to head, neck, and torso

          c. Used most commonly to immobilize noncritical sitting patients

          d. Should only be used to immobilize patient while moving him from a sitting position to a long board

        4. Other immobilization equipment

          a. Backboard straps or cravats

            (1) Place to prevent patient from moving up and down or laterally

          b. Head immobilizer

    B. Immobilization techniques (pp. 892–904)

        1. Immobilizing a supine or prone patient

          a. Move the patient onto the long board by log rolling the patient. **(Figs. 32-17, 32-18, 32-19 and 32-20, pp. 894–898)**

Slides/Videos

Brady Skill Series: EMT-B, "Cervical Collar" "Kendrick Extrication Device (KED)" "Immobilizing a Supine Patient" "Immobilizing a Standing Patient" "Helmet Removal" "Rapid Extrication"

On the Net

Valuable information on KED application and its value in the field. http://home.ica.net/~jwilmot/fire/emnov97.htm

b. Position long spine board under patient.

c. Place padding in spaces between the patient and the board.

   (1) Adult

      (a) Pad under head and torso.

   (2) Infant or child

      (a) Pad under shoulders and anywhere along body as necessary.

d. Immobilize patient's torso to board with straps.

e. Immobilize patient's head to board with a commercial head/cervical immobilization device or with blanket rolls and tape.

f. Secure patient's legs to board with straps.

2. Immobilizing a standing patient **(Figs. 32-21 and 32-22, pp. 899–900)**

a. (1st EMT) Immediately take and maintain normal manual in-line spinal stabilization measures. (2nd and 3rd EMTs perform steps b through g)

b. Apply a cervical collar.

c. Position long board behind patient, examining the back carefully.

d. Stand on either side of patient to support him.

   (1) Each place one arm under patient's armpit and grasp highest reachable handhold on long board with hand of same arm

   (2) Each hold patient's elbow with other hand to steady and support him.

e. Each place a leg behind the board, then slowly tip board backward and begin lowering it to ground while 1st EMT maintains stabilization.

f. Perform necessary assessment and care while 1st EMT maintains manual in-line stabilization.

g. Immobilize patient on backboard.

3. Immobilizing a seated patient **(Fig. 32-23, pp. 901–902)**

a. (1st EMT) Immediately take and maintain normal manual in-line spinal stabilization measures. (2nd and 3rd EMTs perform steps b through i)

b. Apply a cervical collar.

c. Position short spinal device behind patient, examining patient's back carefully.

   (1) Top of board should be level with top of patient's head.

   (2) Bottom of board should not extend past the coccyx.

   (3) Body straps should fit snugly under patient's armpits.

d. Secure device to patient's torso.

e. Pad behind patient's head, ensuring neutral alignment.

f. Secure patient's head to device, while 1st EMT maintains manual in-line stabilization even though the head is secured to the device.

g. Position long backboard under or next to patient's buttocks, and rotate patient until his back is in line with backboard.

h. Lower patient onto backboard while maintaining in-line stabilization.

        i. Immobilize patient to the long backboard.
   4. Special considerations when using a short spinal device
        a. Do any assessment of the back, scapula, arms, or clavicles before you apply the board.
        b. Angle board to fit between arms of 1st EMT, who is stabilizing patient's head, without jarring rescuer's arms.
        c. Push spine board as far down into seat as possible.
        d. Never place a chin cup or chin strap on patient.
        e. Do not apply torso strap so tightly that it could cause abdominal injury or impair breathing.
        f. Always tighten torso and leg straps before securing patient's head to device.
        g. Never allow buckles to be placed midsternum where they would interfere with CPR.
        h. Never pad between cervical collar and board.
        i. Assess pulses and motor and sensory function before and after applying the device.
   5. Rapid extrication (**Fig. 32-24, p. 903–904**)
        a. Use only in the following situations in which movement is permissible:
           (1) The scene is not safe.
           (2) You need to move and transport unstable patient immediately.
           (3) The patient blocks your access to a second, more seriously injured patient.
        b. Know that rapid extrication requires constant in-line stabilization and good communication among EMTs.
        c. Follow procedure described in detail with **Fig. 32-24, page 903–904**.

IV. Special considerations (pp. 904–911)
   A. Helmets (p. 904)
      1. Assessment
        a. Assess patient's airway and breathing.
        b. Assess fit of helmet and likelihood of movement of patient's head within helmet.
        c. Determine your ability to gain access to patient's airway.
      2. Leave helmet in place if assessment reveals the following:
        a. Helmet fits well; there is little or no movement of patient's head inside helmet.
        b. There are no impending airway or breathing problems.
        c. Removal would cause further injury to the patient.
        d. You can properly immobilize spine with helmet in place.
        e. The helmet does not interfere with your ability to assess and reassess airway and breathing.
      3. Remove helmet if assessment reveals the following:
        a. Helmet interferes with your ability to assess or reassess airway and breathing.
        b. Helmet interferes with your ability to adequately manage airway or breathing.
        c. Helmet does not fit well: allows excessive movement of head within it.
        d. Helmet interferes with proper spinal immobilization.
        e. Patient is in cardiac arrest.
   B. Helmet removal (pp. 905–907) (**Figs. 32-25 and 32-26, pp. 905–907**)

1. Take off patient's eyeglasses before you attempt to remove helmet.
2. (1st EMT) Place hands on each side of helmet, fingers on mandible (lower jaw), to provide stabilization.
3. (2nd EMT) Loosen chin strap.
4. (2nd EMT) Assume stabilization responsibility
   a. Place one hand on mandible at angle of jaw, thumb on one side, fingers on other.
   b. Place other hand in occipital region.
5. (1st EMT) Pull sides of helmet apart, gently slip helmet halfway off patient's head, and then stop.
6. (2nd EMT) Reposition, sliding hand under patient's head to keep head from falling back after helmet is completely removed.
7. (1st EMT) Remove helmet completely, and then take over stabilization.
8. (2nd EMT) Apply cervical collar and immobilize patient while 1st EMT maintains in-line stabilization.

C. Football injuries (pp. 907–909) (**Fig. 32-27, pp. 908–909**)
1. Shoulder pads and helmet hold player almost in neutral position.
2. Leave helmet on player unless absolutely necessary to remove it.
3. Remove face mask and establish and maintain airway, leaving player's helmet in place.
4. Attempt to apply a cervical immobilization collar.
5. Log rolling player onto long backboard is difficult; flat lifting is preferable.
6. After patient is secured to backboard, helmet should be taped to backboard to prevent movement.

D. Infants and children (pp. 909–911)
1. Special considerations when immobilizing
   a. Pad from shoulders to heels.
   b. Make sure cervical collar fits properly before applying it.
   c. If you don't have a collar that fits, immobilize neck with a rolled towel, taping towel to backboard, and manually supporting head in a neutral in-line position.
2. Immobilization in a car seat (**Fig. 32-28 and 32-29, pp. 910–913**)
   a. Apply manual in-line stabilization.
   b. Assess to ensure that there are no reasons for removal from car seat.
   c. Place towel rolls on both sides of child's head between head and car seat.
   d. Secure with tape across child's forehead to each side of seat.
   e. Determine that child is secure in seat; there is not a lot of room between child and seat.
   f. Transport in regular seated position with car seat securely belted to ambulance seat.

ENRICHMENT (OPTIONAL)

The following section contains information that is valuable as background for the EMT, but that goes substantially beyond the U.S. Department of Transportation's EMT-Basic National Standard Curriculum.

V. Neurogenic shock (spinal shock) (p. 911)

   A. Signs different from normal signs of shock, but treatment is similar. (p. 911)

CASE STUDY FOLLOW-UP

Ask a student volunteer to read the Case Study that begins on page 869 of the textbook. You may wish to use the following questions to engage the students in a discussion of the Case Study Follow-up that begins on page 914 of the textbook. Provide missing information and clarify ideas as needed.

Q1. How does the coach describe the mechanism of injury?

A1. *The coach says, "She missed a maneuver off the top bar. She fell and hit the bottom bar with the middle of her back, then landed head first on the floor."*

Q2. What does your rapid trauma assessment reveal about Carrie's head and neck?

A2. *There is a contusion along the scalp line above the right eye and tenderness to the cervical region at about the level of the sixth vertebrae.*

Q3. Describe your rapid trauma assessment of Carrie's upper extremities.

A3. *Inspection and palpation of Carrie's arms determines that radial pulses are present bilaterally. Responding to an EMT request, Carrie shows she can wave her hand slightly. Out of Carrie's sight, the EMT touches the little finger of her left hand, which Carrie correctly identifies. The test is repeated successfully on her right hand. Carrie grips the EMT's fingers simultaneously and demonstrates strength to be equal and strong in both upper extremities. Both radial pulses are strong.*

Q4. Describe your rapid trauma assessment of Carrie's lower extremities.

A4. *Inspection and palpation of the lower extremities reveals pedal pulses are present bilaterally. Carrie is able to move both feet, but cannot identify a touch to the big toe on the right foot. That leg is stabilized to avoid unsuspected and exaggerated movement. The top of the left foot is then pinched, which Carrie correctly identifies. The pinch is repeated on the right foot, eliciting a response to the pinch.*

Q5. How do you prepare Carrie for transport?

A5. *The coach, who is familiar with log rolling, is positioned at Carrie's feet. The backboard is positioned next to the patient. One EMT, holding in-line stabilization at Carrie's head, directs and coordinates the coach and other EMT to log roll her up for quick assessment of her back. No deformities are found, but there is some tenderness in the lumbar region. The backboard is positioned under her, and she is rolled back onto it. A void behind the lumbar region is padded, and straps are applied to the torso and legs and secured. A head/cervical immobilization device is applied and secured.*

IN REVIEW

Assess students' ability to apply what they have just learned by discussing the Review Questions on page 916 in the textbook.

Q1. Describe the relationship between the spinal column and the spinal cord.

A1. *The relationship between the spinal column and the spinal cord is the vertebrae of the spinal column sheathe and protect the spinal cord, which carries nerve impulses from the brain to other parts of the body through nerve bundles. (pp. 869–870)*

Q2. Name the most common mechanisms of spine injury.

A2. *The most common mechanisms of spine injury are compression, flexion, extension, rotation, lateral bending, distraction, and penetration. (pp. 871–872)*

Q3. List the signs and symptoms of potential spine injury.

A3. *The signs and symptoms of potential spine injury are tenderness in the area of injury, especially along spinal column; localized pain; pain independent of movement or palpation along the spine or in the lower legs; obvious deformity of the spine; soft tissue injuries; numbness, weakness, tingling, or loss of sensation in arms and/or legs; loss of sensation or paralysis of the extremities; incontinence; priapism; and impaired or diaphragmatic breathing. (pp. 878–879)*

Q4. Explain the types of stabilization and immobilization that must be applied in cases of suspected spine injury.

A4. *The types of stabilization and immobilization that must be applied in cases of suspected spine injury are manual, in-line stabilization from initial patient contact until the patient is fully immobilized with a head/cervical immobilization device and straps to a backboard. (pp. 880–883)*

Q5. Describe how the airway is managed in a patient with a suspected spine injury.

A5. *To manage the airway in a patient with a suspected spine injury, after in-line spinal stabilization is applied, open the airway with a jaw-thrust maneuver. Insert an oropharyngeal or nasopharyngeal airway, if necessary. Suction the airway instead of turning the patient's head for drainage. Because breathing problems are common in such cases, be prepared to provide positive-pressure ventilation. (p. 881)*

Q6. Explain the purpose and use of the cervical spine immobilization collar.

A6. *The cervical spine immobilization collar prevents the head from moving in relation to the spine and reduces compression of the cervical spine during movement of the patient; it does not immobilize the patient. (p. 881)*

Q7. Explain how to assess motor and sensory function in a patient with suspected spine injury.

A7. *To assess motor function, check upper extremities by having a patient grip your fingers with both hands; check lower extremities by having him push both his feet against your hands. To assess sensory function, touch the patient's hands and feet lightly out of his sight; if the patient can't detect the touches, pinch the hand and/or foot. (p. 874 and Fig. 32-4, pp. 875–876)*

Q8. Explain the use of long and short spinal immobilization devices for seated patients with suspected spine injuries.

A8. *For seated patients with suspected spine injuries, the patient is first immobilized to the short device to prevent aggravation of the injury as he is moved to a supine position for full immobilization to a long device. (p. 893–895)*

Q9. Under what circumstances is rapid extrication appropriate?

A9. *Rapid extrication is appropriate only in situations where the scene is not safe; where the patient's condition is so unstable that you need to move and transport him immediately; or where the patient blocks access to others more seriously injured. (p. 902–904)*

Q10. Under what circumstances should you leave a helmet in place on a patient with suspected spine injury?

A10. *A helmet should be left on the patient if it fits well and there's little movement of the patient's head inside the helmet; there are no impending airway or breathing problems; there is no difficulty in accessing the airway if problems arise; there is no interference with patient immobilization; or removing the helmet would cause further injury. (p. 904)*

CRITICAL THINKING

Assess students' ability to respond to real-life emergency situations by discussing the Critical Thinking questions on page 916 in the textbook.

Q1. What initial emergency care would you provide to the patient?

A1. *One EMT should immediately establish manual in-line spine stabilization. A nonrebreather should be applied to the patient and set at 15 lpm.*

Q2. What would you assess in your neurological exam on the patient?

A2. *Motor function and light touch and pain sensation must be assessed in the patient. Motor function must be assessed in both the upper and lower extremities. Have the patient close her eyes and assess for both pain sensation and light in all four extremities.*

Q3. Based on the presentation, what type of spinal cord injury do you suspect?

A3. *The patient presents with loss of motor function in the upper extremities; however, the patient retains good motor function in the lower extremities. This is an indication of an incomplete spinal cord injury involving the central portion of the spinal cord. This injury pattern may occur in elderly patients as a result of a hyperextension mechanism of injury.*

Q4. What other assessment findings would confirm the type of suspected spinal injury?

A4. *Assess for pain and light touch function in all four extremities. The patient should retain pain and some light touch sensation. If this were a complete spinal cord injury, the patient would have no motor function and pain or light touch sensation below the level of injury.*

Q5. How would you manage the spinal injury?

A5. *Because the patient has suffered a spinal cord injury, the patient must be completely immobilized to a backboard. Continue with oxygen therapy and perform ongoing assessments en route to the medical facility.*

SKILLS DEMONSTRATION AND PRACTICE

Write the following on a chalkboard, flipchart, or overhead transparency:

1. Spinal immobilization of a seated patient and rapid extrication procedure
2. Four-rescuer log roll and spinal immobilization of a supine patient
3. Rapid takedown of standing patient
4. Helmet removal from injured patient
5. Immobilizing in a child safety seat and rapid extrication from a child safety seat

Tell students that in just a moment you are going to divide them into teams of four. Each team is to visit the five listed demonstration and practice stations. At each station, there will be a "patient" and a teaching assistant who will demonstrate and help the students practice the skill. Divide the class into teams. If there is an odd number of students, it is acceptable to have a team of three or five, provided that each student practices each skill.

Direct each team to its first practice station. Pay special attention to student safety.

When each team has completed each station, make sure that students return to the main classroom.

ASSIGNMENTS

Assign students to read Chapter 33, "Eye, Face, and Neck Injuries," before the next class. Also ask them to complete Chapter 32 of the Workbook.

EVALUATION

Chapter Quiz Distribute copies of the Chapter Quiz provided in Handout 32-2 to evaluate student understanding of this chapter. Remind students not to refer to their textbooks or notes while taking the quiz.

Test Manager You may wish to create a custom-tailored test using Prentice Hall *TestGen for Prehospital Emergency Care, Eighth Edition* to evaluate student understanding of this chapter.

Online Test Preparation (for students and instructors) Additional test preparation is available through *EMT Achieve: Basic Test Preparation* at http://www.prenhall.com/EMTAchieve. Instructors can also monitor student mastery online.

Reading/Reference
Textbook, pp. 917–940

Workbook
Chapter 32 Activities

Chapter Quiz
Handout 32-2

TestGen
Chapter 32 Test

Online Test Preparation
Send your students to
http://www.prenhall.com/
EMTAchieve

Handouts 32-3 to 32-7
Reinforcement Activities

**Brady Skills Series
EMT-B Videos/CD**
Visual Reinforcement

**PowerPoint
Presentation**
Chapter 32

Student CD
Chapter 32

Companion Website
http://www.prenhall.com/
mistovich

REINFORCEMENT

Handouts If classroom discussions or performance on the quiz indicates that some students have not fully mastered the chapter content, you may wish to assign some or all of the Reinforcement Handouts for this chapter.

TECH EXTRAS

Brady Skills Series EMT-B Videos/CD Have your students watch the skills come to life on either VHS or CD-ROM.

PowerPoint Presentation (for instructors) The PowerPoint material developed for this chapter offers useful reinforcement of chapter content.

Student CD A wide variety of material on this CD-ROM will reinforce and also expand student knowledge and skills.

Companion Website (for students) Additional review quizzes and links to EMS resources will contribute to further reinforcement of this chapter. Please visit http://www.prenhall.com/mistovich.

OBJECTIVES CHECKLIST

Cognitive		Date Mastered
5-4.1	State the components of the nervous system.	
5-4.2	List the functions of the central nervous system.	
5-4.3	Define the structure of the skeletal system as it relates to the nervous system.	
5-4.4	Relate mechanism of injury to potential injuries of the head and spine.	
5-4.5	Describe the implications of not properly caring for potential spine injuries.	
5-4.6	State the signs and symptoms of a potential spine injury.	
5-4.7	Describe the method of determining if a responsive patient may have a spine injury.	
5-4.8	Relate the airway emergency medical care techniques to the patient with a suspected spine injury.	
5-4.9	Describe how to stabilize the cervical spine.	
5-4.10	Discuss indications for sizing and using a cervical spine immobilization device.	
5-4.11	Establish the relationship between airway management and the patient with head and spine injuries.	
5-4.12	Describe a method for sizing a cervical spine immobilization device.	
5-4.13	Describe how to log roll a patient with a suspected spine injury.	
5-4.14	Describe how to secure a patient to a long spine board.	
5-4.15	List instances when a short spine board should be used.	
5-4.16	Describe how to immobilize a patient using a short spine board.	
5-4.17	Describe the indications for the use of rapid extrication.	
5-4.18	List steps in performing rapid extrication.	
5-4.19	State the circumstances when a helmet should be left on the patient.	
5-4.20	Discuss the circumstances when a helmet should be removed.	
5-4.21	Identify different types of helmets.	
5-4.22	Describe the unique characteristics of sports helmets.	
5-4.23	Explain the preferred methods to remove a helmet.	
5-4.24	Discuss alternative methods for removal of a helmet.	
5-4.25	Describe how the patient's head is stabilized to remove the helmet.	
5-4.26	Differentiate how the head is stabilized with a helmet compared to without a helmet.	

OBJECTIVES

Affective		Date Mastered
5-4.27	Explain the rationale for immobilization of the entire spine when a cervical spine injury is suspected.	
5-4.28	Explain the rationale for utilizing immobilization methods apart from the straps on the cots.	
5-4.29	Explain the rationale for utilizing a short spine immobilization device when moving a patient from the sitting to the supine position.	
5-4.30	Explain the rationale for utilizing rapid extrication approaches only when they indeed will make the difference between life and death.	
5-4.31	Defend the reasons for leaving a helmet in place for transport of a patient.	
5-4.32	Defend the reasons for removal of a helmet prior to transport of a patient.	

Psychomotor		Date Mastered
5-4.33	Demonstrate opening the airway in a patient with suspected spinal cord injury.	
5-4.34	Demonstrate evaluating a responsive patient with a suspected spinal cord injury.	
5-4.35	Demonstrate stabilization of the cervical spine.	
5-4.36	Demonstrate the four-person log roll for a patient with a suspected spinal cord injury.	
5-4.37	Demonstrate how to log roll a patient with a suspected spinal cord injury using two people.	
5-4.38	Demonstrate securing a patient to a long spine board.	
5-4.39	Demonstrate using the short board immobilization technique.	
5-4.40	Demonstrate procedure for rapid extrication.	
5-4.41	Demonstrate preferred methods for stabilization of a helmet.	
5-4.42	Demonstrate helmet removal techniques.	
5-4.43	Demonstrate alternative methods for stabilization of a helmet.	
5-4.44	Demonstrate completing a prehospital care report for patients with head and spina injuries.	

CHAPTER 32 QUIZ

Write the letter of the best answer in the space provided.

_____ 1. All of the following are signs and symptoms in patients with spinal injuries *except*
    A. paralysis.   **C.** hyperglycemia.
    B. priapism.   **D.** incontinence.

_____ 2. The part of the nervous system located outside of the brain and spinal cord that detects sensations such as pain is the _____ nervous system.
    A. peripheral   **C.** central
    B. autonomic   **D.** involuntary

_____ 3. The part of the nervous system that controls involuntary functions such as heartbeat and breathing is the _____ nervous system.
    A. peripheral   **C.** central
    B. autonomic   **D.** involuntary

_____ 4. Sports helmets most typically open in the
    A. front.   **C.** left side.
    B. back.   **D.** right side.

_____ 5. In the prehospital environment, the two most likely types of helmets to be encountered are the sports helmet and the _____ helmet.
    A. flight   **C.** football
    B. military   **D.** motorcycle

_____ 6. The mechanism of injury in which the vertebrae and spinal cord are stretched and pulled apart is called
    A. rotation.   **C.** distraction.
    B. flexion.   **D.** extension.

_____ 7. The appropriate time to initiate in-line stabilization of the cervical spine is
    A. prior to opening the airway.
    B. after opening the airway.
    C. during transport.
    D. after insertion of an oropharyngeal airway.

_____ 8. In spinal shock, a patient's skin is
    A. cool and dry.   **C.** flushed and damp.
    B. warm and dry.   **D.** cool and sweaty.

_____ 9. Probably the most common and reliable sign of spinal-cord injury in conscious patients is
    A. Battle's sign.   **C.** raccoon's sign.
    B. pupil dilation.   **D.** paralysis of the extremities.

_____ 10. In the normal extrication of a patient with suspected spinal injury, the device that an EMT would apply first is the
    A. cervical collar.   **C.** Kendrick Extrication Device.
    B. short spine board.   **D.** long spine board.

_____ **11.** The mechanism of injury in which there is severe forward movement of the head or the torso is curved excessively forward is called

    A. rotation.

    B. flexion.

    C. distraction.

    D. extension.

_____ **12.** When applying a short spine board or flexible extrication device, you should first secure the

    A. torso.

    B. chest.

    C. shoulders.

    D. head.

_____ **13.** The move used to shift a supine patient onto a long backboard for immobilization is the

    A. blanket drag.

    B. armpit–forearm drag.

    C. firefighter's lift.

    D. log roll.

_____ **14.** The spinal column is composed of 33 bones called

    A. meninges.

    B. vertebrae.

    C. phalanges.

    D. carpals.

_____ **15.** Which one of the following is *not* an indication for removing a helmet in a case of suspected head or spine injury?

    A. Helmet interferes with assessment of the ABCs.

    B. Helmet fits snugly.

    C. Patient goes into cardiac arrest.

    D. Helmet fits loosely.

IN THE FIELD

Read the following real-life situation. Then answer the questions that follow.

You and your partner are called to the football stadium at the local high school. You arrive to find the quarterback lying in the center of the field at the 30-yard line in a supine position. Coaches are gathered around him, and one of them meets you as you exit the ambulance. This coach tells you that the quarterback has not moved since he was tackled. As you approach, you notice that none of the quarterback's protective gear has been removed.

1. What is your general impression of the mechanism of the patient's injury?

2. As you approach the patient, what should you do?

3. What device would you use for transporting the patient?

4. What continuing emergency care steps would you provide for this patient?

CHAPTER 32 REVIEW

Write the word or words that best complete each sentence in the space provided.

1. Two major functions of the nervous system are _____ and

   _____.

2. The structural divisions of the nervous system are the _____ nervous

   system and the _____ nervous system.

3. The functional divisions of the nervous system are the _____ nervous

   system and the _____ nervous system.

4. The _____ _____ gives the body its framework,

   supports and protects vital organs, and permits motion.

5. The _____ _____ is the principal support system

   of the body.

6. The spinal column is made up of 33 irregularly shaped bones called _____.

7. The first seven vertebrae, which form the neck, are called the _____

   _____.

8. _____ _____ must not be released until the

   patient is securely strapped to a backboard and is completely immobilized.

9. A condition referred to as _____ shock inhibits neural transmissions to the

   arteries and arterioles.

10. If neurogenic shock is caused by spinal-cord injury, it may be called _____

    shock.

11. _____ is a persistent erection of the penis resulting from the damage to the

    spinal nerves to the genitals.

12. Damage to the spinal cord and neck can produce complete paralysis of the entire body, a condition

    called _____.

13. Paralysis to only one side of the body is more common in head injuries and stroke, and it is called

    _____.

14. An EMT will need to _____ _____ a supine

patient to apply the long backboard.

15. Whenever an EMT sees a spider-web-cracked windshield, he or she knows that the driver needs full

_____ _____.

Spine Injuries: Listing

1. List the structural divisions and functional divisions of the nervous system.

2. List four signs or symptoms that suggest a possible spinal injury.

3. List the five divisions of the spinal or vertebral column and the number of vertebra in each.

©2008 by Pearson Education, Inc.
Prehospital Emergency Care, 8th ed.

4. Compression is one mechanism of spinal injury. List six others.

5. List questions that should be asked during assessment of a patient with suspected spine injury.

SPINE INJURIES: TRUE OR FALSE

Indicate if the following statements are true or false by writing T or F in the space provided.

_____ **1.** If the EMT suspects that the patient has a spinal injury, he or she should initiate spinal precautions.

_____ **2.** Your suspicion regarding the presence of a spinal injury should *not* be altered by the patient's ability to walk.

_____ **3.** Until the EMT has completely immobilized the patient, manual stabilization of the head and neck should be maintained.

_____ **4.** Because an improperly fitting immobilization device will do more harm than good, proper sizing is of utmost importance.

_____ **5.** The larger head of the infant or young child will cause the head to flex when the patient is supine.

_____ **6.** If a sports helmet is left in place on the patient, the spine is considered to be properly immobilized.

_____ **7.** Spinal injury cannot exist without external evidence of trauma.

_____ **8.** Spinal shock results specifically from injury to the spinal cord, usually high in the cervical spine.

_____ **9.** A single spinal-cord injury can affect several body organ systems.

_____ **10.** If a patient is responsive, a rapid trauma assessment is *not* indicated.

©2008 by Pearson Education, Inc.
Prehospital Emergency Care, 8th ed.

REINFORCEMENT

IMMOBILIZATION

Review your knowledge of immobilization techniques by putting the steps of the procedures below in proper order. With each procedure, write "1" in the space provided next to the step you would perform first, "2" next to the step you would perform next, and so on.

A. Spinal Immobilization of a Supine Patient

_____ Immobilize patient's torso to the board.

_____ Move patient onto long board without compromising integrity of spine.

_____ Apply appropriately sized cervical collar.

_____ Immobilize patient's head to the long board.

_____ Secure patient's legs to board.

_____ Place head in neutral in-line position and maintain manual stabilization.

_____ Position long spine board.

B. Spinal Immobilization of a Seated Patient

_____ Immobilize to long spine board.

_____ Apply appropriately sized cervical collar.

_____ Rotate patient and lower to long spine board.

_____ Pad behind patient's head as necessary.

_____ Manually stabilize patient's head in neutral in-line position.

_____ Position short immobilization device behind patient.

_____ As needed, secure patient's legs.

_____ Secure patient's head to the device.

_____ Secure device to patient's torso.

Injuries to the Spine

Anatomy and Physiology of Spine Injury

Nervous System

- Functions
- Divisions

Skeletal System

- Skull
- Spinal column
- Mechanisms of spine injury
- Compression
- Flexion
- Extension
- Rotation
- Lateral bending
- Distraction
- Penetration

Assessment and Care Guidelines for Immobilization

Tools

- Cervical spine immobilization collars
- Full-body spinal immobilization devices
- Short spinal immobilization devices
- Other equipment

©2008 by Pearson Education, Inc.
Prehospital Emergency Care, 8th ed.

Immobilization Techniques
- Supine or prone patient
- Standing patient
- Seated patient
- Rapid extrication

Special Considerations
Helmets

Infants and Children

Neurogenic Shock (Spinal Shock)

HANDOUT 32-2: Chapter 32 Quiz

1. C	**5.** D	**9.** D	**13.** D
2. A	**6.** C	**10.** A	**14.** B
3. B	**7.** A	**11.** B	**15.** B
4. A	**8.** B	**12.** A	

HANDOUT 32-3: In the Field

1. The patient possibly suffered an injury to his spinal cord when he was tackled.
2. You should take BSI precautions, approach from the patient's head to prevent movement, provide in-line stabilization of the cervical spine, assess the ABCs and PMS in the extremities, and assess the cervical region and spine. After those steps, you would apply the collar and prepare to immobilize the patient to a long spine board for transport.
3. A long spine board with appropriately sized cervical collar, straps, and head/cervical immobilization device
4. Continuing emergency care steps include providing oxygen, performing a detailed assessment; continuing an ongoing assessment en route to the hospital, monitoring vital signs, and getting additional history, if possible.

HANDOUT 32-4: Chapter 32 Review

1. communication, control
2. central, peripheral
3. voluntary, autonomic
4. skeletal system
5. spinal column
6. vertebrae
7. cervical spine
8. Manual stabilization
9. neurogenic
10. spinal
11. Priapism
12. quadriplegia
13. hemiplegia
14. log roll
15. spinal immobilization

HANDOUT 32-5: Spine Injuries: Listing

1. Structural: central and peripheral. Functional autonomic and voluntary.
2. Paralysis of the extremities, loss of bowel or bladder control, pain independent of movement or palpation along spinal column or in lower legs; localized pain with movement; obvious deformity of spine upon palpation; tenderness anywhere along the spine; soft tissue injuries to the head and neck, shoulders, back, abdomen, or lower extremities; numbness, weakness, tingling, or loss of sensation in extremities; priapism; impaired breathing.
3. Cervical, 7; thoracic, 12; lumbar, 5; sacral, 5; coccyx, 4.
4. Flexion, extension, rotation, lateral bending, distraction, penetration.
5. Does your neck hurt? Does your back hurt? Where does it hurt? Can you move your hands and feet? Do you have any pain or muscle spasms along your back or neck? Is there any numbness or tingling in arms or legs? Was the onset of pain associated with the injury? Did you move or did someone move you before EMTs arrived? Were you walking around before EMTs arrived?

HANDOUT 32-6: Spine Injuries: True or False

1. T	**4.** T	**7.** F	**9.** T
2. T	**5.** T	**8.** T	**10.** F
3. T	**6.** F		

HANDOUT 32-7: Immobilization

The order of steps reading down in each column should be:
A. 5, 4, 2, 6, 7, 1, 3
B. 9, 2, 8, 6, 1, 3, 5, 7, 4

©2008 by Pearson Education, Inc.
Prehospital Emergency Care, 8th ed.

33 Eye, Face, and Neck Injuries

This chapter contains information that is valuable as background for the EMT but that goes substantially beyond the U.S. Department of Transportation (DOT) EMT-Basic curriculum.

OBJECTIVES

Numbered objectives are from the U.S. Department of Transportation's EMT-Basic National Standard Curriculum. Asterisked objectives, if any, pertain to material that is supplemental to the DOT curriculum. Page numbers refer to pages in the textbook.

Cognitive

* * List the major anatomical structures of the eye, face, and neck. (pp. 918–919)
* * Describe the relationship between eye, face, and neck injuries and the personal protection and safety of the EMT-Basic. (p. 920)
* * List the overall assessment procedures for eye, face, and neck injuries. (pp. 920–922)
* * Describe the general assessment procedures for eye injuries, including use of the penlight. (pp. 922–923, 928)
* * List the basic rules for emergency medical care for eye injuries. (pp. 922–923, 928)
* * List specific common eye injuries and describe their appropriate emergency medical care. (pp. 923–927)
* * Describe emergency medical care for eye-injured patients wearing contact lenses. (pp. 917–928)
* * Describe the general assessment and care guidelines for face injuries. (pp. 929–931, 935)
* * List the signs and symptoms and describe the emergency medical care for injuries to the mid-face, upper jaw, and lower jaw. (pp. 931–933)
* * Describe the emergency medical care for an object impaled in the cheek. (p. 933)
* * Describe the emergency medical care for injuries to the nose and ear. (pp. 933–934)
* * List special signs or symptoms of injury to the neck. (p. 936)
* * Describe the emergency medical care for injuries to the neck. (pp. 935–938)

Affective

* * Recognize and respect the feelings of a patient suffering eye, face, or neck injury. (pp. 917, 920)

Total Teaching Time
115 minutes

Resources Needed
* Scored Chapter 32 Quizzes
* Moulage materials for simulating injuries
* Large supply of dressings and bandages

Additional Resources
Larmon/Davis, *Basic Life Support Skills*

Elling, *EMT Achieve: Basic Test Preparation*

Limmer/Mistovich/ O'Keefe, *Audio Lecture & Study Guide: EMT*

Mistovich/Kuvlesky, *SUCCESS! for the EMT, Second Edition*

*   Demonstrate the steps in the emergency medical care of common eye injuries.

*   Demonstrate the steps in the removal of soft and hard contact lenses from eye-injured patients.

*   Demonstrate the steps in the emergency medical care of various types of face, jaw, and neck injuries, including care for avulsed teeth and for severed blood vessels to the neck.

REVIEW

In the last chapter, students learned that spinal injuries are among the most formidable and traumatic they will manage as EMTs. Yet EMTs may face such injuries on almost a daily basis. Automobile crashes, shallow-water diving accidents, motorcycle crashes, and falls are all common causes of spine injury. Likewise, accidents during skiing, sledding, football, and gymnastics can result in spine injury. It is the job of the EMT to recognize injuries that could damage the spinal column or spinal cord and to provide appropriate emergency care. EMTs must also be aware that improper movement and handling of patients in such situations can easily lead to permanent disability or even death.

Distribute the quizzes from the last class. Go over each question on the quiz and handle any concerns students may have about the answers.

INTRODUCTION TO CHAPTER 33

Chapter 33, "Eye, Face, and Neck Injuries," is the eighth chapter in Module 5. If your students have ever experienced a serious eye, facial, or neck injury, they can appreciate a patient's fear and panic associated with one of these emergencies. Aside from the pain, injuries to the eye cause emotional duress as the patient thinks about the possible loss of vision, and the patient who suffers a facial injury may fear permanent scarring or disfigurement. As EMTs, students must remain aware that injuries to the eyes, face, or neck have a high probability of causing airway compromise, severe bleeding, and shock. Additionally, injury to the face and neck is likely to be associated with spinal injury. While caring for the sometimes dramatic or horrific injuries themselves, students must always maintain a high index of suspicion for spinal injury and give first priority to care for life-threatening compromise of the airway and circulation.

Distribute the Chapter 33 Objectives Checklist, and give students a few minutes to look it over. Then briefly paraphrase the objectives for this lesson in your own words.

Handout 33-1
Chapter 33 Objectives Checklist

Lecture Master
You may wish to display Lecture Master 33 when presenting the lecture to the class.

LECTURE

The following suggested lecture outline is based on the Department of Transportation's EMT-Basic National Standard Curriculum. In some places, the DOT curriculum has been rearranged or expanded upon so that it is more complete or easier for the student to understand. The page numbers in parentheses refer to pages in the textbook. The parenthetical references in dark, heavy type are to figures, tables, and scans in the textbook.

EYE, FACE, AND NECK INJURIES

I. Anatomy of the eye, face, and neck (pp. 918–920)
  A. Eye (pp. 918–919) **(Fig. 33-1, p. 919)**
    1. Sclera
       a. Tough outer coat; the "white of the eye"
    2. Cornea
       a. Clear front portion of eye
    3. Pupil
       a. Dark, center opening of eye that expands or contracts to regulate light
    4. Iris
       a. Colored portion of eye
    5. Anterior chamber
       a. Front interior chamber filled with aqueous humor
    6. Aqueous humor
       a. Watery fluid
    7. Vitreous body
       a. Area behind lens
    8. Vitreous humor
       a. Clear jelly that fills vitreous body
  B. Face (p. 919)
    1. Composed of one movable bone (mandible or lower jaw) and 13 immovable bones
    2. Is part of skull and helps protect brain
    3. Compromise of facial structures **(Fig. 33-2, p. 920)** can also cause brain injury
    4. May cause airway compromise when injured
    5. Mechanism of injury is likely to also cause spinal injury
    6. Is extremely vascular so bleeds profusely
  C. Neck (pp. 919–920) **(Fig. 33-3, p. 921)**
    1. Carotid arteries
    2. Jugular veins
    3. Trachea
    4. Larynx
    5. Cervical spine (posterior neck)
    6. Assume that any injury to neck has caused spinal injury.

II. Eye, face, and neck injuries (pp. 920–938)
  A. Assessment and care: eye, face, and neck injuries (pp. 920–922)
    1. Scene size-up
       a. Try to determine mechanism of injury.
       b. Protect your own safety.
    2. Initial assessment
       a. Establish manual in-line stabilization of head and neck.
       b. Open airway with jaw-thrust maneuver.
       c. Suction vomitus and other substances as needed.
       d. Consider advanced life support backup.
       e. Breathing adequate
         (1) Provide oxygen at 15 liters per minute by nonrebreather mask.
       f. Breathing inadequate
         (1) Provide positive-pressure ventilation with supplemental oxygen.
       g. Control severe bleeding.

       h. Determine transport priority, treating the following injuries as high priority:
         (1) Chemical burns to eye
         (2) Impaled object in eye
         (3) Extruded eyeball
         (4) Severe injuries to face or throat
         (5) Respiratory distress
         (6) Major bleeding

  3. Focused history and physical exam
     a. Unresponsive patient/significant mechanism of injury
       (1) Begin with rapid trauma assessment.
     b. Responsive patient
       (1) Conduct focused trauma assessment.
     c. Check for DCAP-BTLS
     d. Check crepitation if facial injury.
     e. Conduct penlight eye exam if eye injury.
     f. Record baseline vitals.
     g. Be prepared to treat for shock.
     h. Obtain a SAMPLE history.
     i. Use OPQRST mnemonic to assess pain.

  4. Detailed physical exam and ongoing assessment
     a. Conduct detailed physical exam if time and patient's condition permit.
     b. Conduct ongoing assessment
       (1) Monitoring for deterioration of mental status, airway, or breathing

B. Injuries to the eye (pp. 922–928) **(Fig. 33-16, p. 929)**
  1. Assessment and care guidelines
     a. Penlight evaluation **(Fig. 33-4, p. 922)**
       (1) Orbits
         (a) Bruising, swelling, laceration, tenderness
       (2) Lids
         (a) Bruising, swelling, laceration
       (3) Conjunctiva
         (a) Redness, pus, foreign bodies
       (4) Globe
         (a) Redness, abnormal coloring, laceration
       (5) Pupils
         (a) Size, shape, equality, reactivity to light
       (6) Eye movements in all directions
         (a) Abnormal gaze, paralysis of gaze, pain on movement
     b. Basic rules for emergency medical eye care
       (1) If eye is swollen shut, avoid unnecessary manipulation.
       (2) Do not force eyelid open unless you need to wash out chemicals.
       (3) Consult medical direction or local protocol before irrigating.
       (4) Do not put salve or medicine in an injured eye.
       (5) Do not remove blood or blood clots from eye.
       (6) Have patient lie down and keep quiet.
       (7) Limit patient's use of uninjured eye.
       (8) Give patient nothing by mouth.
       (9) Transport all patients with eye injuries.
     c. Foreign object in the eye **(Fig. 33-5, p. 923)**

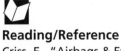

Reading/Reference

Criss, E., "Airbags & Eye Injuries," *JEMS,* May 2005.

On the Net

Eye injuries. http://www.nlm.nih.gov/medlineplus/eyeinjuries.html

On the Net

Preventing eye injuries. http://www.preventblindness.org/safety/prvnt_injuries.html

Point to Emphasize

Do not use anything other than water or saline to irrigate the patient's eyes.

(1) Generally safer to transport than to attempt to remove particles in the field

(2) Attempt removal only of objects in the conjunctiva and only with approval of medical direction and local protocol. **(Fig. 33-6, p. 923)**

    (a) Follow local protocol.

    (b) Flush with clean water.

    (c) Hold eyelids apart, if possible.

(3) Removing particle from white of eye **(Fig. 33-7, p. 923)**

    (a) Pull down lower lid while patient looks up, or pull up upper lid while patient looks down.

    (b) Remove object with a piece of sterile gauze or a swab.

(4) Removing foreign object from upper eyelid **(Fig. 33-8, p. 924)**

    (a) Draw upper lid down over lower lid and release.

    (b) If object remains, grasp upper lid lashes, and turn lid upward over a cotton swab or similar object.

    (c) Carefully remove object with corner of sterile gauze or swab.

(5) Removing foreign object from lower eyelid

    (a) Pull down lower lid.

    (b) Remove object with a piece of sterile gauze or a swab.

d. Injury to the orbits **(Fig. 33-9, p. 925)**

(1) If fracture is suspected, establish and maintain spinal stabilization.

(2) Inspect and palpate for signs and symptoms of injury or orbital fracture.

    (a) Double vision

    (b) Marked decrease in vision

    (c) Loss of sensation above eyebrow, over cheek, or in upper lip

    (d) Nasal discharge

    (e) Tenderness to palpation

    (f) Bony "step-off"

    (g) Paralysis of upward gaze

(3) Uninjured eyeball: place cold packs over injured eye and transport patient in sitting position.

(4) Injured eyeball: avoid using cold packs and transport patient in supine position.

e. Lid injury (include bruising, burns, and lacerations) **(Fig. 33-10, p. 925)**

(1) Control bleeding with light pressure from a dressing; use no pressure at all if eyeball is injured

(2) Cover lid with sterile gauze soaked in saline.

(3) Preserve any avulsed skin and carry it with patient for possible grafting.

(4) Uninjured eyeball—cover injured lid with cold compresses to reduce swelling.

(5) Cover the uninjured eye with a bandage to decrease movement.

        (6) Transport.

    f. Injury to the globe (**Fig. 33-11, p. 925**)

        (1) Recognize signs and symptoms of an injury to the globe

           (a) Obvious bruising, lacerations, foreign objects, abrasions

           (b) Corneal abrasions, inflammation of conjunctiva, corneal ulcers (indicate overnight or extended contact lens wear)

           (c) Pear shaped-irregular eyeball

           (d) Blood in anterior chamber of eye

           (e) Minimal external signs if mechanism of injury was high-speed activity (e.g., grinding)

        (2) Best treated at hospital; if necessary to treat in the field:

           (a) If eyeball not ruptured, apply patches lightly to both eyes.

           (b) Apply an eye shield to injured eye.

           (c) Keep patient supine.

           (d) Transport.

    g. Chemical burn to the eye (**Fig. 33-12, p. 926**)

        (1) Immediately begin irrigation with clean or sterile water or saline.

        (2) Hold eyelids open.

        (3) Continuously irrigate for at least 20 minutes. (**Fig. 33-13, p. 926**)

        (4) If injury due to an alkali, continuously irrigate for at least 60 minutes.

        (5) Use running water or continuously pour water across eye. Run or pour water from inside corner, across eyeball to outside edge, taking care not to contaminate uninjured eye. Use eye wash system if available at the site.

        (6) Remove or flush out contact lenses.

        (7) Remove any solid particles with a moistened cotton swab.

        (8) Place patient on his side on stretcher, with basin or towels under head.

        (9) Continue irrigation throughout transport.

      (10) Following irrigation, wash your own hands thoroughly and clean under your nails with a nail brush.

    h. Impaled object in the eye or extruded eyeball

        (1) Do not remove impaled object and never try to replace eye in socket. (**Figs. 33-14 and 33-15, pp. 927–928**)

        (2) Place patient supine and immobilize head.

        (3) Encircle eye and impaled object with a gauze dressing or soft sterile cloth.

        (4) Do not apply pressure.

        (5) If necessary, cut a hole in a single bulky dressing to accommodate impaled object.

        (6) Place a metal shield, crushed paper cup, or cone over impaled object or extruded eyeball.

        (7) Do not use a Styrofoam cup.

(8) Ensure that impaled object or eyeball does not touch top or sides of cup.

(9) Hold cup and dressing in place with self-adhering or roller bandage that covers both eyes.

(10) Bandage both eyes to prevent eye movement.

(11) If patient is unresponsive, close uninjured eye before bandaging.

(12) Transport immediately.

2. Removing contact lenses

  a. Remove contact lenses if

    (1) Chemical burn to eye

    (2) Patient wearing hard contact lenses is unresponsive and transport will be lengthy or delayed

  b. Do not remove contact lenses if

    (1) Eyeball is injured (other than chemical burn)

    (2) Transport time is short enough to allow emergency department to remove lens

  c. Removing soft contact lenses (**Fig. 33-17, p. 930**)

    (1) Pull the lid down with our fingertip on lower lid.

    (2) Place index fingertip on lower edge of lens.

    (3) Slide lens down to sclera.

    (4) Compress lens gently between your thumb and index finger and remove from eye.

    (5) Store removed lens in water or saline solution.

  d. Removing hard contact lenses (**Figs. 33-18 and 33-19, p. 930**)

    (1) Separate eyelids.

    (2) Position visible lens over cornea by manipulating eyelids.

    (3) Place thumbs gently on top and bottom eyelids and open eyelids wide.

    (4) Gently press eyelids down and forward to edges of lens.

    (5) Press lower eyelid slightly harder and move it under bottom edge of lens.

    (6) Moving eyelids toward each other, slide lens out between them.

C. Injuries to the face (pp. 928–934) (**Fig. 33-20, p. 931**)

  1. Assessment and care guidelines (**Fig. 33-25, p. 935**)

    a. Injury to the mid-face, upper jaw, or lower jaw (**Figs. 33-21 and 33-22, pp. 932–933**)

      (1) Establish and maintain in-line stabilization.

        (a) Inspect mouth for small fragments.

        (b) Pick fragments from mouth or remove them with finger sweeps.

        (c) Leave in place secure and unbroken dentures; remove broken or loose ones.

        (d) Open airway, using jaw-thrust maneuver.

        (e) If necessary, pull tongue forward.

        (f) If possible, insert oral airway.

        (g) Suction blood, vomitus, secretions, or small debris from mouth and throat throughout treatment and transport.

        (h) Request advanced life support backup if needed.

Point to Emphasize

The primary concern with facial fractures is the patient's airway. Be prepared to suction it and remove debris and blood. Because of possible spinal injury, use the jaw-thrust maneuver to open the airway.

On the Net

Causes of facial trauma. http://www.drpaulgeunes.com/Facial_Trauma/facial_trauma.html

(2) Adequate breathing
- **(a)** Provide oxygen by nonrebreather mask at 15 liters per minute.

(3) Inadequate breathing
- **(a)** Begin positive-pressure ventilation with supplemental oxygen.

(4) Control severe bleeding.

(5) Cover any exposed nerves, tendons, or blood vessels with a moist, sterile dressing.

(6) If a tooth has been lost, try to find it.
- **(a)** Rinse tooth with saline.
- **(b)** Transport tooth in a cup of saline or wrapped in gauze soaked in sterile saline.
- **(c)** Seek medical direction and follow local protocol.

(7) Treat for shock and transport.

b. Object impaled in the cheek

(1) Stabilize object with bulky dressings and transport patient.

(2) If object may fall into mouth and obstruct airway, remove it.
- **(a)** Pull or push object out of cheek in same direction it entered.
- **(b)** Pack dressing material between patient's teeth and wound.
- **(c)** Tape end of dressing outside mouth to prevent patient from swallowing it.
- **(d)** Monitor closely to ensure that dressing doesn't come loose and compromise airway.

(3) Dress and bandage outside of wound to control bleeding.

(4) Consider requesting ALS backup if needed.

(5) Suction mouth and throat frequently during transport.

c. Injury to the nose (**Fig. 33-23, p. 934**)

(1) Assess and treat as for other soft tissue injuries.

(2) Take special care to maintain open airway.

(3) Position patient so that blood does not drain into throat.

(4) Never pack an injured nose.

(5) Do not try to remove foreign objects in nose.

(6) Look for swelling and deformity, signs and symptoms of nasal fracture.

(7) If nasal fracture, apply cold compresses and transport.

d. Injury to the ear (**Fig. 33-24, p. 934**)

(1) Assess and treat as for other soft tissue injuries.

(2) Save any avulsed parts, wrapping them in saline-soaked gauze and transporting with patient.

(3) When dressing, place part of dressing between ear and head.

(4) Never pack ear to stop bleeding.

(5) Place loose clean dressing across opening, but do not exert pressure to stop bleeding.

(6) Do not attempt to remove foreign objects from ear.

D. Injuries to the neck (pp. 934–938) **(Figs. 33-26, 33-27, and 33-28, pp. 936–938)**
   1. Signs and symptoms
      a. Obvious swelling or bruising
      b. Difficulty speaking
      c. Loss of voice
      d. Airway obstruction that is not obviously due to other sources
      e. Crepitation heard during speaking or breathing
      f. Displacement of the trachea to one side (also a sign of possible chest injury)
   2. General treatment
      a. Use proper BSI precautions.
      b. Establish and maintain in-line spinal stabilization.
      c. Establish a patent airway.
      d. Provide high-flow oxygen or positive-pressure ventilation with supplemental oxygen.
      e. Consider requesting ALS backup if advanced airway management is needed.
      f. Control severe bleeding.
      g. Treat for shock.
      h. Transport.

Point to Emphasize

A large neck wound presents the danger that air can be sucked into a vein and carried to the heart, a potentially lethal situation. Immediately cover the wound with a gloved hand to control bleeding, and then apply an occlusive dressing.

CASE STUDY FOLLOW-UP

Ask a student volunteer to read the Case Study that begins on page 918 of the textbook. You may wish to use the following questions to engage the students in a discussion of the Case Study Follow-up that begins on page 938 of the textbook. Provide missing information and clarify ideas as needed.

Q1. During your scene size-up, what mechanism of injury do you suspect?

A1. *An exploding car battery.*

Q2. What is Hector's chief complaint?

A2. *That he can't see and that his eyes hurt "really bad."*

Q3. Once it is clear that Hector's injury is due to battery acid, what treatment do you initiate?

A3. *The patient is brought into the kitchen. When it is established that he is not wearing contact lenses, he is positioned leaning over the sink so that water from the faucet runs into his eyes. Hector is also told to turn his head from side to side so that the water runs from the medial to the lateral side of each eye in turn.*

Q4. For how long do you irrigate Hector's eyes before transport?

A4. *For 20 minutes.*

Q5. What treatment do you administer during transport?

A5. *Irrigation is continued with the ambulance's bottled water.*

IN REVIEW

Assess students' ability to apply what they have just learned by discussing the Review Questions on page 939 in the textbook.

Q1. Describe the emergency care that may need to be undertaken during initial assessment of eye, face, or neck injuries.

A1. *Emergency care that may need to be undertaken during initial assessment of eye, face, or neck injuries includes spinal stabilization, care for airway and breathing, and control of severe bleeding. Patients with chemical burns to the eye, an impaled object in the eye, an extruded eyeball, and severe injuries to the neck must be considered a high priority for immediate transport. (pp. 920–922)*

Q2. Explain why you should consider requesting advanced life support backup for injuries to the eyes, face, or neck.

A2. *ALS backup may be needed for injuries to the eyes, face, and neck because advanced airway procedures may be required. (p. 921)*

Q3. Describe how to conduct the physical exam of a patient with an eye injury.

A3. *When you conduct the physical exam of a patient with an eye injury, assess the eyes separately and together with a small penlight to evaluate the orbits, lids, conjunctivae, globe, and pupils (for size, shape, equality, and reactivity to light). Ask the patient to follow movements of your finger in all directions to check for abnormal gaze, paralysis of gaze, or pain on movement. (pp. 922–923)*

Q4. List the basic rules of emergency care for all eye injuries.

A4. *The basic treatment guidelines for all eye injuries are as follows: (1) If the eye is swollen shut, avoid any unnecessary manipulation in examining the eye. (2) Do not try to force the eyelid open unless you have to wash out chemicals. (3) Consult medical direction or local protocol before irrigating. (4) Do not put salve or medicine in an injured eye. (5) Do not remove blood or blood clots from the eye. (6) Have the patient lie down and keep quiet. (7) Limit use of the uninjured eye by covering it along with the injured eye. (8) Give the patient nothing by mouth. (9) Transport every patient with an eye injury for evaluation by a physician. (pp. 922–927)*

Q5. Describe the emergency care steps for a patient with a foreign object (a) located on the white of the eye; (b) located under the upper eyelid; and (c) lodged in the eyeball.

A5. *(a) For a foreign object located on the white of the eye, pull down the lower lid while the patient looks up or pull up the upper lid while the patient looks down. Then remove the foreign object with a piece of sterile gauze. (b) For a foreign object located under the upper eyelid, draw the upper lid down over the lower lid so that, as the lid returns to normal position, the lashes of the lower lid remove the object. If the foreign object remains, grasp the eyelashes of the upper lid and turn the lid upward over a cotton swab or similar object, and remove the object with the corner of a piece of sterile gauze. (c) For a foreign object lodged in the eyeball, do not attempt removal. Place a bandage over both eyes and transport. (pp. 923–927)*

Q6. Describe the emergency care steps for a patient with a chemical burn to the eye.

A6. *In all chemical burns of the eye, begin immediate, continuous irrigation for at least 20 minutes (at least 60 minutes for an alkali burn) with water or saline with water running from inside corner to outside. Continue irrigation en route to the hospital. (p. 926)*

Q7. List the reasons for removing, and the reasons for not removing, contact lenses from a patient with an eye injury.

A7. *Remove contact lenses if there has been a chemical burn to the eye, if the patient is unresponsive, is wearing hard contact lenses, and transport time will be lengthy or delayed. Do not remove contact lenses if the eyeball is injured (other than a chemical burn) or if transport time is short. (pp. 927–928)*

Q7. List the general emergency medical care guidelines for injuries to the face, mouth, and jaw.

A8. *The general emergency medical care guidelines for injuries to the face, mouth, and jaw are the following: Use proper BSI precautions; manually stabilize the spine; establish a patent airway; provide oxygen or positive-pressure ventilation with supplemental oxygen as necessary; control severe bleeding; cover any exposed nerves, tendons, or blood vessels with a moist, sterile dressing; if a tooth has been lost, try to find it, rinse it with saline, and transport in sterile saline-soaked gauze; treat for shock; and transport. Consider requesting ALS backup if advanced airway procedures may be needed. (pp. 930–933)*

Q9. Describe the care for a foreign object in the nose or ear.

A9. *For a foreign object in the nose or ear, reassure the patient (and parents if patient is a child) and transport the patient to the hospital for removal of the object. (p. 933)*

Q10. In addition to obvious lacerations or wounds, list the signs and symptoms of neck injury.

A10. *In addition to obvious lacerations or wounds, signs and symptoms of an injured neck include obvious swelling or bruising, difficulty speaking, loss of the voice, airway obstruction that is not obviously due to other sources, crepitation heard during speaking or breathing as air escapes from an injured larynx, and displacement of the trachea to one side. (p. 935)*

CRITICAL THINKING

Assess students' ability to respond to real-life emergency situations by discussing the Critical Thinking questions on page 940 in the textbook.

Q1. Given this presentation, what is the most important initial step the EMT should perform in the management of this patient?

A1. *One EMT should establish and maintain manual in-line spinal stabilization while opening the airway with a jaw-thrust maneuver. Immediately suction the airway clear of blood, secretions, and any other substances. Begin bag-valve-mask ventilation if the tidal volume or respiratory rate is inadequate. If the patient's respirations are adequate, apply a nonrebreather mask at 15 lpm.*

Q2. Briefly describe three different reasons that may explain why this patient is unresponsive.

A2. *This patient may be unresponsive for numerous reasons including a traumatic brain injury, hypoperfusion, hypoxia due to an occluded airway or even alcohol or drug overdose.*

Q3. If attempts at clearing the airway with suctioning fail, how else may the EMT ensure the adequacy of this patient's airway?

A3. *If suctioning fails to adequately clear this patient's airway, the EMTs should consider placing the patient in a lateral recumbent position while maintaining spinal stabilization to allow the blood to drain from the patient's oropharynx. If the patient is already immobilized on the backboard, it would be appropriate to turn the entire backboard on its side. Continue to suction.*

Q4. After treating all life threats, what would be the specific management for the eye injury?

A4. *The EMT should encircle the extruded eye with a gauze dressing and, without applying any pressure to the injury, cover it with a metal shield, crushed paper cup or cone. The EMT should then gently secure the cover or cup to the patient's face with roller gauze while also covering the uninjured eye.*

Q5. What could be the advantage of calling ALS backup for this patient?

A5. *The probability is very high that this patient will need advanced airway management due to the massive facial trauma and bleeding into the airway. An endotracheal tube will isolate the trachea and prevent any blood from leaking down the trachea past the inflated cuff and entering the lungs.*

SKILLS DEMONSTRATION AND PRACTICE

Ask for several students to serve as volunteers. Use moulage on the volunteers to simulate a variety of injuries to the eyes, face, and neck. Then, step-by-step, describe the procedures that should be used for dressing each type of wound. Give students the opportunity to ask questions or, if it is feasible, practice applying dressings to the "injuries" themselves.

ASSIGNMENTS

Assign students to read Chapter 34, "Chest, Abdomen, and Genitalia Injuries," before the next class. Also ask them to complete Chapter 33 of the Workbook.

EVALUATION

Chapter Quiz Distribute copies of the Chapter Quiz provided in Handout 33-2 to evaluate student understanding of this chapter. Remind students not to refer to their textbooks or notes while taking the quiz.

Test Manager You may wish to create a custom-tailored test using Prentice Hall *TestGen for Prehospital Emergency Care, Eighth Edition* to evaluate student understanding of this chapter.

Online Test Preparation (for students and instructors) Additional test preparation is available through *EMT Achieve: Basic Test Preparation* at http://www.prenhall.com/EMTAchieve. Instructors can also monitor student mastery online.

Reading/Reference
Textbook, pp. 941–970

Workbook
Chapter 33 Activities

Chapter Quiz
Handout 33-2

TestGen
Chapter 33 Test

Online Test Preparation
Send your students to
http://www.prenhall.com/
EMTAchieve

REINFORCEMENT

Handouts If classroom discussions or performance on the quiz indicates that some students have not fully mastered the chapter content, you may wish to assign some or all of the Reinforcement Handouts for this chapter.

TECH EXTRAS

Brady Skills Series EMT-B Videos/CD Have your students watch the skills come to life on either VHS or CD-ROM.

PowerPoint Presentation (for instructors) The PowerPoint material developed for this chapter offers useful reinforcement of chapter content.

Student CD A wide variety of material on this CD-ROM will reinforce and also expand student knowledge and skills.

Companion Website (for students) Additional review quizzes and links to EMS resources will contribute to further reinforcement of this chapter. Please visit http://www.prenhall.com/mistovich.

Handouts 33-3 to 33-6
Reinforcement Activities

Brady Skills Series EMT-B Videos/CD
Visual Reinforcement

PowerPoint Presentation
Chapter 33

Student CD
Chapter 33

Companion Website
http://www.prenhall.com/mistovich

OBJECTIVES CHECKLIST

Cognitive	Date Mastered
* List the major anatomical structures of the eye, face, and neck.	
* Describe the relationship between eye, face, and neck injuries and the personal protection and safety of the EMT.	
* List the overall assessment procedures for eye, face, and neck injuries.	
* Describe the general assessment procedures for eye injuries, including use of the penlight.	
* List the basic rules for emergency medical care for eye injuries.	
* List specific common eye injuries and describe their appropriate emergency medical care.	
* Describe emergency medical care for eye-injured patients wearing contact lenses.	
* Describe the general assessment and care guidelines for face injuries.	
* List the signs and symptoms and describe the emergency medical care for injuries to the mid-face, upper jaw, and lower jaw.	
* Describe the emergency medical care for an object impaled in the cheek.	
* Describe the emergency medical care for injuries to the nose and ear.	
* List special signs or symptoms of injury to the neck.	
* Describe the emergency medical care for injuries to the neck.	

Affective	Date Mastered
* Recognize and respect the feelings of a patient suffering an eye, face, or neck injury.	

Psychomotor	Date Mastered
* Demonstrate the steps in the emergency medical care of common eye injuries.	
* Demonstrate the steps in the removal of soft and hard contact lenses from eye-injured patients.	
* Demonstrate the steps in the emergency medical care of various types of face, jaw, and neck injuries, including care for avulsed teeth and for severed blood vessels to the neck.	

OBJECTIVES

EVALUATION

CHAPTER 33 QUIZ

Write the letter of the best answer in the space provided.

_____ 1. The part of the eye that contains the aqueous humor is the
　　　　　　A. lens.　　　　　　　　　　　C. anterior chamber.
　　　　　　B. cornea.　　　　　　　　　　D. vitreous body.

_____ 2. An eye injury that involves an eye being pulled out of its socket is called a(n)
　　　　　　A. extrusion.　　　　　　　　　C. orbital fracture.
　　　　　　B. evisceration.　　　　　　　　D. periorbital ecchymosis.

_____ 3. The neck contains all of the following structures *except* the
　　　　　　A. carotid arteries.　　　　　　C. jugular veins.
　　　　　　B. mandible.　　　　　　　　　D. trachea.

_____ 4. The facial bone that is *not* fused into immovable joints is the
　　　　　　A. mandible.　　　　　　　　　C. temporal bone.
　　　　　　B. malar.　　　　　　　　　　D. maxillae.

_____ 5. An EMT should only attempt to remove a foreign object from the
　　　　　　A. retina.　　　　　　　　　　C. globe.
　　　　　　B. cornea.　　　　　　　　　　D. conjunctiva.

_____ 6. The globe of the eye, or eyeball, is a sphere approximately 1 inch in diameter that is covered with a tough outer coat called the
　　　　　　A. cornea.　　　　　　　　　　C. sclera.
　　　　　　B. pupil.　　　　　　　　　　D. iris.

_____ 7. A primary treatment for a patient with chemical burns to the eye is
　　　　　　A. plentiful irrigation.
　　　　　　B. bandaging only the injured eye.
　　　　　　C. covering both eyes with dry dressings.
　　　　　　D. covering both eyes with soaked gauze pads.

_____ 8. The signs and symptoms of orbital fracture include all of the following *except*
　　　　　　A. vision improvement.　　　　C. nasal discharge.
　　　　　　B. double vision.　　　　　　　D. tenderness to palpation.

_____ 9. The portion of the eye that focuses light to the retina is the
　　　　　　A. cornea.　　　　　　　　　　C. iris.
　　　　　　B. pupil.　　　　　　　　　　D. lens.

_____ 10. If a patient has sustained a chemical burn to the eye, the EMT should irrigate the eye for at least 20 minutes or, if the injury involves an alkali, for at least
　　　　　　A. 1½ hours.　　　　　　　　　C. 45 minutes.
　　　　　　B. 1 hour.　　　　　　　　　　D. 30 minutes.

_____ 11. An appropriate irrigant for an EMT to use for a chemical burn is
　　　　　　A. diluted vinegar.　　　　　　C. saline.
　　　　　　B. alcohol.　　　　　　　　　　D. sodium bicarbonate.

_____ **12.** The thin covering of the inner eyelids is called the

    A. conjunctiva.   **C.** retina.

    B. sclera.   **D.** orbit.

_____ **13.** The correct emergency treatment for profuse bleeding with facial injuries includes

    A. application of cold packs.

    B. application of heat packs.

    C. application of alum.

    D. application of direct pressure.

_____ **14.** Clear or bloody fluid draining from the ear can indicate a

    A. dangerously high fever.   **C.** foreign body.

    B. skull fracture.   **D.** flexion injury.

_____ **15.** If a nose fracture is suspected, the EMT should

    A. apply direct pressure.

    B. apply cold compresses.

    C. apply warm compresses.

    D. pack the nose with saline gauze.

IN THE FIELD

Read the following real-life situation. Then answer the questions that follow.

Today is a particularly warm day in July. You and your partner respond to a call to a residence not far from your station. A woman is standing in the front yard flagging you down and appears to be quite upset. As you follow her to the back of the house, she explains to you, between sobs, that her 8-year-old son was hosting a pool party for his baseball team. Two of the young boys were scuffling, and her son was inadvertently pushed into a plate glass window into the house.

   You enter the house and you note a very upset and crying child lying just inside the den. You note moderate bleeding from the patient's face and neck. In addition, the boy is holding his hand over his left eye. He complains of pain in that eye. After you convince him to remove his hand and allow you to inspect the injury, you note a 1-inch vertical laceration on the left lower eyelid. There is also a laceration on the left side of the neck.

1. List the basic steps you would take in treating this patient.

2. List your steps in management of the eyelid injury.

3. Name at least four considerations for the assessment and treatment of these face and neck injuries.

REINFORCEMENT

CHAPTER 33 REVIEW

Write the word or words that best complete each sentence in the space provided.

1. The bony structures of the skull that surround the eyes are called the

   _____.

2. The face has _____ bones.

3. The proper medical term for the cheekbones is the _____ bones.

4. When considering an injury to the eye, the EMT must be aware that

   _____ is a critical consideration in the treatment.

5. If a foreign object becomes lodged in the _____, the EMT should not

   attempt to disturb it.

6. The face has many _____ _____, so any facial

   injuries may bleed profusely.

7. Injuries serious enough to cause orbital fractures may also cause trauma to the

   _____ _____.

8. Eyelid injuries include _____, _____, and

   _____.

9. Injuries to the globe are best treated at the _____.

10. A chemical burn to the eye represents a(n) _____

    _____.

11. If an eyeball injury is *not* suspected, the EMT should cover an injured eyelid with

    _____ _____ to help reduce swelling.

12. In all calls involving chemical burns to the eye, the EMT should begin

    _____ with _____ or

    _____ immediately on contact with the patient.

13. The primary concern with facial fractures is _____

    _____.

14. With chemical burns to the eye, the EMT should irrigate the eye for at least

_____ minutes or until arrival at the hospital.

15. Eye injuries are often complicated by the presence of _____

_____.

REINFORCEMENT

EYE, FACE, AND NECK INJURIES: LISTING

1. List five anatomical structures of the eye.

2. List four structures contained in the neck.

3. List four types of facial fractures.

4. List four signs and/or symptoms of orbital fractures.

EYE, FACE, AND NECK INJURIES: TRUE OR FALSE

Indicate if the following statements are true or false by writing T or F in the space provided.

_____ **1.** When treating bleeding wounds to the neck, the EMT should use circumferential bandages.

_____ **2.** When treating an injury to the nose, the EMT should *not* probe for a foreign body.

_____ **3.** Maintaining an airway is extremely important in neck injuries as is maintaining a high index of suspicion for spine injuries.

_____ **4.** When dressing an injured ear, place part of the dressing between the ear and side of the head.

_____ **5.** If the patient has a foreign object impaled in the cheek of the face, the EMT should immediately remove it and transport the patient.

_____ **6.** When assessing and treating a facial fracture, your first priorities should be to establish and maintain a patent airway, support breathing, and control bleeding.

_____ **7.** If a tooth has been lost, the tooth should be wrapped in dry gauze.

_____ **8.** The specialized structures of the face are prone to injury because of their location, but injuries to them are rare.

_____ **9.** Only attempt removal of objects in the conjunctiva; do not attempt removal of objects on or lodged in the cornea.

_____ **10.** Even though they are designed for extended wear, soft contact lenses can cause damage if left in for a long time.

_____ **11.** Generally, you should not remove contact lenses if there has been a chemical burn to the eye.

_____ **12.** The EMT should always attempt to replace an extruded eyeball back into the socket.

_____ **13.** If fracture of the orbits is suspected, you should establish and maintain spinal immobilization.

_____ **14.** In any case of severe facial trauma, suspect cervical-spine injury.

Eye, Face, and Neck Injuries

Anatomy of the Eye, Face, and Neck
Eye

Face

Neck

Eye Injuries
Basic Assessment and Care

Specific Injury Considerations

- Foreign objects in the eye
- Injuries to the orbits
- Injuries to the globe
- Lid injuries
- Chemical burns to the eye
- Impaled object or extruded eyeball

Removing Contact Lenses

Face Injuries
Basic Assessment and Care

Specific Injury Considerations

- Injury to the mid-face, upper jaw, or lower jaw
- Object impaled in cheek
- Injury to nose
- Injury to ear

Neck Injuries
Basic Assessment and Care

HANDOUT 33-2: Chapter 33 Quiz

1.	C	**5.**	D	**9.**	D	**13.**	D
2.	A	**6.**	C	**10.**	B	**14.**	B
3.	B	**7.**	A	**11.**	C	**15.**	B
4.	A	**8.**	A	**12.**	A		

HANDOUT 33-3: In the Field

1. Take BSI precautions; ensure stabilization of the cervical spine; assess and control of airway, breathing, and circulation.
2. Control bleeding with light pressure; cover lid with sterile gauze soaked in saline (if lid skin is avulsed, preserve and transport with the patient); cover lid with cold compresses; patch both eyes.
3. Assess the bleeding wounds and the amount of blood lost. Apply a sterile dressing with direct pressure to the open wounds. Use an occlusive dressing on the neck wound to prevent air from entering. Provide stabilization and later immobilization of the spine in a neutral, in-line position.

HANDOUT 33-4: Chapter 33 Review

1. orbits
2. 14
3. zygomatic
4. time
5. eyeball (or globe)
6. blood vessels
7. cervical spine
8. bruising, burns, lacerations
9. hospital

10. dire emergency
11. cold compresses
12. irrigation, water, saline
13. airway compromise
14. 20
15. contact lenses

HANDOUT 33-5: Eye, Face, and Neck Injuries: Listing

1. Any five: sclera, cornea, pupil, lens, retina, conjunctiva, aqueous humor, vitreous humor, orbit.
2. Any four: carotid arteries, jugular arteries, trachea, larynx, cervical spine.
3. Any four: maxilla fracture, mandible fracture, nasal-orbital fracture, malar (cheek) fracture, maxilla–nasal–orbital fracture.
4. Any four: double vision; marked decrease in vision; loss of sensation above the eyebrow, over the cheek, or in the upper lip; nasal discharge; tenderness upon palpation; bony "step-off"; paralysis of an upward gaze in the involved eye.

HANDOUT 33-6: Eye, Face, and Neck Injuries: True or False

1.	F	**5.**	F	**9.**	T	**12.**	F
2.	T	**6.**	T	**10.**	T	**13.**	T
3.	T	**7.**	F	**11.**	F	**14.**	T
4.	T	**8.**	F				

34 Chest, Abdomen, and Genitalia Injuries

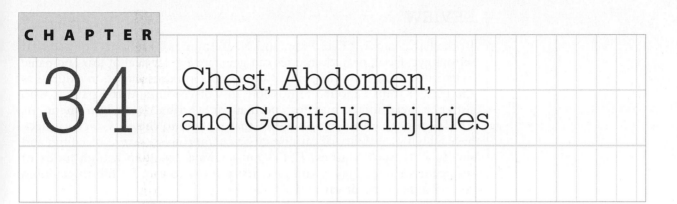

This chapter covers portions of Lesson 5-2 and Lesson 5-5 of the U.S. Department of Transportation's EMT-Basic National Standard Curriculum.

OBJECTIVES

Numbered objectives are from the U.S. Department of Transportation EMT-Basic National Standard Curriculum. Asterisked objectives, if any, pertain to material that is supplemental to the DOT curriculum. Page numbers in parentheses refer to pages in the textbook.

Cognitive

5-2.8 Discuss the emergency medical care considerations for a patient with a penetrating chest injury. (pp. 950–952, 955)

5-2.9 State the emergency medical care considerations for a patient with an open wound to the abdomen. (pp. 958–959, 960, 961)

5-2.10 Differentiate the care of an open wound to the chest from an open wound to the abdomen. (pp. 950–952, 958–959)

   * Review the anatomy of the chest cavity as it pertains to chest injuries. (pp. 942–946)

   * Identify signs and symptoms of possible life-threatening chest injuries. (pp. 949–950)

   * Describe emergency medical care for life-threatening chest injuries. (pp. 950–952, 955)

   * Review the anatomy of the abdomen. (pp. 953, 955)

   * Recognize the common signs and symptoms of abdominal injuries. (p. 958)

   * Describe the emergency medical care for a suspected abdominal injury. (pp. 958–959, 960, 962)

   * Describe the emergency medical care for genitalia injuries (p. 959, 960)

Psychomotor

5-2.31 Demonstrate the steps in the emergency medical care of a patient with an open chest wound.

5-2.32 Demonstrate the steps in the emergency medical care of a patient with open abdominal wounds.

The numbered objectives are also addressed in Chapter 28, "Soft Tissue Injuries."

Total Teaching Time
120 minutes

Resources Needed
- Scored Chapter 33 Quizzes
- Complete jump kit containing BSI equipment, oxygen equipment, cervical spinal collar, bandages, and dressings

Additional Resources
Larmon/Davis, *Basic Life Support Skills*

Elling, *EMT Achieve: Basic Test Preparation*

Limmer/Mistovich/O'Keefe, *Audio Lecture & Study Guide: EMT*

Mistovich/Kuvlesky, *SUCCESS! for the EMT, Second Edition*

REVIEW

In the last chapter, "Eye, Face, and Neck Injuries," students learned that serious eye, facial, or neck injuries can generate a great deal of fear and panic in patients. Aside from the pain, injuries to the eye cause emotional duress as the patient thinks about the possible loss of vision, and the patient who suffers a facial injury may fear permanent scarring or disfigurement. As EMTs, students must remain aware that injuries to the eyes, face, or neck have a high probability of causing airway compromise, severe bleeding, and shock. With such injuries, EMTs must always maintain a high index of suspicion for spinal injury and give first priority to care for life-threatening compromise of the airway and circulation.

Distribute the quizzes from the last class. Go over each question on the quiz and handle any concerns students may have about the answers.

INTRODUCTION TO CHAPTER 34

Chapter 34, "Chest, Abdomen, and Genitalia Injuries," is the ninth chapter in Module 5. Most injuries to the chest or abdomen are not characterized by large, gaping wounds. Unlike some injuries to the extremities, they rarely involve bones protruding through the skin. Injuries to the chest and abdomen, in fact, are often not very dramatic in appearance and can be easily overlooked in the physical assessment. The patient may actually be complaining of much more pain from injuries to bones and joints or from surface lacerations and abrasions. Initially, the patient may not even realize that he has a serious injury to the chest or abdomen.

It is important to understand, however, that the chest and abdomen contain vital organs and that injuries to the chest and abdomen are often lethal. Chest injuries can cause a disturbance in respiration, oxygen exchange, and circulation. Abdominal injuries may produce severe internal bleeding and shock (hypoperfusion). The EMT must rely on the mechanism of injury, a high index of suspicion, and careful physical examination to determine and then care for life-threatening injuries to the chest and abdomen.

Distribute the Chapter 34 Objectives Checklist, and give students a few minutes to look it over. Then briefly paraphrase the objectives for this lesson in your own words.

LECTURE

The following lecture outline is based on Chapter 34, which contains material that goes beyond the DOT curriculum but that will be of great value to your students when they become EMRs. Use the outline to present your lecture. The page numbers in parentheses refer to pages in the textbook. The parenthetical references in dark, heavy type are to figures, tables, and scans in the textbook.

CHEST, ABDOMEN, AND GENITALIA INJURIES

I. **Chest** (pp. 942–953)
    A. Anatomy of the chest (pp. 942–953) **(Fig. 34-1, p. 943)**
    B. Chest injuries (pp. 943–946) **(Figs. 34-2 and 34-3, p. 944)**
        1. Closed
            a. Flail segment

Handout 34-1
Chapter 34 Objectives Checklist

● ➤

Lecture Master
You may wish to display Lecture Master 34 when presenting the lecture to the class.

On the Net
Common chest injuries and treatment. http://www.parasolemt.com.au/Manual/chest injuries.html

On the Net
Abdominal and chest injuries as well as other systems. http://www.surgical-tutor.org.uk/default-home.htm?core/trauma.htm~right

      (1) Two or more adjacent ribs broken in two or more places creating a segment unattached to rib cage **(Fig. 34-4, p. 945)**

   b. Paradoxical movement

      (1) Contrary movement of the flail segment **(Fig. 34-5, p. 946)**

 2. Open

   a. Pneumothorax

      (1) Air in chest cavity

   b. Sucking chest wound

      (1) When open chest wound pulls air into thoracic cavity

   c. Tension pneumothorax

      (1) Air in chest cavity builds enough pressure to collapse lung on uninjured side and to compress heart's large vessels

C. Assessment and care: chest injuries (pp. 946–953) **(Figs. 34-12 and Fig. 34-13, pp. 954–956)**

 1. Scene size-up

   a. Ensure personal safety.

   b. Take all BSI precautions.

   c. Look for evidence of mechanism of injury.

 2. Initial assessment

   a. Establish and maintain in-line stabilization if you suspect chest trauma.

   b. Quickly expose chest and examine it.

   c. Immediately place gloved hand over any open, sucking wound.

   d. If there is paradoxical movement, immediately place gloved hand over flail segment.

   e. Determine patient's mental status.

   f. Visually inspect airway in patient with altered mental status.

   g. Perform jaw-thrust procedure to open airway if necessary.

   h. Note patient's speech pattern.

   i. Carefully assess breathing status.

      (1) Adequate breathing

         (a) Administer oxygen with a nonrebreather mask at 15 liters per minute.

      (2) Inadequate breathing

         (a) Begin positive-pressure ventilation with supplemental oxygen. **(Fig. 34-6, p. 947)**

   j. Transport immediately.

 3. Focused history and physical exam

   a. Perform rapid trauma assessment.

   b. Assess breathing status.

   c. Assess neck for any of the following:

      (1) Subcutaneous emphysema

      (2) Jugular vein distension

      (3) Tracheal deviation

   d. If you suspect spinal injury, apply a cervical collar.

   e. Expose patient's chest and look for signs and symptoms of chest trauma.

   f. Palpate chest, checking for symmetry, paradoxical movement, swelling, and deformities.

⊙

Point to Emphasize

Always suspect chest or abdominal cavity trauma in a patient with multiple injuries.

    g. Note patient's position (with injuries to chest wall or ribs, patient is likely to place an arm over injured area to guard and splint it during breathing)
    h. Auscultate breath sounds bilaterally.
    i. Reevaluate breathing status.
    j. Inspect abdomen for excessive muscle movement during breathing.
    k. Assess baseline vital signs.
    l. Obtain a SAMPLE history.
4. Signs and symptoms (**Fig. 34-7, p. 949**)
    a. Cyanosis to fingernails, fingertips, lips, or face
    b. Dyspnea
    c. Breathing rate slower or faster than normal and usually shallow
    d. Signs of trauma to chest
    e. Coughing up frothy blood (hemoptysis)
    f. Signs of shock (hypoperfusion)
    g. Decreasing blood pressure with pulse becoming faster and weaker
    h. Tracheal deviation
    i. Paradoxical movement of segment in chest wall
    j. Open wound with possible sucking sound
    k. Distended jugular veins
    l. Absent or decreased breath sounds upon auscultation
    m. Pain at injury site, especially if it increases during respiration
    n. Lack of normal chest expansion during inhalation
5. General emergency medical care—chest injury
    a. Maintain an open airway.
    b. Continue oxygen therapy.
    c. Reevaluate breathing status.
    d. Stabilize any impaled object.
    e. Completely immobilize patient with suspected spinal injury.
    f. Treat patient for shock.
6. Emergency medical care—open chest wound
    a. Immediately seal open wound.
    b. Apply occlusive dressing. (**Figs. 34-8 and 34-9, p. 951**)
       (1) Asherman Chest Seal (**Fig. 34-10, p. 952**)
    c. Continuously assess respiratory status; look for
       (1) Difficulty breathing with increased respiratory distress and dyspnea
       (2) Tachypnea
       (3) Severely decreased or absent breath sounds on injured side
       (4) Cyanosis
       (5) Tachycardia
       (6) Decreasing blood pressure with a narrowing pulse pressure
       (7) Jugular vein distension (late sign)
       (8) Tracheal deviation (late sign)
       (9) Unequal movement of chest wall
      (10) Extreme anxiety and apprehension
      (11) Increased resistance to positive-pressure ventilation

7. Emergency medical care—flail segment
    a. Stabilize paradoxical movement. **(Fig. 34-11, p. 952)**
    b. Proceed with steps for general care of chest wound.
8. Detailed physical exam and ongoing assessment
D. Summary: assessment and care—chest injuries (p. 953)
    (Figs. 34-12 and 34-13, pp. 954–956)

II. Abdomen (pp. 953–959)
  A. Anatomy of the abdominal cavity (p. 953)
    1. Hollow organs
    2. Solid organs
    3. Vascular structures
  B. Abdominal injuries (pp. 953–955)
    1. Open
    2. Closed
  C. Assessment and care: abdominal injuries (pp. 955–959)
    (Figs. 34-17 and 34-18, pp. 961–963)
    1. Scene size-up
      a. Look for evidence of mechanism of injury.
      b. Be aware of the agents that can cause penetrating and blunt trauma to the abdomen.
    2. Initial assessment
      a. Form general impression: patients commonly in fetal position **(Fig. 34-15, p. 957)**
      b. Establish in-line spinal stabilization if spinal injury is suspected.
      c. Ensure an open airway and adequate breathing.
        (1) Adequate breathing
          (a) Deliver oxygen by nonrebreather mask at a rate of 15 liters per minute.
        (2) Inadequate breathing
          (a) Begin positive-pressure ventilation with supplemental oxygen.
      d. Assess circulation.
      e. Look for signs of shock.
    3. Focused history and physical exam
      a. Apply cervical collar if spine injury is suspected.
      b. Perform rapid trauma assessment.
        (1) Inspect the abdomen.
        (2) Inspect and provide emergency medical care for any abdominal evisceration. **(Fig. 34-14, p. 957)**
        (3) Assess extremities for injury.
        (4) Log roll patient and inspect entire back and lumbar region.
      c. Assess baseline vital signs.
      d. Obtain a SAMPLE history.
      e. Evaluate pain using the OPQRST mnemonic.
    4. Signs and symptoms
      a. Signs of trauma
      b. Progressively worsening pain
      c. Tenderness on palpation in areas other than site of injury
      d. Rigid abdominal muscles
      e. Fetal position
      f. Distended abdomen
      g. Discoloration around umbilicus or flank (late finding)
      h. Rapid, shallow breathing

Point to Emphasize
Detecting the exact nature of the abdominal trauma patient's injury is less important than developing a reasonable suspicion of trauma.

i. Signs of shock

     j. Nausea and vomiting (possible blood in vomitus)

     k. Possible abdominal cramping

     l. Possible pain radiation to either shoulder

     m. Weakness

  5. General emergency medical care—abdominal injury

     a. Maintain open airway and spinal precautions.

     b. Continue oxygen therapy.

     c. Reassess breathing.

     d. Treat for shock (hypoperfusion).

     e. Control external bleeding.

     f. Position the patient.

       (1) No spinal injury

         (a) Supine position with legs flexed at knees

       (2) Spinal injury suspected

         (a) Immobilize to backboard

     g. Stabilize any impaled object.

     h. Apply PASG if locally approved.

     i. Transport quickly.

  6. Emergency medical care—abdominal evisceration (**Fig. 34-16, p. 960**)

     a. Do not touch or attempt to replace protruding organs.

     b. Expose wound.

     c. Position the patient.

       (1) No spinal injury

         (a) Supine position with legs flexed at knees

       (2) Spinal injury suspected

         (a) Immobilize to backboard

     d. Prepare clean, sterile dressing by soaking it with saline or sterile water.

     e. Apply dressing over protruding organs.

     f. Cover the moist dressing with an occlusive dressing.

     g. Administer high-flow oxygen; be prepared for shock.

III. Genitalia (pp. 959–960)

  A. Injuries to male genitalia (pp. 959–960)

    1. Treat as for soft tissue injury, and apply direct pressure to control bleeding.

    2. Apply cold compresses to scrotum to reduce pain and swelling.

    3. If penis has been avulsed or amputated, take the following steps:

     a. Apply direct pressure to control bleeding.

     b. Locate amputated or avulsed part.

     c. Wrap part in sterile dressing moistened with sterile saline.

     d. Place part in a plastic bag.

     e. Place bagged part on a cold pack or ice that has been wrapped in a towel.

    4. Provide oxygen at 15 liters per minute by nonrebreather mask.

    5. Carefully assess for signs and symptoms of shock.

    6. Transport patient with any amputated parts.

  B. Injuries to female genitalia (p. 960)

    1. Control bleeding with direct pressure, using moistened compresses such as a sanitary napkin.

    2. Do not pack or place dressings inside vagina.

3. Carefully assess for signs and symptoms of shock.
4. Provide oxygen at 15 liters per minute by nonrebreather mask.
5. Transport.

ENRICHMENT (OPTIONAL)

The following section contains information that is valuable as background for the EMT but that goes substantially beyond the U.S. Department of Transportation's EMT-Basic National Standard Curriculum.

IV. Conditions that may result from chest injury (pp. 962–967)
  A. Flail segment (p. 962) **(Fig. 34-19, p. 964)**
  B. Pulmonary contusion (pp. 962–964) **(Fig. 34-20, p. 964)**
  C. Pneumothorax (p. 964)
  D. Open pneumothorax (pp. 964–965) **(Fig. 34-21, p. 965)**
  E. Tension pneumothorax (p. 965) **(Fig. 34-21, p. 965)**
  F. Hemothorax (pp. 965–966) **(Fig. 34-21, p. 965)**
  G. Traumatic asphyxia (p. 966) **(Fig. 34-21, p. 965)**
  H. Cardiac contusion (p. 966) **(Fig. 34-22, p. 966)**
  I. Pericardial tamponade (pp. 966–967) **(Fig. 34-22, p. 966)**
  J. Rib injury (p. 967) **(Figs. 34-23 and 34-24, p. 967)**

CASE STUDY FOLLOW-UP

Ask a student volunteer to read the Case Study that begins on page 942 of the textbook. You may wish to use the following questions to engage the students in a discussion of the Case Study Follow-up that begins on page 968 of the textbook. Provide missing information and clarify ideas as needed.

Q1. Why is in-line spinal stabilization established?

A1. Because of uncertainty over the mechanism of injury or nature of the illness.

Q2. What does your initial assessment yield about the patient's airway and breathing? What do you do in response?

A2. The airway is open and clear of any secretions or vomitus. The breathing is rapid and shallow at a rate of approximately 40 per minute. Ventilations with supplemental oxygen are begun via bag-valve mask.

Q3. Describe the wound you find during your physical exam.

A3. There appears to be a small-caliber gunshot wound to the right anterior aspect of the chest at about the third intercostal rib on the midclavicular line. A bubbly crackle is heard when the patient inhales spontaneously.

Q4. How do you treat this open chest wound?

A4. By immediately placing a gloved hand over the wound. Plastic wrap from the oxygen tubing is applied over the wound, and it is taped on three sides.

Q5. During transport, you notice that it is becoming extremely difficult to ventilate the patient. The heart rate has increased to 148 per minute and the skin is becoming severely cyanotic. What do you do in response?

A5. *Lift a corner of the occlusive dressing off the wound and note the sound of air escaping. Almost immediately the patient's condition improves, allowing replacement of the dressing over the wound.*

IN REVIEW

Assess students' ability to apply what they have just learned by discussing the Review Questions on page 969 in the textbook.

Q1. Identify and describe the two general categories of injuries to the chest.

A1. *Two general categories of injuries to the chest are open and closed. Closed injuries to the chest are the result of blunt trauma applied to the chest cavity, which can cause extensive damage to the ribs and internal organs. An open chest injury is the result of a penetrating chest wound, which can cause damage to tissues and organs along the path of penetration or (in the case of a bullet) cause extensive internal damage throughout the chest cavity. (p. 943)*

Q2. List the signs and symptoms associated with major chest trauma.

A2. *Signs and symptoms associated with major chest trauma are cyanosis to the fingernails or fingertips, lips, or face; dyspnea; breathing rate that is faster or slower than normal; shallow breathing; contusions, lacerations, punctures, swelling, or other obvious signs of trauma; coughing up frothy blood; signs of shock (hypoperfusion); decreasing blood pressure with an increasing pulse that becomes weaker; tracheal deviation; paradoxical movement of a segment of the chest wall; open wound that may or may not produce a sucking sound; distended jugular veins; absent or decreased breath sounds upon auscultation; pain at the injury site, especially pain that increases with inhalation and exhalation; and failure of the chest to rise during inhalation. (pp. 949–950)*

Q3. Describe the general guidelines for emergency medical care of trauma to the chest.

A3. *General guidelines for emergency medical care of trauma to the chest are as follows: Maintain an open airway. Continue oxygen therapy at 15 liters per minute by nonrebreather mask. Reevaluate breathing status, remaining alert for sudden and rapid deterioration. If, at any time, signs of inadequate breathing appear, immediately begin positive-pressure ventilation with supplemental oxygen. Stabilize any impaled object. Completely immobilize the patient if spinal injury is suspected. Treat the patient for shock (hypoperfusion) if signs and symptoms are present. (p. 950)*

Q4. Describe additional emergency medical care required for (a) an impaled object to the chest, (b) an open wound to the chest, and (c) a flail segment (paradoxical movement).

A4. *(a) For an impaled object to the chest, stabilize the object in place with bulky gauze and bandages. (b) An open wound to the chest should be immediately sealed with a gloved hand, and then with an occlusive dressing. Tape the dressing on three sides to allow air from the thoracic cavity to escape during exhalation (or on four sides, lifting a corner to relieve pressure as necessary). Continually assess the patient's* *respiratory status. (c) Flail segment (paradoxical movement) should be splinted in an inward position by placing a hand over the unstable flail segment, or by placing bulky dressings, a pillow, or towels over the unstable segment, or by securing the patient's arm to the body. If the patient's breathing is inadequate, initiate positive-pressure ventilation. (pp. 950–953)*

Q5. List the signs and symptoms associated with trauma to the abdomen.

A5. *Signs and symptoms associated with trauma to the abdomen are contusions, abrasions, lacerations, punctures, or other signs of blunt or penetrating trauma; pain that may initially be mild, then worsening; tenderness on palpation to areas other than the injury site; rigid abdominal muscles; patient lying with legs drawn up to the chest in an attempt to reduce the pain; distended abdomen; discoloration around the umbilicus or to the flank (late finding); rapid, shallow breathing; signs of shock; nausea and vomiting (the vomitus may contain blood); abdominal cramping possibly present; pain may radiate to either shoulder; and weakness. (p. 958)*

Q6. Describe the general guidelines for emergency medical care of both open and closed abdominal injuries.

A6. *General guidelines for emergency medical care of both open and closed abdominal injuries include the following: Take appropriate spinal precautions. Maintain an open airway, performing a jaw-thrust maneuver and inserting an oropharyngeal or nasopharyngeal airway if patient's condition deteriorates. Continue oxygen therapy. Reassess the breathing status and, if inadequate, begin positive-pressure ventilation. Treat for shock (hypoperfusion). Control any external bleeding. Position the patient in a supine position with legs flexed at the knees. Stabilize any impaled objects. Apply a pneumatic antishock garment (PASG) if indicated and allowed by local protocol. Transport as quickly as possible. (pp. 958–959)*

Q7. Describe emergency medical care for an abdominal evisceration.

A7. *Emergency medical care for an abdominal evisceration is to follow the general guidelines for abdominal injury, except dress the evisceration in the following way: Expose the wound, cutting away clothing as necessary. Position the patient on his back and flex the legs up toward the chest if spinal injury is not suspected. Prepare a clean, sterile dressing by soaking it with saline or sterile water. Apply the dressing over the protruding organs. Do not use absorbent cotton or any other material that might cling to the organs when wet, such as paper towels or toilet tissue. Cover the moist dressing with an occlusive dressing to retain moisture and warmth. Administer high-flow oxygen and be prepared to treat for shock. (p. 959)*

Q8. Describe the general emergency care for injuries to the male or female genitalia.

A8. *General emergency care for injuries to male genitalia is as follows: Treat as a soft tissue injury, and control bleeding with direct pressure. Apply cold compresses to the scrotum to reduce pain and swelling. If the penis has been avulsed or amputated, apply direct pressure to control bleeding. Locate amputated or avulsed part, wrap it in sterile dressing moistened with sterile saline, place it in a plastic bag, and keep it cool by placing it on a cold pack or ice that has been wrapped in a towel. Provide oxygen at 15 liters per minute by nonrebreather mask. Carefully* *assess for signs and symptoms of shock. Transport patient with any amputated parts. General emergency care for injuries to female genitalia is as follows: Control bleeding with direct pressure, using moistened compresses such as a sanitary napkin. Do not pack or place dressings inside the vagina. Carefully assess for signs and symptoms of shock. Provide oxygen at 15 liters per minute by nonrebreather mask. Transport. (pp. 950–960)*

CRITICAL THINKING

Assess students' ability to respond to real-life emergency situations by discussing the Critical Thinking questions on page 970 in the textbook.

Q1. What initial immediate emergency care would you provide for the patient?

A1. *Even though the patient is moaning in pain, his respiratory rate is 38 per minute with a shallow tidal volume. This would require ventilation with a bag-valve-mask device. Supplemental oxygen must be connected to the BVM's reservoir and set a 12 to 15 lpm. The high respiratory rate and shallow tidal volume may be due to the severe abdominal pain the patient is experiencing. A patient with severe abdominal pain may intentionally breathe fast and shallow to reduce the excursion of the diaphragm. The deeper the patient breathes, the more the diaphragm moves downward and displaces the abdominal cavity creating more pain.*

Q2. How would you manage the protruding abdominal organs?

A2. *The EMTs should cut away the patient's shirt to expose the wound. Be careful not to injure the exposed organs. Cover the protruding small intestines with a sterile dressing soaked with saline. Be sure all of the exposed abdominal contents are covered by the moist sterile dressing. Place a large occlusive dressing completely over the moist dressing. This is done to keep the eviscerated organs moist and to prevent excessive heat loss.*

Q3. What do the vital signs indicate?

A4. *The tachycardic rate of 126 bpm; weak radial pulse; pale, cool, and clammy skin are all indicators of shock. The shock in this patient is a result of blood loss.*

Q4. How would you position the patient for transport?

A4. *Since there is no suspected spinal injury, this patient should be placed on his back with his knees flexed up toward his chest. This will relieve some of the tension of the abdominal muscles and may reduce the patient's pain.*

ROLE PLAY

Request the assistance of four volunteers, two to play the role of EMTs responding to a 9-1-1 call, one to be the patient, and one to be a coworker of the patient.

Take the two EMT players outside the classroom and provide them with a complete jump kit containing BSI equipment, oxygen equipment, and a cervical spinal collar. Describe the following situation to them:

©2008 by Pearson Education, Inc.
Prehospital Emergency Care, 8th ed.

You have been dispatched to a suburban home where a new garage is being constructed for a man reported injured. You should act appropriately on what you find there. The emphasis of the scenario is dealing with chest, abdominal, or genitalia injuries. However, you should utilize all the skills you have learned to this point. We will call you to the scene in just a minute.

Have the patient and the coworker come to the front of the classroom. Describe the following situation to them and the class:

Tom and Al are builders putting up a new garage. As Tom was moving around the site this morning, he fell and accidentally discharged a nail gun, sending a nail into his chest. Al heard Tom cry out and called 9-1-1 on the cell phone. Tom is awake, but anxious and in obvious pain. He can hear a sucking noise from his chest as he breathes. Tom did not fall or suffer any other injuries during this incident. He has no allergies or any significant medical conditions.

Decide who will play the patient and coworker. (Names may be changed according to the gender of the actors.) You should use moulage on the volunteer playing Tom to simulate a nail protruding about 1 inch from the chest on the left side. (You might mix an effervescent tablet with fake blood to simulate the sucking chest wound.)

Tell Tom and Al to take their places and start acting. Call the EMTs back into the classroom.

Allow the role play to progress naturally. Provide appropriate vital signs—pulse, 104; respirations, 24 with slightly decreased lung sounds on the left side; blood pressure, 100/78; skin, pale, cool, clammy; pupils, normal—and other objective information about the patient if the EMTs assess this information. Intervene only if the players seem to be at a loss for what to do.

End the play when the EMTs are ready to transport the patient. With the entire class, discuss the following:

- What did the EMTs do well?

- What, if anything, should then have done differently?

ASSIGNMENTS

Assign students to read Chapter 35, "Agricultural and Industrial Emergencies," before the next class. Also ask them to complete Chapter 34 of the Workbook.

EVALUATION

Chapter Quiz Distribute copies of the Chapter Quiz provided in Handout 34-2 to evaluate student understanding of this chapter. Remind students not to refer to their textbooks or notes while taking the quiz.

Test Manager You may wish to create a custom-tailored test using Prentice Hall *TestGen for Prehospital Emergency Care, Eighth Edition* to evaluate student understanding of this chapter.

Online Test Preparation (for students and instructors) Additional test preparation is available through *EMT Achieve: Basic Test Preparation* at http://www.prenhall.com/EMTAchieve. Instructors can also monitor student mastery online.

Reading/Reference
Textbook, pp. 971–983

Workbook
Chapter 34 Activities

Chapter Quiz
Handout 34-2

TestGen
Chapter 34 Test

Online Test Preparation
Send your students to
http://www.prenhall.com/
EMTAchieve

Handouts 34-3 to 34-6
Reinforcement Activities

**Brady Skills Series
EMT-B Videos/CD**
Visual Reinforcement

**PowerPoint
Presentation**
Chapter 34

Student CD
Chapter 34

Companion Website
http://www.prenhall.com/
mistovich

REINFORCEMENT

Handouts If classroom discussions or performance on the quiz indicates that some students have not fully mastered the chapter content, you may wish to assign some or all of the Reinforcement Handouts for this chapter.

TECH EXTRAS

Brady Skills Series EMT-B Videos/CD Have your students watch the skills come to life on either VHS or CD-ROM.

PowerPoint Presentation (for instructors) The PowerPoint material developed for this chapter offers useful reinforcement of chapter content.

Student CD A wide variety of material on this CD-ROM will reinforce and also expand student knowledge and skills.

Companion Website (for students) Additional review quizzes and links to EMS resources will contribute to further reinforcement of this chapter. Please visit http://www.prenhall.com/mistovich.

OBJECTIVES CHECKLIST

Cognitive		Date Mastered
5-2.8	Discuss the emergency medical care considerations for a patient with a penetrating chest injury.	
5-2.9	State the emergency medical care considerations for a patient with an open wound to the abdomen.	
5-2.10	Differentiate the care of an open wound to the chest from an open wound to the abdomen.	
*	Review the anatomy of the chest cavity as it pertains to chest injuries.	
*	Identify signs and symptoms of possible life-threatening chest injuries.	
*	Describe emergency medical care for life-threatening chest injuries.	
*	Review the anatomy of the abdomen.	
*	Recognize the common signs and symptoms of abdominal injuries.	
*	Describe the emergency medical care for a suspected abdominal injury.	
*	Describe the emergency medical care for genitalia injuries	

Psychomotor		Date Mastered
5-2.31	Demonstrate the steps in the emergency medical care of a patient with an open chest wound.	
5-2.32	Demonstrate the steps in the emergency medical care of a patient with open abdominal wounds.	

EVALUATION

CHAPTER 34 QUIZ

Write the letter of the best answer in the space provided.

_____ 1. The respiratory and circulatory organs are protected by the
  A. ribs.   C. vena cavae.
  B. mediastinum.   D. clavicles.

_____ 2. A flail segment occurs
  A. when initiated by paradoxical motion.
  B. with fracture of two or more ribs in two or more places.
  C. only from bullet or knife wounds.
  D. after a pneumothorax.

_____ 3. When a patient presents with jugular venous distension, respiratory distress, and hypotension following a closed chest injury, suspect
  A. rib fractures.   C. subcutaneous emphysema.
  B. a sucking chest wound.   D. a tension pneumothorax.

_____ 4. A screwdriver impaled in the chest should be managed by
  A. stabilizing it with a bulky dressing.
  B. removing it and covering with an occlusive dressing.
  C. applying vaseline around the screwdriver to seal the edge.
  D. removing it and covering the wound with a pressure dressing.

_____ 5. If a patient develops respiratory distress after an occlusive dressing has been applied to a chest wound, the EMT should
  A. cover the wound with more dressing.
  B. lift a corner of the dressing to allow pressure to escape.
  C. begin assisting breathing with positive-pressure ventilation.
  D. continue monitoring, as this reaction is to be expected.

_____ 6. To manage an evisceration, place the patient on his back and
  A. gently replace the organs.
  B. cover the organs with a moist dressing.
  C. apply a PASG.
  D. apply a chemical hot pack to prevent heat loss.

_____ 7. The damage that results from ruptured hollow abdominal organs is
  A. treatable in the field.   C. caused by acids and bacteria.
  B. caused by profuse bleeding.   D. non-life-threatening.

_____ 8. Your patient is the driver of a car that was hit head on. You find her lying on the sidewalk with her knees drawn toward her chest. She has no specific complaints. You suspect
  A. little or no injury because she has gotten out of the car.
  B. abdominal trauma due to mechanism of injury and positioning.
  C. cavitational injuries due to mechanism of injury.
  D. paradoxical motion due to patient positioning.

_____ 9. Your patient with an evisceration becomes tachycardic, cool, and hypotensive during transport; your next action should be to
   A. replace the dressing.
   B. support the injury with the patient's arm.
   C. reevaluate priority status and expedite transport.
   D. loosen one corner of the dressing.

_____ 10. Management of an injury caused by blunt trauma to the scrotum may include
   A. direct pressure.   C. oxygen.
   B. cold compresses.   D. all of these.

_____ 11. Management of a female patient who has suffered a laceration to the genital area will include all of the following *except*
   A. direct pressure.   C. vaginal packing.
   B. use of a moistened sanitary pad. D. assessment for hypoperfusion.

_____ 12. A pulmonary contusion can be life-threatening because it can
   A. reduce oxygen exchange via the alveoli.
   B. cause a hemorrhage into the trachea.
   C. take up space needed by the heart to contract.
   D. penetrate the lung.

IN THE FIELD

Read the following real-life situation. Then answer the questions that follow.

You are dispatched to a tavern where a fight has just taken place. The caller had stated that one man was injured and needed an ambulance because he couldn't breathe.

1. Given the reported circumstances, what causes might you expect for this problem?

2. What would you do first upon arrival at the scene?

3. After you are able to enter the scene, you find a 24-year-old male lying on the floor, splinting his right rib area and having some difficulty breathing. Blood is noted on the floor, and a raspy noise is heard each time he takes a breath. What would you do next?

4. What emergency care would you provide?

5. During transport, the young man complains of greater difficulty breathing. He is cool, tachypneic, and his neck veins are distended. Examination reveals no breath sounds on the right side. What is likely to be the cause of the problem?

6. What emergency care would you provide?

CHAPTER 34 REVIEW

Write the word or words that best complete each sentence in the space provided.

1. The _____ is the tube-like structure that connects the stomach with the mouth.

2. The two types of chest injuries are _____ and _____.

3. The aorta, vena cava, esophagus, and trachea are located in the _____, a hollow area in the center of the thoracic cavity.

4. The heart is a special type of _____ muscle that can be damaged by penetrating or blunt trauma.

5. Inhalation occurs when the _____ contracts and drops downward and the _____ _____ pull the ribs outward.

6. A(n) _____ _____ occurs when air trapped in the thoracic cavity expands under pressure.

7. A(n) _____ _____ is an injury that is created by a rib segment unattached to the rest of the rib cage.

8. In _____ _____, the rib segment will move inward during inhalation and outward during exhalation.

9. Stabilize a flail segment in the _____ position.

10. Apply a(n) _____ _____ to seal an open chest wound.

11. If a(n) _____ _____ exists, it will become increasingly difficult to ventilate the patient.

12. An open chest wound can pull air into the thoracic cavity, sometimes with a noticeable sound. This injury is referred to as a(n) _____ _____ _____.

13. Fractured ribs may produce _____, a grating sound or sensation.

14. An impaled object in the chest must be _____ before moving the patient.

15. Solid abdominal organs include the _____,

_____, _____, and the kidneys.

16. Alcohol ingestion, drugs, and _____ _____ can

reduce the patient's perception of pain.

17. Patients with _____ injuries often assume the fetal position.

18. When a large abdominal wound allows organs to protrude, a(n) _____ has

developed.

19. To manage the protrusion of abdominal organs, _____ them, using a(n)

_____ _____.

20. If the penis has been amputated, wrap it in a moist, sterile dressing, place it in a(n)

_____ _____, and keep it

_____.

CHEST, ABDOMEN, AND GENITALIA INJURIES: TRUE OR FALSE

Indicate if the following statements are true or false by writing T or F in the space provided.

_____ **1.** The mediastinum houses the trachea.

_____ **2.** During exhalation, the diaphragm contracts and moves downward.

_____ **3.** A pneumothorax occurs only if there is a break in the skin over the chest cavity.

_____ **4.** An occlusive dressing must be taped on all four sides to protect the chest wound.

_____ **5.** Air in the chest cavity is a hemothorax.

_____ **6.** Penetrating chest trauma occurs most often with violence.

_____ **7.** Gloves and eye protection are considered minimal body substance isolation precautions for an open chest injury.

_____ **8.** Jugular venous distension is an early sign of a tension pneumothorax.

_____ **9.** Crepitation with rib fractures is generally felt over the abdomen.

_____ **10.** When a sucking chest wound is detected, immediate care is to dress and bandage it.

_____ **11.** A patient with a chest injury is considered a high priority.

_____ **12.** A blow to the chest may cause ineffective heart pumping.

_____ **13.** The abdominal cavity is lined by a two-layer sheath-like membrane called the peritoneum.

_____ **14.** The abdomen contains vascular structures as well as solid and hollow organs.

_____ **15.** To control bleeding from the vagina, pack dressings into the vagina until the bleeding stops.

CHEST, ABDOMEN, AND GENITALIA INJURIES: MATCHING

Write the letter of the term in the space provided next to the appropriate definition.

_____ **1.** Air trapped in the thoracic cavity under pressure.

_____ **2.** Protrusion of the abdominal organs.

_____ **3.** Blood in the sac surrounding the heart.

_____ **4.** Contrary chest motion during respiration.

_____ **5.** Engorgement of the neck veins.

_____ **6.** Sudden compression of the thoracic cavity.

_____ **7.** Muscles between the ribs.

_____ **8.** Collapsed lung.

_____ **9.** The space within the chest.

_____ **10.** An open chest wound that permits air entry.

_____ **11.** Slow heart rate.

_____ **12.** Rapid respiratory rate.

_____ **13.** Condition created by the fracture of two or more ribs in two or more places.

_____ **14.** Grating sensation.

_____ **15.** Movement of the primary breathing tube from its usual position.

A. bradycardia

B. crepitation

C. evisceration

D. flail segment

E. intercostal muscles

F. jugular venous distension

G. paradoxical movement

H. pericardial tamponade

I. pneumothorax

J. sucking chest wound

K. tachypnea

L. tension pneumothorax

M. thoracic cavity

N. tracheal deviation

O. traumatic asphyxia

Chest, Abdomen, and Genitalia Injuries

Chest
Anatomy
Common Injuries
General Assessment and Care
Specific Injury Considerations
- Open chest wound
- Flail segment

Abdomen
Anatomy
Common Injuries
General Assessment and Care
Special Considerations with Eviscerations

Genitalia
Injuries to the Male Genitalia
Injuries to the Female Genitalia

Conditions Resulting from Chest Injury
Flail Segment
Pulmonary Contusion
Pneumothorax
Open Pneumothorax
Tension Pneumothorax
Hemothorax
Traumatic Asphyxiation
Cardiac Contusion
Pericardial Tamponade
Rib Injury

HANDOUT 34-2: Chapter 34 Quiz

1. A	**5.** B	**9.** C	**12.** A
2. B	**6.** B	**10.** D	**13.** D
3. D	**7.** C	**11.** C	**14.** D
4. A	**8.** B		

HANDOUT 34-3: In the Field

1. Blunt or penetrating trauma to the chest following the violence of a fight.
2. You should not enter the scene until police have secured it and made it safe to enter.
3. Take BSI precautions including gloves and eye protection. Then begin assessment.
4. Develop a general impression including difficulty in breathing. Perform an initial assessment. Provide manual in-line stabilization. Assess responsiveness. Assess airway; look for any current of potential obstructions including blood or broken teeth. Assess breathing. Be ready to administer oxygen. Examine for a wound and immediately cover it with a gloved hand. Search the underarm and posterior of the body for an exit wound. Ready and apply an occlusive dressing and tape on three sides. Be ready to assist breathing with positive-pressure ventilation if necessary. Assess circulation. Control breathing. Make this patient a high priority due to chest injury and expedite transport.
5. A developing tension pneumothorax.
6. Lift one edge of the dressing to allow pressure to escape and then reassess.

HANDOUT 34-4: Chapter 34 Review

1. esophagus
2. open, closed
3. mediastinum
4. contractile
5. diaphragm, intercostal muscles
6. tension pneumothorax
7. flail chest
8. paradoxical motion
9. inward
10. occlusive dressing
11. tension pneumothorax
12. sucking chest wound
13. crepitation

14. stabilized
15. spleen, liver, pancreas
16. head injury
17. abdominal
18. evisceration
19. cover, moist dressing
20. plastic bag, cool

HANDOUT 34-5: Chest, Abdomen, and Genitalia Injuries: True or False

1. T	**5.** F	**9.** F	**13.** T
2. F	**6.** T	**10.** F	**14.** T
3. F	**7.** T	**11.** T	**15.** F
4. F	**8.** F	**12.** T	

HANDOUT 34-6: Chest, Abdomen, and Genitalia Injuries: Matching

1. L	**5.** F	**9.** M	**13.** D
2. C	**6.** O	**10.** J	**14.** B
3. H	**7.** E	**11.** A	**15.** N
4. G	**8.** I	**12.** K	

CHAPTER

35 Agricultural and Industrial Emergencies

The chapter contains information that is valuable as background for the EMT but that goes substantially beyond the U.S. Department of Transportation (DOT) EMT-Basic curriculum.

OBJECTIVES

Numbered objectives are from the U.S. Department of Transportation's EMT-Basic National Standard Curriculum. Asterisked objectives, if any, pertain to material that is supplemental to the DOT curriculum. Page numbers refer to pages in the textbook.

Cognitive

* Describe the general guidelines for emergency care of agricultural injuries and related industrial injuries. (p. 974)
* Identify the mechanisms of injury responsible for the majority of agricultural accidents. (pp. 975–976)
* List the general guidelines for stabilizing and shutting down agricultural equipment and other machinery. (p. 976)
* List the common accidents/mechanisms of injury associated with various types of agricultural machinery, storage devices, and livestock. (pp. 974–980)
* List the general guidelines for industrial rescue. (pp. 980–981)

REVIEW

In the last chapter, students learned that most injuries to the chest or abdomen are not characterized by large, gaping wounds. Unlike some injuries to the extremities, they rarely involve bones protruding through the skin. Injuries to the chest and abdomen, in fact, are often not very dramatic in appearance and can be easily overlooked in the physical exam. The patient may actually be complaining of much more pain from injuries to bones and joints or from surface lacerations and abrasions. Initially, the patient may not even realize that he has a serious injury to the chest or abdomen.

It is important to understand, however, that the chest and abdomen contain vital organs and that injuries to those areas are often lethal. Chest injuries can cause a disturbance in respiration, oxygen exchange, and circulation. Abdominal injuries may produce severe internal bleeding and shock (hypoperfusion). EMTs must rely on the mechanism of injury, a high index of suspicion, and careful physical examination to determine and then to care for life-threatening injuries to the chest and abdomen.

Total Teaching Time
155 minutes

Resources Needed
* Scored Chapter 34 Quizzes
* Complete jump kit
* Stretcher

Additional Resources

Larmon/Davis, *Basic Life Support Skills*

Elling, *EMT Achieve: Basic Test Preparation*

Limmer/Mistovich/ O'Keefe, *Audio Lecture & Study Guide: EMT*

Mistovich/Kuvlesky, *SUCCESS! for the EMT, Second Edition*

©2008 by Pearson Education, Inc.
Prehospital Emergency Care, 8th ed.

839

Distribute the quizzes from the last class. Go over each question on the quiz and handle any concerns students may have about the answers.

INTRODUCTION TO CHAPTER 35

Chapter 35, "Agricultural and Industrial Emergencies," is the 10th and last chapter in Module 5. There is some form of agricultural activity in every state in the United States. Agriculture-related accidents usually involve heavy machinery and specialized equipment, which can present unique challenges to EMTs and other emergency care personnel. However, injuries that occur on a farm also can occur in urban areas, since farm-type machinery is used for many applications. The equipment in many industries is similar. The pizza dough roller works on the same principles as the printing press or the agricultural combine, for example. Workers who do snow removal, construction work, and factory work also use similar machinery—and are prone to similar accidents. Distribute the Chapter 35 Objectives Checklist, and give students a few minutes to look it over. Then briefly paraphrase the objectives for this lesson in your own words.

LECTURE

The following suggested lecture outline is based on the Department of Transportation's EMT-Basic National Standard Curriculum. In some places, the DOT curriculum has been rearranged or expanded upon so that it is more complete or easier for the student to understand. The page numbers in parentheses refer to pages in the textbook. The parenthetical references in dark, heavy type are to figures, tables, and scans in the textbook.

AGRICULTURAL AND INDUSTRIAL EMERGENCIES

I. **Response to agricultural and industrial emergencies** (pp. 972–974)
   A. Assessment and care: agricultural and industrial emergencies (pp. 972–974) **(Fig. 35-1, p. 973)**
      1. Scene size-up
         a. Wait for specialized rescue personnel, if necessary.
         b. Call the fire department if there has been a tractor accident.
         c. Do not attempt solo rescues in agricultural storage areas.
         d. Wear the appropriate personal protective clothing and equipment.
      2. Initial assessment
         a. Always assume spinal injury.
         b. Assess patient's mental status.
         c. Manage life-threatening problems with airway, breathing, and circulation.
         d. Make priority decision for further care and transport.
      3. Focused history and physical exam
         a. With significant MOI or unresponsive patient, perform rapid trauma assessment.
         b. Be aware that chest and abdominal injuries, and bone and joint injuries to extremities, are common.
         c. Record baseline vital signs.

Handout 35-1
Chapter 35 Objectives Checklist

Lecture Master
You may wish to display Lecture Master 35 when presenting the lecture to the class.

Point to Emphasize
Remember that personal safety is the EMT's first priority at any rescue scene.

On the Net
Agricultural EMS.
www.farmedic.com

On the Net
Farm accident response.
http://www.cdc.gov/nasd/docs/d001001-d001100/d001070/d001070.html

  d. Gather the SAMPLE history from the patient or bystanders.
 4. Emergency medical care
  a. Establish patent airway.
  b. Adequate breathing
   (1) Administer oxygen via nonrebreather mask at 15 liters per minute.
  c. Inadequate breathing
   (1) Initiate positive-pressure ventilation with supplemental oxygen.
  d. Control severe bleeding.
  e. If patient was exposed to chemicals or manure, remove exposed clothing and flush patient with water.
  f. Preserve all avulsed body parts.
  g. Stabilize all injuries.
  h. Immobilize patient to long backboard.
  i. Treat for shock.
  j. Transport.
 5. Detailed physical exam and ongoing assessment
  a. Perform if time and patient's condition permit.
  b. Be prepared to adjust care if patient's condition deteriorates.

II. Characteristics of agricultural accidents (pp. 974–980)
 A. Factors contributing to agricultural accidents (pp. 974–975)
  1. Long work hours
  2. Unstable weather conditions
  3. Old equipment
  4. Independent equipment maintenance
  5. Complicated equipment **(Fig. 35-2, p. 975)**
 B. Contributing factors that often make agricultural injuries serious (pp. 974–975)
  1. Little use of personal protective equipment
  2. Lengthy extrication processes
  3. Delayed discovery (working alone in remote areas)
  4. Long transport times
 C. Mechanisms of injury (pp. 975–976)
  1. Pinch points
  2. Wrap points
  3. Shear points
  4. Crush points
  5. Stored energy
 D. Stabilizing and shutting down agricultural equipment (pp. 976–978)
  1. General guidelines
   a. Stabilize equipment
    (1) Block or chock wheels and set brake
   b. Locate ignition switch, key, or throttle; if there are doubts about them, wait for help.
   c. Slow engine, then shut it off.
   d. If engine cannot be shut down from cab, try fuel tank shut-off valve.
   e. If that doesn't work, try clamping fuel line shut.
   f. If situation is life-threatening and all shut-off attempts have failed, discharge a 20-pound CO_2 fire extinguisher into air intake.
  2. Tractors

        a. Stabilizing techniques
        b. Lifting techniques
      3. Power takeoff shafts (**Fig. 35-3, p. 977**)
        a. Types of entrapment/injuries
        b. Extricating the patient
        c. Removing the PTO shaft
      4. Combines
        a. Sources of injury
        b. Extricating the patient
      5. Corn pickers
        a. Operation
        b. Types of injuries
        c. Dismantling the machine
      6. Hay balers
        a. Operation
        b. Types of entrapment
        c. Extricating the patient
    E. Agricultural storage devices (pp. 978–980)
      1. Grain tanks
        a. Personal safety before entering
        b. Patient rescue
      2. Silos (**Fig. 35-4, p. 979**)
        a. Signs of presence of silo gas
        b. Personal safety before entering
        c. Patient rescue
      3. Manure storage
        a. Signs and symptoms of hydrogen sulfide intoxication
        b. Personal safety before entering
        c. Treating the patient
      4. Agricultural chemicals
        a. Common symptoms of pesticide poisoning
        b. Personal safety before entering
        c. Treating the patient
    F. Injuries from livestock (p. 980)
      1. Common types of trauma
      2. Common mechanisms of injury
      3. Personal safety
  III. Industrial rescue (pp. 980–981) (**Fig. 35-5, p. 980**)
    A. Preparing for emergency care (pp. 980–981)
    B. Rescue guidelines (p. 981)

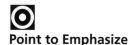

Point to Emphasize
Only personnel trained in a particular type of rescue operation should participate in dangerous rescue techniques.

CASE STUDY FOLLOW-UP

Ask a student volunteer to read the Case Study that begins on page 972 of the textbook. You may wish to use the following questions to engage the students in a discussion of the Case Study Follow-up that begins on page 981 of the textbook. Provide missing information and clarify ideas as needed.

  Q1. What does your scene size-up reveal about the nature of the emergency?

  A1. *That there is a man sitting on the ground in a field near a tractor. It is not clear whether the patient is suffering from a medical problem or trauma.*

Q2. When Mr. Fenwick's granddaughter tells you that he was working by the silo, what do you begin to suspect?

A2. *Inhalation of noxious gases.*

Q3. What other potential causes of Mr. Fenwick's illness do you discover during your initial assessment?

A3. *A history of heart problems and hunger because he skipped lunch.*

Q4. Regardless of the cause of the problem, how do you treat Mr. Fenwick?

A4. *By administering oxygen and transporting him to the hospital.*

Q5. Assuming that silo gas is present, what do you tell the family and what do you tell dispatch?

A5. *The family is told to keep everyone away from the silo until it can be checked out. Dispatch is contacted to request a hazmat expert to check out the silo at the Fenwick farm.*

IN REVIEW

Assess students' ability to apply what they have just learned by discussing the Review Questions on page 982 in the textbook.

Q1. Briefly describe sizing up the scene of an agricultural accident. Describe what you can do to ensure scene safety.

A1. *To size up the scene of an agricultural accident, check for potential exposure to gases, fumes, chemicals, unstable equipment, and livestock; make sure machinery is stabilized and shut down and other hazards such as leaking fuel have been controlled by specialized rescue personnel. All rescuers at the scene should also wear the appropriate personal protective equipment, such as self-contained breathing apparatus and lifeline, before attempting rescue. (pp. 972–974)*

Q2. List the specialized personnel that may be necessary to control the scene of an agricultural accident.

A2. *Specialized personnel that may be necessary to control the scene of an agricultural accident are fire personnel and hazardous materials teams. (pp. 972–974)*

Q3. List mechanisms of injury associated with agricultural machinery.

A3. *Mechanisms of injury associated with agricultural machinery are pinch points, wrap points, shear points, crush points, and stored energy. (pp. 975–976)*

Q4. List the general guidelines for stabilizing and shutting down agricultural equipment.

A4. *General guidelines for stabilizing and shutting down agricultural equipment are the following: To stabilize agricultural equipment, block or chock the wheels, set the parking brake, or tie it to another vehicle. To shut down agricultural equipment, slow the engine down with the throttle, and then switch off the ignition key. If the engine uses diesel fuel, use a fuel or air shut-off lever instead. Alternatively, try the shut-off valve at the bottom of the fuel tank, vise-grip pliers to clamp the fuel line shut, or as a last resort discharge a 20-pound CO_2 fire extinguisher into the air intake. (p. 976)*

Q5. Describe accidents/mechanisms of injury associated with tractors, power takeoff shafts (PTOs), combines, corn pickers, and hay balers.

A5. *Accidents/mechanisms of injury specific to these machinery are as follows: Tractor—Fuel leaks; fires; explosions; tractor turning over backward or rolling to the side over the worker. Power takeoff (PTO) shaft—Clothing caught in the spinning shaft pulls the worker in. Combine—Rotating auger pulls victims in; oscillating cutting bars; impalement on reels, with hardened steel tines; and crushing injuries from snapping rollers. Corn picker—Entrapment and possible amputation of the hands and arms. Hay baler—Header assembly picks up and pulls worker in, injuries caused by tines and cross auger. (pp. 976–978)*

Q6. Describe accidents/mechanisms of injury associated with storage areas and storage devices.

A6. *Accidents/mechanisms of injury associated with storage areas and storage devices are suffocation and inhalation of toxic gases in or around grain tanks, silos, and manure storage areas and structures; and poisoning by pesticides. (pp. 978–980)*

Q7. Describe accidents/mechanisms of injury associated with farm animals.

A7. *Accidents/mechanisms of injury associated with farm animals include falling on slippery floors and getting bitten, thrown, knocked down, stepped on, kicked, or punctured. (p. 980)*

Q8. List the general guidelines that should be applied to rescue in an industrial setting.

A8. *The general guidelines that should be applied to rescue in an industrial setting are the following: Check with staff to determine potential hazards at the scene. Verify that all valves, switches, and levers that allow a machine to operate have been padlocked to the off position. If the patient is in a confined space or has been injured by an airborne or spilled agent, wait for specialized personnel or hazardous materials teams to arrive and decontaminate the scene and the patient. (p. 981)*

CRITICAL THINKING

Assess students' ability to respond to real-life emergency situations by discussing the Critical Thinking questions on page 983 in the textbook.

Q1. What immediate care would you provide for the patient?

A1. *Establish and maintain manual in-line spinal stabilization. Open the airway using a jaw thrust maneuver. Insert and oropharyngeal airway and begin bag-valve-mask ventilation. Reassess the pulses. Because the patient was likely in cardiac arrest for more than 4 to 5 minutes, immediately begin chest compressions.*

Q2. Would the use of an AED be appropriate for this patient?

A2. *The AED is indicated in this patient since this is likely a medical causes of the cardiac arrest. It appears the patient has been in cardiac arrest for more than 4 to 5 minutes; thus, it is necessary to perform 5 cycles of CPR at a ratio of 30 compressions and 2 ventilations. Following the 5 cycles of CPR, apply the AED and follow the prompts. The only other consideration would be to consider the hypothermia AED protocol if you suspect hypothermia in this patient.*

Q3. What special considerations would you include in your emergency care of the patient?

A3. *It is unknown whether the patient has suffered a mechanism of injury that may have caused a spinal injury; thus, take the necessary spinal precautions to include complete spinal immobilization. Another consideration is the possibility of silo gases that may have contributed or caused the patient to lose consciousness. The other consideration is the possibility of the patient being hypothermic. Grain retains a cold temperature even in the summer months. If the patient was entrapped in the grain for a long period of time, his body temperature may have been reduced while in contact with the cold grain.*

ROLE PLAY

Tell students that they will now have a chance to apply the information they have learned to a real-life situation encountered by EMS personnel. Call for two volunteers to play the role of EMTs who are responding to a 9-1-1 call, one volunteer to be a bystander, and one volunteer to be the patient. Take the two EMT players outside the classroom and provide them with a complete jump kit and a stretcher. Describe the following situation to them:

You are dispatched to the Triangle-Q Ranch on a weekday morning. The dispatcher said that the patient is a woman who has been injured by a horse.

Remind the EMT players that the emphasis of the scene is on dealing with agricultural emergencies. However, they should use all the skills they have learned to date. Return to the classroom after telling the EMT players that you will call them to the scene as soon as you have prepared it and the other players.

Have the bystanders and the patient come to the front of the classroom. Describe the following situation to them and the class:

Twenty-two-year-old Tina Suarez was attempting to break a new horse. Although she was usually quite successful, the stallion with which she was currently working was proving to be a challenge. As she attempted to put a bit in his mouth, the stallion kicked her in the chest. She was knocked to the ground, winded. She now has a very sore sternum and difficulty breathing. Her uncle, Hernando Suarez, who was helping Tina with the horse, promptly called 9-1-1.

Tell the patient and bystanders to take their places and to start acting. Call the EMTs back into the classroom. Allow the role play to progress naturally. Provide appropriate vital signs and other objective information about the patient if the EMTs assess this information. Intervene only if the players seem to be at a loss for what to do.

End the play when the EMTs have prepared the patient for transport to the ambulance or have obtained a signed refusal.

Discuss the following with the entire class:

- What did the EMTs do well?
- What, if anything, should they have done differently?

ASSIGNMENTS

Assign students to read Chapter 36, "Infants and Children," before the next class. Also ask them to complete Chapter 35 of the Workbook.

Reading/Reference
Textbook, pp. 986–1048

Workbook
Chapter 35 Activities

Chapter Quiz
Handout 35-2

TestGen
Chapter 35 Test

Online Test Preparation
Send your students to
http://www.prenhall.com/
EMTAchieve

Handouts 35-3 to 35-5
Reinforcement Activities

**Brady Skills Series
EMT-B Videos/CD**
Visual Reinforcement

**PowerPoint
Presentation**
Chapter 35

Student CD
Chapter 35

Companion Website
http://www.prenhall.com/
mistovich

EVALUATION

Chapter Quiz Distribute copies of the Chapter Quiz provided in Handout 35-2 to evaluate student understanding of this chapter. Remind students not to refer to their textbooks or notes while taking the quiz.

Test Manager You may wish to create a custom-tailored test using Prentice Hall *TestGen for Prehospital Emergency Care, Eighth Edition* to evaluate student understanding of this chapter.

Online Test Preparation (for students and instructors) Additional test preparation is available through *EMT Achieve: Basic Test Preparation* at http://www.prenhall.com/EMTAchieve. Instructors can also monitor student mastery online.

REINFORCEMENT

Handouts If classroom discussions or performance on the quiz indicates that some students have not fully mastered the chapter content, you may wish to assign some or all of the Reinforcement Handouts for this chapter.

TECH EXTRAS

Brady Skills Series EMT-B Videos/CD Have your students watch the skills come to life on either VHS or CD-ROM.

PowerPoint Presentation (for instructors) The PowerPoint material developed for this chapter offers useful reinforcement of chapter content.

Student CD A wide variety of material on this CD-ROM will reinforce and also expand student knowledge and skills.

Companion Website (for students) Additional review quizzes and links to EMS resources will contribute to further reinforcement of this chapter. Please visit http://www.prenhall.com/mistovich.

OBJECTIVES CHECKLIST

Cognitive	Date Mastered
* Describe the general guidelines for emergency care of agricultural injuries and related industrial injuries.	
* Identify the mechanisms of injury responsible for the majority of agricultural accidents.	
* List the general guidelines for stabilizing and shutting down agricultural equipment and other machinery.	
* List the common accidents/mechanisms of injury associated with various types of agricultural machinery, storage devices, and livestock.	
* List the general guidelines for industrial rescue.	

OBJECTIVES

CHAPTER 35 QUIZ

Write the letter of the best answer in the space provided.

_____ 1. At the scene of a tractor accident, the scene would be declared safe when
  A. the EMTs can reach the patient.
  B. the tractor is shut down, stabilized, and fuel and hydraulic fluids are controlled.
  C. all rescuers are wearing SCBA.
  D. a technical rescue unit has reached the scene.

_____ 2. With a patient who has been injured while using farm machinery, the EMT's first action upon reaching the patient's side would be to
  A. apply high-flow oxygen.   C. establish in-line stabilization.
  B. record baseline vital signs.   D. flush the patient with water.

_____ 3. To remove a patient trapped in a combine unit, the rescuer may need to do all of the following *except*
  A. use the self-reversing mechanism.   C. spread the snapping rollers.
  B. set a pry bar in place.   D. lock the hydraulic system.

_____ 4. A patient caught in a grain storage tank for an extended period is likely to suffer from
  A. hyperthermia.   C. crush injuries.
  B. hypothermia.   D. poisoning.

_____ 5. An EMT who arrives at the scene of a "man down" outside a silo and notes a smell of bleach and yellow stains on equipment and clothing should suspect the presence of
  A. cleaning fluids.   C. pesticides.
  B. hydraulic fuel.   D. silo gas.

_____ 6. Signs and symptoms of pesticide exposure include all of the following *except*
  A. hot, dry skin.   C. drooling.
  B. abdominal cramps.   D. tearing (crying).

_____ 7. Treatment for a patient who has been bitten on the arm by an animal and who has then slipped on the barn floor should include
  A. application of an occlusive dressing.
  B. packing of the arm in ice or cold packs.
  C. flushing of the wound with water before it is dressed.
  D. assistance in administration of the patient's Epi-Pen®.

_____ 8. The EMT must be aware that pesticides can
  A. decompose when exposed to air.
  B. be absorbed through the eyes.
  C. increase intensity over time.
  D. cause the release of carbon monoxide.

_____ 9. In an industrial accident, the EMT knows that
  A. by law, all machinery must be automatically shut down.
  B. the patient must be removed from the scene immediately.
  C. specialized personnel or hazmat teams may be necessary.
  D. the equipment in one facility is not like equipment anywhere else.

EVALUATION

IN THE FIELD

Review the following real-life situation. Then answer the questions that follow.

You are called to a local industrial park for a "man trapped." You arrive to find coworkers surrounding a grain storage bin. They tell you that John, a 40-year-old man, was trying to get the grain to flow and didn't come back out.

1. What are the possible scene hazards?

2. What would you do first?

3. After you are able to enter the scene, you find a middle-age male in the center of the tank. What would you do next?

4. What emergency care would you provide?

REINFORCEMENT

CHAPTER 35 REVIEW

Write the word or words that best complete each sentence in the space provided.

1. Before you begin an agricultural accident rescue, perform a thorough

   _____ _____ _____.

2. In an agricultural storage area, all rescuers must wear _____

   _____ _____ _____ in

   addition to appropriate _____ _____

   _____.

3. If the patient was exposed to chemicals or manure, remove his _____ and

   _____ the patient with copious amounts of

   _____.

4. Before a patient can be extricated from agricultural equipment, _____

   _____ and _____ the equipment.

5. If you are concerned that you do not know the correct controls to shut down equipment,

   _____ _____ _____ and

   _____ _____ _____.

6. Accidents with power takeoff shafts occur when _____ gets

   _____ in the spinning shaft.

7. A common source of agricultural injury is from a(n) _____, which is the

   rotating part of a screw conveyer.

8. Most injuries from a corn picker involve _____ of the hands and arms.

9. When crops are stored in silos, they can ferment and release _____

   _____, _____ and oxides of _____.

10. Signs of silo gas include a(n) _____ odor, _____

    or _____ vapor, or dead insects or birds near the structure.

AGRICULTURAL AND INDUSTRIAL EMERGENCIES: LISTING

1. List five factors that contribute to agricultural accidents.

2. List five mechanisms of injury associated with agricultural equipment accidents.

3. List five ways to shut down agricultural equipment.

4. List two problems associated with accidents in agricultural storage devices.

Agricultural and Industrial Emergencies

Response to Agricultural and Industrial Emergencies

Basic Assessment and Care Considerations

Characteristics of Agricultural Accidents

Mechanisms of Injury

- Pinch points
- Wrap points
- Shear points
- Crush points
- Stored energy

Stabilizing and Shutting Down Equipment

- Tractors
- Power takeoff shafts
- Combines
- Corn pickers
- Hay balers

Agricultural Storage Devices

Injuries from Livestock

Industrial Rescue

HANDOUT 35-2: Chapter 35 Quiz

1.	B	**4.**	B	**6.**	A	**8.**	B
2.	C	**5.**	D	**7.**	C	**9.**	C
3.	A						

HANDOUT 35-3: In the Field

1. Burial by the grain, hypothermia, grain in the airway, equipment, grain explosions.

2. Call for specialized extrication teams and the fire department. Be sure that all rescuers have assistance including lifelines and disposable mechanical filter respirators rated for dust particles. Turn off the electricity, but keep fans working until the actual rescue. Breach the wall of the storage bin by cutting triangles on opposing sides below the level of the grain and opening them up at the same time to allow grain to flow out. Be sure the fire department is ready with a charged line before any cuts are made.

3. Secure the patient with a lifeline. Shore grain away from him.

4. Airway management will be the top priority. Aggressively suction and clear the airway. Be prepared to ventilate as needed. Take spinal precautions and secure the patient to a long spine board before removing him from the storage bin. Apply oxygen once extricated form the bin. Continue with further assessment and treatments.

HANDOUT 35-4: Chapter 35 Review

1. scene size-up
2. self-contained breathing apparatus, personal protective equipment
3. clothing, flush, water
4. shut down, stabilize
5. leave them alone; wait for help
6. clothing, caught
7. auger
8. entrapment
9. carbon monoxide, methane, nitrogen
10. bleach, yellow, red

HANDOUT 35-5: Agricultural and Industrial Emergencies: Listing

1. Any five: long hours; unstable weather; excessive noise and vibration; old equipment; complicated maintenance; nonuse of PPE; lengthy extrication times; working alone; long transport times.

2. Pinch points, wrap points, shear points, crush points, stored energy.

3. Locate and turn off the ignition switch. (If you are unsure, leave it alone and wait for help.) Slow the engine with the throttle and switch-off key. Try the shut-off switch at the bottom of the fuel tank if the ignition switch didn't work. Clamp the fuel line. If the patient is in a life-threatening situation, destroy the engine by discharging a 20-pound CO_2 fire extinguisher into it through the air-intake valve.

4. Suffocation and inhalation of toxic gases.

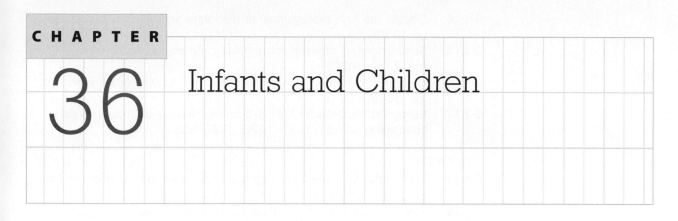

36 Infants and Children

This chapter covers Lessons 6-1 and 6-2 of the U.S. Department of Transportation's EMT-Basic National Standard Curriculum.

OBJECTIVES

Numbered objectives are from the U.S. Department of Transportation's EMT-Basic National Standard Curriculum. Asterisked objectives, if any, pertain to material that is supplemental to the DOT curriculum. Page numbers refer to pages in the textbook.

Cognitive

6-1.1 Identify the developmental considerations for the following age groups: (pp. 989–990)
— infants
— toddlers
— preschool
— school age
— adolescent

6-1.2 Describe the differences in anatomy and physiology of the infant, child, and adult patient. (pp. 990–994)

6-1.3 Differentiate the response of the ill or injured infant or child from that of an adult. (pp. 989–990, 994)

6-1.4 Indicate various causes of respiratory emergencies. (pp. 996–999)

6-1.5 Differentiate between respiratory distress and respiratory failure. (pp. 997–998)

6-1.6 List the steps in the management of foreign body airway obstruction. (pp. 1014–1016)

6-1.7 Summarize emergency medical care strategies for respiratory distress and respiratory failure. (pp. 1008–1018)

6-1.8 Identify the signs and symptoms of shock (hypoperfusion) in the infant and child patient. (pp. 1023–1024)

6-1.9 Describe the method of determining end organ perfusion in the infant and child patient. (pp. 995, 1002)

6-1.10 State the usual causes of cardiac arrest in infants and children versus adults. (p. 996)

6-1.11 List the common causes of seizures in the infant and child patient. (p. 1016)

6-1.12 Describe the management of seizures in the infant and child patient. (p. 1020)

6-1.13 Differentiate between the injury patterns in adults, infants, and children. (pp. 1028–1030)

Total Teaching Time
240 minutes

Resources Needed
- Scored Chapter 35 Quizzes
- Complete jump kit with BSI equipment and assorted cervical collars
- Oxygen equipment
- Portable suction unit
- Stretcher

Additional Resources

Larmon/Davis, *Basic Life Support Skills*

Elling, *EMT Achieve: Basic Test Preparation*

Limmer/Mistovich/O'Keefe, *Audio Lecture & Study Guide: EMT*

Mistovich/Kuvlesky, *SUCCESS! for the EMT, Second Edition*

6-1.14 Discuss the field management of the infant and child trauma patient. (p. 1030)

6-1.15 Summarize the indicators of possible child abuse and neglect. (pp. 1031–1032)

6-1.16 Describe the medical legal responsibilities in suspected child abuse. (pp. 1032, 1034)

6-1.17 Recognize the need for EMT debriefing following a difficult infant or child transport. (pp. 1027–1028, 1034, 1038)

Affective

6-1.18 Explain the rationale for having knowledge and skills appropriate for dealing with the infant and child patient. (p. 988)

6-1.19 Attend to the feelings of the family when dealing with an ill or injured infant or child. (p. 988)

6-1.20 Understand the provider's own response (emotional) to caring for infants or children. (pp. 1027–1028,1034, 1038)

Psychomotor

6-1.21 Demonstrate the techniques of foreign body airway obstruction removal in the infant.

6-1.22 Demonstrate the techniques of foreign body airway obstruction removal in the child.

6-1.23 Demonstrate the assessment of the infant and child.

6-1.24 Demonstrate bag-valve-mask artificial ventilations for the infant.

6-1.25 Demonstrate bag-valve-mask artificial ventilations for the child.

6-1.26 Demonstrate oxygen delivery for the infant and child.

REVIEW

In the last lesson, "Agricultural and Industrial Emergencies," students learned that there is some form of agricultural activity in every state in the United States. Agriculture-related accidents usually involve heavy machinery and specialized equipment, which can present unique challenges to EMTs and other emergency care personnel. However, injuries that occur on a farm also occur in urban areas and in many industries, since farm-type machinery is used for many applications. The pizza dough roller works on the same principles as the printing press or the agricultural combine, for example. Workers who do snow removal, construction work, and factory work also use similar machinery—and are prone to similar accidents.

Distribute the quizzes from the last class. Go over each question on the quiz and handle any concerns students may have about the answers. Explain to students that they have now completed Module 5, Trauma. In Module 5, they learned that trauma is the leading cause of death in the United States for people between the ages of 1 and 44. They also learned about the kinetics of trauma; bleeding control and shock; soft tissue injuries; burns; injuries to the muscles and bones; injuries to the head and spine; injuries to eyes, face, neck, chest, abdomen, and genitalia; and farm and industrial emergencies.

INTRODUCTION TO MODULE 6/CHAPTER 36

Explain that this next module is a single chapter, "Infants and Children." Children are our greatest resource. Unfortunately, nearly 45,000 children die in the United States each year. Approximately one in four children will sustain an injury during their childhood that will require medical attention. Trauma is the leading cause of fatal injuries in children under the age of 14, particularly in motor vehicle crashes, drownings, burns, poisonings, and falls. Of medical problems, respiratory problems are the most serious. Approximately 10 percent of an EMT's patients will be children.

If asked, experienced EMS providers would probably concur that dealing with infants and children is one of the most (if not *the* most) stressful situations they encounter during their EMS careers. This is mainly due to the relative infrequency of dealing with pediatric patients, the particularities of assessment and treatment, and having to deal with the emotions of the pediatric patient, the distressed parents, and probably the feelings the EMTs have themselves. Very few things can evoke an emotional charge in people like a critically ill or injured child. Despite this, EMTs must be able to prevent the emotions they experience from interfering with the task at hand: assessing and treating the young patient. To help focus on this task, the EMT needs to remember that despite the patient's age, a breathing problem is a breathing problem, a bleeding wound is a bleeding wound, and an unresponsive patient is an unresponsive patient. While the EMT's assessment approach to the ill or injured child is somewhat different from the approach to an adult, the basic treatment goals are the same.

Distribute the Chapter 36 Objectives Checklist, and give students a few minutes to look it over. Then briefly paraphrase the objectives for this lesson in your own words.

LECTURE

The following suggested lecture outline is based on the Department of Transportation's EMT-Basic National Standard Curriculum. In some places, the DOT curriculum has been rearranged or expanded upon so that it is more complete or easier for the student to understand. The page numbers in parentheses refer to pages in the textbook. The parenthetical references in dark, heavy type are to figures, tables, and scans in the textbook.

INFANTS AND CHILDREN

  I. Dealing with caregivers (p. 988)
 II. Dealing with the child (pp. 988–1016)
   A. Developmental characteristics (pp. 988–990)
    1. Neonates (0 to hospital discharge)
     a. Totally dependent upon others
     b. Present no special assessment problems
    2. Infants (0–1 year)
     a. Exhibit minimal stranger anxiety up to 6 months
     b. Do not like to be separated from caregiver. Allow familiar person to hold infant while you complete examination.
     c. Should be kept warm; warm your hands, stethoscope, and examining surface.
     d. Are frightened by initial stimulation around the face. Begin assessment at feet or trunk and end with head.
    3. Toddlers (1–3 years)
     a. Do not like to be touched
     b. Do not like being separated from parents
     c. Do not like having clothing removed. Remove, examine, replace.

Handout 36-1
Chapter 36 Objectives Checklist

Lecture Master
You may wish to display Lecture Master 36 when presenting the lecture to the class.

Reading/Reference
Markenson, D., *Pediatric Prehospital Care,* Upper Saddle River, NJ: Brady/ Pearson Education, 2002.

    d. Do not like having an oxygen mask over face and will resist

    e. Afraid of needles; fear pain

    f. May believe that injury or illness they have is form of punishment

    g. Are frightened by initial stimulation around the face. Use toe-to-head or trunk-to-head examination approach.

    h. Can be distracted. Try to distract child with favorite toy.

4. Preschoolers (3–6 years)

    a. Are concrete thinkers who interpret literally

    b. Have vivid imaginations and dramatize events

    c. Still believe that accident or injury is their fault and view it as punishment

    d. Are modest

    e. Are aware of death

    f. Are afraid of blood

    g. Fear pain

    h. Fear permanent injury

5. School age (6–12 years)

    a. Are usually more cooperative, even curious

    b. Are able to rationalize

    c. Have understanding of what EMS is about

    d. Have simple understanding of their bodies

    e. Are curious and interested in their surroundings. They will be fascinated by the contents of each ambulance cabinet.

    f. May regress emotionally or act exceptionally mature

    g. May become anxious if you cut their clothes

    h. Still fear pain, the sight of blood, permanent injuries, and disfigurement. Explain their physical injuries to them.

6. Adolescents (12–18 years)

    a. Are developing abstract thinking skills

    b. Think they are invincible; thus, may take risks that lead to injury

    c. Fear the possibility of disfigurement and disability

    d. Will be reluctant to disclose information about their sexual history, drug use, personal habits, illegal activities

    e. Sometimes find the presence of a peer, caregiver, or close friend physically and emotionally reassuring

    f. Are preoccupied by their bodies and extremely concerned about modesty

    g. May occasionally overreact and are capable of having a hysterical reaction

B. Anatomical differences (p. 991) **(Fig. 36-1, p. 991; Table 36-1, p. 992)**

1. Airway

    a. Infants have proportionally larger airways

    b. The diameter of a newborn's trachea is only about 4 to 5 mm or about one-third the diameter of a dime, or the size of a straw

    c. The pediatric trachea is much more pliable

    d. Pressure on the soft tissue under the chin can easily cause the tongue to be displaced

    e. Newborns and infants are obligate nose breathers.

    f. The smallest area of the upper airway is at the level of the cricoid

    g. The epiglottis is much higher in the airway

2. Head

    a. Children's heads are proportionally larger **(Fig. 36-2, p. 993)**

    b. Infants younger than 9 months typically cannot fully support their own heads.

    c. Infants have a "soft spot" on their head

3. Chest and lungs

    a. The child's ribs are much more pliable

    b. The child's ribs are more horizontal than they are rounded

    c. Lung tissue is much more fragile

    d. The chest will move minimally with respiration

    e. It is normal for the abdomen to rise with inhalation and the abdomen to fall with exhalation.

    f. The chest muscles are underdeveloped and used more as accessory muscles

4. Respiratory system

    a. The breathing is inadequate once the respiratory rate reaches 60 breaths per minute or greater in children

    b. Infants and children less than 5 years of age will breathe at a rate 2–3 times faster than the adult patient

5. Cardiovascular system

    a. The heart rate will increase in response to fear, fever, anxiety, hypoxia, activity, and hypovolemia.

    b. In infants and children, bradycardia is a late response to hypoxia.

    c. In newborns, bradycardia is the initial response to hypoxia.

    d. Infants and children have a smaller circulating blood volume

    e. Hypotension will not usually develop in infants and children until greater than 20 percent of the blood volume has been lost.

    f. The onset of the hypotension is sudden once the compensation falls.

    g. Infants and young children have a limited ability to increase the strength of cardiac contraction.

6. Abdomen

    a. The child's abdominal musculature is less well developed.

    b. Until the child reaches puberty, the liver and spleen are more exposed and less protected.

7. Extremities

    a. The bones of the extremities in a child will fracture more often by bending and splintering.

    b. The infant and young child's motor development occurs from the head to the toes.

8. Metabolic rate

    a. Infants and children have a faster metabolic rate

9. Skin and body surface area

    a. A child's skin surface is large compared to his body mass.

b. The skin is thinner and much more delicate than in an adult.

C. Pediatric assessment triangle (pp. 994–996) **(Fig. 36-3, p. 994; Fig. 36-4, p. 996)**

    1. Appearance

    2. Work of breathing

    3. Circulation

D. Airway and breathing problems in infants and children (pp. 996–999)

    1. Early respiratory distress (compensated respiratory distress) **(Fig. 36-5 and 36-6, p. 997)**

        a. Increase in respiratory rate above normal rate for child

        b. Nasal flaring

        c. Intercostal reactions on inspiration

        d. Supraclavicular and subcostal retractions on inspiration

        e. Neck muscle retractions

        f. Audible breathing noises: stridor, wheezing, grunting

        g. "Seesaw" respirations

    2. Decompensated respiratory failure **(Fig. 36-8, p. 998)**

        a. Respiratory rate over 60/minute

        b. Cyanosis

        c. Decreased muscle tone

        d. Severe use of accessory muscles to aid respirations

        e. Poor peripheral perfusion

        f. Altered mental status

        g. Grunting

        h. Head bobbing

    3. Respiratory arrest **(Fig. 36-9, p. 998)**

        a. Respiratory rate less than 10/minute or absent breathing

        b. Irregular respirations

        c. Limp muscle tone

        d. Unresponsiveness

        e. Slower than normal or absent heart rate

        f. Weak or absent peripheral pulses

        g. Hypotension in patients over 3 years old

    4. Airway obstruction

        a. Indications of partial airway obstruction

            (1) May be alert, pink, and with peripheral perfusion

            (2) Normal or slightly pale skin with peripheral perfusion

            (3) Stridor

            (4) Retractions of intercostal, supraclavicular, and subcostal tissues

            (5) Possible crowing or other noisy respirations

            (6) Possible crying

            (7) Forceful cough

        b. Indications of complete airway obstruction

            (1) No crying or talking

            (2) Ineffective or absent cough

            (3) Altered mental status, including possible loss of responsiveness

            (4) Probable cyanosis

E. Assessment and care: respiratory emergencies (pp. 999–1016) **(Figs. 36-26, pp.1017–1018; Fig. 36-27, p. 1019)**

    1. Initial assessment

a. Visually assess patient from across the room before approaching.
b. Form general impression based on overall appearance.
c. Be acutely aware of alterations in respiratory effort.
d. Be alert for the following clues to respiratory status:
   (1) Rapid breathing
   (2) Noisy breathing
e. Assess circulation (quality of pulse, skin, and capillary refill). **(Fig. 36-11, p. 1003)**
f. Assess for signs of inadequate perfusion (shock).
g. Interventions
   (1) Clear an unclear airway.
   (2) If breathing is adequate, provide oxygen by nonrebreather mask; if inadequate, immediately provide positive-pressure ventilation with supplemental oxygen. **(Fig. 36-7, p. 997)**
   (3) Assess circulation.
      (a) Control bleeding.
      (b) Treat for shock, if necessary.
   (4) Determine priority for transport.
2. Focused history and physical exam **(Table 36-4, p. 1004; Fig. 36-12, pp. 1005–1008)**
   a. Begin at the scene.
   b. Gather history first and then perform examination.
   c. Complete SAMPLE history using OPQRST.
   d. If trauma is suspected, perform a complete rapid trauma assessment, using DCAP-BTLS on each part of the body.
   e. Assess baseline vital signs. **(Table 36-3, p. 995)**
   f. Look for signs and symptoms of respiratory distress.
3. Emergency medical care—respiratory emergencies
   a. Establish and maintain a patent airway.
      (1) Perform the head-tilt, chin-lift, extending head only enough to ensure a patent airway. **(Fig 36-13, p. 1009)**
      (2) If there is possible spinal injury, perform the jaw-thrust maneuver. **(Fig. 36-14, p. 1009)**
   b. Suction any secretions, vomitus, or blood. **(Fig. 36-15, p. 1009)**
   c. If you need to assist ventilations, maintain a patent airway with an oropharyngeal or nasopharyngeal airway. **(Figs. 36-16, p. 1010 and 36-17, p. 1011)**
   d. Initiate positive-pressure ventilation if infant or child is in decompensated respiratory failure or respiratory arrest.
      (1) Use one-way valve on mouth-to-mask valve.
      (2) Use appropriately sized bag on bag-valve-mask device.
      (3) Select appropriately sized mask that fits over bridge of nose and into cleft of chin. **(Fig. 36-18, p. 1012 and Fig. 36-19, p. 1012)**
      (4) Ensure good mask seal by using one or two hands.
      (5) Ventilate at a minimum rate of 12–20 per minute.
      (6) Press on cricoid cartilage to help alleviate regurgitation if it is a problem.

Point to Emphasize
For an infant or a child, the oropharyngeal airway is inserted with the tip pointing toward the tongue, in the same position in which it will be after insertion.

e. Maintain oxygen therapy; if patient will not tolerate mask, try "blow-by" method. **(Fig. 36-20, p. 1013)**

f. Position the patient.

g. Transport.

4. Emergency medical care—foreign body airway obstruction

    a. Unresponsive infant (<1 year of age) **(Figs. 36-21, 36-22 and 36-23, pp. 1014–1015)**

        (1) If the infant is unresponsive and a foreign body airway obstruction is suspected, or if the infant with a mild or severe foreign body airway obstruction becomes unresponsive during your treatment, immediately perform the following steps.

        (2) Open the airway using a head-tilt, chin-lift maneuver.

        (3) Open the mouth and look for the foreign body. If the foreign body is seen in the oropharynx, attempt to remove it. Do not perform a blind finger sweep. Doing so may push the obstruction further down the pharynx or may damage the oropharynx.

        (4) Provide two ventilations over a one-second period.

        (5) Using the same landmarks and techniques for CPR, provide 30 chest compressions at a rate of 100 per minute followed.

        (6) After the chest compressions, look in the mouth for the obstruction. If it can be seen in the oropharynx, attempt to remove it.

        (7) Provide two ventilations followed by another set of 30 compressions.

        (8) Continue this sequence until the foreign body is removed. The patient should be transported without delay. Be sure to connect oxygen to the bag-valve-mask device via a reservoir to deliver the highest possible concentration of oxygen.

    b. Child (>1 year of age)

        (1) If the patient is older than 1 year of age and has a severe foreign body airway obstruction and is no longer able to cough or make sounds, perform subdiaphragmatic abdominal thrusts (Heimlich maneuver) as follows:

        (2) Assure the patient that you are there to help.

        (3) Position yourself behind the child, and reach your arms around his abdomen **(Figure 36-24, p. 1015)**.

        (4) Locate the navel and place the thumb side of one clenched fist midway between the navel and the xiphoid process (cartilage below the sternum).

        (5) Wrap the other hand over the clenched hand.

        (6) Deliver five abdominal thrusts inward and upward, at a 45-degree angle toward the head

        (7) Continue to deliver sequential series of five abdominal thrusts until the object is dislodged, you arrive at the medical facility, or the patient becomes unresponsive.

    c. Unresponsive child (>1 year of age) **(Fig. 36-25, p. 1016)**

(1) If the child is unresponsive and a foreign body airway obstruction is suspected, or if the child with a mild or severe foreign body airway obstruction becomes unresponsive during your treatment, immediately perform the following steps:

(2) Open the airway using a head-tilt, chin-lift maneuver.

(3) Open the mouth and look for the foreign body. If the foreign body is seen in the oropharynx, attempt to remove it. Do not perform a blind finger sweep. Doing so may push the obstruction further down the pharynx or may damage the oropharynx.

(4) Provide two ventilations over a one-second period.

(5) Using the same landmarks and techniques for CPR, provide 30 chest compressions at a rate of 100 per minute followed.

(6) After the chest compressions, look in the mouth for the obstruction. If it can be seen in the oropharynx, attempt to remove it.

(7) Provide two ventilations followed by another set of 30 compressions.

(8) Continue this sequence until the foreign body is removed. The patient should be transported without delay. Be sure to connect oxygen to the bag-valve-mask device via a reservoir to deliver the highest possible concentration of oxygen.

d. Detailed physical exam and ongoing assessment

e. Perform for unresponsive or trauma patient

f. Repeat ongoing assessment every 5 minutes or as frequently as possible for patient with respiratory distress.

III. **Medical problems common to infants and children** (pp. 1016–1028)

   A. Seizures (pp. 1016–1020)

      1. Assessment considerations

         a. While obtaining SAMPLE history, find out whether child has had previous seizures.

         b. If so, find out whether this is the child's normal seizure pattern.

         c. Determine whether child has been taking antiseizure medication.

      2. Emergency medical care (**Fig. 36-28, p. 1020**)

   B. Altered mental status (pp. 1020–1021)

      1. Assessment considerations (**Fig. 36-29, p. 1020**)

         a. Child's level of maturity greatly influences assessment.

         b. AVPU (**Table 36-2, p. 995**)

            (1) A—curious, alert and awake

            (2) V—turns head to sounds

            (3) P—moans or cries to pain

            (4) U—does not respond or displays nonactivity

         c. Pediatric Glasgow Coma Scale (**Table 36-5, p. 1021**)

         d. Shout or pinch an unresponsive patient to elicit a response.

         e. Never shake an infant or child for any reason.

2. Emergency medical care (**Fig. 36-30, p. 1022**)
C. Poisonings (pp. 1021–1022)
  1. Assessment considerations
    a. Perform thorough focused history and physical exam.
    b. Gather as much information as possible about type of overdose.
  2. Emergency medical care (**Fig. 36-31, p. 1023**)
D. Fever (pp. 1022–1023)
  1. Assessment considerations
    a. How quickly fever "spikes" is greater concern than how high the fever.
    b. Not all high temperatures produce seizures.
    c. Dehydration is a common result of fever.
    d. Signs and symptoms of dehydration in infants and children
      (1) Nausea
      (2) Lack of appetite
      (3) Vomiting and possible fainting
      (4) Weak, rapid pulse
      (5) Pale skin and sunken eyes
      (6) Dry, parched mucous membranes
      (7) Skin that stays 'tented" when pinched
      (8) Possible sunken fontanelle in infant
  2. Emergency medical care (**Fig. 36-32, p. 1024**)
E. Shock (hypoperfusion) (pp. 1023–1025) (**Table 36-3, p. 995**)
  1. Assessment considerations
    a. Signs and symptoms in children (**Fig. 36-33, p. 1024; Table 36-6, p. 1025**)
      (1) May be sudden
      (2) Rapid respiratory rate
      (3) Pale, cool, clammy skin
      (4) Decreased mental status
      (5) Prolonged capillary refill
      (6) Weak or absent peripheral pulses
    b. Hypoperfused pediatric patients deteriorate faster and more severely than adults.
  2. Emergency medical care (**Fig. 36-34, p. 1025**)
F. Drowning (pp. 1025–1026)
  1. Assessment considerations
    a. Be aware of the possibility of trauma and/or hypothermia.
    b. Be on the alert for the occurrence of secondary drowning syndrome (a deterioration that takes place after normal breathing is restored) from minutes to hours after event.
  2. Emergency medical care (**Fig. 36-35, p. 1026**)
G. Sudden infant death syndrome (pp. 1026–1028)
  1. Assessment considerations
    a. Condition cannot be diagnosed in the field.
    b. Proceed with care as for any patient in cardiac arrest.
    c. As practical, obtain a brief SAMPLE history and observe surroundings:
      (1) Physical appearance of baby
      (2) Position of baby in crib
      (3) Physical appearance of crib
      (4) Presence of objects in crib
      (5) Unusual or dangerous objects in room

Point to Emphasize

A mild fever can quickly turn into a high fever, indicating a serious problem. If the infant or child feels very warm or hot to the touch, prepare the patient for immediate transport. Transport as quickly as possible all children who have suffered a seizure, protecting the patient from temperature extremes.

Point to Emphasize

Infants and children are able to compensate for shock for a long time. Then the compensating mechanisms fail at approximately 30 percent blood loss, and decompensated shock develops very rapidly. This means that a child may appear fine, then "go sour" in a hurry.

On the Net

For more on sudden infant death syndrome, go to: www.sids-network.org

    (6) Appearance of room/house
    (7) Presence of medication, even if for adults
    (8) Circumstances concerning discovery of unresponsive child
    (9) Time baby was put to bed or fell asleep
    (10) Problems at birth
    (11) General health
    (12) Any recent illnesses
    (13) Date and result of last physical exam
  2. Emergency medical care **(Fig. 36-36, p. 1028)**
  3. Aiding family members in SIDS emergencies
 H. Presence of parents during pediatric resuscitation (p. 1028)

IV. Trauma in infants and children (pp. 1028–1035)
 A. Common patterns of injury (pp. 1028–1029)
  1. Unrestrained children in cars
   a. Head and neck injuries
  2. Restrained children in cars
   a. Abdominal and/or lumbar injuries
  3. Child struck while riding a bike
  4. Head, spinal, and abdominal injuries
  5. Child struck by car
   a. Head, chest, and lower extremity injuries
  6. Diving or falls
   a. Head and spinal injuries
  7. Heat/fire
   a. Burns may be more severe; smoke inhalation will cause swelling of airway more rapidly than in adults
  8. Sports injuries
   a. Head and neck injuries
 B. Trauma and the infant's or child's anatomy (pp. 1029–1030)
  1. Assessment considerations
   a. Head
    (1) Common in children because of the relatively large size of head **(Fig. 36-37, p. 1029)**
    (2) Common findings of head injury
     (a) Nausea and vomiting
     (b) Respiratory arrest
     (c) Facial and scalp injuries (Blood loss can be profound enough to cause hypoperfusion.) **(Fig. 36-38, p. 1030)**
    (3) Most common cause of hypoxia is tongue obstruction airway
    (4) If hypoperfusion present with closed head injury, suspect other injuries.
   b. Chest
    (1) Infants and children are less likely to suffer rib fractures but more likely to suffer internal damage.
    (2) Suspect intrathoracic injuries when you see even minimal signs of external trauma.
   c. Abdomen
    (1) More common site of injury in children than in adults
    (2) Often a source of hidden injury
    (3) Always consider abdominal injury if patient is deteriorating rapidly without external signs.

On the Net
Pediatric soft tissue injuries.
http://www.musckids.com/
health_library/poison/
wounds.htm

(4) Consider any trauma to the abdomen a serious injury.

(5) Air in stomach can distend abdomen and interfere with artificial ventilation efforts.

2. Emergency medical care—trauma in infants and children (**Fig. 36-30, p. 1022**)

    a. Establish and maintain in-line stabilization and airway, using jaw-thrust.

    b. Suction as necessary.

    c. Adequate breathing—provide oxygen at 15 liters per minute by nonrebreather mask.

    d. Inadequate breathing—initiate positive-pressure ventilation with supplemental oxygen.

    e. Provide complete spinal immobilization.

    f. Transport. (**Table 36-7, p. 1031; Fig. 36-39, p. 1032**)

C. Child abuse and neglect (pp. 1030–1035) (**Fig. 36-40, pp. 1033–1034**)

  1. Abuse

    a. Improper or excessive action so as to injure or cause harm

  2. Neglect

    a. Giving insufficient attention or respect to someone who has a claim to that attention

  3. Abuser rarely shows guilt and may show hostility toward the child or toward another caregiver in the household.

  4. Abused child will usually show fear when asked to describe the injury.

  5. In many cases, the child will be the victim of physical, emotional, and sexual abuse and neglect.

  6. Signs and symptoms of abuse

    a. Multiple abrasions, lacerations, incisions, bruises, broken bones

    b. Multiple injuries or bruised in various stages of healing

    c. Injuries on both front and back or on both sides of child's body

    d. Unusual wounds (such as cigarette burns)

    e. A fearful child

    f. Injuries to the genitals

    g. Injuries, often lethal, to brain or spinal cord that occur when infant or child is violently shaken ("shaken baby syndrome")

    h. Situations in which injuries do not match mechanism of injury described by caregivers or patient

    i. Lack of adult supervision

    j. Untreated chronic illnesses

    k. Malnourishment and unsafe living environment

    l. Delay in reporting injuries

  7. Emergency medical care guidelines for child abuse and neglect (Fig. 36-41, p. 1035)

V. Infants and children with special needs (pp. 1035–1038)

  A. Tracheostomy tubes (pp. 1035–1036) (**Figs. 36-42, 36-43, and 36-44, p. 1036**)

    1. Common problems

      a. Accumulation of mucus obstructing the airway

      b. Bleeding

      c. Infection around the site

      d. An air leak around the tube

      e. Dislodgment of the tube

Point of Interest

It is estimated that 3–5 percent of children in the United States are abused or neglected. Over 7,000 children will die as a result of child abuse. Only one-third of all abuse cases in children over 3 years of age are reported.

Teaching Tip

Identify local policies regarding reporting cases of suspected child abuse. Have a member of the local Human Services Department come to answer questions about child abuse.

Point to Emphasize

Always report suspicions of child abuse to Emergency Department staff. Keep accurate records of possible child abuse. State all objective findings.

On the Net

For more on child abuse, go to: www.childabuse.org

---

2. General care guidelines

    a. Maintain a patent airway.

    b. Suction out any foreign material or fluid.

    c. Provide supplemental oxygen. (Attach bag-valve-mask device directly to the standard fitting on the tracheostomy tube.)

    d. Maintain a position of comfort for the patient.

    e. Transport for evaluation at the hospital.

B. Home artificial ventilators (pp. 1036–1037)

  1. Causes of home ventilator malfunction

    a. Mechanical failure

    b. Power outages

    c. Diminished oxygen supply

    d. Failure of backup batteries

  2. General care guidelines

    a. Establish and maintain an open airway.

    b. Provide positive-pressure ventilation with supplemental oxygen at a rate of one every 3 seconds

    c. Transport to the hospital.

C. Central lines (p. 1037) **(Fig. 36-45, p. 1037)**

  1. Long-term venous access device

  2. Normally outside the area of practice for EMTs

  3. Reasons for calls to EMS about central lines

    a. Device has become infected

    b. Device clotted off because it is not flushing properly

    c. Device has cracked or ruptured

    d. Device has cracked or ruptured beneath the skin with significant bleeding

  4. General care guidelines

    a. Correct and maintain any inadequacies to child's airway, breathing, and circulation.

    b. Apply pressure directly to device to control bleeding, if necessary.

    c. Transport child to hospital.

D. Gastrostomy tubes (p. 1037)

  1. Gastrostomy tube

    a. Tube placed in stomach through abdominal wall for patients who cannot be fed by mouth

  2. Feeding button

    a. Small silicon device that protrudes slightly from abdominal wall and accepts a feeding tube through its one-way valve

  3. Reasons for calls about gastrostomy tubes

    a. Tube has become dislodged

    b. Area around tube has become infected

  4. General care guidelines

    a. Maintain adequate airway and breathing status.

    b. Be prepared to suction.

    c. Be alert for changes in mental status.

    d. Provide oxygen as necessary.

    e. Transport patient in a Fowler's position or on right side with the head elevated.

E. Shunts (pp. 1037–1038)

  1. Shunt

    a. Surgically placed device extending from the brain to the abdomen in order to drain extra cerebrospinal fluid

2. Signs of shunt malfunction
   a. Changes in mental status
   b. Seizures
   c. Loss of motor or sensory function
   d. Vomiting
   e. Respiratory depression
3. General care guidelines
   a. Manage the airway.
   b. Be alert for occlusion by the tongue if mental status is decreased.
   c. Initiate positive-pressure ventilation if the breathing is inadequate. (Respiratory arrest is common.)
   d. Position patient on left side and be prepared to suction.
   e. Provide rapid transport to hospital.

VI. **Taking care of yourself** (p. 1038)
  A. Causes of stress and anxiety (p. 1038)
     1. Lack of experience in treating children
     2. Fear of failure
     3. Identifying patients with own children
  B. Steps to alleviating stress (p. 1038)
     1. Know that much of what you learned about adults applies to children.
     2. Know that often it is not what you do but how you do it that varies.
     3. Be prepared; learn and practice equipment and exam skills.
     4. Focus on the task at hand; momentarily separate how you feel from what you must do.
  C. Critical incident stress debriefing (CISD) (p. 1038)
     1. Seek the help of the CISD team.
     2. If your system does not have such a team, share your feelings with a trusted friend.

ENRICHMENT (OPTIONAL)

The following sections contain information that is valuable as background for the EMT, but that goes substantially beyond the U.S. Department of Transportation's EMT-Basic National Standard Curriculum.

VII. **More on pediatric emergencies** (pp. 1038–1045)
  A. Respiratory emergencies (pp. 1038–1041)
     1. Croup (**Fig. 36-46, p. 1039**)
        a. Common infection of upper airway
     2. Epiglottitis
        a. Condition that resembles croup caused by bacterial infection that inflames and swells epiglottis
     3. Asthma (**Fig. 36-47, p. 1040**)
        a. Bronchioles spasm and constrict, swelling bronchial membranes, reducing airway size, and producing mucus
     4. Bronchiolitis
        a. Easily confused with asthma but caused when bronchioles in the lungs become inflamed by viral infection
     5. Cardiac arrest
        a. Almost all result from airway obstruction and respiratory arrest; most of remaining are caused by shock

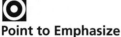

Point to Emphasize

If you cannot resolve the impact of a stressful event, contact the local CISD team for assistance before the problem compounds.

Point to Emphasize

All cases of epiglottitis must be considered life-threatening, no matter how early the detection. The child must be handled gently since rough handling and stress could lead to a total airway obstruction from spasms of the larynx and swelling tissues.

CASE STUDY FOLLOW-UP

Ask a student volunteer to read the Case Study that begins on page 988 of the textbook. You may wish to use the following questions to engage the students in a discussion of the Case Study Follow-up that begins on page 1046 of the textbook. Provide missing information and clarify ideas as needed.

Q1. What does your initial assessment reveal about the baby's condition?

A1. *It reveals cyanosis, flaccid muscles, and an absence of any response to the environment. It is obvious that this child is terribly ill, with ominous signs of respiratory arrest.*

Q2. Describe your attempts to secure Jason's airway and breathing.

A2. *Immediate opening of Jason's airway does not result in spontaneous respirations. Because Jason's mother says he was not ill (which tends to indicate the problem is not related to a respiratory disease), and because repositioning the airway was unsuccessful, there is a high index of suspicion that Jason's airway is obstructed by a foreign body. Jason is positioned facedown on the EMT's forearm and given five back blows. His condition does not improve, so he is turned over into a supine position on the forearm and given five chest thrusts. After the next reassessment, Jason is still not breathing, and ventilations are still impossible. The sequence of five back blows and five chest thrusts is repeated. Inspection of Jason's mouth reveals what looks like a peanut in the back of the throat. It is hooked out with the EMT's little finger.*

Q3. Since Jason is still not breathing, what do you do?

A3. *An oropharyngeal airway is inserted and positive-pressure ventilations provided using a BVM with oxygen attached.*

Q4. What change occurs in Jason's condition as a result of securing his airway and assisting breathing?

A4. *Jason's color changes from blue to a normal pink. His muscle tone returns and he moves around actively. When ventilations are stopped to assess Jason's spontaneous respiratory effort, it is found to be at a rate of 30 per minute and with a normal depth. At this point, Jason is provided with oxygen at 15 liters per minute via a nonrebreather mask.*

IN REVIEW

Assess students' ability to apply what they have just learned by discussing the Review Questions on page 1047 in the textbook.

Q1. Describe differences in anatomy and physiology of the infant and child as compared to the adult patient.

A1. *Differences in anatomy and physiology of the infant and child as compared to adult patients are numerous. (See textbook, pages 000–000.) However, the most significant to the EMT typically concerns the airway. Those differences include: Infants have proportionally larger tongues, making it easier to occlude the airway; the diameter of a newborn's trachea is only about 4–5 mm, which means life-threatening swelling occurs faster than in an adult; pressure on the soft tissue under the chin can easily displace the tongue back into the pharynx, leading to airway obstruction; newborns and infants are obligate nose breathers, which means an obstructed nose can cause respiratory distress; the smallest area of the upper airway is at the level of the cricoid cartilage, and not at the level of the vocal cords as seen in an adult; the epiglottis is much higher in the airway than in an adult, leading to a higher incidence of aspiration, especially when the neck is hyperextended. (pp. 990–994)*

Q2. Differentiate between early (compensated) respiratory distress and decompensated respiratory failure.

A2. *The patient in early respiratory distress presents with adequate respiratory depth and minute volume but has an above-normal respiratory rate; nasal flaring; intercostal, supraclavicular, and subcostal retractions on inspiration; neck muscle use; audible breathing noises such as stridor, wheezing, or grunting; and "seesaw" respirations. Decompensated respiratory failure presents with signs of early respiratory distress and any of the following: respiratory rate over 60/minute, cyanosis, decreased muscle tone, severe use of accessory muscles to aid in respirations, poor peripheral perfusion, altered mental status (in relation to the patient's developmental stage), grunting, or head bobbing. (pp. 997–998)*

Q3. List the signs of an obstructed airway.

A3. *Signs of an obstructed airway include no crying or talking, ineffective or absent cough, altered mental status including possible loss of responsiveness, and probable cyanosis. (pp. 998–999)*

Q4. Describe the methods of determining end organ perfusion in the infant and child patient.

A4. *End organ perfusion is adequate if all of the following assessment determinations are normal (or acceptable): capillary refill, pulse rate and strength, strength of peripheral versus core pulses, warmth and color of the hands and feet, urinary output, and mental status. (pp. 1024–1024)*

Q5. List the common causes of seizures in the infant and child patient and describe the management of seizures for the pediatric patient.

A5. *Seizures are commonly caused in children by fever (febrile seizures) plus any condition that would also produce seizures in adults: epilepsy, head injury, meningitis, oxygen deficiency, drug overdose, and low blood sugar (hypoglycemia). If the child has a single seizure, ensure airway patency, position the patient on his side (if there is no possibility of spine trauma) and make sure he doesn't injure himself, be prepared to suction, provide oxygen and ventilate as appropriate, and transport. If seizures last longer than 10 minutes or recur without a recovery period (status epilepticus), provide positive-pressure ventilation with supplemental oxygen. Transport rapidly, monitoring the airway. (pp. 1016, 1020)*

Q6. Describe the patterns of injury most likely to occur when pediatric patients are victims of trauma.

A6. *Patterns of injury most likely to occur when pediatric patients are victims of trauma are as follows: In motor-vehicle crashes, unrestrained infants and children are likely to have head and neck injuries, while restrained pediatric patients will have abdominal and lumbar spine injuries. Pediatric patients struck while riding bicycles are likely to suffer head, spinal, and/or abdominal injuries, whereas those struck by vehicles as pedestrians will probably have head injuries, chest injuries, and lower extremity injuries. In falls from height or diving into water, suspect head and neck injuries. When pediatric patients suffer burns, expect them to be more severe since their skin is not as thick or durable as adult skin, and inhalation of smoke, toxic fumes, or super-heated air can cause airway swelling more rapidly and severely in pediatric patients. In sports injuries, suspect head and neck injuries. Finally, maintain a high index of suspicion for child abuse when the child's injury does not match her or the caregiver's description of what happened. (pp. 1028–1029)*

Q7. List the indicators of possible child abuse and neglect.

A7. *Indicators of possible child abuse and neglect include multiple abrasions, lacerations, incisions, bruises, broken bones; multiple injuries or bruises in various stages of healing; injuries on both the front and back or on both sides of the child; unusual wounds (such as curricular burns); a fearful child; injuries to the genitals; injuries to the CNS system that occur when the infant or child is violently shaken; situations in which the injuries do not match the mechanism of injury described by the caregivers or the patient; lack of adult supervision; untreated chronic illnesses; and malnourishment, an unsafe living environment, and a delay in reporting injuries. (pp. 1030–1034)*

Q8. List five advanced support devices for children who receive home care; for each device, briefly state its general purpose, one or more problems that may prompt a call to EMS, and appropriate emergency care steps.

A8. *Five advanced support devices for children who receive home care (with description of purpose, problems, and emergency care) are the following:*

- *Tracheostomy tubes. Purpose: Placed through opening into trachea to secure airway. Problems: Mucus obstruction, bleeding, infection, air leak, dislodgment. Care: Maintain patent airway, suction mucous or blood, maintain position of comfort, transport. (pp. 1035–1036)*

- *Home artificial ventilators. Purpose: Assist ventilations. Problems: Mechanical failure, power outage, battery failure, diminished oxygen supply. Care: Ensure airway, assist ventilations, administer oxygen, assist caregiver in troubleshooting the problem and/or transport. (pp. 1036–1037)*

- *Central lines. Purpose: Deliver medications or substances intravenously. Problems: Infection, blocked line, cracked or ruptured device with bleeding. Care: Ensure airway, breathing, and circulation, apply pressure to device to control bleeding, transport. (p. 1037)*

- *Gastrostomy tubes. Purpose: Feeding through a tube into the stomach. Problems: Infection, dislodgment. Care: Maintain airway and breathing, suction if necessary, monitor for changes in mental status (e.g., if patient is hypoglycemic), provide oxygen as necessary, transport. (p. 1037)*

- **Shunts.** *Purpose: Draining CSF from skull. Problems: Any malfunction resulting in signs typical of head injury including altered mental status, seizures, loss of motor or sensory function, or respiratory depression. Care: Manage airway, provide positive-pressure ventilation if respiration is inadequate, transport. (pp. 1037–1038)*

Q9. Discuss ways the EMT can deal with the emotional consequences of a difficult infant or child transport.

A9. *The EMT can deal with the emotional consequences of a difficult infant or child transport by making use of the services of a CISD team or talking things over with a trusted friend or family member. Emotions that are ignored or suppressed can lead to burnout. (p. 1038)*

CRITICAL THINKING

Assess students' ability to respond to real-life emergency situations by discussing the Critical Thinking questions on page 1048 in the textbook.

Q1. What emergency care would you immediately provide for the toddler?

A1. *One EMT should immediately position the toddler on the floor. Open the airway using a head-tilt chin-lift maneuver. Insert an oropharyngeal airway and begin ventilation. Another EMT should find the proper landmark and begin chest compressions.*

Q2. What special anatomical characteristics would you consider when establishing an airway and ventilating the toddler as compared to the adult?

A2. *The EMTs should be aware that the pediatric patient's trachea will be softer and more pliable than an adult; therefore, hyperextending the neck while opening the airway can actually kink the trachea and result in an occluded airway at the level of the trachea. The head and neck should be placed in a neutral position and extended only until the airway is open and ventilation is delivered without resistance. The head is disproportionately large as compared to the body. When the toddler is placed supine, the large occiput of the head causes the head and neck to flex forward resulting in an airway obstruction. To alleviate this problem, it is necessary to pad under the shoulders to elevate the body so that the large head and neck is brought into an in-line position with the torso. Also, placing pressure on the soft tissue under the chin (during head-tilt, chin-lift, for example) can displace the tongue and cause airway compromise.*

Q3. How would you perform CPR on this toddler?

A3. *The child should be placed on a flat hard surface. Open the airway using a head-tilt chin-lift maneuver being careful not to hyperextend the head and neck. Chest compressions and ventilations should then be initiated at a ratio of 30 compressions to 2 ventilations when doing one-person or two-person CPR. In the infant and child, it is acceptable to perform two-person CPR at a ratio of 15 compressions and 2 ventilations. It is important to compress deep, approximately 1/2 to 1/3 the depth of the chest and to compress fast at a rate of at least 100 compressions per minute.*

Q4. Would you apply the AED? If so, what special considerations must you contemplate when using the AED on a 2-year-old?

A4. *It is acceptable to apply the AED to children older than one year of age. Pediatric or child electrode pads with a dose attenuating resistor or an AED with a child key or switch should be used if possible. If these pads or child AED dose device is not available, apply adult AED pads to the chest. The electrode pads of the AED should be placed on the anterior chest to the right of the sternum just below the right clavicle and to the left apex following 5 cycles (approximately two minutes) of CPR.*

ROLE PLAY

Tell students that they will now have the opportunity to apply what they have learned to a real-life situation encountered by EMS personnel. Call for two volunteers to play the role of EMTs who are responding to a 9-1-1 call, two volunteers to be bystanders, and one volunteer to be the patient.

Take the two EMT players outside the classroom and provide them with a complete jump kit containing BSI equipment, assorted cervical collars, oxygen equipment, a portable suction unit, and a stretcher. Make sure that pediatric sizes of all equipment are provided. Describe the following situation to the volunteers:

You are dispatched to an apartment complex at 2100 hours on a Sunday night. The dispatcher said that the patient is an injured toddler. Tell student volunteers that they should act appropriately on what they find at the scene. Remind them that the emphasis at the scene should be on dealing with the pediatric patient, but that they may use all the skills they have learned to date.

Reenter the classroom, first telling those volunteers in the hall that you will call them to the scene shortly. Have the bystanders and the patient come to the front of the classroom. Describe the following situation to them and the class:

Two-year-old Felicia lives with her mother, Tracey Smith, and her grandmother, Rita Smith, in a one-bedroom apartment. Tracey is single and unemployed. Rita reluctantly supports Tracey for the sake of the child. One evening after supper, Rita and Tracey are watching TV. Suddenly they hear a piercing scream from the kitchen. Little Felicia has somehow gotten hold of a knife and cut her hand. She is sitting on the floor and bleeding. Rita accuses Tracey of being a bad mother for not watching her child and a loud argument develops. Rita runs the child's hand under the kitchen faucet and calls 9-1-1. The argument is still in progress when the EMTs arrive. By this time the child is starting to get a little shocky.

Tell the patient and bystanders to take their places and to start acting. Call the EMTs back into the classroom.

Allow the role play to progress naturally. Provide appropriate vital signs and other objective information about the patient if the EMTs assess this information. Intervene only if the players seem to be at a loss for what to do.

Discuss the following with the entire class:

- What did the EMTs do well?

- What, if anything, should they have done differently?

Reading/Reference
Textbook, pp. 1049–1073

Workbook
Chapter 36 Activities

Chapter Quiz
Handout 36-2

TestGen
Chapter 36 Test

Online Test Preparation
Send your students to
http://www.prenhall.com/
EMTAchieve

Handouts 36-3 to 36-6
Reinforcement Activities

**Brady Skills Series
EMT-B Videos/CD**
Visual Reinforcement

**PowerPoint
Presentation**
Chapter 36

Student CD
Chapter 36

Companion Website
http://www.prenhall.com/
mistovich

ASSIGNMENTS

Assign students to read Chapter 37, "Geriatrics," before the next class. Also ask them to complete Chapter 36 of the Workbook.

EVALUATION

Chapter Quiz Distribute copies of the Chapter Quiz provided in Handout 36-2 to evaluate student understanding of this chapter. Remind students not to refer to their textbooks or notes while taking the quiz.

Test Manager You may wish to create a custom-tailored test using Prentice Hall *TestGen for Prehospital Emergency Care, Eighth Edition* to evaluate student understanding of this chapter.

Online Test Preparation (for students and instructors) Additional test preparation is available through *EMT Achieve: Basic Test Preparation* at http://www.prenhall.com/EMTAchieve. Instructors can also monitor student mastery online.

REINFORCEMENT

Handouts If classroom discussions or performance on the quiz indicates that some students have not fully mastered the chapter content, you may wish to assign some or all of the Reinforcement Handouts for this chapter.

TECH EXTRAS

Brady Skills Series EMT-B Videos/CD Have your students watch the skills come to life on either VHS or CD-ROM.

PowerPoint Presentation (for instructors) The PowerPoint material developed for this chapter offers useful reinforcement of chapter content.

Student CD A wide variety of material on this CD-ROM will reinforce and also expand student knowledge and skills.

Companion Website (for students) Additional review quizzes and links to EMS resources will contribute to further reinforcement of this chapter. Please visit http://www.prenhall.com/mistovich.

OBJECTIVES CHECKLIST

Cognitive		Date Mastered
6-1.1	Identify the developmental considerations for the following age groups: — infants — toddlers — preschool — school age — adolescent	
6-1.2	Describe the differences in anatomy and physiology of the infant, child, and adult patient.	
6-1.3	Differentiate the response of the ill or injured infant or child from that of an adult.	
6-1.4	Indicate various causes of respiratory emergencies.	
6-1.5	Differentiate between respiratory distress and respiratory failure.	
6-1.6	List the steps in the management of foreign body airway obstruction.	
6-1.7	Summarize emergency medical care strategies for respiratory distress and respiratory failure.	
6-1.8	Identify the signs and symptoms of shock (hypoperfusion) in the infant and child patient.	
6-1.9	Describe the method of determining end organ perfusion in the infant and child patient.	
6-1.10	State the usual causes of cardiac arrest in infants and children versus adults.	
6-1.11	List the common causes of seizures in the infant and child patient.	
6-1.12	Describe the management of seizures in the infant and child patient.	
6-1.13	Differentiate between the injury patterns in adults, infants, and children.	
6-1.14	Discuss the field management of the infant and child trauma patient.	
6-1.15	Summarize the indicators of possible child abuse and neglect.	
6-1.16	Describe the medical legal responsibilities in suspected child abuse.	
6-1.17	Recognize the need for EMT-Basic debriefing following a difficult infant or child transport.	

Affective		Date Mastered
6-1.18	Explain the rationale for having knowledge and skills appropriate for dealing with the infant and child patient.	
6-1.19	Attend to the feelings of the family when dealing with an ill or injured infant or child.	
6-1.20	Understand the provider's own response (emotional) to caring for infants or children.	

Psychomotor		Date Mastered
6-1.21	Demonstrate the techniques of foreign body airway obstruction removal in the infant.	
6-1.22	Demonstrate the techniques of foreign body airway obstruction removal in the child.	
6-1.23	Demonstrate the assessment of the infant and child.	
6-1.24	Demonstrate bag-valve-mask artificial ventilations for the infant.	
6-1.25	Demonstrate bag-valve-mask artificial ventilations for the child.	
6-1.26	Demonstrate oxygen delivery for the infant and child.	

CHAPTER 36 QUIZ

Write the letter of the best answer in the space provided.

_____ 1. The leading medical cause of cardiac arrest in infants and children is
   A. seizure.   C. anaphylactic shock.
   B. respiratory failure.   D. fever.

_____ 2. In caring for a sick child, the EMT should have the parent or caregiver
   A. step out of the room.
   B. assist in the care of the child when appropriate.
   C. follow the ambulance to the hospital.
   D. speak only with the doctor about the child.

_____ 3. Artificial ventilations should be performed on an infant or a child at a minimal rate of
   _____ breaths per minute.
   A. 10   C. 20
   B. 15   D. 30

_____ 4. The EMT recognizes that a normal developmental characteristic of toddlers is that they
   A. do not like to be touched.
   B. are very accepting of an oxygen mask.
   C. are eager to show independence from caregivers.
   D. need detailed explanations.

_____ 5. The first step in emergency care for a pediatric patient in shock is
   A. providing oxygen.   C. keeping the patient warm.
   B. managing bleeding.   D. ensuring an open airway.

_____ 6. Children develop hypothermia more easily than adults because of their
   A. lower metabolisms.
   B. slower heart rates.
   C. smaller lung capacity.
   D. larger surface area in proportion to body mass.

_____ 7. In assessing a toddler, the EMT knows that the rib cage is
   A. more susceptible to fracture than in adults.
   B. much more pliable than in adults.
   C. a likely spot for fractures.
   D. composed of incomplete skeletal plates.

_____ 8. Signs of early respiratory distress in an infant include all of the following *except*
   A. retractions.   C. fontanels.
   B. "seesaw" respirations.   D. nostril flaring.

_____ 9. Approximately 5 percent of children have seizures caused by
   A. fever.   C. head injuries.
   B. epilepsy.   D. shock.

_____ 10. After a pediatric submersion patient has been removed from the water, you should provide _____ while establishing an airway.

A. suctioning

B. chest thrusts

C. back blows

D. immobilization

_____ 11. The leading cause of death in children ages 1–14 is

A. fever.

B. drowning.

C. trauma.

D. respiratory arrest.

_____ 12. The most common injuries sustained by children who are struck by a car while riding a bike are to the

A. leg, hand, and back.

B. head, spine, and abdomen.

C. head, spine, and lower extremity.

D. upper extremity, lower extremity, and abdomen.

_____ 13. The most common cause of hypoxia in the unconscious pediatric patient with a head injury is

A. the tongue.

B. intracranial pressure.

C. intercranial pressure.

D. Kussmaul's respirations.

_____ 14. When using the PASG in a pediatric patient, do *not*

A. inflate both legs.

B. worry about accurate sizing.

C. use if hypoperfusion or pelvic instability is suspected.

D. inflate the abdominal compartment.

_____ 15. One complication that pediatric burn patients are especially susceptible to is

A. hyperthermia.

B. febrile seizure.

C. hypothermia.

D. hypoxia.

_____ 16. The only major cause of infant and child death to have increased in the last 30 years is

A. vehicular trauma.

B. poisoning.

C. child abuse.

D. burns.

_____ 17. Central lines are intravenous lines that are placed

A. in the center of the extremities.

B. close to the dermis.

C. close to the heart.

D. in the groin.

_____ 18. When a child who an EMT has cared for dies, it can be a good idea for the EMT to turn for assistance to the

A. ALS crew.

B. CISD team.

C. QI manual.

D. ICS plan.

©2008 by Pearson Education, Inc.
Prehospital Emergency Care, 8th ed.

IN THE FIELD

Review the following real-life situations. Then answer the questions that follow.

(A) You are dispatched to a home where you find an 8-month-old child in her mother's arms. The mother says the child is lethargic. She is breathing at a rate of 46 times a minute, and her pulse rate is 190. Her skin is cool to the touch, and she is pale. The mother states that the child has been sick for 2 days. This afternoon she became worse. The mother adds that the child has been vomiting and has had diarrhea.

1. What is likely to be the cause of the problem?

2. What emergency care would you provide?

(B) You are called to the home of a frantic mother of a 4-year-old girl. Her daughter is normally active, and this morning was no exception. After putting her daughter to bed for a morning nap, the mother went downstairs and returned a little later to find the child in the bathroom, lethargic and unresponsive, with several empty prescription pill bottles nearby. The mother immediately called for the ambulance.

1. What is likely to be the cause of the problem?

2. What emergency care would you provide?

(C) You are at the home of a family with a 10-month-old child. The father explains he called because the child had a seizure that lasted about a minute. The child appears flushed. You touch her skin, which is extremely hot to the touch. The father says the child has been running a fever all day. He put her to bed about an hour ago. About 10 or 15 minutes ago he heard a crash in the infant's room and went to investigate. When he entered, the child was convulsing in the crib. That's when he called 9-1-1.

1. What is likely to be the cause of the problem?

2. What emergency care would you provide?

CHAPTER 36 REVIEW

Write the word or words that best complete each sentence in the space provided.

1. During the assessment and treatment of a young child, you will, if possible, want the child to sit in

   the _____ _____.

2. When opening a child's airway, it is important not to _____ the child's

   neck.

3. Use _____ _____ alternating with

   _____ _____ to clear a complete airway

   obstruction in an infant 1-year-old or younger.

4. In infants and children, the _____ system is usually an early indicator of

   other medical problems.

5. For infants and young children who are frightened by the oxygen mask, provide oxygen using the

   _____ technique.

6. For infants and children, provide artificial ventilations at a minimum rate of

   _____ breaths per minute.

7. Diarrhea and/or vomiting, dehydration, infection, abdominal injuries, and blood loss are common

   causes of _____ in infants and children.

8. Because children have a large surface area in proportion to their body mass, they are especially prone

   to _____.

9. Fever, epilepsy, meningitis, drug overdose, hypoglycemia, head trauma, and decreased levels of

   oxygen can bring on _____ in children.

10. If a pediatric patient has a seizure and there is no possibility of spinal injury, position the patient

    _____ _____ _____.

11. In the case of a submersion, assume that _____

    _____ has occurred and fully immobilize the child.

12. The diagnosis of SIDS is made _____.

13. Inflation of the abdominal compartment of the PASG with a pediatric patient may compromise

    _____.

14. Cases of _____ trauma exceed those of _____

trauma in infants and children.

15. When dealing with suspected foreign body airway obstruction in an infant or a child, never perform

_____ _____ _____.

16. If you suspect abuse as the cause of injury with a child trauma patient, do not

_____ the caregivers about abuse or _____ them.

17. If there is bleeding in a pediatric patient with a central intravenous line, your emergency care will

consist of _____ _____ to the device and

_____ the patient.

18. Pediatric calls are among the most _____ for EMTs.

19. For children with special airway needs, the most common problems that EMS will encounter are

with _____ tubes, _____

_____, central lines, and feeding tubes.

20. _____ tubes are placed into the stomach to assist with feeding.

REINFORCEMENT

INFANTS AND CHILDREN: TRUE OR FALSE

Indicate if the following statements are true or false by writing T or F in the space provided.

_____ **1.** The term "toddler" refers to a child between 2 and 4 years old.

_____ **2.** Modesty and body image are very important issues for school-age children.

_____ **3.** With children, padding under the shoulders is often necessary to maintain an open airway during immobilization to a spine board.

_____ **4.** Because children have a smaller blood volume than adults, issues of blood loss are less serious in those patients.

_____ **5.** Determining the cause of respiratory distress in a pediatric patient is an important part of an EMT's assessment.

_____ **6.** Provide an initial series of six back blows to any infant or child patient suffering a partial airway obstruction.

_____ **7.** Capillary refill can be a useful tool in assessing circulation in pediatric patients.

_____ **8.** Infants and children need a respiratory tidal volume of approximately 10 mL/kg.

_____ **9.** In a pediatric patient with a foreign body airway obstruction, perform a "blind" finger sweep of the oral cavity if back blows do not dislodge the obstruction.

_____ **10.** Seizures that last longer than 10 minutes or recur without interruption represent a true medical emergency.

_____ **11.** To assess an unresponsive child, give him or her a gentle shake.

_____ **12.** With any infant or child poisoning patient, administer activated charcoal once you determine that the airway is open.

_____ **13.** A sunken fontanel is a sign of dehydration in an infant.

_____ **14.** A drop in blood pressure is a late sign of shock in children.

_____ **15.** With submersion patients in whom normal breathing is restored, deterioration can still take place from minutes to hours after the event.

_____ **16.** Explaining to parents that SIDS is a relatively common occurrence is one way the EMT can help them cope with the loss of a child.

_____ **17.** With child patients, slow delivery of ventilations and cricoid pressure can help reduce gastric distension.

_____**18.** Use a single leg of the PASG to control serious bleeding in an infant.

_____**19.** Never ask a suspected victim of child abuse to explain the circumstances of an incident while the possible abuser is present.

_____**20.** CISD is one way EMTs can defuse the stress created by dealing with pediatric emergencies.

REINFORCEMENT

INFANTS AND CHILDREN: LISTING

1. List at least five signs of respiratory distress in pediatric patients.

2. List the emergency care steps for a child with fever and seizures.

3. List the basic emergency care steps for the pediatric trauma patient.

4. List four signs of possible child abuse.

Infants and Children

Dealing with Caregivers
Dealing with the Child

Developmental Characteristics

- Neonates
- Infants
- Toddlers
- Preschoolers
- School age
- Adolescents

Anatomical Differences

Airway and Breathing Problems

Early Respiratory Distress

Decompensated Respiratory Failure

Airway Obstruction

Assessment and Care

Assessment and Care: Common Medical Problems

Seizures

Altered Mental Status

Poisonings

Fever

Shock

Submersion

Sudden Infant Death Syndrome

HANDOUT 36-2: Chapter 36 Quiz

1. B	**6.** D	**11.** C	**15.** C
2. B	**7.** B	**12.** B	**16.** C
3. C	**8.** C	**13.** A	**17.** C
4. A	**9.** A	**14.** D	**18.** B
5. D	**10.** D		

HANDOUT 36-3: In the Field

A. 1. The child is likely in the early stages of shock (hypoperfusion) from infection and hypovolemia.

2. Ensure an open airway. Provide oxygen at 15 liters per minute by nonrebreather mask and be prepared to provide positive-pressure ventilations. Keep the child warm. Expedite transport.

B. 1. The child may be suffering from poisoning.

2. Establish and maintain an airway. Be prepared to suction. Provide high-flow oxygen and be prepared to provide positive-pressure ventilation with supplemental oxygen as needed. Expedite transport. Perform a rapid trauma assessment.

C. 1. The child may have suffered a febrile seizure.

2. Maintain the airway and provide oxygen at 15 liters per minute by nonrebreather mask. (Provide positive-pressure ventilation, if necessary.) Lower the infant's body temperature. Be alert for possible vomiting and the need to suction. Transport.

HANDOUT 36-4: Chapter 36 Review

1. parent's (caregiver's) lap
2. hyperextend
3. back blows, chest thrusts
4. respiratory
5. "blow-by"
6. 20
7. shock (hypoperfusion)
8. hypothermia
9. seizures
10. on his side
11. spinal injury
12. postmortem
13. respirations
14. blunt, penetrating
15. blind finger sweeps
16. question, accuse
17. applying pressure, transporting
18. stressful
19. tracheostomy, mechanical ventilators
20. Gastrostomy

HANDOUT 36-5: Infants and Children: True or False

1. F	**6.** F	**11.** F	**16.** F
2. T	**7.** T	**12.** F	**17.** T
3. T	**8.** T	**13.** T	**18.** F
4. F	**9.** F	**14.** T	**19.** T
5. F	**10.** T	**15.** T	**20.** T

HANDOUT 36-6: Infants and Children: Listing

1. Any five: nasal flaring, retractions; neck muscle use; "seesaw" respirations; breathing noises such as stridor, wheezing, or grunting; breathing rate above normal for child's age. Additional: cyanosis, decreased muscle tone, poor peripheral perfusion, altered mental status, head bobbing.

2. Establish and maintain an airway. Protect patient from injury. Suction secretions for no longer than 5–10 seconds at a time. Provide positive-pressure ventilations with supplemental oxygen at 20/minute if breathing is inadequate; administer oxygen; consider blow-by oxygen in very young children. Remove clothing and cool by fanning or sponging with tepid water. Consider Advanced Life Support. Transport. Ongoing assessment every 5 minutes.

3. Establish and maintain in-line spinal stabilization and open the airway using the jaw-thrust maneuver. Suction as necessary, no more than 5–10 seconds at a time. Provide oxygen by nonrebreather mask at 15 liters per minute or provide positive-pressure ventilation with supplemental oxygen for inadequate breathing. Provide occlusive dressings for any open wound to the chest. Cover any eviscerations with moist, sterile gauze dressing and secure. Provide complete spinal immobilization. Consider request for ALS support. Apply PASG if pelvic injury is suspected and local protocols direct. Transport. Splint fractures and dress open wounds. Perform ongoing assessment every 5 minutes.

4. Any four of the following: multiple abrasions, lacerations, incisions, bruises, broken bones; multiple injuries or bruises in various stages of healing; injuries on both sides or both front and back of child's body; unusual wounds; a fearful child; injuries to the genitalia; injuries to spinal cord and brain when child is violently shaken; situations in which the injuries are not consistent with the story; lack of adult supervision; untreated chronic illness; malnourishment; delay in reporting injuries.

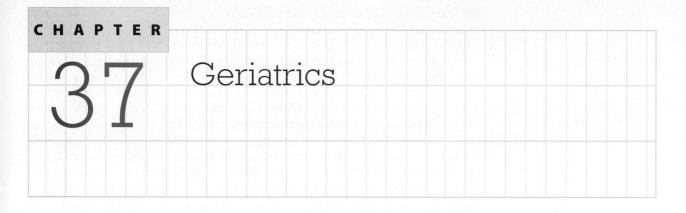

37 Geriatrics

The chapter contains information that is valuable as background for the EMT but that goes substantially beyond the U.S. Department of Transportation's EMT-Basic National Standard Curriculum.

OBJECTIVES

Numbered objectives are from the U.S. Department of Transportation's EMT-Basic National Standard Curriculum. Asterisked objectives, if any, pertain to material that is supplemental to the DOT curriculum. Page numbers refer to pages in the textbook.

Cognitive

* * Discuss at least four factors that contribute to the geriatric patient being at a higher risk for medical emergencies. (pp. 1050–1055)
* * Discuss the general physiological changes in the body systems of the geriatric patient that are due to the normal aging process. (pp. 1050–1055)
* * Discuss special considerations for assessing the geriatric patient suffering from a medical or traumatic emergency. (pp. 1055–1063)
* * Outline the special considerations for obtaining an accurate medical history from a geriatric patient. (pp. 1059–1062)
* * List the emergency care steps and considerations for the geriatric patient suffering either a medical or a traumatic emergency. (pp. 1062–1063)
* * Discuss positioning, immobilization, and packaging of the elderly trauma patient with consideration of physical deformity. (pp. 1053–1054, 1062)
* * Recite and explain common disease processes that cause generalized complaints in the elderly. (pp. 1063–1070)

Affective

* * Explain why the EMT-B should use special communication skills when assessing a geriatric patient. (pp. 1059–1062)

Psychomotor

* * Demonstrate various immobilization techniques that would be necessary for packaging an elderly patient with degenerative skeletal deformities.

REVIEW

In the last lesson, "Infants and Children," students learned that nearly 45,000 children die in the United States each year. Approximately one in four children will sustain an injury that will require medical attention.

Total Teaching Time
100 minutes

Resources Needed
* Scored Chapter 36 Quizzes
* Cotton balls
* Eyeglasses
* Vaseline or other petroleum jelly
* Elastic bandages

Additional Resources
Larmon/Davis, *Basic Life Support Skills*

Elling, *EMT Achieve: Basic Test Preparation*

Limmer/Mistovich/ O'Keefe, *Audio Lecture & Study Guide: EMT*

Mistovich/Kuvlesky, *SUCCESS! for the EMT, Second Edition*

Approximately 10 percent of an EMT's patients will be children. If asked, experienced EMS providers would probably concur that dealing with infants and children is one of the most stressful situations they encounter during their EMS careers. This is mainly due to the relative infrequency of dealing with pediatric patients, the differences in assessment and treatment, and having to deal with the emotions of the pediatric patient, the distressed parents, and probably the feelings the EMTs have themselves. Very few things can evoke an emotional charge in people like a critically ill or injured child. Despite this, EMTs must be able to prevent the emotions they experience from interfering with the task at hand: assessing and treating the young patient. To help focus on this task, the EMT needs to remember that despite the patient's age, a breathing problem is a breathing problem, a bleeding wound is a bleeding wound, and an unresponsive patient is an unresponsive patient. While the EMT's assessment approach to the ill or injured child is somewhat different from the approach to an adult, the basic treatment goals are the same.

Distribute the quizzes from the last class. Go over each question on the quiz and handle any concerns students may have about the answers.

INTRODUCTION TO CHAPTER 37

Chapter 37, "Geriatrics," is the second and final chapter in Module 6. It is an optional chapter that you may choose to include in your course. Geriatric patients—those over the age of 65—differ from their younger counterparts. The elderly are at greater risk of nearly all types of injuries and illnesses. Also, they present with different signs and symptoms because of the changing physiology of the geriatric body system. Additionally, the geriatric patient often has one or more coexisting long-term conditions that can mask or change the presentation of the emergency problem. In the United States, people over age 65 make up the fastest growing segment of the population. In fact, the majority of EMS calls involve geriatric patients. Therefore, it is important that students understand the characteristics of geriatric patients and how to tailor assessment to the special needs of these patients.

Distribute the Chapter 37 Objectives Checklist and give students a few minutes to look it over. Then briefly paraphrase the objectives for this lesson in your own words.

LECTURE

The following suggested lecture outline is based on the Department of Transportation's EMT-Basic National Standard Curriculum. In some places, the DOT curriculum has been rearranged or expanded upon so that it is more complete or easier for the student to understand. The page numbers in parentheses refer to pages in the textbook. The parenthetical references in dark, heavy type are to figures, tables, and scans in the textbook.

ASSESSMENT OF GERIATRIC PATIENTS

I. Effects of aging on body systems (pp. 1050–1055) **(Fig. 37-1, p. 1051)**
  - **A.** Cardiovascular system (pp. 1051–1052)
  - **B.** Respiratory system (pp. 1052–1053)
  - **C.** Musculoskeletal system (p. 1053) **(Fig. 37-2, p. 1054)**
  - **D.** Neurological system (p. 1053)
  - **E.** Gastrointestinal system (p. 1053)

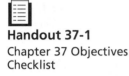

Handout 37-1
Chapter 37 Objectives Checklist

Lecture Master
You may wish to display Lecture Master 37 when presenting the lecture to the class.

Point of Interest
By 2030, it is estimated that 70 percent of all ambulance transports will be of patients 65 or older.

On the Net
For eldercare information and links on aging, go to: www.elderweb.com

On the Net
Information about osteoporosis can be found at: http://www.cinn.org

x

F. Renal system (pp. 1053–1055)

G. Integumentary system (p. 1055)

II. Assessment: Geriatric patient (pp. 1055–1063)

A. Scene size-up (p. 1056) **(Table 37-1, p. 1057)**

B. Initial assessment (pp. 1057–1058) **(Table 37-2, p. 1058)**

1. Mental status

2. Airway and breathing

3. Circulation

4. Skin condition and temperature

C. Focused history and physical exam and detailed physical exam (pp. 1059–1062) **(Figs. 37-3 and 37-4, pp. 1060–1061) (Table 37-3, p. 1060)**

1. Geriatric trauma patient

2. Geriatric medical patient

D. Emergency medical care and ongoing assessment (pp. 1062–1063)

III. Special geriatric assessment findings (pp. 1063–1070) **(Table 37-4, p. 1063)**

A. Chest pain or absence of chest pain (pp. 1063–1064) **(Fig. 37-5, p. 1064)**

1. "Silent heart attack."

2. Congestive heart failure (CHF)

B. Shortness of breath (pp. 1064–1066) **(Fig. 37-6, p. 1065)**

1. Pulmonary edema

2. Pulmonary embolism

3. Pneumonia

4. Aspiration pneumonia

5. Chronic obstructive pulmonary diseases (COPD) **(Fig. 37-7, p. 1066)**

C. Altered mental status (pp. 1066–1069) **(Fig. 37-8, p. 1067)**

1. Stroke

2. Transient ischemic attack (TIA, or "mini stroke")

3. Seizure

4. Syncope (fainting)

5. Drug toxicity **(Fig. 37-9, p. 1068)**

6. Dementia and delirium

7. Alzheimer's disease

D. Signs of trauma or shock (pp. 1069–1070)

E. Environmental temperature extremes (p. 1070)

1. Hypothermia

2. Hyperthermia

F. Geriatric abuse (p. 1070)

CASE STUDY FOLLOW-UP

Ask a student volunteer to read the Case Study that begins on page 1050 of the textbook. You may wish to use the following questions to engage students in a discussion of the Case Study Follow-up that begins on page 1071 of the textbook. Provide missing information and clarify ideas as needed.

Q1. During your initial assessment, how do you enhance communication with Mrs. Vaughn?

A1. *By assisting her in placing her hearing aid.*

Reading/Reference

Nixon, R., "Geriatrics and Their Meds: Problems and Perils," *EMS Magazine,* Feb. 2003.

Point of Interest

Some 49 percent of falls in the elderly are due to factors like slipping or tripping. The remaining 60 percent are due to factors such as poor health, acute illness, or chronic illness.

Teaching Tip

Contact your state's office of adult protective services or office on aging to obtain additional information on geriatric patients.

Reading/Reference

Nixon, Robert G., *Geriatric Prehospital Care.* Brady/Prentice Hall Health, 2002.

Reading/Reference

Northington, et al., "Caring for the Aged," *JEMS,* July 2005.

Reading/Reference

Eder, S., "The Alzheimer's Challenge," *EMS Magazine,* June 2005.

Q2. Mrs. Vaughn does not appear to be in serious distress. Why do you decide to treat her as a priority patient?

A2. *Because of her age.*

Q3. Mrs. Vaughn is a medical patient with no signs of trauma; why do you conduct a detailed physical exam?

A3. *As a precautionary measure, because Mrs. Vaughn is a geriatric patient.*

Q4. In what position do you place Mrs. Vaughn to make it easier for her to breathe during transport?

A4. *In a Fowler's position on the stretcher.*

Q5. What diagnosis is made at the hospital of Mrs. Vaughn's condition? Why did the signs and symptoms differ in Mrs. Vaughn versus younger patients?

A5. *The doctor said that Mrs. Vaughn has pneumonia even though she did not display signs that are classic in younger pneumonia patients such as high fever, chills, and chest pain. Instead, because of physiological changes due to aging, she displayed increased breathing difficulty, rapid respirations, and a cough.*

IN REVIEW

Assess students' ability to apply what they have just learned by discussing the Review Questions on page 1073 in the textbook.

Q1. A 79-year-old male patient is crossing the street to get his mail when he is struck by a vehicle traveling at 45 miles per hour. Discuss the changes in the following body systems from the normal aging process that would increase his susceptibility to injury and the after-effects of injury: cardiovascular system, respiratory system, and musculoskeletal system.

A1. *Changes in the following body systems that would increase susceptibility to trauma of an elderly person include the following: (1) Cardiovascular system—Degenerative processes decrease the ability of the heart to pump blood. There is a general decline in the maximum heart rate, which means that the heart rate may not increase in response to shock. Arteries lose their elasticity and tear easily, resulting in additional bleeding. The blood vessels also do not react as fast (or as efficiently) in response to stimulation from the central nervous system. (2) Respiratory system— Due to changes in respiratory musculature and a change in the normal elasticity and recoil of the thorax, the thorax is not as effective in moving the air in and out of the lungs. A progressive decrease in gas diffusion across the alveolar membrane causes poorer oxygenation, which leads to poorer compensation in traumatic chest injuries. The body's response to hypoxia is blunted. Dampened cough and gag reflexes decrease the ability to clear substances from the airway. (3) Musculoskeletal system— Osteoporosis causes the bones to weaken and become brittle, thereby increasing the likelihood of fracturing. The disks that are located between each vertebrae in the spine start to narrow, causing kyphosis, which can complicate normal immobilization techniques. Joints begin to lose their flexibility, and there is a general and progressive loss of skeletal muscle mass. In all, skeletal fractures take longer to heal and may precipitate secondary medical emergencies. (pp. 1051–1053)*

Q2. Describe communication challenges caused by sensory degeneration in an elderly patient, and outline strategies for overcoming these challenges.

A2. *Challenges caused by sensory degeneration and strategies for overcoming them include diminished eyesight (place yourself where the patient can see you; explain what is happening; make sure the patient is wearing eyeglasses if he has them); diminished hearing (speak louder, not higher; assist the patient in using a hearing aid if he has one; possibly speak into a stethoscope placed into the patient's ears; determine if the patient can lip read; try note-writing). Never assume a patient is hard of hearing or has diminished eyesight. (p. 1059)*

Q3. List questions you should ask the elderly patient in order to help obtain an accurate history.

A3. *Questions you should ask the elderly patient in order to help obtain an accurate history include: Have you had any trouble breathing? Have you had a cough lately? (If so, have you been coughing up anything like mucus or blood?) Have you had any chest pain? Did you get dizzy? (If so, what were you doing when this occurred?) Have you fainted? Have you had any headaches lately? Have you been eating and drinking normally? Have there been any changes in your bowel or bladder habits? Have you fallen lately? (p. 1061)*

Q4. Explain the reasons why a detailed physical exam should always be performed on all geriatric patients, whether trauma or medical, unresponsive or alert.

A4. *A detailed physical exam should always be performed on all geriatric patients as an extra precaution because a geriatric patient may be unable or unwilling to reveal all of her problems in describing her chief complaint; also, a geriatric patient's condition can deteriorate very rapidly. (pp. 1060, 1062)*

Q5. Give emergency care guidelines for positioning and packaging the following geriatric patients: the alert medical patient, the patient with altered mental status, and the patient with suspected spinal injury. Also explain procedures for immobilizing a patient with spinal curvature.

A5. *Emergency care guidelines for positioning and packaging the geriatric patient include: (1) If the emergency run is medical in nature and the patient is alert and able to protect his own airway, place the patient in a position that is comfortable for him, typically a Fowler's position. (2) If the patient has an altered mental status and is unable to protect his own airway, the patient should be placed on his left side to avoid aspiration. (3) If spinal injury is suspected, the patient needs immediate stabilization of the cervical spine during initial airway assessment. The patient should also be immobilized to a long spine board, using appropriate immobilization devices. (4) The patient with severe curvature should not be forced into the usual immobilization position but should be immobilized using blankets or other devices that can accommodate the spinal curvature. (pp. 1062–1063)*

Q6. Discuss how an assessment finding of denial of chest pain in the geriatric patient differs from the same finding in a younger adult patient.

A6. *An assessment finding of denial of chest pain in the geriatric patient differs from the same finding in a younger adult patient because a geriatric patient has depressed pain perception and may be suffering a "silent heart attack." Other signs and symptoms such as weakness or fatigue, breathing difficulty, aching shoulders, or indigestion should be considered signs of possible cardiac difficulty or heart attack. Also, the patient may be experiencing pain but denying it to the EMT for fear of hospitalization. (pp. 1063–1064)*

Q7. List factors that make the elderly more likely to fall.

A7. *Factors that make the elderly more likely to fall include altered mental status, slower reflexes, failing eyesight and hearing, activities that exceed physical limitations, arthritis, and general loss in muscle tone and strength. (p. 1069)*

Q8. List at least five possible causes of altered mental status in the geriatric patient and discuss special treatment considerations for the geriatric patient with altered mental status.

A8. *Possible causes of altered mental status in the geriatric patient include stroke, TIA, seizures, syncope, drug toxicity, and dementia or Alzheimer's disease. Treatment considerations include the following: Never assume that a geriatric patient's altered mental status is "normal" for him or that it is "senility." Inquire of family members or others who know the patient if the mental status is, indeed, normal for him or if it represents a significant change. Remember also that the noise of a radio, a siren, or strange voices may add to the patient's confusion. Attempt to explain or reduce the noise. In addition, when treating patients with dementia and, particularly, dementia caused by Alzheimer's disease, do not take personally the uncooperativeness or hostility that may result from the disease. (pp. 1066–1069)*

Q9. Explain why geriatric patients are predisposed to environmental heat or cold emergencies.

A9. *Geriatric patients are predisposed to environmental heat or cold emergencies because the aging process diminishes the body's ability to create heat when cold, or dissipate heat when hot. These factors include a smaller insulating layer of fat, reduced muscle mass, the body's metabolic rate slowing with age, impaired reflexes, decreasing blood flow (especially to the extremities), and a reduced shivering response. Also, because of impaired perception, geriatric patients simply may not realize how cold or hot it is. It is also likely that elderly patients on a fixed income may be unable to afford keeping their homes adequately heated or cooled. (p. 1070)*

Q10. List signs and symptoms of geriatric abuse and discuss emergency care procedures when there is a high index of suspicion for geriatric abuse.

A10. *Signs and symptoms of geriatric abuse include bruises, bite marks, bleeding beneath the scalp (indicative of hair-pulling), lacerations on the face, trauma to the ears, broken bones, deformities of the chest, cigarette burns, and rope marks. If abuse is suspected, pay attention to inconsistencies when you get your history from the patient and from the provider or family. Treatment elements for normal wound/injury* *management would apply. Do not confront the family or care provider with your suspicion of abuse. Instead, if you do suspect geriatric abuse, you should make your suspicion known to the receiving hospital's staff or follow local protocols or state law with regard to reporting suspected abuse. (p. 1070)*

CRITICAL THINKING

Assess students' ability to respond to real-life emergency situations by discussing the Critical Thinking questions on page 1073 in the textbook.

Q1. What action would you immediately take to manage this patient's airway?

A1. *The pillows should be removed from under the patient's head and her airway should be opened with the head-tilt chin-lift maneuver.*

Q2. What other emergency care would you provide in the initial assessment?

A2. *If the snoring sounds are not relieved by manually positioning the airway, it may be necessary to insert an oropharyngeal airway. If the patient does not accept the oropharyngeal airway, insert a nasopharyngeal airway. That patient should be placed on 15 lpm of oxygen by a nonrebreather mask if the ventilation rate and tidal volume is adequate. If the ventilation rate or tidal volume is inadequate, immediately begin bag-valve-mask ventilation and connect supplemental oxygen to the BVM reservoir.*

Q3. What is your interpretation of the SpO$_2$ reading?

A3. *An SpO2 reading of 95% on room air indicates that the patient is currently not hypoxic.*

Q4. What is your interpretation of the blood glucose reading?

A4. *The blood glucose reading of 98 mg/dL falls within a normal range. It is therefore unlikely that the altered mental status is due to either a hypoglycemic or hyperglycemic event.*

Q5. What conditions might cause this patient to experience an altered mental status?

A5. *Many answers are possible but based on the assessment findings, this patient's altered mental status could be caused by stroke, head injury, medication interaction, or infection. This is an acute condition and must not be mistaken for a normal part of the aging process.*

AGING SIMULATION EXERCISE

To help students empathize with the feelings and perceptions of older patients, try having one or more students pretend they are geriatric patients by doing the following:

- Place cotton balls in both ears to simulate hearing loss.
- Put on a pair of eyeglasses that have been coated with petroleum jelly to simulate blurred vision and vision loss.
- Stand and walk with their legs approximately 12 inches apart to simulate the gait of an aging person.
- Stand slightly bent over to simulate curvature of the spine.

Reading/Reference
Textbook, pp. 1076–1100

Workbook
Chapter 37 Activities

Chapter Quiz
Handout 37-2

TestGen
Chapter 37 Test

Online Test Preparation
Send your students to
http://www.prenhall.com/
EMTAchieve

Handouts 37-3 to 37-5
Reinforcement Activities

**Brady Skills Series
EMT-B Videos/CD**
Visual Reinforcement

**PowerPoint
Presentation**
Chapter 37

Student CD
Chapter 37

Companion Website
http://www.prenhall.com/
mistovich

■ Wrap elastic bandages around the knees and medical tape around the fingers to simulate arthritis and the difficulty found in walking.

Once students have had the chance to experience all of these effects, ask them to describe their reactions. You might ask questions such as the following:

■ How does it feel to walk with all of these limitations?
■ Is it easy to walk? To perform normal life activities?
■ Does this experience change your perspective on the geriatric patient?

ASSIGNMENTS

Assign students to read Chapter 38, "Ambulance Operations," before the next class. Also ask them to complete Chapter 37 of the Workbook.

EVALUATION

Chapter Quiz Distribute copies of the Chapter Quiz provided in Handout 37-2 to evaluate student understanding of this chapter. Remind students not to refer to their textbooks or notes while taking the quiz.

Test Manager You may wish to create a custom-tailored test using Prentice Hall *TestGen for Prehospital Emergency Care, Eighth Edition* to evaluate student understanding of this chapter.

Online Test Preparation (for students and instructors) Additional test preparation is available through *EMT Achieve: Basic Test Preparation* at http://www.prenhall.com/EMTAchieve. Instructors can also monitor student mastery online.

REINFORCEMENT

Handouts If classroom discussions or performance on the quiz indicates that some students have not fully mastered the chapter content, you may wish to assign some or all of the Reinforcement Handouts for this chapter.

TECH EXTRAS

Brady Skills Series EMT-B Videos/CD Have your students watch the skills come to life on either VHS or CD-ROM.

PowerPoint Presentation (for instructors) The PowerPoint material developed for this chapter offers useful reinforcement of chapter content.

Student CD A wide variety of material on this CD-ROM will reinforce and also expand student knowledge and skills.

Companion Website (for students) Additional review quizzes and links to EMS resources will contribute to further reinforcement of this chapter. Please visit http://www.prenhall.com/mistovich.

OBJECTIVES CHECKLIST

Cognitive	Date Mastered
* Discuss at least four factors that contribute to the geriatric patient being at a higher risk for medical emergencies.	
* Discuss the general physiological changes in the body systems of the geriatric patient that are due to the normal aging process.	
* Discuss special considerations for assessing the geriatric patient suffering from a medical or traumatic emergency.	
* Outline the special considerations for obtaining an accurate medical history from a geriatric patient.	
* List the emergency care steps and considerations for the geriatric patient suffering either a medical or a traumatic emergency.	
* Discuss positioning, immobilization, and packaging of the elderly trauma patient with consideration of physical deformity.	
* Recite and explain common disease processes that cause generalized complaints in the elderly.	

Affective	Date Mastered
* Explain why the EMT-Basic should use special communication skills when assessing a geriatric patient.	

Psychomotor	Date Mastered
* Demonstrate various immobilization techniques that would be necessary for packaging an elderly patient with degenerative skeletal deformities.	

OBJECTIVES

CHAPTER 37 QUIZ

Write the letter of the best answer in the space provided.

_____ 1. The best place to check for signs of dehydration in the elderly patient is/are the
   A. scalp.
   B. skin of the forearms.
   C. palms of the hands or soles of the feet.
   D. mucous membranes of the eyes and mouth.

_____ 2. If an elderly patient has altered mental status and is unable to swallow, position him
   A. on a backboard, using pillows to support the head.
   B. in the left lateral recumbent position.
   C. in a Fowler's position.
   D. supine.

_____ 3. When assessing an elderly patient in a nursing home or extended-care facility who shows
   signs and symptoms of a respiratory disorder, the EMT should
   A. put a surgical mask on the patient.
   B. make the patient a high priority for transport.
   C. immediately begin positive-pressure ventilations.
   D. put on a HEPA or N-95 respirator.

_____ 4. Which one of the following should be performed for an elderly trauma patient regardless
   of mechanism of injury or level of responsiveness?
   A. focused medical exam   C. focused trauma exam
   B. rapid trauma assessment   D. historical exam

_____ 5. Ongoing assessment of an elderly patient who is alert but has an injured arm should take
   place every _____ minutes.
   A. 5   C. 15
   B. 10   D. 20

_____ 6. When obtaining a history from an elderly patient, the EMT should
   A. shout loudly, as the patient is probably deaf.
   B. use terms of endearment like "honey" to break the ice.
   C. address the patient as "Mr." or "Mrs." unless asked to do otherwise.
   D. speak first to family members, as they are most likely to have accurate information.

_____ 7. With an elderly patient who has aching in her shoulders, fatigue, and trouble breathing,
   an EMT should suspect
   A. kyphosis.   C. arteriosclerosis.
   B. a heart attack.   D. degenerative spinal changes.

_____ 8. Efforts to save money by elderly people living on fixed incomes may lead to cases of
   A. lordosis.   C. hypothermia.
   B. pulmonary embolus.   D. stroke.

©2008 by Pearson Education, Inc.
Prehospital Emergency Care, 8th ed.

_____ **9.** Emergency care for an elderly patient experiencing a seizure includes
      A. suctioning the airway as necessary.
      B. restraining the patient to prevent injury.
      C. placing the patient in the prone position.
      D. oxygen at 21 liters per minute via nasal cannula.

_____ **10.** Inconsistencies in a patient's history as supplied by the patient and caregivers should increase suspicions of the possibility of
      A. TIA.   **C.** COPD.
      B. geriatric abuse.   **D.** "silent heart attack."

REINFORCEMENT

IN THE FIELD

Review the following real-life situation. Then answer the questions that follow.

You and your partner are dispatched to a senior citizen's apartment complex in the center of town. The caller stated that her husband is "talking gibberish" and not acting right. Your partner, a new EMT, says, "What does she expect? He's old!" Since the complex was now less than a minute away, you decide to explore that comment later.

Upon arrival, you are met by Mrs. Heisler, a spry 80-year-old, who tells you that about 20 minutes ago her husband began speaking in a slurred voice and not making sense. She didn't know how to help him, and so she called 9-1-1. "I'm really sorry. I hope I'm not bothering you people." After looking for hazards, putting on BSI, and reassuring Mrs. Heisler that she had done the right thing, you approach the patient. He is an elderly man, sitting slouched in a chair and drooling. You introduce yourself and ask his name. The reply is garbled.

1. During the scene size-up and initial assessment, what special considerations must be kept in mind?

2. How should the EMTs address the patient? How can they obtain a chief complaint and a history?

3. After performing the initial assessment and rapid medical assessment, the EMTs note the following results:

   • Unequal pupils
   • Weakness on the right side of the body
   • Slurred speech
   • Alterations in respiratory patterns and pulse

What is the likely cause of these signs and symptoms? How should the EMTs manage them?

CHAPTER 37 REVIEW

Write the word or words that best complete each sentence in the space provided.

1. With age, degenerative changes decrease the ability of the heart to _____

   _____.

2. The net effect of changes in the respiratory systems of elderly people is that

   _____ air enters the system, _____ gas exchange

   takes place, and there is _____ likelihood of an infection.

3. In the elderly, there is a decrease in _____ and

   _____ of the brain, leading to more cerebrospinal fluid to fill the space.

4. A decrease in the size of the liver with aging means that many elderly patients who take prescription

   medication suffer from drug _____.

5. Aging decreases the effectiveness of the _____ as a protective barrier that

   keeps microorganisms out of the body.

6. The geriatric patient's mental status may be influenced by chronic illness, the present illness or

   _____, _____, or by familiarity with

   surroundings.

7. Perform a _____ _____

   _____ on any elderly trauma victim regardless of responsiveness or

   mechanism of injury.

8. Exercise extreme caution in _____ the geriatric patient for transport.

9. Due to changes in pain perception, the elderly may experience a(n) _____

   heart attack.

10. _____ _____ _____ is

    caused by a heart that has become weakened over time.

11. Fluid that has leaked into the space between the capillaries and alveoli causes

    _____ _____.

12. _____ pneumonia results from inhaled food or vomitus.

13. If a patient with COPD becomes fatigued from the effort of breathing, be prepared to provide

_____ _____ _____.

14. _____ is a temporary loss of responsiveness that is caused by a reduced

flow of blood to the brain.

15. In the case of suspected geriatric abuse, your first priority is to provide

_____ _____ for the injuries.

GERIATRIC PATIENTS: LISTING

1. List six factors that make a geriatric patient especially at risk for a medical/trauma emergency.

2. List at least five conditions commonly responsible for an assessment finding of altered mental status in geriatric patients.

3. List at least six signs that may indicate geriatric abuse.

Assessment of Geriatric Patients

Effects of Aging on Body Systems

Cardiovascular

Respiratory

Musculoskeletal

Neurological

Gastrointestinal

Renal

Integumentary

Special Considerations of Geriatric Assessment

Scene Size-up

Initial Assessment

Focused History and Physical Exam
- Medical
- Trauma

Detailed Physical Exam

Emergency Care

Ongoing Assessment

Special Geriatric Assessment Findings

Chest Pain or Absence of Chest Pain

Shortness of Breath

Altered Mental Status

Signs of Trauma or Shock

Environmental Temperature Extremes

Geriatric Abuse

HANDOUT 37-2: Chapter 37 Quiz

1.	D	**4.**	B	**7.**	B	**9.**	A
2.	B	**5.**	C	**8.**	C	**10.**	B
3.	D	**6.**	C				

HANDOUT 37-3: In the Field

1. Special considerations include: Be aware of environmental concerns (too hot or too cold). Consider the possibility of TB. During the initial assessment, remember that mental status can be affected by chronic illness, medications, or changes in the surroundings. Any diminished gag reflex leaves the patient at risk for aspiration. Be prepared to maintain the airway and assist breathing if the patient is tiring. Assess both peripheral and central pulses. Note irregularities. Keep in mind the differences in the skin of the elderly. Look for hydration status in the mucous membranes of the mouth or eyes.

2. The EMT should call the patient "Mr. Heisler." They should speak to the patient while his wife is available to listen also. If they cannot get satisfactory answers from the patient himself, they should then ask the wife directly. At all times, they must treat the patient with respect.

3. Stroke may be the most likely cause. The EMT should provide aggressive oxygenation and ventilation, continue to protect the airway and prevent aspiration, and transport in a Fowler's position (change to left lateral recumbent if the patient loses consciousness).

HANDOUT 37-4: Chapter 37 Review

1. pump blood
2. less, less, greater
3. mass, weight
4. toxicity
5. skin
6. injury, drugs
7. rapid trauma assessment
8. packaging
9. silent
10. Congestive heart failure
11. pulmonary edema
12. Aspiration
13. positive-pressure ventilations
14. Syncope
15. emergency care

HANDOUT 37-5: Geriatric Patients: Listing

1. The patient lives alone, is incontinent, is immobile, has recently been hospitalized, has recently been bereaved, has an altered mental status.
2. Any five: stroke, transient ischemic attack, seizure, syncope, drug toxicity, dementia, Alzheimer's disease.
3. Any six: bruises, bite marks, bleeding beneath the scalp (indicates hair-pulling), lacerations on the face, trauma to the ears, broken bones, deformities of the chest, cigarette burns, rope marks, inconsistencies in patient history.

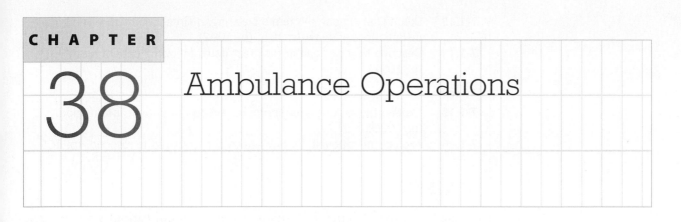

CHAPTER

38 Ambulance Operations

This chapter covers Lesson 7-1 of the U.S. Department of Transportation's EMT-Basic National Standard Curriculum.

OBJECTIVES

Numbered objectives are from the U.S. Department of Transportation's EMT-Basic National Standard Curriculum. Asterisked objectives, if any, pertain to material that is supplemental to the DOT curriculum. Page numbers refer to pages in the textbook.

Cognitive

7-1.1 Discuss the medical and nonmedical equipment needed to respond to a call. (p. 1084)

7-1.2 List the phases of an ambulance call. (p. 1082)

7-1.3 Describe the general provisions of state laws relating to the operation of the ambulance and privileges in any or all of the following categories: (pp. 1077–1078, 1080–1081)
— Speed
— Warning lights
— Sirens
— Right-of-way
— Parking
— Turning

7-1.4 List contributing factors to unsafe driving conditions. (pp. 1079–1080, 1096–1098)

7-1.5 Describe the considerations that should be given to: (pp. 1079–1080)
— Request for escorts
— Following an escort vehicle
— Intersections

7-1.6 Discuss "Due Regard for Safety of All Others" while operating an emergency vehicle. (p. 1078)

7-1.7 State what information is essential in order to respond to a call. (p. 1084)

7-1.8 Discuss various situations that may affect response to a call. (pp. 1079–1080, 1096–1098)

7-1.9 Differentiate between the various methods of moving a patient to the unit based on injury or illness. (pp. 1085, 1087)

7-1.10 Apply the components of the essential patient information in a written report. (p. 1090)

7-1.11 Summarize the importance of preparing the unit for the next response. (pp. 1090–1092)

7-1.12 Identify what is essential for completion of a call. (pp. 1090–1092)

Total Teaching Time
210 minutes

Resources Needed
- Scored Chapter 37 Quizzes
- Inspection checklists for the BLS ambulances students will inspect, one copy for each student
- BLS ambulances, at least one or as many as you can get, each with a two-EMT crew.

Additional Resources
Larmon/Davis, *Basic Life Support Skills*

Elling, *EMT Achieve: Basic Test Preparation*

Limmer/Mistovich/O'Keefe, *Audio Lecture & Study Guide: EMT*

Mistovich/Kuvlesky, *SUCCESS! for the EMT, Second Edition*

7-1.13 Distinguish among the terms cleaning, disinfection, high-level disinfection, and sterilization. (p. 1092)

7-1.14 Describe how to clean or disinfect items following patient care. (p. 1092)

Affective

7-1.15 Explain the rationale for appropriate report of patient information. (p. 1090)

7-1.16 Explain the rationale for having the unit prepared to respond. (p. 1090)

REVIEW

In the last lesson, "Geriatrics," students learned about various ways geriatric patients—those over age 65—differ from their younger counterparts and about how those differences impact assessment. At greater risk of nearly all types of injuries and illnesses, the elderly also present with different signs and symptoms due to the physiology of the geriatric body system. Additionally, the geriatric patient often has one or more coexisting long-term conditions that can mask or change the presentation of the current emergency problem. Students who understand these characteristics of geriatric patients and know how to tailor their assessments to meet their patients' special needs will be well suited to provide care for this fastest growing segment of the population.

Distribute the scored quizzes from the last class. Go over each question on the quiz and handle any concerns students may have about the answers.

INTRODUCTION TO MODULE 7

In Module 7, "Operations," students will learn how to package and move patients, how to operate an ambulance, how to gain access to entrapped patients, and how to deal with hazardous materials and multiple-casualty incidents.

INTRODUCTION TO CHAPTER 38

Chapter 38, "Ambulance Operations," is the first lesson of Module 7. The ambulance is the vehicle that brings care to the patient in times of emergency and transports the patient to a medical receiving facility for follow-up care. It is a crucial part of the EMS system. An ambulance should be a place of comfort and support to patients suffering from life-threatening problems. It should not pose additional hazards to them. But statistics tell a different story. According to national data, about 10 percent of all ambulances are involved in a collision each year. To keep from adding to these statistics, the EMT must learn to drive an ambulance skillfully and safely. The process takes time. But the regulations and guidelines can be learned before getting behind the wheel. This chapter describes how to operate an ambulance safely. It also details other procedures to help ensure the most efficient operation of a properly equipped ambulance.

Distribute the Chapter 38 Objectives Checklist, and give students a few minutes to look it over. Then briefly paraphrase the objectives for this lesson in your own words.

Handout 38-1
Chapter 38 Objectives Checklist

The following suggested lecture outline is based on the Department of Transportation's EMT-Basic National Standard Curriculum. In some places, the DOT curriculum has been rearranged or expanded upon so that it is more complete or easier for the student to understand. The page numbers in parentheses refer to pages in the textbook. The parenthetical references in dark, heavy type are to figures, tables, and scans in the textbook.

AMBULANCE OPERATIONS

I. **Driving the ambulance** (pp. 1077–1080)
   A. Laws, regulations, and ordinances (pp. 1077–1078)
      1. Ambulance operator privileges in most states
         a. May exceed posted speed limit as long as not endangering lives
         b. May drive wrong way on one-way street or down opposite side of road
         c. May turn in any direction at an intersection
         d. May park anywhere as long as not endangering lives or property
         e. May leave ambulance standing in middle of street or intersection
         f. May cautiously proceed through a red light or red flashing signal
         g. May pass other vehicles in a no-passing zone
      2. Ambulance driver qualifications
         a. Must have valid driver's license
         b. May have to attend an approved driving course
         c. Must use warning devices in manner prescribed by law
         d. Must exercise due regard for the safety of others; if EMT does not, he or she is liable for consequences
         e. May be additional local/agency qualifications (e.g., top speed cannot be more than 10 mph over traffic)
   B. Driving excellence (pp. 1078–1080)
      1. Basics of good driving
         a. Make sure that you and all team members wear the ambulance's seatbelts.
         b. Hold the steering wheel with both hands at all times.
         c. Place your hands at 9 o'clock and 3 o'clock positions on steering wheel.
         d. Practice accelerating and decelerating, parking, braking, and cornering.
         e. Recognize and respond to changes in weather and road conditions.
         f. Adjust your speed to allow for decreased visibility.
         g. Select an alternate route to avoid being caught in a traffic jam when responding to a motor-vehicle collision.
         h. Select a transport route best suited for safe travel.
         i. Become familiar with the roads, streets, and routes in your community.
         j. Maintain a safe following distance.
         k. Use headlights to improve vehicle's visibility.
         l. Exercise caution when using red lights and siren.
      2. Maintaining control

Lecture Master
You may wish to display Lecture Master 38 when presenting the lecture to the class.

Point to Emphasize
If an emergency vehicle operator does not drive with due regard for the safety of others, he or she must be prepared to pay such consequences as fines, lawsuits, and even jail time.

On the Net
Ambulance accidents. http://www.emsnetwork .org/ambulance_crashes .htm

a. Braking
- **(1)** Avoid sudden braking.
- **(2)** Never brake on a curve.
- **(3)** Know that your stopping distance is the time it takes you to stop plus your braking time.

b. Railroads
- **(1)** Plan alternative routes when possible.
- **(2)** If you must wait for a train, monitor patient and keep calm.

c. School buses
- **(1)** Be especially alert when approaching stopped bus with red lights flashing.
- **(2)** Follow your state laws regarding stopping.

d. Bridges and tunnels
- **(1)** If in congested traffic near bridge or tunnel, consider an alternate route.
- **(2)** If there's no way around, you will probably not be able to pass, so "go with the flow" until you emerge.

e. Day of the week
- **(1)** Expect less traffic on weekends than on work days, particularly on commuter routes.
- **(2)** Traffic around shopping centers is heaviest on Saturdays.
- **(3)** Traffic to and from resort areas is heaviest on Fridays and Sundays.

f. Time of day
- **(1)** Plan for rush-hour traffic.
- **(2)** Watch for school zones and industrial plant shift changes.

g. Road surface
- **(1)** Goal is to give patient smoothest ride possible.
- **(2)** Be on the lookout for potholes and bumps.
- **(3)** Two inner lanes on four-lane highway are generally smoothest.

h. Backing up
- **(1)** Backing up is source of many ambulance accidents.
- **(2)** Use all resources.
- **(3)** Back up slowly and carefully.

i. Higher speeds
- **(1)** Be especially careful on curves that lead into population pockets, curves that lead to intersections, and those that crest hills.
- **(2)** Brake to proper speed before you enter a curve.
- **(3)** Accelerate carefully and gradually as you leave a curve.
- **(4)** Keep your exit from the curve slow and steady.
- **(5)** Instead of riding the brake, use lower gear when descending long hills.
- **(6)** Always use a smooth braking motion.

j. Escorts
- **(1)** Use only as last resort.
- **(2)** Escort is dangerous to the escort, driver, patient, and others on road.

(3) Use an escort only if unfamiliar with how to get to the hospital or if you cannot find victim's location.
    k. Intersection collisions (main causes of)
       (1) Motorist approaches just as light is changing, so speeds through.
       (2) There are two emergency vehicles and motorists expect only one.
       (3) Vehicles waiting at intersection block the ambulance driver's view of people in crosswalk.

II. Warning devices (pp. 1080–1081)
  A. Colors and markings (p. 1080) **(Fig. 38-1, p. 1080)**
  B. Warning lights and emergency lights (pp. 1080–1081)
    1. Activate emergency lights at all times when responding.
    2. Turn on headlights during daytime.
    3. Place emergency lights high enough to cast a beam above the traffic and low enough to be seen in rear-view mirror of vehicle ahead.
    4. Use emergency lights that revolve or flash for a longer duration in addition to strobe lights.
    5. Know that white lights can be seen from a greater distance than can red or blue.
    6. Do not assume that drivers are aware of you.
    7. Flash a spotlight quickly across the rear-view mirror of a driver who is unaware of you, but do not panic him.
    8. Use only minimal lighting when there is fog or when you are parked.
    9. Use your emergency lights only when needed.
  C. Using your siren (p. 1081)
    1. Do not assume that drivers are aware of you even with lights and siren.
    2. Insulation on newer automobiles can reduce the interior decibel level of an approaching siren by 35–40 percent.
    3. Never pull directly behind a car and blast your siren; this can panic the driver.
    4. Siren can create emotional and physical stress for the patient.
    5. Always let patient know when you are going to use the siren.
    6. Know the effects of the siren on your driving.
      a. Tends to increase ambulance driver speed by 15 mph.
      b. Can easily hypnotize driver
      c. Can prevent driver from hearing sirens and horns of other emergency vehicles responding to same incident
  D. Using your air horn (p. 1081)
    1. Avoid overuse.
    2. Do not sound when you are close to other vehicles.

III. Roadway incident scene safety (pp. 1081–1082)
  A. Do not trust approaching traffic (p. 1081)
  B. Do not turn your back to approaching traffic (p. 1082)
  C. Position the first arriving emergency vehicle to create a block and a physical barrier between upstream traffic and the scene (p. 1082)
  D. Wear appropriate personal protective equipment and ANSI high-visibility vests (p. 1082)
  E. At nighttime, turn off vision-impairing lights, including headlights and spotlights on emergency vehicles that are positioned to oncoming traffic (p. 1082)
  F. Use other emergency vehicles, such as police and fire apparatus, to initially slow down and redirect the flow of traffic (p. 1082)

Slides/Videos
"Intersection Crashes,"
Pulse, Oct. 1998.

On the Net
Code 3 driving. http://
www.tempe.gov/fire/docs/
211.01.htm

G. Use advance warning signs and other traffic control measures upstream of the scene to reduce the speed of the oncoming traffic (p. 1082)

H. Use traffic cones for traffic control (p. 1082)

I. Assign a person to monitor oncoming traffic. (p. 1082)

IV. **Phases of an ambulance call** (pp. 1082–1092)

A. Daily prerun preparation (p. 1082–1084) **(Fig. 38-2, p. 1083)**

  1. Ambulance maintenance (benefits)

  2. Daily inspection of vehicle **(Table 38-1, p. 1084)**

  3. Inspection and stocking of ambulance equipment **(Table 38-2, p. 1084)**

  4. Personnel

B. Dispatch (pp. 1084–1085)

  1. Information dispatcher should provide

    a. Location of call

    b. Nature of call

    c. Name, location, and callback number of caller

    d. Location of patient

    e. Number of patients and severity of problem

    f. Any other special problems or circumstances

C. En route to the scene (p. 1085)

  1. Check vehicle before departure.

  2. Fasten seatbelt.

  3. Write down information from dispatcher.

  4. Confirm dispatch information.

  5. Listen for status reports from other units on-scene.

  6. Think about what equipment you will want to take into the scene.

  7. Remain relaxed yet focused.

  8. Drive responsibly, maintaining a 3- to 4-second following distance.

  9. Determine what the responsibilities of the team members will be.

  10. Call for ALS, if necessary.

D. At the scene (pp. 1086–1087) **(Fig. 38-3, p. 1086)**

  1. Notify dispatch of arrival.

  2. Park the ambulance safely.

    a. In front or behind but never alongside collision

    b. Taking up entire road on narrow, no-parking road (so no one will try to squeeze past)

    c. In driveway or on shoulder whenever possible

    d. Minimum of 100 feet from wreckage or burning vehicle

    e. At least 2,000 feet from hazardous materials spill

    f. Uphill and upwind of fires and hazardous materials spills **(Fig. 38-4, p. 1087)**

  3. Take necessary BSI precautions.

  4. Identify and control hazards.

  5. Call dispatcher immediately if you need additional resources.

  6. Carefully observe and size up scene.

    a. Determine patient's mechanism of injury.

    b. Determine total number of patients.

    c. Determine priority of care.

  7. Extricate patient, if necessary.

  8. Take time to splint and immobilize extremities before moving patient.

  9. Move patient to ambulance, using suitable technique.

Reading/Reference
Harkins, S., "Vehicle Maintenance and Inspections," *EMS Magazine,* Nov. 2003.

On the Net
EMS equipment.
www.alliedhpi.com

10. Transfer patient to ambulance and lock stretcher in place.
E. En route to the receiving facility (pp. 1087–1089) **(Fig. 38-5, pp. 1088–1089)**
   1. Check and ensure patient well-being and comfort.
   2. Check vehicle to ensure it is ready for transport.
   3. Begin ongoing assessment.
   4. Notify dispatch of departure to receiving facility.
   5. Check patient interventions.
   6. Drive prudently.
   7. Keep driver informed of patient condition.
   8. Notify receiving facility.
   9. Continue to reassess patient's condition.
F. At the receiving facility (p. 1090)
   1. Notify dispatch of your arrival.
   2. Transfer care of patient to emergency department personnel.
   3. Transfer all records and information to emergency department personnel.
   4. Give a complete oral report to emergency department personnel at patient's bedside:
      a. Introduce patient by name (if known).
      b. Repeat patient's chief complaint.
      c. Provide additional vital signs taken en route.
      d. Report any history not given previously.
      e. Report any additional treatment you provided.
   5. Assist emergency department personnel in lifting and moving patient to hospital gurney or bed, if requested.
   6. Transfer any valuables or personal effects with patient.
   7. Exchange any linens, spine boards, and other equipment to be left at hospital.
   8. Complete the written prehospital care report and leave a copy at the emergency department.
   9. Ask hospital personnel if you are needed further before you leave.
G. En route to the station (p. 1090)
   1. Clean and inspect ambulance, patient care equipment, reusable supplies, and patient compartment before notifying dispatch of your availability.
   2. Wash your hands.
   3. Radio dispatcher that you are returning to the station **(Fig. 38-6, p. 1090)**
   4. Buckle your seatbelt; drive in a safe, cautious manner.
   5. Have compartment team member continue to clean from seated, buckled position.
   6. Refuel according to local protocol.
H. Postrun (pp. 1090–1092) **(Fig. 38-7, p. 1091)**
   1. General guidelines
      a. Fill out and file required reports.
      b. Fill fuel tank if it is approaching half empty.
      c. Inventory and replenish equipment and supplies.
      d. Wash ambulance exterior, if necessary.
      e. Change soiled uniforms.
      f. Notify dispatch that you are in service, available for calls.
   2. Infection control procedures
      a. Dispose of sharps.
      b. Wash hands.

Point to Emphasize
Under no circumstances should an EMT simply wheel a patient into a hospital, place the patient in a bed, and leave. Unless the EMT transfers care of the patient directly to a member of the hospital staff, he or she may be open to a charge of abandonment.

     c. Clean, disinfect, or sterilize contaminated equipment.
       (1) Clean up visible spills of blood, vomitus, or other body fluids first.
         (a) Put on protective gloves.
         (b) Wear impervious shoe coverings if there is a great deal of blood.
         (c) Use disposable towels and other materials.
         (d) After use, place cleaning towels and materials in plastic bag of contaminated laundry.
         (e) After clean-up of visible spills, decontaminate surfaces with a germicide.
         (f) Use clean towels with germicide. Let area air dry.
         (g) After area has been decontaminated, place shoe coverings, gloves, and other contaminated items in a sealed plastic bag for disposal.
       (2) Disinfect reusable patient care equipment.
         (a) Low-level disinfection
           (i) Routine housekeeping; no visible blood or body fluid contamination; no suspicion of TB
           (ii) 1:100 solution of household bleach and water or EPA-registered "hospital disinfectant" with no tuberculocidal claim on label
         (b) Intermediate-level disinfection
           (i) Surfaces that come into contact with skin
           (ii) 1:10 solution of household bleach and water or EPA-registered "hospital disinfectant" with a claim on its label that it is a tuberculocidal
         (c) High-level disinfection
           (i) For reusable instruments that come in contact with mucous membranes
           (ii) Hot-water pasteurization for 30 minutes or EPA-registered chemical sterilant for 10–45 minutes
         (d) Sterilization
           (i) Equipment that will be used invasively
           (ii) Immerse in EPA-registered chemical sterilant for 6–10 hours (if heat sterilization not available), or expose to steam (autoclave), gas, or dry-heat sterilization.
     d. Launder soiled clothing and linens.
     e. Dispose of infectious wastes according to local protocol.
V. Air medical transport (pp. 1092–1094)
    A. When to request air medical transport (p. 1093)
      1. Operational guidelines
        a. Patient needs transport to facility distant from present location
        b. High-priority patient facing prolonged extrication
        c. Air transport will clearly save time.
        d. Patient cannot be reached by ground vehicles

Teaching Tip
Have a flight unit arrive at the class facility and discuss various aspects of air medical transport.

   e. Air transport crew possesses medical skills not possessed by ambulance crew

  2. Medical guidelines

   a. Shock

   b. Head injury with altered mental status

   c. Chest or abdominal trauma with signs of respiratory distress or shock

   d. Serious mechanism of injury with alteration of vital signs

   e. Penetrating injury to body cavity

   f. Other time-critical illnesses or injuries

 B. Information needed when requesting air medical transport (p. 1093)

  1. Your name

  2. Department name

  3. Call-back number

  4. Nature of incident

  5. Exact location of incident

  6. Radio frequency you use

  7. Exact location of landing zone

 C. Setting up a landing zone (pp. 1093–1094) **(Fig. 38-8, p. 1093; Figs. 38-9 and 38-10, pp. 1095–1096)**

  1. Clear area of obstructions.

  2. If site is highway, stop traffic in both directions.

  3. Consider wind direction.

  4. Mark each corner of landing area with highly visible device.

  5. Put a fifth warning device on upwind side to designate wind direction.

  6. Wet down dry, dusty areas, if possible.

  7. Keep patient and crew clear of air down-wash area.

  8. Assign one person to guide pilot in.

  9. Follow instructions of pilot and crew exactly.

  10. Be extremely cautious about rotor blades.

  11. Always crouch when approaching or leaving a helicopter.

  12. Never approach helicopter until pilot indicates that it is safe.

  13. Secure all loose items so that nothing will blow into rotor blades.

  14. Ensure that no one smokes within 50 feet of the aircraft.

  15. If helicopter lands on incline, approach from downhill side, never from uphill side.

ENRICHMENT (OPTIONAL)

The following sections contain information that is valuable as background for the EMT, but that goes substantially beyond the U.S. Department of Transportation's EMT-Basic National Standard Curriculum.

VI. Operational security measures (pp. 1094–1096)

 A. Personnel (p. 1094)

  1. Security briefings are held at beginning of each shift.

  2. EMS crews are involved in development of operational security measures and situation awareness.

 B. Vehicle (p. 1094)

  1. All EMS vehicles are tracked at all times.

  2. Vehicles are never left running.

3. Vehicles are never left unattended with keys inside.
C. Tracking of vehicle access (pp. 1094–1096)
   1. All off-service vehicles must be secured.
   2. Randomized and routine vehicle audits are conducted.
   3. Comprehensive key log must be kept.
   4. Security measures must be strongly enforced when EMS vehicle is off premises for repairs or other work.
   5. Any vehicles sold to non-EMS must have all EMS markings and warning devices removed.
D. Uniforms and identification items (p. 1096)
   1. EMS patches and ID cards or badges must be safeguarded.
   2. IDs should be counterfeit resistant.
   3. IDs should include a photo of owner.
   4. Uniform stores must verify the identification of any person seeking to purchase any EMS uniform or ID.

VII. Changing conditions (pp. 1096–1098)
A. Driving at night (pp. 1096–1097)
B. Driving in bad weather (pp. 1097–1098)
   1. Winter driving
   2. Fog, mist, dust storms, smog

VIII. Carbon monoxide in ambulances (p. 1098)
A. Sources (p. 1098)
B. Prevention (p. 1098)

CASE STUDY FOLLOW-UP

Ask a student volunteer to read the Case Study that begins on page 1077 of the textbook. You may wish to use the following questions to engage the students in a discussion of the Case Study Follow-up that begins on page 1099 of the textbook. Provide missing information and clarify ideas as needed.

Q1. Prior to receiving this call, what did you do to make sure you would be ready for it?

A1. *Used the patient compartment checklist to make sure the OB kit (and the rest of the ambulance) was stocked.*

Q2. How do you safely park your ambulance at the scene?

A2. *By setting the parking brake and then putting the transmission in park. The vehicle is parked so that it will not be necessary to back into traffic when leaving.*

Q3. Where do you ask Mr. Austin to ride?

A3. *In the front seat of the ambulance.*

Q4. How fast does your partner drive the ambulance to the hospital?

A4. *The posted speed limit.*

Q5. What does your partner do while you complete the prehospital care report?

A5. *Gets clean linen and disinfects the cot.*

IN REVIEW

Assess students' ability to apply what they have just learned by discussing the Review Questions on page 1100 in the textbook.

Q1. List some of the privileges that may be granted to an ambulance operator. List the qualifications necessary for using these privileges.

A1. *Privileges that may be granted to an ambulance driver include exceeding the speed limit; driving the wrong way on a one-way street or opposite side of the road; turning in any direction at an intersection; parking anywhere; leaving the ambulance in the middle of a street or intersection; cautiously proceeding through a red light; and passing in a no-passing zone. Qualifications for these privileges include having a valid driver's license; having gone through a training program; responding to a true emergency; using warning devices; and exercising due regard for the safety of others. (p. 1078)*

Q2. Explain when an ambulance operator should use a police escort.

A2. *An ambulance driver should use a police escort only if he or she doesn't know how to get to a patient's location or to the hospital. When using an escort, the driver should keep a safe distance between the ambulance and the escort vehicle. (pp. 1079–1080)*

Q3. List the major causes of intersection collisions.

A3. *The major causes of intersection collisions are vehicle coming from a side street hurrying through a changing light or not seeing the ambulance that is proceeding through a red light; vehicle from a side street encountering two emergency vehicles when only one is expected; vehicles blocking the ambulance driver's view of pedestrians in the crosswalk. (p. 1080)*

Q4. Explain the problems use of a siren can pose for ambulance safety.

A4. *The problems use of a siren can pose for ambulance safety are incorrect assumption that driver of another vehicle can hear you; causing the other driver to panic and suddenly brake or swerve; emotional stress for the patient; hypnotic effect on ambulance driver with increase of speed; and inability of ambulance driver to hear other emergency vehicles. (p. 1081)*

Q5. List the phases of an ambulance run.

A5. *The phases of an ambulance run are prerun preparation, dispatch, en route to the scene, at the scene, en route to the receiving facility, at the receiving facility, en route to the station, and postrun. (p. 1082)*

Q6. List information an ambulance crew should receive from dispatch before beginning a run.

A6. *Information an ambulance crew should receive from dispatch before beginning a run includes the nature of the call; name, location, and call-back number of the caller; location of the patient; number of patients and severity of problem; and any other special problems or pertinent information. (p. 1084)*

Q7. Describe the procedures you should follow in turning a patient over to a receiving facility.

A7. *The procedures for turning a patient over to a receiving facility are as follows: notify dispatch of arrival at medical facility; present the patient to emergency department personnel; turn over all records; give an oral report (introduce patient by name, chief complaint, update vital sign readings, history, administration of treatment); assist in lifting and moving the patient; turn over valuables; exchange supplies* *and equipment; complete written prehospital care report; ask if you will be needed any further before leaving. (p. 1090)*

Q8. Explain when cleaning and restocking of an ambulance after a run should begin, and why.

A8. *Cleaning and restocking of an ambulance after a run should begin at the hospital and continue en route to the station and at the station in order to be ready as quickly as possible for return to service. (pp. 1090–1092)*

Q9. List the infection control procedures that should be followed.

A9. *The infection control procedures that should be followed are disposal of sharps; wash hands; clean, disinfect, or sterilize contaminated equipment; launder soiled clothing and linens; and dispose of infectious wastes. (p. 1092)*

Q10. Explain how you should mark a landing area for air ambulance use.

A10. *To mark a landing area for air ambulance, mark each corner of the landing area with a highly visible device, such as a flag or surveyor's tapes by day and a flashing or rotating light at night; use flares either by day or night, but only if there is no danger of fire; and put a fifth warning device on the upwind side to designate the wind direction. (pp. 1093–1094)*

CRITICAL THINKING

Assess students' ability to respond to real-life emergency situations by discussing the Critical Thinking questions on page 1100 in the textbook.

Q1. What emergency vehicle driving practices would you use to ensure a safe response to the scene?

A1. *The EMTs should always follow the basics of safe driving and exercise due regard for the safety of others. In this situation, the rain, the slick roadways, and the high-traffic call location should all be taken into consideration when operating the ambulance. It may be necessary to reduce your speed and be cautious when braking to avoid hydroplaning and loss of traction.*

Q2. What other resources may you request to respond to the scene?

A2. *Additional law enforcement for traffic control, rescue crews for extrication, fire personnel for fires or fluid leaks, additional ambulances (ALS if available), and possibly air medical transport may be needed at the scene.*

Q3. What specific steps would you take to improve your safety while on the scene of the crash?

A3. *Position the ambulance out of the flow of traffic. Do not allow the loading entrance of the patient compartment to be exposed to approaching traffic. Use a fire truck, police car, or other vehicle to block the scene. When doing so, have the vehicle turn its wheels away from the scene. Reduce any unnecessary emergency lighting to avoid blinding oncoming traffic. Set cones or other markers out to direct traffic away from the immediate accident scene. If any spills are present, have the fire department available with a charged hose line in case of any ignition.*

Q4. What personal protective equipment should you wear while on the scene?

A4. *The EMTs should be wearing highly visible clothing or vests and stay away from traffic lanes that are still open. The standard precautions must also be taken to include examination gloves and eye protection. At the scene of an accident, the EMTs should also wear a helmet, turnout gear, and heavy gloves if they are to enter the crashed vehicles.*

Q5. If a helicopter is requested, how would you prepare a landing zone?

A5. *First, all traffic should be stopped in both directions and an appropriately sized landing area should be cleared and marked with either highly visible flags or flares/lights (depending on lighting conditions). Then place a flag or flare on the upwind side of the landing zone and notify the flight crew of any hazards in the area such as power lines, tree limbs, antennas, etc.*

ROLE PLAY: AMBULANCE FAMILIARIZATION

Divide students into teams of two and provide each team with an ambulance inspection checklist. Explain to students that there are several ambulances parked outside and that you want them to pretend that it is a shift change. Tell students that they are to inspect an ambulance completely, using the checklist you have provided. Explain that no more than one team at a time should be in the front cab or patient care compartment. If a team cannot locate an item, they may ask the EMTs who are on-scene. Tell students to make sure that they return every item to its original location. Instruct students to return to this classroom when they are finished so that you can review their checklists.

Help students locate the ambulances and observe students in their ambulance inspections.

Review the ambulance inspection checklists as students turn them in. Return checklists to students.

FIELD TRIP (OPTIONAL)

Explain to students that because the next chapter is concerned with vehicle stabilization and patient access, all or part of the next class will be held at an alternate location so that these principles can be demonstrated. Provide students with directions to the site where the demonstration will take place. Provide the date and the time.

ASSIGNMENTS

Assign students to read Chapter 39, "Gaining Access and Extrication," before the next class. Also ask them to complete Chapter 38 of the Workbook.

EVALUATION

Chapter Quiz Distribute copies of the Chapter Quiz provided in Handout 38-2 to evaluate student understanding of this chapter. Remind students not to refer to their textbooks or notes while taking the quiz.

Reading/Reference
Textbook, pp. 1101–1118

Workbook
Chapter 38 Activities

TestGen
Chapter 38 Test

Online Test Preparation
Send your students to
http://www.prenhall.com/
EMTAchieve

Handouts 38-3 to 38-6
Reinforcement Activities

**Brady Skills Series
EMT-B Videos/CD**
Visual Reinforcement

**PowerPoint
Presentation**
Chapter 38

Student CD
Chapter 38

Companion Website
http://www.prenhall.com/
mistovich

Test Manager You may wish to create a custom-tailored test using Prentice Hall *TestGen for Prehospital Emergency Care, Eighth Edition* to evaluate student understanding of this chapter.

Online Test Preparation (for students and instructors) Additional test preparation is available through *EMT Achieve: Basic Test Preparation* at http://www.prenhall.com/EMTAchieve. Instructors can also monitor student mastery online.

REINFORCEMENT

Handouts If classroom discussions or performance on the quiz indicates that some students have not fully mastered the chapter content, you may wish to assign some or all of the Reinforcement Handouts for this chapter.

TECH EXTRAS

Brady Skills Series EMT-B Videos/CD Have your students watch the skills come to life on either VHS or CD-ROM.

PowerPoint Presentation (for instructors) The PowerPoint material developed for this chapter offers useful reinforcement of chapter content.

Student CD A wide variety of material on this CD-ROM will reinforce and also expand student knowledge and skills.

Companion Website (for students) Additional review quizzes and links to EMS resources will contribute to further reinforcement of this chapter. Please visit http://www.prenhall.com/mistovich.

OBJECTIVES CHECKLIST

Cognitive		Date Mastered
7-1.1	Discuss the medical and nonmedical equipment needed to respond to a call.	
7-1.2	List the phases of an ambulance call.	
7-1.3	Describe the general provisions of state laws relating to the operation of the ambulance and privileges in any or all of the following categories: — Speed — Warning lights — Sirens — Right-of-way — Parking — Turning	
7-1.4	List contributing factors to unsafe driving conditions.	
7-1.5	Describe the considerations that should be given to: — Request for escorts — Following an escort vehicle — Intersections	
7-1.6	Discuss "Due Regard for Safety of All Others" while operating an emergency vehicle.	
7-1.7	State what information is essential in order to respond to a call.	
7-1.8	Discuss various situations that may affect response to a call.	
7-1.9	Differentiate between the various methods of moving a patient to the unit based on injury or illness.	
7-1.10	Apply the components of the essential patient information in a written report.	
7-1.11	Summarize the importance of preparing the unit for the next response.	
7-1.12	Identify what is essential for completion of a call.	
7-1.13	Distinguish among the terms cleaning, disinfection, high-level disinfection, and sterilization.	
7-1.14	Describe how to clean or disinfect items following patient care.	

Affective		Date Mastered
7-1.15	Explain the rationale for appropriate report of patient information.	
7-1.16	Explain the rationale for having the unit prepared to respond.	

CHAPTER 38 QUIZ

Write the letter of the best answer in the space provided.

_____ **1.** The EMT's first duty to the patient is to arrive at the scene
  A. quickly.   **C.** safely.
  B. by the most direct route.   **D.** with red lights, horn, and siren.

_____ **2.** The EMT should not exceed the posted speed limit unless
  A. traffic is light.   **C.** the situation is critical.
  B. traveling on holidays.   **D.** using a police escort.

_____ **3.** Using a police or other emergency vehicle escort en route to the collision or the hospital should be
  A. a last resort.   **C.** used with all critical patients.
  B. standard procedure.   **D.** only used at night.

_____ **4.** The standard color for ambulances is
  A. orange.   **C.** yellow.
  B. red.   **D.** white.

_____ **5.** The most common collisions in which ambulances are involved are those at
  A. intersections.   **C.** interstate off-ramps.
  B. railroad crossings.   **D.** pedestrian crosswalks.

_____ **6.** Most states allow an emergency vehicle operator to do all of the following *except*
  A. pass a school bus whose lights are flashing.
  B. pass other vehicles in a no-passing zone.
  C. proceed past red lights.
  D. exceed the speed limits.

_____ **7.** A reason for using the siren sparingly is that it signals "emergency," and it can create emotional and physical stress for
  A. bystanders.   **C.** the patient.
  B. EMTs.   **D.** dispatchers.

_____ **8.** The daily inspection of the ambulance should include all of the following *except*
  A. checking emergency lights.   **C.** inspecting tie rods.
  B. checking power systems.   **D.** testing the horn.

_____ **9.** En route to an emergency call, EMTs should do all of the following *except*
  A. think about what equipment will be carried to the scene.
  B. determine crew responsibilities.
  C. call for ALS support.
  D. decontaminate essential equipment.

_____ **10.** A common danger when an ambulance follows an escort vehicle is
  A. losing contact with the escort.
  B. creating additional stress for the patient.
  C. confusion for the emergency dispatchers.
  D. following the escort too closely.

_____11. The minimum distance an ambulance should be parked from wreckage or a burning
vehicle is _____ feet.
- A. 100
- B. 200
- C. 300
- D. 400

_____12. At the receiving facility, the complete oral report to appropriate emergency department
personnel should include all of the following *except*
- A. the patient's chief complaint.
- B. any history not given previously.
- C. diagnosis of patient's illness.
- D. vital signs taken en route.

_____13. Once a helicopter has set down and the pilot has indicated it is safe, you should approach
a helicopter that has landed on an incline from the
- A. front.
- B. uphill side.
- C. rear.
- D. downhill side.

_____14. If tires are worn, hydroplaning on a wet road can begin at speeds as low as _____ mph.
- A. 30
- B. 15
- C. 20
- D. 35

_____15. The level of disinfection required for reusable instruments that have come into contact
with mucous membranes is
- A. low level.
- B. intermediate level.
- C. high level.
- D. sterilization.

_____16. When the ambulance is ready to return to quarters, one of the first steps should be to
- A. inform the dispatcher.
- B. complete the log entry.
- C. refuel the vehicle.
- D. check the lights and siren.

_____17. When cleaning ambulance surfaces where there is no visible blood or body fluid
contamination, the EMT should use
- A. a high-pressure hose.
- B. an infrared lamp.
- C. soap and water.
- D. an EPA-approved germicide.

_____18. Equipment that will be used invasively should be treated with
- A. a 1:100 bleach-to-water mixture.
- B. sterilization techniques.
- C. Lysol.
- D. a 1:10 bleach-to-water mixture.

_____19. An operational reason to request air rescue is
- A. a Glasgow Coma Scale score of less than 13.
- B. prolonged extrication.
- C. head injury with altered mental status.
- D. penetrating injury to the body cavity.

_____20. If you have to set up a helicopter landing zone at night, its minimum size should be
_____ feet.
- A. 50 × 50
- B. 75 × 75
- C. 100 × 100
- D. 200 × 200

REINFORCEMENT

IN THE FIELD

Read the following real-life situation. Then answer the questions that follow.

"I am an experienced emergency vehicle operator. I took the defensive driving courses, the emergency vehicle operator's course, and everything else I could get my hands on. And my supervisor still put me through an extensive driver's training program. So I was proud to be a driver, and I took my job seriously. At least I thought I did. But here I am, in court, getting ready to tell a grand jury what happened. Let me tell you, first.

"It was a sunny day. Business was brisk, but not too busy. We'd had a couple of runs, and we thought we'd take a break. My partner, Jan, and I liked to go to the coffee shop on the other end of town. It was a little out of the way, but we liked the company there.

"Wouldn't you know it! As soon as we sat down, the tones go out. 'Ambulance 60: respond Code 3 to a person down, unconscious, possible cardiac arrest. Citizen CPR in progress. Address: Oak Crest Apartments, Apartment 222. Time out is 1245 hours.'

"We grabbed our coffees and hauled out fast. Traffic was heavy, and I had to make time being on the other side of the district and all. So I didn't 'spare the horses' as they say.

"Then up ahead I saw a police car. The police in our town first respond to medical emergencies when they can. To tell the truth, they've pulled us out of jams more than once, so I'm usually glad to see them. Anyway, I got right in behind him, following him carefully. I'd changed my siren to yelp so that other drivers could hear the difference as we came up to the intersection.

"I couldn't have been doing more than 30 when we went through the intersection. She must have run the light or something. I had the red, but it should have changed by the time I was in the intersection. And I thought it was OK because the police car got through.

"Next thing, there's a crash and Jan's on top of me and the rig's rolling on its side. My arm was busted and a few of Jan's ribs. We were lucky, though, luckier than the lady who hit us. The ER did what they could, but she was too far gone.

"Anyway, a couple of days later, I'm back at the station. That police officer I followed comes in. He arrests me for reckless endangerment. Now, I'm waiting to talk to the grand jury."

1. List the factors that contributed to this incident.

2. Did the driver make a mistake in following the police car into the intersection? Why or why not?

3. Did the ambulance driver show "due regard for the safety of others"?

4. If you were on the grand jury, would you find sufficient cause to indict the driver on the charges of reckless endangerment?

REINFORCEMENT

CHAPTER 38 REVIEW

Write the word or words that best complete the following sentences in the space provided.

1. The General Services Administration and the U.S. Department of _____ have published federal specifications for ambulances.

2. Always wear _____ _____ when driving or riding in an ambulance.

3. Activate _____ _____ on the ambulance at all times when responding to an emergency call.

4. All emergency-vehicle operators must demonstrate _____ _____ for the safety of others when driving their vehicles.

5. During transport, select the route best suited for _____ _____.

6. In some states, one _____ in the patient compartment is considered the minimum standard; however, two are preferred.

7. At the scene, determine if it is _____ to approach the patient.

8. During an emergency call, ambulance headlights should always be _____.

9. Take the time needed to properly immobilize injured extremities _____ you move the patient, unless he or she is a high priority for immediate transport.

10. Use ordinary _____ and _____ to wash your hands at the end of the run and after all cleaning procedures have been completed.

AMBULANCE OPERATIONS: LISTING

1. List at least six factors other than speed that affect the ability to control the ambulance during a call and that the EMT must be alert to.

2. List the eight major phases of an ambulance call.

3. List four activities commonly performed while en route to a receiving facility.

4. List five medical conditions that would justify a request for air medical transport.

REINFORCEMENT

AMBULANCE OPERATIONS: TRUE OR FALSE

Indicate if the following statements are true or false by writing T or F in the space provided.

_____ **1.** As an ambulance operator, you should be familiar only with the laws and regulations that apply on the local level.

_____ **2.** During transport, select the shortest route—this is not necessarily the least congested route.

_____ **3.** The most common collisions in which ambulances are involved are head-ons.

_____ **4.** The General Services Administration and the DOT developed and published federal specifications for ambulances.

_____ **5.** Most states allow ambulances to be parked anywhere if they do not damage personal property or endanger lives.

_____ **6.** If an ambulance operator acts without due regard for the safety of others, he or she is still protected by Good Samaritan laws.

_____ **7.** The insulation in a newer automobile can reduce the interior decibel level of an approaching siren by 35–40 percent when the car is parked.

_____ **8.** Upon arrival at a vehicle collision, the EMT should park the ambulance in front of or behind the collision, but never alongside it.

_____ **9.** At a car wreck, the ambulance should be parked as close to the wreckage as possible to speed the loading of patients.

_____ **10.** If, en route to the hospital, you are the EMT with the patient, you should keep the driver informed of the patient's condition.

_____ **11.** If the patient vomits en route, clean up the vomitus with paper towels and dispose of them as soon as you arrive at the receiving facility.

_____ **12.** As a rule, the dispatcher should know the amount of time it takes to travel to a medical facility so there is no need to notify dispatch when you arrive there.

_____ **13.** A mixture of 1:100 bleach-to-water is equivalent to an EPA-registered "hospital disinfectant."

_____ **14.** Stopping an ambulance on wet pavement takes approximately twice the distance as stopping on dry pavement.

_____ **15.** When choosing a landing site for a helicopter, the site should *not* be more than 40 yards from the vehicles involved in a collision in order to facilitate patient loading.

Ambulance Operations

Driving the Ambulance

Laws, Ordinances, and
Regulations

Basics of Good Driving

Maintaining Control

- Braking
- Railroads
- School buses
- Bridges and tunnels
- Day of week and time of day
- Road surface
- Backing up
- Higher speeds
- Escorts
- Intersections

Warning Devices

Colors and Markings

Warning Lights and Emergency
Lights

Using Sirens and Air Horns

Phases of an Ambulance Call

Daily Prerun Preparation

Dispatch

En Route to the Scene

At the Scene

En Route to Receiving Facility

At the Receiving Facility

En Route to the Station

Postrun

Air Medical Transport

Requesting Air Medical Transport

- Operational guidelines
- Medical guidelines

Information Needed When Requesting Air Medical Transport

Setting Up a Landing Zone

Operational Security Measures

Changing Conditions

Carbon Monoxide in Ambulances

HANDOUT 38-2: Chapter 38 Quiz

1. C	**6.** A	**11.** A	**16.** A
2. C	**7.** C	**12.** C	**17.** D
3. A	**8.** C	**13.** D	**18.** B
4. D	**9.** D	**14.** D	**19.** B
5. A	**10.** D	**15.** C	**20.** C

HANDOUT 38-3: In the Field

1. Contributing factors: distance between the ambulance and patrol car; speed entering the intersection; failure to yield in the intersection.
2. Yes, following the patrol car too closely raised the risk that the ambulance wouldn't be identified by other drivers.
3. No, his actions directly contributed to a fatality.
4. Student responses may vary, but at least the grounds for indicting are here, whether or not they believe he was actually guilty.

HANDOUT 38-4: Chapter 38 Review

1. Transportation
2. seat belts
3. emergency lights
4. due regard
5. safe travel
6. EMT
7. safe
8. on
9. before
10. soap, water

HANDOUT 38-5: Ambulance Operations: Listing

1. Any six: braking; railroads; school buses; bridges and tunnels; day of the week; time of day; road surface; backing up; higher speeds; escorts; intersections.
2. Prerun vehicle and equipment preparation; dispatch; en route to the scene; at the scene; en route to the receiving facility; at the receiving facility; en route to the station; postrun.
3. Any four of the following: Give calming reassurance. Make sure that the patient is stabilized and settled. Collect patient information with a standard report. Continue your ongoing assessment; reassess vital signs. Review patient priorities. Check your medical interventions. The driver should drive prudently. Advise the driver of any changing conditions in the patient. Notify dispatch and the hospital of the number of patients you are transporting and the condition of the patient(s).
4. Any five: shock; head injury with altered mental status; chest or abdominal trauma with signs of respiratory distress or shock; serious mechanism of injury with alteration of vital signs; penetrating injury to the body cavity; other time-critical illnesses such as severe carbon monoxide poisoning, digit or limb amputation, or heart attack.

HANDOUT 38-6: Ambulance Operations: True or False

1. F	**5.** T	**9.** F	**13.** T
2. F	**6.** F	**10.** T	**14.** T
3. F	**7.** T	**11.** F	**15.** F
4. T	**8.** T	**12.** F	

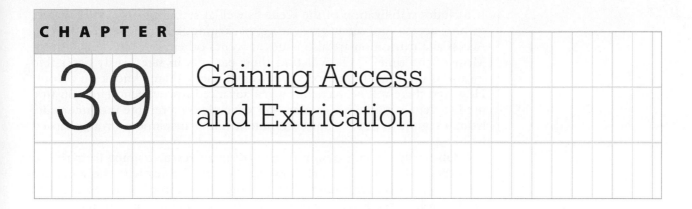

This chapter covers Lesson 7-2 and portions of Lesson 7-4 of the U.S. Department of Transportation's EMT-Basic National Standard Curriculum.

OBJECTIVES

Numbered objectives are from the U.S. Department of Transportation's EMT-Basic National Standard Curriculum. Asterisked objectives, if any, pertain to material that is supplemental to the DOT curriculum. Page numbers refer to pages in the textbook.

Cognitive

7-2.1   Describe the purpose of extrication. (p. 1108)

7-2.2   Discuss the role of the EMT-Basic in extrication. (pp. 1108–1110)

7-2.3   Identify what equipment for personal safety is required for the EMT-Basic. (p. 1103)

7-2.4   Define the fundamental components of extrication. (p. 1108)

7-2.5   State the steps that should be taken to protect the patient during extrication. (pp. 1108–1110)

7-2.6   Evaluate various methods of gaining access to the patient. (pp. 1106–1108)

7-2.7   Distinguish between simple and complex access. (p. 1106)

REVIEW

In the last chapter, "Ambulance Operations," students learned that the ambulance is the vehicle that brings care to the patient in times of emergency and transports the patient to a medical receiving facility for follow-up care. It is a crucial part of the EMS system. An ambulance should be a place of comfort and support to patients suffering from life-threatening problems. It should not pose additional hazards to them. But statistics tell a different story. According to national data, about 10 percent of all ambulances are involved in a collision each year. To keep from adding to these statistics, the EMT must learn to drive an ambulance skillfully and safely.

Distribute the quizzes from the last class. Go over each question on the quiz and handle any concerns students may have about the answers.

INTRODUCTION TO CHAPTER 39

Chapter 39, "Gaining Access and Extrication," is the second lesson of Module 7. By far the most common rescue situations encountered by the EMT are motor-vehicle collisions. Patient rescue begins with the scene size-up.

Total Teaching Time
150 minutes

Resources Needed
- Scored Chapter 39 Quizzes
- Assistance of local fire and rescue squad in demonstrations of vehicle stabilization and access

Additional Resources
Larmon/Davis, *Basic Life Support Skills*

Elling, *EMT Achieve: Basic Test Preparation*

Limmer/Mistovich/ O'Keefe, *Audio Lecture & Study Guide: EMT*

Mistovich/Kuvlesky, *SUCCESS! for the EMT, Second Edition*

It includes stabilization of the scene as well as stabilization of the vehicle, gaining access, and safely extricating, packaging, and moving the patient. Access and extrication are also issues at scenes other than vehicle collisions. Most of the time EMTs will find their patients in safe, easily accessible locations where gaining access requires no more than a knock on a door. However, there will be occasions when advanced rescue techniques must be used to get to and help a patient—for example on a remote mountainside, from a raging river, or from entrapment under machinery or a collapsed building.

Obviously students cannot receive advanced rescue training from this or any other EMT text. They can, however, become familiar with the situations in which patients are found and the roles they can play in rescue. The primary role of the EMT in a rescue situation is gaining access to the patient as quickly as can be safely accomplished in order to perform patient assessment and care, even as the rescue operation proceeds. The EMT's two major priorities in a rescue situation are (1) to keep himself and his partner safe, and (2) to prevent further harm to the patient.

Distribute the Chapter 39 Objectives Checklist, and give students a few minutes to look it over. Then briefly paraphrase the objectives for this lesson in your own words.

LECTURE

The following suggested lecture outline is based on the Department of Transportation's EMT-Basic National Standard Curriculum. In some places, the DOT curriculum has been rearranged or expanded upon so that it is more complete or easier for the student to understand. The page numbers in parentheses refer to pages in the textbook. The parenthetical references in dark, heavy type are to figures, tables, and scans in the textbook.

GAINING ACCESS AND EXTRICATION

I. Planning ahead (pp. 1102–1103)
  A. Dispatch (p. 1102)
    1. Evaluate obstacles to patient access as soon as you receive dispatch.
    2. Begin to plan for access and extrication problems.
  B. Location (pp. 1102–1103)
    1. Know your local area.
    2. Identify locations and occupations that may present difficulties.
    3. Be prepared. Have strategies for gaining access in mind.
  C. Motor-vehicle collisions (p. 1103)
    1. Consider factors such as time of day and location.
    2. Begin to mentally weigh odds of patient entrapment and difficult access.
II. Sizing up the scene (pp. 1103–1106)
  A. Personal protective equipment (PPE) (p. 1103)
    1. Wear appropriate proper protective clothing and equipment at every incident.
    2. Minimum PPE for the EMT includes eye and head protection, disposable gloves, and any other protection needed to prevent contact with blood and body fluids.
    3. Work uniforms do not provide adequate protection for access/extrication activities.

Handout 39-1
Chapter 39 Objectives Checklist

● ➤

Lecture Master
You may wish to display Lecture Master 39 when presenting the lecture to the class.

✓

Teaching Tip
Identify how many agencies represented by the students have written safety protocols. Encourage students to take a critical look at their agency's procedures with a keen eye toward safety.

◆

Slides/Videos
"Safety in Rescue," *Pulse*, June 2001.

Reading/Reference
Czajkowski, J., and Kidd, S., "Ten Tips for EMS Crews Working at Extrication Scenes," *JEMS*, Aug. 2001.

4. Personnel involved in patient extrication process must wear full turnout gear.

5. Know local protocols.

B. Scene safety (p. 1104)

    1. Rescuer's safety is always highest priority.

    2. Electrical lines

        a. Always assume line is electrically alive.

        b. Call electric company.

        c. Secure area against accidental contact, making radius of safe area greater in all directions than length of downed line.

        d. If power lines are in contact with vehicle, stay away.

        e. Advise any patients in vehicle that electric company is en route and to stay inside vehicle.

    3. Traffic

        a. Traffic control responsibility of police

        b. Rescue personnel should have prior training in traffic control.

        c. Safest method is to stop and reroute all traffic.

        d. Traffic should be routed at least 50 feet from wrecked cars.

        e. Take extreme care when directing traffic away from scene.

            (1) Enlist the help of additional personnel and use warning devices.

            (2) Wear adequate reflective clothing or tape to be clearly seen.

            (3) Make visual signals clear.

            (4) Set flares and cones far enough from scene so that driver can stop. **(Fig. 39-1, p. 1105)**

C. Locating all patients (pp. 1104–1106)

    1. Always locate the patient before trying to gain access.

    2. Look for patients both at site of emergency and in immediate vicinity.

    3. Look for clues to "missing" patients.

    4. Get information from witnesses and patients about others who may be hurt at the scene.

    5. When in doubt, have the police contact relatives in an attempt to learn who might have been in the vehicle.

    6. Conduct a thorough search of the area for all victims before leaving the scene.

D. Vehicle safety (p. 1106)

    1. If engine company is not on-scene, remove a fire extinguisher and place it near the collision in case of fire.

    2. Trained rescue personnel stabilize vehicle after all hazards are addressed and scene is secure.

    3. If vehicle is in unstable or unsafe position and you cannot stabilize it with available equipment, do not enter it and do not put any weight on it.

III. Gaining access (pp. 1106–1108)

A. Simple access (p. 1106)

    1. Access in which tools are not required

B. Complex access (p. 1106)

    1. Access that requires the use of tools and specialized equipment

C. Residential access (pp. 1106–1107) **(Fig. 39-2, p. 1107)**

    1. Check windows and doors for one that is unlocked or open.

On the Net
Extrication procedure.
http://www.extrication
.com/modifiedash1.htm

On the Net
New extrication tools.
http://www.nfrmag.com/
backissues/JulAug2002/
feature1.asp

2. Look through and shout through windows to try to locate patient and check for hazards.
3. If window is open but blocked by a screen, cut through the screen.
4. If you must break a window, locate the smallest and least expensive window that will allow you access.
5. Inform patient of what you are going to do.
6. Wear eye protection, heavy work gloves, and a coat.
7. Stand alongside the window to be broken. (**Fig. 39-3, p. 1109**)
8. Strike the top corner of the pane nearest you with an object such as a flashlight.
9. Use striking object to clear broken pieces of glass from frame before reaching in to unlock window or door.

D. Motor-vehicle access (pp. 1107–1108)
1. Walk once around vehicle to identify mechanism of injury.
2. Approach facing the patient.
3. If patient is responsive, tell him repeatedly not to move his head or neck.
4. Tell patient everything you and others are going to do before you do it.
5. Try the doors first.
6. If doors are locked and windows up and intact, say to patient, "Without moving your head or neck, try to unlock a door."
7. If none of these methods work, break a window.
   a. Wear personal protective equipment, heavy gloves, and eye protection.
   b. Tell patient what you are going to do.
   c. Locate window farthest from patient.
   d. Cover window with contact paper strips or broad masking tape if time allows.
   e. Place sharp tool, such as a screwdriver, against lower corner of window and place hand holding tool against the car, then strike tool with a hammer.
   f. Rescue personnel often use a spring-loaded punch.
   g. Carefully remove broken glass from window frame with striking tool, not with gloved hand.
8. Attempt to unlock and open the door.
9. If you cannot get the door open, cover the window opening with a blanket or tarp before crawling into vehicle.

IV. Extrication (pp. 1108–1110)
A. Role of the EMT (p. 1108)
1. Patient-care provider
2. Should cooperate in every way with extrication personnel
3. EMS provider may be both medical care provider and rescuer.
4. When both medical care provider/rescuer, a chain of command should be established to ensure patient care priorities.
5. Patient care always precedes removal from the vehicle unless delay would endanger the life of the patient, EMS personnel, or other rescuers.
B. Caring for the patient (pp. 1108–1110)

1. Perform assessment, stabilization, and resuscitation efforts as for any trauma patient.
2. Establish rapport, and prepare patient for rescue operation.
3. Protect patient from glass, sharp metal, or other hazards off-scene.
4. Continually monitor patient's condition and position in relation to extrication tools and procedures.
5. Give patient some control over process.

Point to Emphasize
The principles of spinal precautions remain the same whether the patient is a low or high priority, but the requirements for speed of removal will dictate the specific techniques used.

ENRICHMENT (OPTIONAL)

The following sections contain information that is valuable as background for the EMT, but that goes substantially beyond the U.S. Department of Transportation's EMT-Basic National Standard Curriculum.

V. **Stabilizing a vehicle** (pp. 1110–1112) **(Table 39-1, p. 1110)**
   A. Upright vehicle (p. 1110) **(Fig. 39-4, p. 1111)**
   B. Vehicle on its side (pp. 1110–1111) **(Fig. 39-5, p. 1111)**
   C. Vehicle on its roof (pp. 1111–1112)
VI. **Extricating a patient** (pp. 1112–1116) **(Fig. 39-6, pp. 1113–1114)**
   A. Rip and blitz disentanglement (p. 1112)
   B. Side-impact or head protection airbags (p. 1112)
   C. Other methods of access and disentanglement (pp. 1112–1115)
      1. Door removal
      2. Windshield removal and roof rolling
   D. Special disentanglement procedures (pp. 1115–1156) **(Fig. 39-7, p. 1116)**

CASE STUDY FOLLOW-UP

Ask a student volunteer to read the Case Study that begins on page 1102 of the textbook. You may wish to use the following questions to engage the students in a discussion of the Case Study Follow-up that begins on page 1117 of the textbook. Provide missing information and clarify ideas as needed.

Q1. Upon arriving at the scene, you determine that it is a complex rescue operation. Since no other emergency personnel are present, what do you do?

A1. *Call for rescue crews.*

Q2. How do you position your ambulance?

A2. *It is positioned 100 feet from the wreckage—the minimum safe distance since there are no electrical lines down or other visible hazards—to provide easy access to equipment while being out of the way of rescue operations.*

Q3. What is your plan for dealing with this scene?

A3. *If the patient access is prevented or hampered, attempt to assess the patients' condition based on the findings of whatever portion of the initial assessment can be performed. If possible, establish and maintain an airway, stabilize the cervical spine, and control any serious bleeding from outside the vehicle. Provide direction to other responding units as to what the situation is and what is needed from them.*

Q4. Since this is a complex rescue operation, what approach is used to help ensure success?

A4. *An Incident Command System with one commander.*

Q5. Why do you avoid giving all of your attention to the patients in the sports car?

A5. *The driver of the truck may also be injured and any potential hazards must not be overlooked.*

IN REVIEW

Assess students' ability to apply what they have just learned by discussing the Review Questions on page 1117 in the textbook.

Q1. Name your first priority in this and any other type of emergency situation.

A1. *The first priority in any emergency is personal safety (safety of yourself and your partner). (p. 1104)*

Q2. Describe the role of the EMT in vehicle stabilization and patient extrication.

A2. *The role of the EMT in vehicle stabilization and patient extrication is that of patient care provider. It includes assessment, necessary emergency medical care including spinal stabilization, plus making certain that the patient is removed from the vehicle in a way that minimizes risk of further injury. It also includes remaining with the patient throughout the rescue and assisting him or her through the process. (p. 1107)*

Q3. Identify the first step you should take upon arriving at the site of a motor-vehicle collision.

A3. *The first step you should take on arriving at the site of a motor-vehicle collision is sizing up the scene to identify real and potential hazards. (p. 1104)*

Q4. Explain how you can locate all the patients involved in an emergency such as a motor-vehicle collision.

A4. *To locate all the patients involved in an emergency such as a motor-vehicle collision, you should do the following: Search thoroughly, both at the site of the emergency and in the immediate vicinity. Question witnesses, bystanders, and other patients. Look for clues such as a child's coat in the backseat of a car. When in doubt, have the police contact relatives in an attempt to learn who might have been in the vehicle. (pp. 1104–1106)*

Q5. Explain why it is important to approach a motor-vehicle collision from the front.

A5. *It is important to approach a motor-vehicle collision from the front to prevent patients from trying to turn their heads to see you, thereby possibly aggravating a spinal injury. (p. 1107)*

Q6. Identify which process comes first—patient care or patient extrication—and describe the exceptions.

A6. *Patient care always precedes removal from the vehicle unless delay would endanger the life of the patient, EMS personnel, or other rescuers. (p. 1108)*

Q7. Describe how you can protect the patient from further physical injury during extrication.

A7. *Protect the patient from glass and other flying debris by covering him or her with a heavy blanket, tarp, or salvage cover, and in some cases with an object such as a short spine board between the working area and the patient. (pp. 1108–1110)*

Q8. Describe the minimum level of personal protective equipment required at a motor-vehicle collision site.

A8. *The minimum level of personal protective equipment required at a motor-vehicle collision site includes eye and head protection, disposable gloves, and any additional protection necessary to prevent direct contact with any blood or bodily fluid. (p. 1103)*

Q9. Describe the steps that may be taken after you identify downed electrical lines at the scene.

A9. *Steps that may be taken after identifying downed electrical lines at the scene are as follows: Assume a downed power line is electrically alive. The area must be secured to avoid accidental contact. Request special assistance from the local electric service company. If patients are still in the vehicle, tell them to stay there. If the situation is immediately threatening to life or the electric company is unable to respond, rescue personnel specially trained in handling electrical emergencies may move the downed line using special equipment and techniques designed for that purpose. (p. 1104)*

Q10. Describe a "stable" vehicle. Then name some simple steps that you can take to stabilize a vehicle in danger of rolling until rescue crews can properly and completely stabilize it.

A10. *A vehicle is considered stable when it is in a secured position and can no longer move, rock, or bounce. To stabilize a vehicle in danger of rolling until rescue crews can properly and completely stabilize it, shut off the engine, set the parking brake, shift the automatic to "park" or the manual to any gear, and place firm objects such as a spare tire in front of and behind a wheel to minimize vehicle movement. (pp. 1110–1112)*

CRITICAL THINKING

Assess students' ability to respond to real-life emergency situations by discussing the Critical Thinking questions on page 1118 in the textbook.

Q1. Do you need to gain immediate access to the patient or should you wait for the extrication crew to arrive?

A1. *The patient is not responding appropriately; thus, it is necessary to gain immediate access to the vehicle. However, the first consideration is whether the scene, including the vehicle itself, is safe for you to enter. If the scene or the vehicle is not safe, do not enter.*

Q2. What methods could be used to gain immediate access to the patient?

A2. *If the EMTs determine that the scene is safe and the patient is in need of immediate access, breaking a side window and either opening a door from the inside or climbing through the window opening would be the best methods.*

Q3. Once access has been gained, what is your primary role?

A3. *Once the patient has been accessed, the EMT's primary responsibility is to assess the patient and provide emergency care. Extrication of the patient should be left to the fire department or rescue crew on the scene designated to do so.*

Q4. How can you assist the extrication crew while providing care to the patient?

A4. *There are numerous ways for the EMT to assist both the patient and the extrication crew, including explaining to the patient everything that is happening, keeping the patient calm, helping to protect the patient during extrication procedures, and helping to extricate the patient in ways that will minimize the risk of further injury.*

FIELD TRIP (OPTIONAL)

If possible, make arrangements with your local fire-rescue service for an off-site demonstration. Fire-rescue personnel should demonstrate the following principles to students: vehicle stabilization, simple access, and complex access.

ASSIGNMENTS

Assign students to read Chapter 40, "Hazardous Materials Emergencies," before the next class. Also ask them to complete Chapter 39 of the Workbook.

EVALUATION

Chapter Quiz Distribute copies of the Chapter Quiz provided in Handout 39-2 to evaluate student understanding of this chapter. Remind students not to refer to their textbooks or notes while taking the quiz.

Test Manager You may wish to create a custom-tailored test using Prentice Hall *TestGen for Prehospital Emergency Care, Eighth Edition* to evaluate student understanding of this chapter.

Online Test Preparation (for students and instructors) Additional test preparation is available through *EMT Achieve: Basic Test Preparation* at http://www.prenhall.com/EMTAchieve. Instructors can also monitor student mastery online.

REINFORCEMENT

Handouts If classroom discussions or performance on the quiz indicates that some students have not fully mastered the chapter content, you may wish to assign some or all of the Reinforcement Handouts for this chapter.

Reading/Reference
Textbook, pp. 1119–1139

Workbook
Chapter 39 Activities

Chapter Quiz
Handout 39-2

TestGen
Chapter 39 Test

Online Test Preparation
Send your students to http://www.prenhall.com/ EMTAchieve

Handouts 39-3 to 39-5
Reinforcement Activities

TECH EXTRAS

Brady Skills Series EMT-B Videos/CD Have your students watch the skills come to life on either VHS or CD-ROM.

PowerPoint Presentation (for instructors) The PowerPoint material developed for this chapter offers useful reinforcement of chapter content.

Student CD A wide variety of material on this CD-ROM will reinforce and also expand student knowledge and skills.

Companion Website (for students) Additional review quizzes and links to EMS resources will contribute to further reinforcement of this chapter. Please visit http://www.prenhall.com/mistovich.

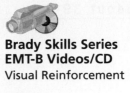

**Brady Skills Series
EMT-B Videos/CD**
Visual Reinforcement

**PowerPoint
Presentation**
Chapter 39

Student CD
Chapter 39

Companion Website
http://www.prenhall.com/
mistovich

OBJECTIVES

OBJECTIVES CHECKLIST

Cognitive		Date Mastered
7-2.1	Describe the purpose of extrication.	
7-2.2	Discuss the role of the EMT-Basic in extrication.	
7-2.3	Identify what equipment for personal safety is required for the EMT-Basic.	
7-2.4	Define the fundamental components of extrication.	
7-2.5	State the steps that should be taken to protect the patient during extrication.	
7-2.6	Evaluate various methods of gaining access to the patient.	
7-2.7	Distinguish between simple and complex access.	

CHAPTER 39 QUIZ

Write the letter of the best answer in the space provided.

_____ 1. The majority of electric current and associated hazards in vehicle collisions can be eliminated most easily by
   A. grounding the vehicles.
   B. disconnecting the battery.
   C. flooding the engine compartment with CO_2.
   D. turning off the engine.

_____ 2. Upon arrival at the scene of a collision, the EMT's first task is to
   A. stabilize the vehicle.
   B. gain access to the patient.
   C. perform a scene size-up.
   D. provide manual in-line stabilization for the patient.

_____ 3. Which article of protective equipment provides an acceptable level of head protection?
   A. bump cap   **C.** uniform cap
   B. firefighter's helmet   **D.** bicyclist's helmet

_____ 4. The role of the EMT in vehicle stabilization and patient extrication is that of
   A. a public information officer.   **C.** a rescuer.
   B. traffic control.   **D.** patient care provider.

_____ 5. The safest shoes to wear when involved in the patient extrication process of a vehicle collision are
   A. rubber boots.   **C.** deck shoes.
   B. high-top cross-training shoes. **D.** steel-toed boots.

_____ 6. In general, approach a vehicle that has been involved in a collision and contains a patient from the
   A. front.   **C.** passenger side.
   B. driver's side.   **D.** rear.

_____ 7. Traffic at the scene of a motor-vehicle collision should be routed away a minimum distance of _____ feet.
   A. 50   **C.** 150
   B. 100   **D.** 200

_____ 8. Before entering a vehicle that was involved in a collision, it must be
   A. removed.   **C.** ticketed.
   B. stabilized.   **D.** marked.

_____ 9. The least costly method of forceful entry into a residence is
   A. calling a locksmith.   **C.** breaking a window.
   B. using the jaws of life.   **D.** breaking a door.

_____ 10. By far, the most common access problems encountered by the EMT involve
   A. crime scenes.   **C.** pets.
   B. children.   **D.** motor-vehicle collisions.

_____ **11.** The easiest method of properly stabilizing a vehicle that is upright and on its wheels is to
  A. use parallel step chocks.
  B. use jacks at the front and rear bumpers.
  C. place two wheel chocks.
  D. put the car in park.

_____ **12.** The most common tool used in vehicle extrication and patient disentanglement is the
  A. airbag.   **C.** power hydraulic rescue tool.
  B. come-along.   **D.** axe.

_____ **13.** Complex access requires the use of
  A. specialized tools.   **C.** no special tools or equipment.
  B. protective equipment.   **D.** heavy gloves.

_____ **14.** All windows in modern automobiles are made of tempered safety glass that will break into rounded pieces rather than sharp shards *except* the
  A. windshield.   **C.** driver's window.
  B. rear windows.   **D.** sunroof.

_____ **15.** Excluding motor-vehicle collisions, most injuries are the result of
  A. hunting.   **C.** electricity.
  B. gravity.   **D.** weather.

IN THE FIELD

Read the following real-life situation. Then answer the questions that follow.

Dispatch: Medic Three, Ambulance 1701, respond Code 3 to a car off the road. Time is now 0315 hours.

"We roll out of our bunks and grab our boots. In minutes, we are on the road, running lights and sirens into the dark night. Trying to shake the sleep from my head, I'm wondering what happened. As we pull up to the scene, we see the State Trooper's patrol car with its lights on up ahead. His spotlight is slowly panning the scene, but we can't see a car.

"Getting out of the ambulance, making sure that there are no downed wires nearby, I walk toward the trooper. He points down a steep embankment and there is the vehicle, resting on its roof. Looking around, I see no other access but down the 65-foot embankment."

1. What would your initial report from this scene say?

2. What special rescue equipment/assistance would be needed?

3. Suppose that once you got down to the patients, they tell you the driver ran off and that they think he was hurt and probably intoxicated. What would you do then?

CHAPTER 39 REVIEW

Write the word or words that best complete each sentence in the space provided.

1. A(n) _____ patient may be found anywhere under any circumstances.

2. The most important point to remember in an emergency is that your own

   _____ as an EMT is always your highest priority.

3. Once the scene is secure and it is safe to approach the vehicle, walk around it once to identify

   mechanisms of injury, and approach _____ the patient.

4. _____ _____ always precedes removal from the

   vehicle unless delay would endanger the life of the patient, EMS personnel, or other rescuers.

5. Stabilize and, if possible, immobilize the patient's _____ securely before

   you remove the patient from the vehicle by normal or rapid extrication procedures.

6. The first step to properly stabilize an upright vehicle is to immobilize the

   _____.

7. The primary goal of patient disentanglement is to remove the _____ from

   around the _____.

8. The _____ posts are the front posts supporting a vehicle's roof.

9. When the patient is pinned between the dash, steering wheel, and seat, the technique known as a(n)

   _____ _____ may provide the safest and easiest

   disentanglement.

10. An EMT should consider all vehicles involved in a collision to be _____.

11. The _____ is always the access of choice because it is the largest

    uncomplicated opening into the passenger compartment of a vehicle.

12. Getting into a vehicle by opening a door or rolling down a window is called

    _____ _____.

13. If the _____ cable on a battery is removed first, a spark may occur that

    could ignite acid fumes or gasoline spilled from the accident.

14. All ambulances should be equipped with _____ so that scenes can be

    assessed from a safe distance and position.

15. When called to a motor-vehicle collision, look for _____ both at the site of the emergency and in the immediate vicinity.

16. A vehicle is considered _____ when it is in a secured position and can no longer move, rock, or bounce.

17. There are two types of window glass in modern vehicles: laminated and

_____.

18. When using chocks to stabilize an upright vehicle, they should be pushed in until they touch the

_____.

GAINING ACCESS AND EXTRICATION: LISTING

REINFORCEMENT

1. List five of the questions the EMT should ask upon receiving a call from dispatch to evaluate whether there may be obstacles to the patient access and extrication.

2. List the personal protective equipment required for personnel involved in the patient extrication process.

3. List the two common hazards at motor-vehicle collisions.

4. List three means of stabilizing an upright vehicle.

5. List the two types of access to a patient involved in a motor-vehicle collision.

Gaining Access and Extrication

Planning Ahead
Dispatch
Location
Motor-Vehicle Collisions

Sizing Up the Scene
Personal Protective Equipment
Scene Safety
  • Electrical lines
  • Traffic
Locating All Patients
Vehicle Safety

Gaining Access
Residential Access
Motor Vehicle Access

Extrication
Role of the EMT
Caring for the Patient

Stabilizing a Vehicle
Upright Vehicle
Vehicle on Its Side
Vehicle on Its Roof

Extricating a Patient
Disentanglement
Special Disentanglement
  Procedures

HANDOUT 39-2: Chapter 39 Quiz

1. D	**5.** D	**9.** C	**13.** A
2. C	**6.** A	**10.** D	**14.** A
3. B	**7.** A	**11.** A	**15.** B
4. D	**8.** B	**12.** C	

HANDOUT 39-3: In the Field

1. That you established EMS Command and that you are requesting lights, heavy rescue, and high-angle rescue personnel and equipment.
2. Ropes, possibly heavy hydraulic tools, even air medical rescue.
3. Inform the trooper and have him form a search party and proceed with a lost person wilderness search while you continue to triage and care for the patients on-scene.

HANDOUT 39-4: Chapter 39 Review

1. trauma
2. safety
3. facing
4. Patient care
5. spine
6. suspension
7. vehicle, patient
8. A

9. dash roll
10. unstable
11. door
12. simple access
13. positive
14. binoculars
15. patients
16. stable
17. tempered
18. undercarriage

HANDOUT 39-5: Gaining Access and Extrication: Listing

1. Any five of the following: Is the patient ill or injured? What is the mechanism of injury? What is the location of the incident? What time of day is it? What is the weather? Is there a report of entrapment? Is there a report of a leak or spill?
2. Full turnout gear: bunker coat, bunker pants, steel-toed boots, head protection (i.e., standard fire helmet), eye protection (goggles or safety glasses), and heavy leather gloves; in addition, appropriate BSI gear would be needed for patient contact.
3. Electrical lines, traffic
4. Step chocks, box crib with wedges, cutting valve stems/tires
5. Complex access, simple access

40 Hazardous Materials Emergencies

This chapter covers portions of Lesson 7-3 and 7-4 of the U.S. Department of Transportation's EMT-Basic National Standard Curriculum.

OBJECTIVES

Numbered objectives are from the U.S. Department of Transportation's EMT-Basic National Standard Curriculum. Asterisked objectives, if any, pertain to material that is supplemental to the DOT curriculum. Page numbers refer to pages in the textbook.

Cognitive

7-3.1	Explain the EMT-Basic's role during a call involving hazardous materials. (p. 1128)
7-3.2	Describe what the EMT-Basic should do if there is reason to believe that there is a hazard at the scene. (p. 1129)
7-3.3	Describe the actions that an EMT-Basic should take to ensure bystander safety. (p. 1129)
7-3.4	State the role the EMT-Basic should perform until appropriately trained personnel arrive at the scene of a hazardous materials situation. (p. 1129)
7-3.5	Break down the steps to approaching a hazardous situation. (p. 1129)
7-3.6	Discuss the various environmental hazards that affect EMS. (pp. 1129–1134)
7-3.11	Describe basic concepts of incident management. (pp. 1129–1132)
7-3.12	Explain the methods for preventing contamination of self, equipment, and facilities. (pp. 1129–1134)

Additional objectives from DOT Lesson 7-3 are addressed in Chapter 41, "Multiple-Casualty Incidents."

REVIEW

In the last chapter, "Gaining Access and Extrication," students learned that motor-vehicle collisions are by far the most common rescue situations encountered by the EMT. Patient rescue begins with scene size-up. It includes stabilization of the scene as well as stabilization of the vehicle, gaining access, and safely extricating, packaging, and moving the patient. Access and extrication are also issues at scenes other than vehicle collisions. Most of the time EMTs will find their patients in safe, easily accessible locations where gaining access requires no more than a knock on a door.

Total Teaching Time
120 minutes

Resources Needed
- Scored Chapter 39 Quizzes
- DOT *Emergency Response Guidebook*
- OSHA publication "29 CFR 1910.120—Hazardous Waste Operations and Emergency Response Standards (1989)"
- *NFPA 473 Competencies for EMS Personnel Responding to Hazardous Materials Incidents*
- A member of a local or regional hazardous materials team to serve as guest speaker

Additional Resources
Larmon/Davis, *Basic Life Support Skills*

Elling, *EMT Achieve: Basic Test Preparation*

Limmer/Mistovich/ O'Keefe, *Audio Lecture & Study Guide: EMT*

Mistovich/Kuvlesky, *SUCCESS! for the EMT, Second Edition*

However, there will be occasions when advance rescue techniques must be used to get to and help a patient.

Obviously students cannot receive advanced rescue training from this or any other EMT text. They can, however, become familiar with the situations in which patients are found and the roles they can play in rescue. The primary role of the EMT in a rescue situation is gaining access to the patient as quickly as can be safely accomplished in order to perform patient assessment and care, even as the rescue operation proceeds. The two major priorities of EMTs in a rescue situation are (1) to keep themselves and their partners safe, and (2) to prevent further harm to the patient.

Distribute the quizzes from the last class. Go over each question on the quiz and handle any concerns students may have about the answers.

INTRODUCTION TO CHAPTER 40

Chapter 40, "Hazardous Materials Emergencies," is the third chapter in Module 7. More than 50 billion tons of hazardous materials are manufactured in the United States annually. More than 4 billion tons are shipped within this country every year, most commonly including explosives, compressed and poisonous gases, flammable liquids and solids, oxidizers (substances that give off oxygen and stimulate combustion of organic matter), corrosives, and radioactive materials. Hazardous materials spills and other accidents are common problems, the exact extent of which is unknown. The EMT is not required to deal with hazardous materials, which takes specialized training. It is more important for the EMT to recognize that a hazardous materials emergency exists.

Distribute the Chapter 40 Objectives Checklist, and give students a few minutes to look it over. Then briefly paraphrase the objectives for this lesson in your own words.

LECTURE

The following suggested lecture outline is based on the Department of Transportation's EMT-Basic National Standard Curriculum. In some places, the DOT curriculum has been rearranged or expanded upon so that it is more complete or easier for the student to understand. The page numbers in parentheses refer to pages in the textbook. The parenthetical references in dark, heavy type are to figures, tables, and scans in the textbook.

HAZARDOUS MATERIALS EMERGENCIES

  I. Identifying hazardous materials (pp. 1120–1128) **(Table 40-1, pp. 1121–1124)**
    A. What is a hazardous material? (p. 1120) **(Fig. 40-1, p. 1124)**
    B. Placards and shipping papers (pp. 1120–1125)
      1. DOT placards **(Figs. 40-2, 40-3, p. 1125)**
      2. NFPA 704 placards **(Fig. 40-4, p. 1126)**
      3. Shipping papers **(Fig. 40-5, p. 1127)**
    C. Clues to presence of hazardous materials
      1. Signs restricting entry **(Fig. 40-6a, p. 1128)**
      2. Storage tanks **(Fig. 40-6b, p. 1128)**
      3. Containers with placards
      4. Smoking or self-igniting materials
      5. Extraordinary fire conditions

Handout 40-1
Chapter 40 Objectives Checklist

Lecture Master
You may wish to display Lecture Master 40 when presenting the lecture to the class.

Point of Interest
Recent studies by the Office of Technology Assessment have shown that some states report 25–50% of identification placards are incorrect, and that many shipping documents are also inaccurate or incomplete.

On the Net
U.S. DOT's Emergency Response Guidebook. http://hazmat.dot.gov/gydebook.htm

Teaching Tip
Have a copy of the *U.S. DOT's Emergency Response Guidebook* available so that students can see what it looks like and how it works. Suggest that students go back to their agencies and see where a copy is kept on their ambulances.

6. Boiling or spattering of materials that have not been heated
7. Wavy or unusually colored vapors over a container of liquid material
8. Characteristically colored vapor clouds
9. Frost near a container leak (liquid coolants)
10. Unusual condition or deterioration of containers

D. Resources for identifying and dealing with hazmat emergencies (pp. 1126–1128)
  1. State and local specialized hazmat teams
  2. U.S. DOT's Emergency Response Guide
  3. CHEMTREC (Chemical Transportation Emergency Center), 800-424-9300
  4. Chemtrel, Inc., 800-255-3924
  5. Regional poison control center

E. Training required by law (p. 1128)
  1. OSHA, EPA, and NFPA regulations
    a. OSHA publication 29 CFR 1910.120
      (1) *Hazardous Waste Operations and Emergency Response Standards* (1989)
    b. *NFPA 473: Competencies for EMS Personnel Responding to Hazardous Materials Incidents*
  2. Training levels
    a. First Responder Awareness
    b. First Responder Operations
    c. Hazardous Materials Technician
    d. Hazardous Materials Specialist

II. **Guidelines for hazardous materials rescues** (pp. 1129–1134)
  A. General rules (p. 1129)
    1. Protect the safety of all rescuers. (**Fig. 40-7, pp. 1130–1131**)
    2. Provide patient care.
    3. Decontaminate clothing, equipment, and the vehicle.
    4. Avoid contact with any unidentified material.
    5. Avoid risking your life or health. Do not enter the scene if no victims are involved.
  B. Incident management (Incident Management Systems are also discussed in Chapter 41. You may choose to discuss them at length here, then briefly review them in the next lecture, or introduce them briefly here and discuss them at length in the next lecture.) (pp. 1129–1132)
    1. Preincident planning
      a. One command officer
      b. Clear chain of command
      c. Established system of communications
      d. Predesignated receiving facilities
    2. Implementing the plan—determine best plan of action based on:
      a. Nature of problem
      b. ID of hazardous materials
      c. Kind and condition of containers
      d. Existing weather conditions
      e. Presence or absence of fire
      f. Elapsed time since emergency occurred
      g. What has already been done at the scene
      h. Number of victims
      i. Danger of victimizing more people
    3. Establishing safety zones (**Fig. 40-8, p. 1132**)

On the Net
CHEMTREC can be found at: www.cmahg.com/cmawebsite.nsf/pages/chemtrec

Teaching Tip
Make copies of OSHA's "29 CFR 1910.120," and *NFPA Standard 47: Competencies for EMS Personnel Responding to Hazardous Materials Incidents* available to students during the lecture.

On the Net
For a copy of "29 CFR 1910.120," go to: www.osha-slc.gov/OshStd_toc/OSHA_Std_toc.html

Slides/Videos
"EMS Response to Hazardous Materials," *Pulse,* Oct. 2000.

       a. Hot zone (exclusion zone)

       b. Warm zone (contamination reduction zone)

          (1) Decontamination **(Fig. 40-9 and 40-10, pp. 1133–1134)**

       c. Cold zone (support zone)

   C. Emergency procedures (pp. 1132–1137)

      1. Hot zone

        a. Wear proper protective equipment in all zones.

        b. Remove patient from accident site.

        c. Perform initial (gross) decontamination.

        d. Leave patient's clothing, tools, and equipment in hot zone.

      2. Warm zone

        a. Perform initial assessment.

        b. Perform complete decontamination.

        c. Perform rapid assessment.

        d. Treat patient's major injuries.

        e. Immobilize spine as appropriate.

        f. Splint where needed.

        g. Move patient to cold zone.

      3. Decontamination area

        a. Remove all protective equipment.

      4. Cold zone

        a. Take vital signs.

        b. Take SAMPLE history.

        c. Prepare patient for transport.

      5. Protect vehicle and equipment from contamination during transport.

      6. Decontaminate yourself if you are accidentally exposed to hazardous material during the rescue. **(Fig 40-9, p. 1133)**

      7. Follow-up exposure with a thorough medical examination and medical surveillance.

      8. Decontaminate your equipment and vehicle.

ENRICHMENT (OPTIONAL)

The following sections contain information that is valuable as background for the EMT, but that goes substantially beyond the U.S. Department of Transportation's EMT-Basic National Standard Curriculum.

III. Radiation emergencies (pp. 1134–1137)

   A. Exposure and contamination (p. 1134)

      1. Exposure

        a. Patient is in presence of radioactive material without material actually touching patient's clothing or body, is not radioactive, and does not pose major threat to rescue personnel.

      2. Contamination

        a. Patient has come into direct contact with radioactive gas, liquid, or particles; patient's clothes and skin contain radioactive material; and patient poses major hazard to rescuers and self.

   B. Guidelines for radiation emergencies (pp. 1134–1135)

      1. Make your first priority the protection of yourself and others from contamination.

      2. Never attempt to decontaminate a radiation patient.

        a. Wait for a Radiation Safety Officer (RSO).

b. If not RSO, transport patient to hospital for decontamination experts there.
- **C.** Procedures for radiation emergencies (pp. 1135–1136)
  - **1.** Ensure scene safety and take personal protection measures. **(Fig. 42-11, p. 1135)**
    - **a.** Time
    - **b.** Distance
    - **c.** Shielding
  - **2.** Patient care
  - **3.** Personal decontamination
  - **4.** Vehicle/equipment decontamination
- **D.** Problems caused by radiation (p. 1135)
  - **1.** Radiation sickness
    - **a.** Starts day after exposure to large amounts of radiation and lasts from few days to 8 weeks
    - **b.** Signs and symptoms
      - **(1)** Nausea
      - **(2)** Vomiting
      - **(3)** Diarrhea
      - **(4)** Hemorrhage
      - **(5)** Weight loss
      - **(6)** Appetite loss
      - **(7)** Malaise
      - **(8)** Fever
      - **(9)** Sores in throat and mouth
      - **(10)** Lowered resistance to disease and infection
  - **2.** Radiation injury
    - **a.** Caused by exposure to large amounts of alpha particles
    - **b.** Signs and symptoms
      - **(1)** Hair loss
      - **(2)** Skin burns **(Fig. 42-12, p. 1136)**
      - **(3)** Generalized skin lesions
  - **3.** Radiation poisoning
    - **a.** Caused by exposure to dangerous amounts of internal radiation and results in host of serious diseases including cancer and anemia
- **E.** Protection from radiation (pp. 1135–1136)
  - **1.** Factors determining the amount of radiation damage you may sustain
    - **a.** Amount and type of personal shielding you use
    - **b.** Strength of radiation source
    - **c.** Distance from radiation source
    - **d.** Type of radiation
      - **(1)** Alpha rays—can be stopped by clothing
      - **(2)** Beta rays—require lead shielding
    - **e.** Length of exposure
    - **f.** Percent of body exposed
  - **2.** Reducing risk
    - **a.** Divide rescue work among many rescuers; work in small teams for short periods.
    - **b.** Shield the radiation source itself.
    - **c.** Know your community's plan for hazardous materials emergencies.
    - **d.** Know how to reach your RSO.
    - **e.** Always wear your protective gear and SCBA as soon as you suspect radiation.

      f. Never smoke or eat food at a radiation emergency site.
  F. Terrorist attacks involving weapons of mass destruction
     (p. 1137)

CASE STUDY FOLLOW-UP

Ask a student volunteer to read the Case Study that begins on page 1120 of the textbook. You may wish to use the following questions to engage the students in a discussion of the Case Study Follow-up that begins on page 1137 of the textbook. Provide missing information and clarify ideas as needed.

Q1. Realizing that the tanker may pose a possible hazardous materials emergency, what do you do?

A1. *Decide on a safe place to park—uphill, upwind, and away from the potential danger. Check the* Emergency Response Guidebook *and find that the size and shape of the tank and a "Flammable Liquid" placard indicate that danger can come from fire or explosion, which reinforces caution about introducing open flames, heat, or sparks at the scene. Further inspection of the container reveals a small leak and vapors. All this data is reported to Incident Command before the fire department arrives and begins to set up an entry and decon area.*

Q2. As two patients begin walking from the crash site to your ambulance, what does Incident Command instruct them to do?

A2. *To stop where they are. Their clothes are contaminated, and they must strip.*

Q3. What do you do once the patients have been decontaminated and are in clean clothes?

A3. *The initial assessment is completed while a First Responder continues to hold manual in-line stabilization.*

Q4. Prior to transporting the patients, what is done by each ambulance crew?

A4. *The stretchers and other items in the ambulance are covered with thick plastic.*

Q5. What do you do after you have transferred the patients to emergency department personnel and completed your verbal and written reports?

A5. *Decontaminate yourselves and the ambulance.*

IN REVIEW

Assess students' ability to apply what they have just learned by discussing the Review Questions on page 1139 in the textbook.

Q1. List clues that tell you a hazardous material may be present at an accident scene.

A1. *Clues that a hazardous material may be present at an accident scene include identifying signs restricting entry, storage tanks, containers with placards, smoking or self-igniting materials, extraordinary fire conditions, boiling or spattering of materials that have not been heated, wavy or unusually colored vapors over a container of liquid material, characteristically colored vapor clouds, frost near a container leak,* *unusual condition of containers such as peeling or discoloration of finishes, unexpected deterioration, deformity, or the unexpected operation of pressure-relief valves. (pp. 1125–1126)*

Q2. Name the first thing an EMT should do after recognizing that hazardous materials might be involved in an accident.

A2. *As soon as you recognize or suspect a hazardous materials emergency, radio immediately for help. (p. 1129)*

Q3. Explain what qualifies the EMT to attempt a hazardous materials rescue.

A3. *An EMT should never attempt a hazardous materials rescue unless he or she has had the necessary specialized training to the hazardous materials technician level or better and proper training in the use of self-contained breathing apparatus. (p. 1129)*

Q4. List specific actions you can take to protect bystanders.

A4. *Specific actions to protect bystanders are securing the scene and, if necessary, cordoning off the whole area and appointing people to keep bystanders away. (p. 1129)*

Q5. If you have had no specialized training, explain what you should do while waiting for expert help to arrive.

A5. *While waiting for help to arrive, you should protect yourself and bystanders by keeping uphill, upwind, and away from the danger. (p. 1129)*

Q6. List the resources available to the EMT at the site of a hazardous materials emergency.

A6. *Resources for proper identification and handling a hazardous materials emergency is available through state and local agencies including specialized hazmat teams, and can be found in the Emergency Response Guidebook and other print references, or can be obtained from CHEMTREC or Chemtrel, Inc., through their toll-free numbers, or from a regional poison control center. (pp. 1126–1127)*

Q7. Explain what you can do to protect yourself, others, and your vehicle from contamination.

A7. *To protect yourself, others, and your vehicle from contamination, do the following: Wear all proper protective clothing including SCBA and make sure all other rescuers do the same. Establish "safety zones" to keep contamination from spreading. Prior to transport, cover the benches, floor, and other exposed areas with thick plastic sheeting secured with duct tape. Decontaminate all patients before transport. Before removing them from the scene, seal all contaminated clothing and equipment in plastic bags or metal containers with tightly fitting lids. Decontaminate yourself by washing with mild detergent or green soap and plenty of running water for at least 20 minutes or until the burning stops. Following rescue, decontaminate equipment and vehicle by washing them thoroughly inside and out. (pp. 1132–1133)*

Q8. List the "safety zones" and describe what work should be done in each.

A8. *The "safety zones" are the hot or contamination zone, the warm or control zone, and the cold or safe zone. In the hot zone, which is immediately adjacent to the accident site and where contamination* *can still occur, perform actual rescue, initial (gross) decontamination, and necessary treatment for life-threatening conditions. In the warm zone, which is immediately adjacent to the hot zone, continue to wear appropriate protective gear. Administer life-saving emergency care to the patient. When the patient is stabilized, perform complete decontamination. Perform a rapid trauma assessment. In the cold zone, shed all contaminated protective gear. Take vital signs and SAMPLE history, complete emergency care of the patient, and prepare for transport. (pp. 1131–1132)*

Q9. List the information that is necessary for trained personnel to decide on a course of action at a hazardous materials emergency.

A9. *Information necessary for trained personnel to decide on a course of action includes nature of the problem, identification of the hazardous materials, the kind and condition of containers, existing weather conditions, whether or not there is presence of fire, time that has elapsed since the emergency occurred, what already has been done by people at the scene, the number of victims, and the potential danger to more people. (pp. 1129–1131)*

Q10. Name the required elements of an incident management plan.

A10. *The required elements of an incident management plan are one command officer who is responsible for all rescue decisions, a clear chain of command, one established system of communications, and predesignated receiving facilities. (p. 1129)*

CRITICAL THINKING

Assess students' ability to respond to real-life emergency situations by discussing the Critical Thinking questions on page 1139 in the textbook.

Q1. What would be your first action?

A1. *The first immediate action would be to leave the scene to avoid any contact with the potentially hazardous substance.*

Q2. How would you manage the scene?

A2. *The area should be cleared of all personnel until the HAZMAT crew is able to determine scene safety. No one should be allowed to enter the scene unless specifically trained to do so. There should be no attempts at a patient rescue until trained personnel are available.*

Q3. Would you call for any additional resources? If so, who?

A3. *The EMTs should immediately call for the fire department or a hazardous materials response team.*

Q4. When would you begin your emergency care for the patient?

A4. *Care for this patient would begin once the HAZMAT team has either determined that there is no danger in entering the area or once they have removed the patient from the toxic environment and the patient has been appropriately decontaminated.*

GUEST LECTURER (OPTIONAL)

Arrange to have a member of a local or regional hazardous materials team visit the class to describe some of the situations that EMT might face during a hazmat emergency. The guest should be prepared to answer student questions about hazmat operations and dangers.

ASSIGNMENTS

Assign students to read Chapter 41, "Multiple-Casualty Incidents," before the next class. Also ask them to complete Chapter 40 of the Workbook.

EVALUATION

Chapter Quiz Distribute copies of the Chapter Quiz provided in Handout 40-2 to evaluate student understanding of this chapter. Remind students not to refer to their textbooks or notes while taking the quiz.

Test Manager You may wish to create a custom-tailored test using Prentice Hall *TestGen for Prehospital Emergency Care, Eighth Edition* to evaluate student understanding of this chapter.

Online Test Preparation (for students and instructors) Additional test preparation is available through *EMT Achieve: Basic Test Preparation* at http://www.prenhall.com/EMTAchieve. Instructors can also monitor student mastery online.

REINFORCEMENT

Handouts If classroom discussions or performance on the quiz indicates that some students have not fully mastered the chapter content, you may wish to assign some or all of the Reinforcement Handouts for this chapter.

TECH EXTRAS

Brady Skills Series EMT-B Videos/CD Have your students watch the skills come to life on either VHS or CD-ROM.

PowerPoint Presentation (for instructors) The PowerPoint material developed for this chapter offers useful reinforcement of chapter content.

Student CD A wide variety of material on this CD-ROM will reinforce and also expand student knowledge and skills.

Companion Website (for students) Additional review quizzes and links to EMS resources will contribute to further reinforcement of this chapter. Please visit http://www.prenhall.com/mistovich.

Reading/Reference
Textbook, pp. 1140–1159

Workbook
Chapter 40 Activities

Chapter Quiz
Handout 40-2

TestGen
Chapter 40 Test

Online Test Preparation
Send your students to
http://www.prenhall.com/
EMTAchieve

Handouts 40-3 to 40-6
Reinforcement Activities

**Brady Skills Series
EMT-B Videos/CD**
Visual Reinforcement

**PowerPoint
Presentation**
Chapter 40

Student CD
Chapter 40

Companion Website
http://www.prenhall.com/
mistovich

OBJECTIVES CHECKLIST

Cognitive		Date Mastered
7-3.1	Explain the EMT-Basic's role during a call involving hazardous materials.	
7-3.2	Describe what the EMT-Basic should do if there is reason to believe that there is a hazard at the scene.	
7-3.3	Describe the actions that an EMT-Basic should take to ensure bystander safety.	
7-3.4	State the role the EMT-Basic should perform until appropriately trained personnel arrive at the scene of a hazardous materials situation.	
7-3.5	Break down the steps to approaching a hazardous situation.	
7-3.6	Discuss the various environmental hazards that affect EMS.	
7-3.11	Describe basic concepts of incident management.	
7-3.12	Explain the methods for preventing contamination of self, equipment, and facilities.	

CHAPTER 40 QUIZ

Write the letter of the best answer in the space provided.

_____ **1.** According to the Department of Transportation, a hazardous material is a substance that
  A. can explode.
  B. can cause death.
  C. poses a threat or unreasonable risk to health, safety, and property if not properly controlled.
  D. does not meet OSHA guidelines for workplace and product safety.

_____ **2.** According to OSHA, EMS responders likely to witness or discover a hazardous materials emergency should have what minimum level of training?
  A. Hazardous Materials Specialist   **C.** Hazardous Materials Technician
  B. First Responder Operations   **D.** First Responder Awareness

_____ **3.** The level of training required of rescuers who actually plug, patch, or stop the release of a hazardous material is
  A. Hazardous Materials Specialist.   **C.** Hazardous Materials Technician.
  B. First Responder Operations.   **D.** First Responder Awareness.

_____ **4.** Normal triage, stabilization, and treatment are performed in the _____ zone.
  A. warm   **C.** cold
  B. control   **D.** hot

_____ **5.** Initial (gross) patient decontamination should be carried out in the _____ zone.
  A. warm   **C.** cold
  B. hot   **D.** triage

_____ **6.** The first and primary concern of the EMT at a hazardous materials incident is for
  A. his or her own personal safety.   **C.** the safety of the public.
  B. the safety of the hazmat team.   **D.** the patient's medical needs.

_____ **7.** The blue color of the NFPA 704 system indicates a _____ hazard.
  A. chemical   **C.** heath
  B. fire   **D.** reactivity

_____ **8.** The U.S. Department of Transportation requires that vehicles carrying hazardous materials display
  A. specific hazard labels or placards.   **C.** red and yellow flashers.
  B. red warning flags.   **D.** a CHEMTREC number.

_____ **9.** A public service division of the Chemical Manufacturer's Association that can answer any questions and advise you on how to handle any emergency involving hazardous materials is called:
  A. CHEMTREC.   **C.** OSHA.
  B. CHEMSAT.   **D.** MSDS.

_____10. A U.S. DOT publication that lists more than a thousand hazardous materials, each with an identification number cross-referenced to complete emergency instructions, is
A. *OSHA Emergency Response Standards.*
B. NFPA Standard #473.
C. Material Safety Data Sheets.
D. *Emergency Response Guidebook.*

_____11. The first course of action that should be taken by the EMT at a hazardous materials incident is
A. securing the scene.
B. limiting exposure of rescuers.
C. beginning rescue of victims.
D. contacting an ALS team.

_____12. The most essential part of hazardous materials rescue operations is
A. the training of EMTs.
B. use of SCBA.
C. effective preincident planning.
D. use of specialized hazmat suits

_____13. Receiving facilities handling patients from hazardous materials incidents should be
A. the closest to the scene.
B. designated in the incident plan.
C. OSHA approved.
D. specialized chemical centers.

_____14. Life-saving emergency care, such as airway management and immobilization, should be performed in the _____ zone.
A. hot
B. containment
C. warm
D. cold

_____15. Radiation contamination occurs when the patient comes into direct contact with radioactive
A. gases.
B. particles.
C. liquids.
D. all of these.

IN THE FIELD

Read the following real-life situation. Then consult the Material Safety Data Sheet on the next page to help you answer the following questions.

Returning to the station after several back-to-back calls, you and your partner, Juan, start to clean up. You begin on the inside of the ambulance, while Juan agrees to wash down the backboards. The backboards are particularly dirty after a couple of tough extrication calls. There is dried blood as well as grease and antifreeze on the boards.

Juan takes the backboards into the dirty utility room off the main bays. It has a deep sink, as well as brushes and cleaners to clean equipment. He reviews the cleaning procedures for washing down a dirty backboard. He then dons a pair of heavy gloves, a plastic gown, and a pair of goggles.

Juan is having a tough time cleaning off the grease from the board, so he decides to mix a little bleach into the ammonia and soapy water mixture he was using. Smelling the mixture, he thinks to himself, "Boy is that strong!" He then continues to scrub the boards.

Soon he realizes that his eyes are watering and burning. But he wants to get the job done, so he keeps on working. Pretty soon he is breathing heavily, more heavily than he should be considering how much work he is doing. He feels a funny tightness in his chest and gets a little apprehensive.

Having completed washing down the inside of the rig, you go see if you can help Juan out. One look tells you that something is wrong with Juan. Juan tells you he is having trouble breathing. You call out for the supervisor and go to work helping your partner.

1. What caused Juan's problem?

2. What health hazards may be present on the scene?

3. What first aid would you provide in this case?

4. Do you need to wear any special protection?

5. Who could you call for more instructions on first aid?

THE Clorox Company
7200 Johnson Drive
Pleasanton, California 94566
Tel. (415) 847-6100

Material Safety Data Sheets

Health	2+
Flammability	0
Reactivity	1
Personal Protection	B

I – CHEMICAL IDENTIFICATION

Name	regular Clorox Bleach	CAS No.	N/A
Description	clear, light yellow liquid with chlorine odor	RTECs No.	N/A

Other Designations	Manufacturer	Emergency Procedure
EPA Reg. No. 5813-1 Sodium hypochlorite solution Liquid chlorine bleach Clorox Liquid Bleach	The Clorox Company 1221 Broadway Oakland, CA 94612	• Notify your supervisor • Call your local poison control center OR • Rocky Mountain Poison Center (303)573-1014

II – HEALTH HAZARD DATA

• Causes severe but temporary eye injury. May irritate skin. May cause nausea and vomiting if ingested. Exposure to vapor or mist may irritate nose, throat and lungs. The following medical conditions may be aggravated by exposure to high concentrations of vapor or mist: heart conditions or chronic respiratory problems such as asthma, chronic bronchitis or obstructive lung disease. Under normal consumer use conditions the likelihood of any adverse health effects are low. FIRST AID: EYE CONTACT: Immediately flush eyes with plenty of water. If irritation persists, see a doctor. SKIN CONTACT: Remove contaminated clothing. Wash area with water. INGESTION: Drink a glassful of water and call a physician. INHALATION: If breathing problems develop remove to fresh air.

III – HAZARDOUS INGREDIENTS

Ingredients	Concentration	Worker Exposure Limit
Sodium hypochlorite CAS# 7681-52-9	5.25%	not established

None of the ingredients in this product are on the IARC, NTP or OSHA carcinogen list. Occasional clinical reports suggest a low potential for sensitization upon exaggerated exposure to sodium hypochlorite if skin damage (e.g., irritation) occurs during exposure. Routine clinical tests conducted on intact skin with Clorox Liquid Bleach found no sensitization in the test subjects.

IV – SPECIAL PROTECTION INFORMATION

Hygienic Practices: Wear safety glasses. With repeated or prolonged use, wear gloves.

Engineering Controls: Use general ventilation to minimize exposure to vapor or mist.

Work Practices: Avoid eye and skin contact and inhalation of vapor or mist.

V – SPECIAL PRECAUTIONS

Keep out of reach of children. Do not get in eyes or on skin. Wash thoroughly with soap and water after handling. Do not mix with other household chemicals such as toilet bowl cleaners, rust removers, vinegar, acid or ammonia containing products. Store in a cool, dry place. Do not reuse empty container; rinse container and put in trash container.

VI – SPILL OR LEAK PROCEDURES

Small quantities of less than 5 gallons may be flushed down drain. For larger quantities wipe up with an absorbent material or mop and dispose of in accordance with local, state and federal regulations. Dilute with water to minimize oxidizing effect on spilled surface.

VII – REACTIVITY DATA

Stable under normal use and storage conditions. Strong oxidizing agent. Reacts with other household chemicals such as toilet bowl cleaners, rust removers, vinegar, acids or ammonia containing products to produce hazardous gases, such as chlorine and other chlorinated species. Prolonged contact with metal may cause pitting or discoloration.

VIII – FIRE AND EXPLOSION DATA

Not flammable or explosive. In a fire, cool containers to prevent rupture and release of sodium chlorate.

IX – PHYSICAL DATA

Boiling point...................................212°F/100°C (decomposes)
Specific Gravity (H_2O = 1).............1.085
Solubility in Water..........................complete
pH..11.4

CHAPTER 40 REVIEW

Write the word or words that best complete each sentence in the space provided.

1. Any substance that in any quantity poses a threat or an unreasonable risk to health, safety, and property if not properly controlled is considered a(n) _____

   _____.

2. The EMT should never attempt a hazardous materials rescue unless he or she has had the necessary

   _____ _____.

3. Regulations developed by the federal agencies _____ and

   _____ spell out requirements for hazmat training.

4. All emergency responders likely to witness or discover a hazardous materials emergency must be minimally trained to the _____ _____

   _____ level.

5. Generally, in the preplanning of incident management, you should prepare for the

   _____ _____ scenario.

6. There should be a clear chain of command from each rescuer to the _____

   _____.

7. The only work done in the _____ _____ is actual rescue, initial decontamination, and treatment for life-threatening conditions by specially trained personnel who are wearing appropriate protective clothing.

8. Before entering the _____ _____ from the warm zone, rescuers should shed all contaminated protective gear and patients should be as fully decontaminated as possible.

9. The area immediately adjacent to the contamination zone is called the

   _____ _____.

10. The 24-hour emergency chemical information and assistance center reachable at 800-424-9300 is

    _____.

11. The NFPA 704 Hazard Identification System identifies potential danger with the use of numbers ranging from _____ to _____.

12. _____ occurs when the patient is in the presence of radioactive material without any of the radioactive material actually touching his or her clothing or body.

13. _____ occurs when the patient has come into direct contact with the source of radioactivity or with radioactive gases, liquids, or particles.

14. A(n) _____ _____

   _____ is an expert specifically trained under federal government provisions to handle radiation-related accidents.

15. _____ is the critical factor in managing radiation emergencies.

Analyzing a Hazmat Incident

Review the following situation.

It's an early Thursday morning when you are dispatched to a reported overturned truck in the Guilderland Industrial Park near the sewage treatment plant. Upon arrival, you can clearly see smoke and vapors coming from an overturned tank truck.

You stay back and view the scene with your binoculars from the cab of the ambulance. On the side of the overturned truck, you can read the UN identification placard number 1017.

Review your hazardous materials information (accompanying pages) and your map and answer the following questions. You should also know that the winds are from the east at 5–10 mph. The top of the map is north and the scale is printed on the map.

1. What material does the tank truck contain?

2. This is a potentially large spill of material that is a highlighted substance. How large an isolation zone should be set up at first? How should that zone be changed later?

3. What basic public safety guidelines apply in this situation?

4. Will evacuation be necessary? What are areas of major concern in this incident?

ID No.	Guide No.	Name of Material
1014	122	Oxygen and Carbon dioxide mixture
1014	122	Oxygen and Carbon dioxide mixture, compressed
1015	126	Carbon dioxide and Nitrous oxide mixture
1015	126	Nitrous oxide and Carbon dioxide mixture
1016	119	Carbon monoxide
1016	119	Carbon monoxide, compressed
1017	124	Chlorine
1018	126	Chlorodifluoromethane
1018	126	Refrigerant gas R-22
1020	126	Chloropentafluoroethane
1020	126	Refrigerant gas R-115
1021	126	1-Chloro-1,2,2,2-tetraflourethane
1021	126	Chlorotetrafluoroethane
1021	126	Refrigerant gas R-124
1022	126	Chlorotrifluoromethane
1022	126	Refrigerant gas R-13
1023	119	Coal gas
1023	119	Coal gas, compressed
1026	119	Cyanogen
1026	119	Cyanogen, liquefied
1026	119	Cyanogen gas
1027	115	Cyclopropane
1027	115	Cyclopropane, liquefied
1028	126	Dichlorodifluoromethane
1028	126	Refrigerant gas R-12
1029	126	Dichlorofluoromethane
1029	126	Refrigerant gas R-21
1030	115	1, 1-Difluoroethane
1030	115	Difluoroethane
1030	115	Refrigerant gas R-152a
1032	118	Dimethylamine, anhydrous
1033	115	Dimethyl ether
1035	115	Ethane
1035	115	Ethane, compressed
1036	118	Ethylamine
1037	115	Ethyl chloride
1038	115	Ethylene, refrigerated liquid (cryogenic liquid)
1039	115	Ethyl methyl ether
1039	115	Methyl ethyl ether
1040	119	Ethylene oxide
1040	119	Ethylene oxide with Nitrogen
1041	115	Carbon dioxide and Ethylene oxide mixture, with more than 9% but not more than 87% Ethylene oxide
1041	115	Carbon dioxide and Ethylene oxide mixture, with more than 6% Ethylene oxide
1041	115	Ethylene oxide and Carbon dioxide mixture, with more than 9% but not more than 87% Ethylene oxide
1041	115	Ethylene oxide and Carbon dioxide mixtures, with more than 6% Ethylene oxide
1043	125	Fertilizer, ammoniating solution, with free Ammonia
1044	126	Fire extinguishers with compressed gas
1044	126	Fire extinguishers with liquefied gas
1045	124	Fluorine
1045	124	Fluorine, compressed
1046	121	Helium
1046	121	Helium, compressed
1048	125	Hydrogen bromide, anhydrous
1049	115	Hydrogen
1049	115	Hydrogen, compressed
1050	125	Hydrogen chloride, anhydrous
1051	117	Hydrocyanic acid, aqueous solutions, with more than 20% Hydrogen cyanide
1051	117	Hydrocyanic acid, liquefied
1051	117	Hydrogen cyanide, anhydrous, stabilized
1051	117	Hydrogen cyanide, stabilized
1052	125	Hydrogen fluoride, anhydrous
1053	117	Hydrogen sulfide
1053	117	Hydrogen sulfide, liquefied
1053	117	Hydrogen sulphide
1053	117	Hydrogen sulphide, liquefied
1055	115	Isobutylene
1056	121	Krypton
1056	121	Krypton, compressed
1057	115	Cigarette lighter, with flammable gas
1057	115	Flammable gas in lighter for cigars, cigarettes, etc.
1057	115	Lighter refills (cigarettes) (flammable gas)
1057	115	Lighters (cigarettes) (flammable gas)
1058	121	Liquefied gas (nonflammable)
1058	121	Liquefied gases, non-flammable, charged with Nitrogen, Carbon dioxide or Air
1060	116P	Methylacetylene and Propadiene mixture, stabilized
1060	116P	Propadiene and Methylacetylene mixture, stabilized
1061	118	Methylamine, anhydrous
1062	123	Methyl bromide
1063	115	Methyl chloride
1063	115	Refrigerant gas R-40
1064	117	Methyl mercaptan
1065	121	Neon
1065	121	Neon, compressed
1066	121	Nitrogen
1066	121	Nitrogen, compressed
1067	124	Dinitrogen tetroxide
1067	124	Dinitrogen tetroxide, liquefied
1067	124	Nitrogen dioxide
1067	124	Nitrogen dioxide, liquefied
1067	124	Nitrogen peroxide, liquid
1067	124	Nitrogen tetroxide, liquid
1067	124	Nitrogen tetroxide, liquefied
1069	125	Nitrosyl chloride
1070	122	Nitrous oxide
1070	122	Nitrous oxide, compressed
1071	119	Oil gas
1071	119	Oil gas, compressed
1072	122	Oxygen
1072	122	Oxygen, compressed
1073	122	Oxygen, refrigerated liquid (cryogeneic liquid)
1075	115	Butane
1075	115	Butane mixture
1075	115	Butylene
1075	115	Isobutane
1075	115	Isobutane mixture
1075	115	Isobutylene
1075	115	Liquefied petroleum gas
1075	115	LPG
1075	115	Petroleum gases, liquefied

GUIDE 124

NAERG96 GASES-TOXIC AND/OR CORROSIVE-OXIDIZING

EMERGENCY RESPONSE

FIRE

Small Fires: Water only; no dry chemical, CO₂ or Halon®.

- Contain fire and let burn. If fire must be fought, water spray or fog is recommended.
- Do not get water inside containers.
- Move containers from fire area if you can do it without risk.
- Damaged cylinders should be handled only by specialists.

Fire involving Tanks

- Fight fire from maximum distance or use unmanned hose holders or monitor nozzles.
- Cool containers with flooding quantities of water well after fire is out.
- Do not direct water at source of leak or safety devices; icing may occur.
- Withdraw immediately in case of rising sound from venting safety devices or discoloration of tank.
- ALWAYS stay away from the ends of tanks.
- For massive fire, use unmanned hose holders or monitor nozzles; if this is impossible, withdraw from area and let fire burn.

SPILL OR LEAK

- Fully encapsulating, vapor protective clothing should be worn for spills and leaks with no fire.
- Do not touch or walk through spilled material.
- Keep combustibles (wood, paper, oil, etc.) away from spilled material.
- Stop leak if you can do it without risk.
- Use water spray to reduce vapors or direct vapor cloud drift.
- Do not direct water at spill or source of leak.
- If possible, turn leaking containers so that gas escapes rather than liquid.
- Prevent entry into waterways, sewers, basements or combined areas.
- Isolate area until gas has dispersed.
- Ventilate the area.

FIRST AID

- Move victim to fresh air. • Call emergency medical care.
- Apply artificial respiration if victim is not breathing.
- Do not use mouth-to-mouth method if victim ingested or inhaled the substance; induce artificial respiration with the aid of a pocket mask equipped with a one-way valve or other proper respiratory medical device.
- Administer oxygen if breathing is difficult.
- Clothing frozen to the skin should be thawed before being removed.
- Remove and isolate contaminated clothing and shoes.
- In case of contact with substance, immediately flush skin or eyes with running water for at least 20 minutes.
- Keep victim warm and quiet. • Keep victim under observation.
- Effects of contact or inhalation may be delayed.
- Ensure that medical personnel are aware of the material(s) involved, and take precautions to protect themselves.

GUIDE 124

NAERG96 GASES-TOXIC AND/OR CORROSIVE-OXIDIZING

POTENTIAL HAZARDS

HEALTH

- **TOXIC; may be fatal if inhaled or absorbed through skin.**
- Fire will produce irritating, corrosive and/or toxic gases.
- Contact with gas or liquefied gas may cause burns, severe injury and/or frostbite.
- Runoff from fire control may cause pollution.

FIRE OR EXPLOSION

- Substance does not burn but will support combustion.
- Vapors from liquefied gas are initially heavier than air spread along ground.
- These are strong oxidizers and will react vigorously or explosively with many materials including fuels.
- May ignite combustibles (wood, paper, oil, clothing, etc.).
- Some will react violently with air, moist air and/or water.
- Containers may explode when heated.
- Ruptured cylinders may rocket.

PUBLIC SAFETY

- **CALL Emergency Response Telephone Number on Shipping Paper first. If Shipping Paper not available or no answer, refer to appropriate telephone number listed on the inside back cover.**
- Isolate spill or leak area immediately for at least 100 to 200 meters (330 to 660 feet) in all directions.
- Keep unauthorized personnel away.
- Stay upwind.
- Many gases are heavier than air and will spread along ground and collect in low or confined areas (sewers, basements, tanks).
- Keep out of low areas.
- Ventilate closed spaces before entering.

PROTECTIVE CLOTHING

- Wear positive pressure self-contained breathing apparatus (SCBA).
- Wear chemical protective clothing which is specifically recommended by the manufacturer. It may provide little or no thermal protection.
- Structural firefighters' protective clothing is recommended for fire situations ONLY; it is not effective in spill situations.

EVACUATION

Spill

- See the Table on Initial Isolation and Protective Action Distances for highlighted substances. For non-highlighted substance, increase, in the downwind direction, as necessary, the isolation distance under "PUBLIC SAFETY."

Fire

- If tank, rail car or tank truck is involved in a fire, ISOLATE for 800 meters (1/2 mile) in all directions; also, consider initial evacuation for 800 meters (1/2 mile) in all directions.

TABLE OF INITIAL ISOLATION AND PROTECTIVE ACTION DISTANCES

ID No.	NAME OF MATERIAL	First ISOLATE in all Directions Meters	(Feet)	Then PROTECT persons Downwind during– DAY Kilometers (Miles)		NIGHT Kilometers (Miles)		First ISOLATE in all Directions Meters	(Feet)	Then PROTECT persons Downwind during– DAY Kilometers (Miles)		NIGHT Kilometers (Miles)	
		SMALL SPILLS (From a small pagage or small leak from a large package)						LARGE SPILLS (From a large package or from many small packages)					
1005 1005	Ammonia, anhydrous Ammonia, anhydrous, liquefied	30 m	(100 ft)	0.2 km	(0.1 mi)	0.3 km	(0.2 mi)	95 m	(300 ft)	0.3 km	(0.2 mi)	0.8 km	(0.5 mi)
1005	Ammonia solution, with more than 50% Ammonia	30 m	(100 ft)	0.2 km	(0.1 mi)	0.2 km	(0.1 mi)	60 m	(200 ft)	0.2 km	(0.1 mi)	0.3 km	(0.2 mi)
1005 1005	Anhydrous ammonia Anhydrous ammonia liquefied	30 m	(100 ft)	0.2 km	(0.1 mi)	0.3 km	(0.2 mi)	95 m	(300 ft)	0.3 km	(0.2 mi)	0.8 km	(0.5 mi)
1008 1008	Boron trifiuoride Boron trifluoride, compressed	60 m	(200 ft)	0.2 km	(0.1 mi)	0.6 km	(0.4 mi)	185 m	(600 ft)	0.6 km	(0.4 mi)	2.4 km	(1.5 mi)
1016 1016	Carbon monoxide Carbon monoxide, compressed	30 m	(100 ft)	0.2 km	(0.1 mi)	0.2 km	(0.1 mi)	95 m	(300 ft)	0.2 km	(0.1 mi)	0.6 km	(0.4 mi)
1017	Chlorine	60 m	(200 ft)	0.3 km	(0.2 mi)	0.8 km	(0.5 mi)	185 m	(600 ft)	0.8 km	(0.5 mi)	3.1 km	(1.9 mi)
1023 1023	Coal gas Coal gas, compressed	30 m	(100 ft)	0.2 km	(0.1 mi)	0.2 km	(0.1 mi)	30 m	(100 ft)	0.3 km	(0.2 mi)	0.8 km	(0.5 mi)
1026 1026 1026	Cyanogen Cyanogen, liquefied Cyanogen gas	60 m	(200 ft)	0.3 km	(0.2 mi)	1.0 km	(0.6 mi)	215 m	(700 ft)	0.8 km	(0.5 mi)	3.5 km	(2.2 mi)
1040 1040	Ethylene oxide Ethylene oxide with Nitrogen	60 m	(200 ft)	0.2 km	(0.1 mi)	0.3 km	(0.2 mi)	125 m	(400 ft)	0.3 km	(0.2 mi)	1.0 km	(0.6 mi)
1045 1045	Fluorine Fluorine compressed	60 m	(200 ft)	0.2 km	(0.1 mi)	0.8 km	(0.5 mi)	185 m	(600 ft)	0.6 km	(0.4 mi)	2.7 km	(1.7 mi)
1048	Hydrogen bromide, anhydrous	60 m	(200 ft)	0.2 km	(0.1 mi)	0.3 km	(0.2 mi)	125 m	(400 ft)	0.3 km	(0.2 mi)	1.1 km	(0.7 mi)
1050	Hydrogen chloride, anhydrous	60 m	(200 ft)	0.2 km	(0.1 mi)	0.5 km	(0.3 mi)	155 m	(500 ft)	0.5 km	(0.3 mi)	1.8 km	(1.1 mi)
1051 1051 1051 1051	Hydrocyanic acid, aqueous solutions, with more than 20% Hydrogen cyanide Hydrocyanic acid, liquefied Hydrogen cyanide, anhydrous, stabilized Hydrogen cyanide stabilized	60 m	(200 ft)	0.2 km	(0.1 mi)	0.8 km	(0.5 mi)	185 m	(600 ft)	0.6 km	(0.4 mi)	2.7 km	(1.7 mi)
1052	Hydrogen fluoride, anhydrous	60 m	(200 ft)	0.2 km	(0.1 mi)	0.6 km	(0.4 mi)	155 m	(500 ft)	0.5 km	(0.3 mi)	2.3 km	(1.4 mi)
1053 1053 1053 1053	Hydrogen sulfide Hydrogen sulfide, liquefied Hydrogen sulphide Hydrogen sulphide, liquefied	60 m	(200 ft)	0.2 km	(0.1 mi)	0.5 km	(0.3 mi)	125 m	(400 ft)	0.3 km	(0.2 mi)	1.4 km	(0.9 mi)
1062	Methyl bromide	30 m	(100 ft)	0.2 km	(0.1 mi)	0.3 km	(0.2 mi)	95 m	(300 ft)	0.2 km	(0.1 mi)	0.6 km	(0.4 mi)
1064	Methyl mercaptan	60 m	(200 ft)	0.2 km	(0.1 mi)	0.5 km	(0.3 mi)	125 m	(400 ft)	0.3 km	(0.2 mi)	1.3 km	(0.8 mi)
1067 1067 1067 1067 1067 1067	Dinitrogen tetroxide Dinitrogen tetroxide, liquefied Nitrogen dioxide Nitrogen dioxide, liquefied Nitrogen peroxide, liquid Nitrogen tetroxide, liquid	60 m	(200 ft)	0.2 km	(0.1 mi)	0.6 km	(0.4 mi)	155 m	(500 ft)	0.5 km	(0.3 mi)	2.1 km	(1.3 mi)
1069	Nitrosyl chloride	60 m	(200 ft)	0.3 km	(0.2 mi)	1.0 km	(0.6 mi)	185 m	(600 ft)	0.8 km	(0.5 mi)	3.2 km	(2.0 mi)
1071 1071	Oil gas Oil gas, compressed	30 m	(100 ft)	0.2 km	(0.1 mi)	0.2 km	(0.1 mi)	30 m	(100 ft)	0.3 km	(0.2 mi)	0.8 km	(0.5 mi)
1076 1076	Diphosgene (when "Inhalation Hazard" is on a package or shipping paper) Phosgene	125 m	(400 ft)	0.6 km	(0.4 mi)	2.7 km	(1.7 mi)	335 m	(1100 ft)	2.3 km	(1.4 mi)	10.0 km	(6.2 mi)
1079 1079 1079 1079	Sulfur dioxide Sulfur dioxide, liquefied Sulphur dioxide Sulphur dioxide, liquefied	125 m	(400 ft)	0.8 km	(0.5 mi)	3.4 km	(2.1 mi)	365 m	(1200 ft)	2.7 km	(1.7 mi)	11.0+ km	(7.0+ mi)

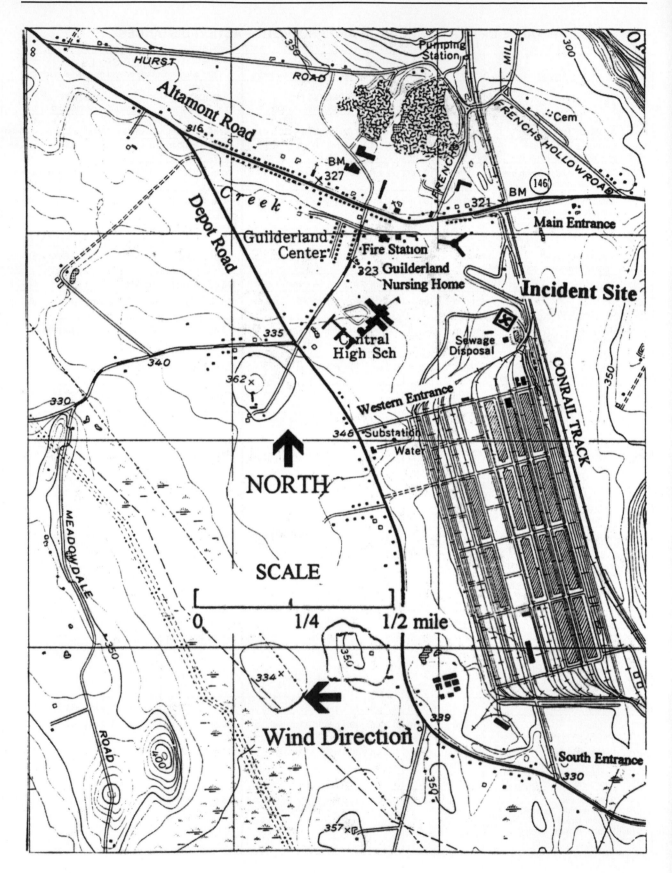

HAZARDOUS MATERIALS: LISTING

1. List the three routes of potential exposure to oxidizers and organic peroxides.

2. List the colors included in the NFPA 704 system and identify the hazard each identifies.

3. List the levels of training identified by the EPA and OSHA in "29 CFR 1910.120—Hazardous Waste Operations and Emergency Response Standards."

4. List the three general priorities for hazardous materials emergencies.

LECTURE MASTER 40

Hazardous Materials Emergencies

Identifying Hazardous Materials

Definition

Placards and Shipping Papers

Clues to Hazardous Materials Emergencies

Resources

- *Emergency Response Guidebook*
- CHEMTREC
- Chemtrel

Training

- First Responder Awareness
- First Responder Operations
- Hazardous Materials Technician
- Hazardous Materials Specialist

Guidelines for Hazardous Materials Rescues

General Rules

Incident Management

Safety Zones

- Hot zone
- Warm zone
- Cold zone

Emergency Procedures

Radiation Emergencies
Exposure and Contamination
Guidelines and Procedures
Problems Caused by Radiation
Protection from Radiation
Weapons of Mass Destruction

CHAPTER 40 ANSWER KEY

HANDOUT 40-2: Chapter 40 Quiz

1. C	**5.** B	**9.** A	**13.** B
2. D	**6.** A	**10.** D	**14.** C
3. C	**7.** C	**11.** A	**15.** D
4. C	**8.** A	**12.** C	

HANDOUT 40-3: In the Field

1. Juan probably created a chlorine gas or other chlorinated species by mixing the bleach and ammonia.
2. The resulting product is severely irritating to the skin and eyes on contact. If inhaled, it may induce asthma-like symptoms including bronchospasm.
3. Move him to fresh air immediately. Call poison control.
4. At a minimum, wear safety glasses and gloves.
5. Either your regional local poison control center or the Rocky Mountain Poison Center.

HANDOUT 40-4: Chapter 40 Review

1. hazardous material
2. specialized training
3. OSHA, EPA
4. First Responder Awareness
5. worst possible
6. command officer
7. hot zone
8. cold zone
9. warm zone

10. CHEMTREC
11. 0, 4
12. Exposure
13. Contamination
14. Radiation Safety Officer (RSO)
15. Time

HANDOUT 40-5: Analyzing a Hazmat Incident

1. Chlorine
2. Initially isolate the spill 600 feet in all directions. Later expand the isolation area downwind to 0.5 miles.
3. Keep unauthorized personnel away. Stay upwind. Keep out of low areas. Ventilate any closed spaces before entering them.
4. Yes. The major area of immediate concern is the school. But if the winds shift slightly, the fire station and nursing home could be threatened.

HANDOUT 40-6: Hazardous Materials: Listing

1. Skin and eyes; inhalation; ingestion
2. Red—flammability; Yellow—reactivity; Blue—health hazard; White—special hazards
3. First Responder Awareness; First Responder Operations; Hazardous Materials Technician; Hazardous Materials Specialist
4. Protect the safety of all rescuers and victims; provide patient care; decontaminate clothing, equipment, and the vehicle.

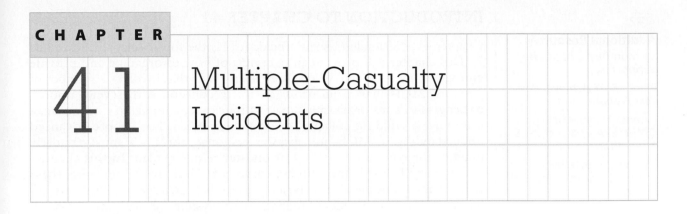

CHAPTER

41 Multiple-Casualty Incidents

This chapter covers portions of Lesson 7-3 and 7-4 of the U.S. Department of Transportation's EMT-Basic National Standard Curriculum.

OBJECTIVES

Numbered objectives are from the U.S. Department of Transportation's EMT-Basic National Standard Curriculum. Asterisked objectives, if any, pertain to material that is supplemental to the DOT curriculum. Page numbers refer to pages in the textbook.

Cognitive

7-3.7	Describe the criteria for a multiple-casualty situation. (p. 1141)
7-3.8	Evaluate the role of the EMT-Basic in the multiple-casualty situation. (pp. 1141–1145)
7-3.9	Summarize the components of basic triage. (pp. 1145–1150)
7-3.10	Define the role of the EMT-Basic in a disaster operation. (p. 1154–1155)
7-3.11	Describe basic concepts of incident management. (pp. 1142–1145)
7-3.13	Review the local mass-casualty incident plan. (pp. 1141–1145)
*	Outline the ways to get help in a multiple-casualty incident. (pp. 1142, 1155–1156)
*	Describe various approaches for reducing rescue personnel stress during an MCI or disaster. (pp. 1153–1154)

Psychomotor

7-3.16	Given a scenario of a mass-casualty incident, perform triage.

Additional objectives from DOT Lesson 7-3 are addressed in Chapter 40, "Hazardous Materials Emergencies."

REVIEW

In the last chapter, "Hazardous Materials Emergencies," students learned that hazardous materials spills and other accidents are common problems, the exact extent of which is unknown. The EMT is not required to deal with hazardous materials, which takes specialized training. It is more important for the EMT to recognize that a hazardous materials emergency exists and react appropriately in such a situation. Distribute the quizzes from the last class. Go over each question on the quiz and handle any concerns students may have about the answers.

Total Teaching Time
180 minutes

Resources Needed

- Scored Chapter 40 Quizzes

- Enough jump kits (including triage tags), oxygen equipment, portable suction units, and stretcher for every other student

- Two two-way radios or cellular phones

- Firefighter to serve as incident commander during the role-play exercise

- Enough patients to challenge but not overwhelm the EMT students. (A ratio of 0.50 to 0.75 patients per student is recommended.) A natural gas explosion has occurred. Each patient should be assigned injuries, which should range across all four triage categories. You may wish to use moulage on patients to appear realistic.

- Have a BLS ambulance close to the scene that can be used as a resource for additional supplies as needed.

INTRODUCTION TO CHAPTER 41

Chapter 41, "Multiple-Casualty Incidents," is the fourth chapter in Module 7. This chapter will provide an overview of how to organize and provide emergency medical care when there is an event that involves a number of patients. MCIs may range from a vehicle collision with several injured passengers to a major disaster such as a hurricane, a flood, an earthquake, a bombing, a building collapse, or an airliner crash. For a more advanced understanding of MCIs and disaster response, the EMT must regularly practice the community's MCI or disaster response plan. In this chapter, students will learn the fundamentals of MCI response, but these fundamentals must necessarily be adapted to their own regions. Students will learn about the incident management system, EMS units, triage, components of a disaster response plan, and—most importantly—how to "get the right patient, to the right hospital, in the right amount of time."

Distribute the Chapter 41 Objectives Checklist, and give students a few minutes to look it over. Then briefly paraphrase the objectives for this lesson in your own words.

LECTURE

The following suggested lecture outline is based on the Department of Transportation's EMT-Basic National Standard Curriculum. In some places, the DOT curriculum has been rearranged or expanded upon so that it is more complete or easier for the student to understand. The page numbers in parentheses refer to pages in the textbook. The parenthetical references in dark, heavy type are to figures, tables, and scans in the textbook.

Note that the concept of Incident Management Systems was introduced in Chapter 40. If you discussed the topic at length in the lecture for that chapter, simply review it now, highlighting links to multiple-casualty incidents. If you discussed it only briefly earlier, present the topic in depth at this time.

MULTIPLE-CASUALTY INCIDENTS

I. Multiple-casualty incidents (MCIs) (pp. 1141–1145)
    A. Multiple-casualty incident (pp. 1141–1142)
        1. Any event that places excessive demands on personnel and equipment; typically involves three or more patients
    B. Key to MCI emergency care is to call for plenty of help early (p. 1142) **(Fig. 41-1, p. 1142)**
    C. Establishing incident management (p. 1142)
        1. Unified command system
            a. EMS, fire service, and law enforcement collaborate to manage incident.
        2. Single command system
            a. One agency manages all emergency response resources.
    D. National Incident Management System (NIMS) (pp. 1142–1145) **(Fig. 41-2, p. 1143)**
        1. Common terminology
            a. Standardization of titles for facilities and positions
            b. Plain English is used for all communications
        2. Common designations are assigned to all organizational resources including personnel, facilities, equipment, and supplies

3. Manageable spans of control
4. Incident facilities are identified by common terminology with specific activities and functions performed at each facility
5. Identify which members of the ICS can be found at each facility
   a. Command post
   b. Staging areas
   c. Base
   d. Camp
   e. Helibase
   f. Helispots
6. Only the facilities needed to manage the incident will be established
7. Distinct titles are used
   a. Only the incident commander is called "commander" **(Figure 41-3, p. 1144)**
   b. Section leaders or heads are called "chiefs."
8. Incident action plans (IAPs) identify the objectives to be accomplished during the incident
   a. IAPs are used to issue assignments, plans, procedures, and protocols
   b. Results of the objectives are documented and reported so that they can be used in further planning.
9. An integrated communications approach is organized so that information can be transferred within the command structure and outside of the command structure
10. Accountability applies at all levels and within all functional areas.
    a. Knowing in advance who is accountable to whom provides an orderly chain of command and makes it easier for responders to check in, regardless of their home agency
    b. Each responder is assigned to only one designated supervisor, the person to whom that responder is accountable
11. Incident Command System sections
    a. Command
    b. Finance/administration
    c. Logistics
    d. Operations
    e. Planning
12. EMS unit responsibilities **(Figs. 41-4, p. 1145 and 41-5, p. 1146)**
    a. Triage unit
    b. Treatment unit
    c. Transport unit
    d. Staging unit
    e. Morgue unit

II. Triage (pp. 1145–1154)
A. Triage unit (pp. 1145–1146)
   1. Place where triage is performed (Triage is a system of sorting patients to determine the order in which they will receive medical care and transportation to definitive care.) **(Fig. 41-6, p. 1147)**
B. Primary and secondary triage (p. 1146)
   1. Primary triage officer

On the Net
Overview of MCIs, from personnel coordination to triage tags. http://www.collegeofparamedics.org/con_ed/2001/mci.htm

    a. Performs initial triage assessments

  2. Secondary triage officer

    a. Tags patients in order of priority

C. Triage systems (pp. 1146–1150)

  1. START (pp. 1146–1147) **(Fig. 41-7, p. 1148)**

    a. Ability to get up and walk (ambulatory)

    b. Respiratory status

    c. Perfusion status

    d. Mental status

  2. JumpSTART (pp. 1148–1150) **(Fig. 41-8, p. 1149)**

    a. Ability to get up and walk (ambulatory)

    b. Respiratory status

    c. Perfusion status

    d. Mental status

D. Initial assessment (pp. 1147–1150)

  1. Airway not open

    a. Open with manual maneuver

  2. Airway open, responsive patient

    a. Move on to next patient

  3. Unresponsive patient

    a. Check for breathing and pulse

  4. No breathing or no pulse

    a. Move on to next patient

  5. Pulse

    a. Check for severe bleeding

  6. Severe bleeding

    a. Apply a pressure dressing and move on to next patient

  7. Continue in this manner, providing only airway management and controlling bleeding as long as there are others still waiting.

  8. If immediate and obvious danger, immediately move patients, regardless of their injuries.

E. Patient tagging (pp. 1150–1151) **(Figs. 41-9, 41-10 and 40-11, pp. 1150–1152)**

  1. Highest priority = red/immediate

  2. Second priority = yellow/delayed

  3. Lowest priority = green/minor

  4. Fourth level = gray or black/deceased

F. Treatment (p. 1151)

  1. Locate treatment unit close to area where ambulances arrive. **(Fig. 41-12, p. 1153)**

  2. Move patients from triage to treatment in order of priority.

  3. Position patients in flagged rows while they await treatment (flags same color as triage tags).

  4. Ensure that each treatment unit has an officer responsible for ongoing assessment.

  5. Set up a morgue in a separate, out-of-sight area.

  6. Remember the key concept: Take shortcuts with non-life-threatening injuries.

  7. Remain in constant communication with transportation unit.

G. Staging and transportation (pp. 1151–1153)

  1. Staging unit

    a. Place where a staging unit officer monitors, inventories, and directs available ambulances to treatment unit at the request of the transportation unit officer **(Fig. 41-13, p. 1154)**

  2. Transportation unit officer

    a. Ensures that ambulances are accessible and that transportation does not occur without the direction of the EMS incident commander

    b. Coordinates patient transportation with triage officer

H. Communications (p. 1153)

    1. Initial oral communication may appear chaotic: tasks may not always be clear and duties may not have been assigned.

    2. Radio communications may face unavailable frequencies ("dead spots") and channel "gridlock."

I. Follow-through (p. 1153)

    1. After all patients have been removed from incident scene, emergency personnel should go to hospital.

    2. Incident commander and an assistant remain at scene to supervise clean-up.

    3. If EMT's services not needed at hospital, prepare the vehicle and equipment for other EMS calls, and update dispatch.

J. Reducing stress (pp. 1153–1154) **(Fig. 41-14, p. 1154)**

    1. Try not to get overwhelmed.

    2. Rest at regular intervals.

    3. Rotate rest periods.

    4. Have a well-designed plan.

    5. Circulate staff among rescue workers to watch for signs of exhaustion and stress.

    6. Make sure that rescue workers are assigned tasks appropriate for their skills.

    7. Provide plenty of nourishing food and beverages.

    8. Encourage workers to talk among themselves, but discourage light-hearted conversation and joking.

    9. Make sure that rescuers have the opportunity to talk to CISD team members or trained counselors after the incident.

III. Disaster management (pp. 1154–1155)

  A. Disaster (p. 1154)

    1. Sudden catastrophic event that overwhelms natural order and causes great loss of property and/or life

  B. Usually a great disparity between casualties and resources (p. 1155)

  C. Natural disasters (p. 1155)

    1. Hurricanes, earthquakes, tornados, etc.

  D. Human-made disasters (p. 1155)

    1. Airline crashes, bombings, explosions, fires, etc.

ENRICHMENT (OPTIONAL)

The following sections contain information that is valuable as background for the EMT but that goes substantially beyond the U.S. Department of Transportation's EMT-Basic National Standard Curriculum.

IV. Requirements of effective disaster assistance (p. 1155)

  A. Preparation of entire community

  B. Careful preplanning

  C. Ability to implement the plan quickly

  D. Application of triage skills

  E. Ability to organize quickly and to utilize fully all emergency personnel

  F. Ability to adapt plan to meet special conditions

On the Net

Lessons learned after 9/11/01. http://www.disasterrelief.org/Disasters/011115wtc lessons/

On the Net

Law Enforcement/EMS response to the MCI at Columbine High School. http://www.911dispatch.com/columbine/managing.html

G. Contingency plan that provides for shelter and transportation of people in an entire area

H. Ability to do greatest good for greatest number

I. Plan that avoids simply relocating the disaster from the scene to the local hospital

V. **Warning and evacuation** (p. 1155)

VI. **Disaster communication systems** (pp. 1155–1156)

A. Establish details of system ahead of time.

B. Appoint only one person at scene who will report to those outside disaster area.

C. Communicator at scene should stay in touch with local hospitals and rescue units.

D. Set up area-wide communications.

E. If area-wide phone service is out, set up central location where people can register.

F. Constantly monitor and communicate road conditions, alternative routes, and closed roads.

G. Constantly monitor and link all hospitals, trauma centers, and clinics in the area.

H. Do not allow en route emergency vehicle operators or EMTs to communicate with the hospital via radio unless an emergency occurs en route.

I. Equip individual rescuers with portable radios if incident is large.

J. Include a recorder or some other device that will allow you to record crucial communications.

VII. **Psychological impact of disasters** (pp. 1156–1157)

A. Assign several rescue workers to gather information and disseminate it to local radio and television stations.

B. Reunite families as soon as possible.

C. If large number of people, group patients with their families and neighbors.

D. Encourage patients to do necessary chores.

E. Provide structure for the emotionally injured and let them know your expectations.

F. Help patients confront the reality of the situation.

G. Don't give false assurances.

H. Reassure those who do not want to accept help that acceptance is not a sign of weakness.

I. Identify high-risk patients.

J. Identify people who are in a unique position to help people in need, and recruit them for psychological emergency care.

K. Arrange follow-up care and support for all involved (including rescuers).

CASE STUDY FOLLOW-UP

Ask a student volunteer to read the Case Study that begins on page 1141 of the textbook. You may wish to use the following questions to engage the students in a discussion of the Case Study Follow-up that begins on page 1157 of the textbook. Provide missing information and clarify ideas as needed.

*Q*1. What role are you assigned by your local MCI plan?

*A*1. *Incident commander.*

Q2. What units do you establish?

A2. *A mobile command unit, an extrication unit, a treatment unit, a transportation unit, a staging unit, a supply unit, and a triage unit.*

Q3. As additional emergency personnel are en route to the raceway, how does your partner conduct the initial triage?

A3. *Using a bullhorn, she directs those patients who are able to walk (Priority 3) to a safe area away from the bleachers. She counts at least ten people who are able to walk away. She knows that, for now, these patients have adequate airways and circulation.*

Q4. What does the treatment officer request of the supply unit officer?

A4. *More blood pressure cuffs, bandages, and oxygen.*

Q5. Who contacts the receiving hospitals?

A5. *The transportation officer, not the EMTs transporting the patients.*

IN REVIEW

Assess students' ability to apply what they have just learned by discussing the Review Questions on page 1159 in the textbook.

Q1. Name the criteria for determining that an emergency is a multiple-casualty incident.

A1. *A multiple-casualty incident is any traumatic or medical incident that places excessive demands on personnel or equipment. Typically, more than three patients are involved. (p. 1141)*

Q2. List the five sections of the incident command system.

A2. *Command*
Finance/Administration
Logistics
Operations
Planning (p. 1144)

Q3. Define the role of the EMT in a multiple-casualty incident or a disaster operation.

A3. *Upon arrival, the EMT should report to the mobile command unit for instructions. If one of the first EMTs on-scene, he or she will probably be asked to perform triage. However, the EMT may also be called upon to provide treatment or assist with moving equipment. (p. 1144)*

Q4. Name the five units of the EMS branch and describe their responsibilities.

A4. • *Triage unit. This unit sorts patients by criticality and assigns priorities for emergency care and transport.*

   • *Treatment unit. Emergency care is provided to patients in this unit. This is done based on the priority assigned to the patient by the triage unit.*

   • *Transport unit. In this unit, patients are moved to ambulances or helicopters for transportation to a medical facility, and communications are organized to notify the receiving medical facilities.*

   • *Staging unit. Ambulances, helicopters, and additional equipment are held in this area until they are assigned to a particular task.*

Sometimes a supply unit is established as part of or separately from the staging unit to gather and distribute supplies and equipment required by all units.

- *Morgue unit. Deceased casualties are moved to this unit where they are held and processed. (p. 1144)*

Q5. Explain how to perform the initial assessment of a patient during initial triage.

A5. *The initial triage of a patient is performed very quickly. For example, in the START system, any patient who is able to walk, despite injuries, is tagged "green" or lowest priority. If a patient is not able to walk, his respirations are quickly assessed and then, if appropriate, perfusion and mental status. At the end of the initial assessment, the patient is tagged with the appropriate priority number/color. (pp. 1146–1148)*

Q6. Identify the appropriate triage level (in a system with three levels of triage) for each of the following: (a) a patient with inadequate breathing; (b) a patient who is in cardiac arrest with insufficient EMS personnel to provide care; (c) a patient found with a painful, swollen, and deformed forearm; (d) a patient with a laceration to his back.

A6. *Appropriate triage levels (in a system with three levels of triage) are as follows: (a) a patient with inadequate breathing—highest priority, or Priority 1; (b) a patient who is in cardiac arrest with insufficient EMS personnel to provide care—lowest priority, or Priority 3; (c) a patient found with a painful, swollen, and deformed forearm—lowest priority, or Priority 3; (d) a patient with a lacerated back—second priority, or Priority 2. (pp. 1150–1151)*

Q7. Explain the reasons for using a patient identification or tagging system and give the criteria for a successful patient identification system.

A7. *Reasons for using a patient identification or tagging system include the following: Tagging the sick or injured helps arriving EMTs to quickly and efficiently identify treatment priorities. Also, arriving EMTs know untagged patients will still need initial triage. The criteria for a successful patient identification system are that the tagging system should be easy to understand, standardized, and easily affixed to the patient. (pp. 1150–1151)*

Q8. List guidelines for effective transport of patients in a multiple-casualty incident.

A8. *To effectively transport patients in a multiple-casualty incident, highest-priority patients should be transported first immediately after treatment and evenly distributed among available hospitals. As each ambulance leaves, the transportation officer should radio the hospital to which the ambulance is en route, briefly describing the injuries involved and giving an estimated time of arrival. Individual EMTs should not try to communicate with the hospital unless an emergency develops during transport. When the only patients left at the site are ambulatory, load them onto a bus with properly equipped EMTs and follow an ambulance to a hospital. (pp. 1151–1153)*

Q9. List at least five ways for reducing stress on EMTs during a multiple-casualty incident or disaster operation.

A9. *Any five of the following guidelines may help to reduce stress: Try not to get overwhelmed by the immensity of the incident and care for patients one by one. Rest at regular intervals upon reporting back to the staffing area for assignment, maybe as often as once every 1–2 hours (but follow local protocol). Make sure that each rescue worker is fully aware of his or her exact assignment. Have several workers in the staffing area circulate among the rescue workers and watch for signs of physical exhaustion or stress. Require workers with problems to return to the staffing area and rest for a longer period than usual. Make sure that rescue workers are assigned to tasks appropriate for their skills and experience. Provide plenty of nourishing drinks and food. Encourage rescue workers to talk among themselves. Make sure that rescuers have the opportunity to talk with trained counselors after the incident. (pp. 1153–1154)*

CRITICAL THINKING

Assess students' ability to respond to real-life emergency situations by discussing the Critical Thinking questions on page 1159 in the textbook.

Q1. What responsibilities would you have as the EMS branch director?

A1. *The EMS branch director is responsible for all triage, treatment, and transportation during the incident.*

Q2. What units would you establish?

A2. *The EMS branch director would set up a triage unit, a treatment unit, a transport unit, a staging unit, and possibly a morgue unit.*

Q3. How should triage be conducted?

A3. *The uninjured and lightly injured individuals (walking wounded) should initially be separated from the more seriously injured patients. The remaining patients should then be evaluated for criticality and labeled with red, yellow, or black tags according to the level of priority.*

Q4. What patients would be moved into the treatment unit first and moved out of the treatment unit first?

A4. *The patients who were red-tagged during triage would be the first ones moved to and treated in the treatment unit. These patients will also be the first ones to be transported. As the red-tagged patients are treated and transported, the yellow-tagged patients become move up, and become the next priority for treatment and transport. Following the yellow, the remaining green-tagged patients would then be treated and transported.*

Q5. How would you manage all of the responding EMS units?

A5. *The EMS branch director would most likely assign the first responding EMS unit to begin triaging the patients. Then, as more units arrive, the responders would be directed into unit leader positions. Once the units are organized, most of the remaining EMS responders would be directed into the treatment and transportation sectors, based on need. The transportation unit officer would be responsible for staging the EMS units to prevent a jam of units at the scene. The treatment unit officer communicates and coordinates vehicles needed in the treatment unit for transport with the transportation unit officer.*

Tell students that they will now have a chance to apply what they have just learned as they role-play EMS response to a multiple-casualty incident.

Note: Use the multiple-casualty incident organizational structure approved for your area if it is different from the one outlined below. Assign about three-quarters of the students in the class to act as victims of a multiple-casualty incident. Divide the remaining students into teams of two, each team to represent one EMS unit staffed by EMTs. Ask for one team to volunteer to be the initial EMS response team. Provide this team with a two-way radio or cellular phone. The first responding team will size up the incident and decide if additional EMS units are needed. Additional units will respond, if summoned, and will act appropriately on what they find at the incident. Explain that while the focus of the scene is on multiple-casualty incidents, students should use all the knowledge and skills they have learned to date.

Arrange for a firefighter to visit the class and play the role of firefighter incident commander for this activity. The incident commander will designate one of the first arriving EMTs as EMS incident commander. The firefighter should inform the EMS commander that fire and gas company personnel are working to control the leak and which patients are in the safe area and which are in the danger area. The two areas should be clearly marked. After the leak has been controlled, the incident commander may declare all patients to be in the safe area. The firefighter incident commander should carefully monitor the scene to ensure that patients and rescuers are not injured during this exercise. The incident commander should intervene in any situation where there is a potential for injury.

Provide each team with a jump kit (which should include triage tags), oxygen equipment, portable suction, and a stretcher. Inform students that they may also use any resources they find at the scene. Explain the following scenario:

You have been dispatched to a local adult education facility. An explosion has been reported. Fire and police departments are en route. Act appropriately on what you find there. Once you have evaluated the scene, call the base station regarding any additional needs you have. Provide the initial response team with the location of the scene. Make sure that all patients are in place and in character when the initial EMS team arrives. The firefighter/incident commander should also be in place and in character.

Take the multiple-casualty incident report when it is called in by the EMS commander. Dispatch the additional units requested at one-minute intervals. Once all units have been dispatched, relocate to the scene and assume the role of EMS commander. Direct students to care for and evacuate patients.

When all patients have been evacuated, regroup students to the main classroom.

Discuss the following questions:

- What was done well during this multiple-casualty incident?
- What could have been done better?

Note: If this is the last class of the course—that is, if you will not be teaching the electives or appendixes—discuss student answers at this time.

ASSIGNMENTS

If you will be teaching it as an elective, assign students to read Chapter 42, "EMS Response to Weapons of Mass Destruction," before the next class. Also ask them to complete Chapter 41 of the Workbook.

EVALUATION

Chapter Quiz Distribute copies of the Chapter Quiz provided in Handout 41-2 to evaluate student understanding of this chapter. Remind students not to refer to their textbooks or notes while taking the quiz.

Test Manager You may wish to create a custom-tailored test using Prentice Hall *TestGen for Prehospital Emergency Care, Eighth Edition* to evaluate student understanding of this chapter.

Online Test Preparation (for students and instructors) Additional test preparation is available through *EMT Achieve: Basic Test Preparation* at http://www.prenhall.com/EMTAchieve. Instructors can also monitor student mastery online.

REINFORCEMENT

Handouts If classroom discussions or performance on the quiz indicates that some students have not fully mastered the chapter content, you may wish to assign some or all of the Reinforcement Handouts for this chapter.

TECH EXTRAS

Brady Skills Series EMT-B Videos/CD Have your students watch the skills come to life on either VHS or CD-ROM.

PowerPoint Presentation (for instructors) The PowerPoint material developed for this chapter offers useful reinforcement of chapter content.

Student CD A wide variety of material on this CD-ROM will reinforce and also expand student knowledge and skills.

Companion Website (for students) Additional review quizzes and links to EMS resources will contribute to further reinforcement of this chapter. Please visit http://www.prenhall.com/mistovich.

Reading/Reference
Textbook, pp. 1160–1177

Workbook
Chapter 41 Activities

Chapter Quiz
Handout 41-2

TestGen
Chapter 41 Test

Online Test Preparation
Send your students to
http://www.prenhall.com/
EMTAchieve

Handouts 41-3 to 41-5
Reinforcement Activities

Brady Skills Series EMT-B Videos/CD
Visual Reinforcement

PowerPoint Presentation
Chapter 41

Student CD
Chapter 41

Companion Website
http://www.prenhall.com/
mistovich

OBJECTIVES

OBJECTIVES CHECKLIST

Cognitive		Date Mastered
7-3.7	Describe the criteria for a multiple-casualty situation.	
7-3.8	Evaluate the role of the EMT-Basic in the multiple-casualty situation.	
7-3.9	Summarize the components of basic triage.	
7-3.10	Define the role of the EMT-Basic in a disaster operation.	
7-3.11	Describe basic concepts of incident management.	
7-3.13	Review the local mass casualty incident plan.	
*	Outline the ways to get help in a multiple-casualty incident.	
*	Describe various approaches for reducing rescue personnel stress during an MCI or disaster.	

Psychomotor		Date Mastered
7-3.16	Given a scenario of a mass-casualty incident, perform triage.	

CHAPTER 41 QUIZ

Write the letter of the best answer in the space provided.

_____ 1. Any event that places excessive demands on emergency response personnel and equipment is called a

    A. catastrophe.   **C.** multiple-casualty incident.
    B. disaster.   **D.** tragedy.

_____ 2. The senior EMT who arrives at the scene of an MCI or disaster assumes responsibility as the _____ commander.

    A. unified   **C.** incident mobile
    B. sole   **D.** EMS incident

_____ 3. The unit responsible for distributing the medical materials and equipment necessary to render care is called the _____ unit.

    A. staging   **C.** supply
    B. extrication   **D.** triage

_____ 4. A system used for sorting patients to determine the order in which they will receive medical care or transportation to definitive care is called

    A. staging.   **C.** triage.
    B. assessment.   **D.** treatment.

_____ 5. In the four-priority triage system, patients who are dead receive what priority level?

    A. Priority 3   **C.** Priority 1
    B. Priority 4   **D.** Priority 2

_____ 6. The unit responsible for the monitoring, overseeing of inventories, and direction of available ambulances to the treatment unit is called the _____ unit.

    A. incident command   **C.** staging
    B. transportation   **D.** communication

_____ 7. As an EMT at an MCI, do *not* let communication difficulties distract you from

    A. patient care.
    B. contacting the incident commander.
    C. using radio codes.
    D. direct communication with the receiving hospital.

_____ 8. A sudden catastrophic event that overwhelms natural order and causes great loss of property and/or life is called a

    A. disaster.   **C.** calamity.
    B. Force 10 event MCI.   **D.** tragedy.

_____ 9. Critical to any successful rescue effort is an efficient communications system that includes

    A. multiple frequencies.   **C.** E9-1-1 capabilities.
    B. EMT dispatchers.   **D.** a back-up system.

_____ 10. A typical color-coding system for triage tags assigns high-priority patients the color:

    A. yellow.   **C.** red.
    B. green.   **D.** black.

©2008 by Pearson Education, Inc.
Prehospital Emergency Care, 8th ed.

EVALUATION

_____ **11.** A key to dealing with non-life-threatening injuries in the treatment unit is
  A. detailed tagging.
  B. taking treatment shortcuts.
  C. frequent consultation with medical direction.
  D. performing detailed assessments.

_____ **12.** After an incident commander is determined, he or she should begin to establish all of the following EMS units _except_
  A. triage.   **C.** finance.
  B. transportation.   **D.** supply.

_____ **13.** EMTs arriving at an MCI should first report to the _____ unit.
  A. mobile command   **C.** staging
  B. supply   **D.** transportation

_____ **14.** Patients should be moved from the triage unit to the treatment unit in order of their
  A. age.   **C.** seniority.
  B. priority.   **D.** complaints.

_____ **15.** During an MCI, radio communications from the scene of the incident to the receiving hospitals should be handled by the
  A. Incident Commander.   **C.** transportation officer.
  B. individual EMTs.   **D.** EMD.

IN THE FIELD

Read the following real-life situation. Then answer the following questions.

Our fire department does not make that many EMS calls; however, we are all EMTs. I still remember the day that we were toned out to a two-car collision with multiple patients. This wasn't your regular car crash, at least not in our town. Upon our arrival, Captain Schultz noted one car with severe front-end damage sitting upright in the intersection with two patients still in the car. The other vehicle was on its side with the driver still in his seatbelt. There was a little girl in the back seat and another child sitting up crying on the ground.

Captain Schultz immediately requested three more ambulances and another engine company for assistance and then took charge of the triage. He took two firefighters with him to assist. In accordance with our SOP for multiple-casualty incidents, the lieutenant took control of getting the responding units and personnel to the patients that Captain Schultz identified as priority.

When the ambulances started to arrive, Captain Schultz directed firefighters to load the priority patients and waited for additional ambulances for the stable patients. All in all, we transported six patients in five ambulances.

1. Did this event meet the criteria of a multiple-casualty event?

2. Who was the EMT incident commander in this scenario?

3. Who was the staging unit officer in this scenario?

REINFORCEMENT

CHAPTER 41 REVIEW

Write the word or words that best complete each sentence in the space provided.

1. A multiple-casualty incident (MCI) is any event that places _____
   _____ on personnel and equipment.

2. Multiple-casualty incidents do *not* always involve victims of _____.

3. Effective management of multiple-casualty incidents consists of getting enough help, positioning
   vehicles properly, giving appropriate _____ _____
   _____, transporting patients efficiently, and providing
   _____ - _____ _____ at
   receiving facilities.

4. The _____ _____ _____
   is responsible for seeing that the multiple-casualty incident is responded to in a controlled and
   orderly way and that all responsibilities are carried out.

5. A(n) _____ _____ system works best when the
   multiple-casualty incident involves more that one emergency response agency.

6. The _____ _____ should be stationed in a
   command center located in a safe area near or at the area where patients will be loaded for transport.

7. The incident commander _____ duties to the various unit officers.

8. EMTs responding to the scene of an MCI should first report to the _____
   _____ _____ for instructions.

9. The _____ _____ is responsible for distributing
   the medical materials and equipment necessary to render care.

10. _____ is a system used for sorting patients to determine the order in which
    they will receive medical care or transportation to definitive care; it is performed in the
    _____ _____.

11. In triage, the _____ priority involves patients with severe injuries but who
    should still survive even if care is somewhat delayed.

12. The _____ _____ officer ensures that ambulances are accessible and that transportation does not occur without the direction of the EMS incident commander.

13. As each ambulance leaves, the _____ _____ _____ should radio the hospital that the ambulance is en route, briefly describing the injuries involved and giving an estimated time of arrival.

14. Effective _____ among emergency responders is one of the most difficult aspects of a multiple-casualty incident.

15. A(n) _____ is a sudden catastrophic event that overwhelms natural order and causes great loss of property and/or life.

16. Faced with the grim physical injuries that can accompany a disaster, it is difficult to remember that the _____ injuries can be severe—even among those *not* _____ _____.

17. In a disaster, the families of patients need and deserve _____ _____—something that is too often overlooked in the rush to begin emergency medical care.

18. Arrange for all those involved in a disaster—including _____—to get good follow-up care and support.

REINFORCEMENT

ANALYZING AN MCI

Attached you will find an example of a typical incident tactical worksheet. Given the following scene size-up information plus reports from the unit officers, answer the questions and complete as much of the sheet as you are able to.

The Southcross apartment complex is on fire. Starting as a small kitchen fire, the fire has spread to five other units and displaced at least 30 people. At least five volunteer fire companies are on the scene, each with at least five firefighters.

Reports of victims are streaming in. As EMS command on-scene, you have coordinated with fire and police command to establish a perimeter. You have also instructed the next senior EMT on the scene to establish a forward triage point near the front door of the building. His first report reveals the following:

- 1 patient that firefighters have started CPR on—Priority 0
- 2 seriously burned adult patients—Priority 1
- 2 elderly people, a married couple, both with extensive medical histories, both complaining of shortness of breath—Priority 1
- 1 person with bilateral broken ankles from jumping from the third story—Priority 2
- 3 persons with burns to the hands from helping victims escape—Priority 3

Police also report about 15 residents who are out of the building and exposed to the elements. A roll call of available receiving facilities shows the following:

St. Mary's Hospital—5 minutes away

- 5 critical care beds
- 10 emergency department beds
- 5 clinic rooms
- no morgue

Memorial Hospital (regional trauma center)—10 minutes away

- 5 critical care beds
- 10 emergency department beds
- 5 clinic rooms
- 5 morgue openings

Galivan Hospital—20 minutes away

- no critical care beds
- 5 emergency department beds
- 5 clinic rooms
- no morgue

1. There are two major missions that EMS command must cope with at this scene. What are they?

2. Is this a multiple-casualty incident (MCI)? Why?

3. Assume you are the staging officer. How many ambulances will be needed?

4. Assume you are the transportation officer. Based on the initial triage report, which patients would you send to which hospital?

Multiple-Casualty Incidents

Basics of Multiple-Casualty Incidents

Definition

National Incident Management System (NIMS)

Establishing Incident Management

- Mobile command unit
- Supply unit
- Extrication unit
- Triage unit
- Treatment unit
- Staging unit
- Transportation unit

Positioning Arriving Vehicles

Triage

Primary and Secondary Triage

Priority Levels

Patient Tagging

Treatment

Staging and Transportation

Communications

Follow-Through

Reducing Stress

Disaster Management

Requirements of Effective Disaster Assistance

Warning and Evacuation

Disaster Communications Systems

Psychological Impact of Disasters

CHAPTER 41 ANSWER KEY

HANDOUT 41-2: Chapter 41 Quiz

1. C	**5.** B	**9.** D	**13.** A
2. D	**6.** C	**10.** C	**14.** B
3. C	**7.** A	**11.** B	**15.** C
4. C	**8.** A	**12.** C	

HANDOUT 41-3: In the Field

1. This event, although not a disaster, met the definition of a multiple-casualty incident in that it placed excessive demands on the small fire department. Six patients involved in one collision may be routine in a large metropolitan area, but in this case overwhelmed a small department.
2. The engine company Captain (Schultz), being the senior EMS on the scene, assumed the responsibilities of the EMS incident commander.
3. The lieutenant, following standard procedures for his department, took responsibility for monitoring and directing ambulances at the scene.

HANDOUT 41-4: Chapter 41 Review

1. excessive demands
2. trauma
3. emergency medical care, follow-up care
4. EMS incident commander
5. unified command
6. incident commander
7. delegates
8. mobile command unit
9. supply unit
10. Triage, triage unit
11. second
12. transportation unit
13. transportation unit officer
14. communications
15. disaster
16. psychological, physically injured
17. accurate information
18. rescuers

HANDOUT 41-5: Analyzing an MCI

1. Emergency medical care and transportation
2. Yes, multiple priority patients—obviously already stressing existing personnel and equipment resources
3. At least six. Each Priority 1 patient needs one ambulance, while two Priority 2 and 3 patients can ride in one ambulance.
4. Student answers will vary, but the Priority 1 patients would go to the regional trauma center. Review completed worksheets.

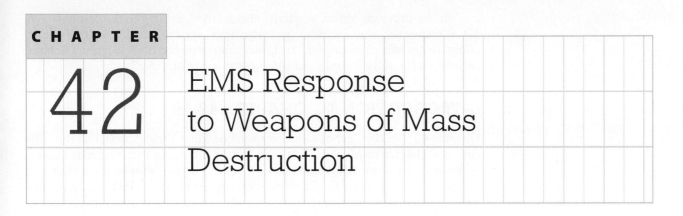

42 EMS Response to Weapons of Mass Destruction

This chapter contains information that is valuable as background for the EMT but that goes substantially beyond the U.S. Department of Transportation's EMT-Basic National Standard Curriculum.

OBJECTIVES

Asterisked objectives pertain to material that is supplemental to the DOT curriculum. Page numbers in parentheses refer to pages in the textbook.

Cognitive

* * Define weapons of mass destruction. (p. 1161)
* * Discuss the role of EMS, particularly the role of the EMT-Basic, in response to weapons of mass destruction attack. (pp. 1163–1165)
* * Describe the primary, secondary, and tertiary effects of an explosive detonation. (p. 1165)
* * Describe the characteristics of and the signs and symptoms and emergency medical care for the following chemical agents: nerve agents, vesicants, cyanide, pulmonary agents, riot-control agents, and industrial chemicals. (pp. 1166–1170)
* * List agents and specific findings for the following types of biological agents and emergency medical care for biological agents: pneumonia-like agents, encephalitis-like agents, biological toxins, and other biological agents. (pp. 1170–1172)
* * Discuss the types of radiation (x-ray and gamma, neutron, beta, and alpha), types of radiation exposure (primary and fallout), types of radiation injuries, assessment, and medical care for radiation injuries. (pp. 1173–1175)
* * Describe appropriate personal protection and patient decontamination for chemical, biological, and nuclear weapons exposure. (p. 1175)

REVIEW

In the last lesson, "Multiple-Casualty Incidents," students received an overview of how to organize and provide emergency medical care when there is an event that involves a number of patients: a multiple-casualty incident, or MCI. MCIs may range from a vehicle collision with several injured passengers to a major disaster such as a hurricane, flood, earthquake, bombing, building collapse, or airliner crash. Point out that to gain a better understanding of MCIs and disaster response, EMTs should regularly practice their community's MCI or disaster response plan.

Total Teaching Time
90 minutes

Resource Needed
Scored Chapter 41 Quizzes

Additional Resources
Larmon/Davis, *Basic Life Support Skills*

Elling, *EMT Achieve: Basic Test Preparation*

Limmer/Mistovich/ O'Keefe, *Audio Lecture & Study Guide: EMT*

Mistovich/Kuvlesky, *SUCCESS! for the EMT, Second Edition*

In the previous lesson, students also learned about the fundamentals of MCI response, the incident management system, EMS units, triage, components of a disaster plan, and, most importantly, how to "get the right patient, to the right hospital, in the right amount of time."

INTRODUCTION TO CHAPTER 42

Chapter 42, "EMS Response to Weapons of Mass Destruction," is the fifth and final chapter in Module 7. It is an optional chapter that you may choose to include in your course. Response to terrorism is now an important mission for EMS. Historically there is an urgent need for EMS to "rush in" to situations to rescue and treat victims. Terrorism is a situation where responders must pause and evaluate the risk, first to themselves and second to the victims of the event. Since the onset of symptoms of biological agents is even more delayed, the investigative skills of EMS personnel are essential and may be the key to protecting an entire community if the agent is identified early. The instructor must reinforce these concepts in this section. There is also a tendency for the EMT student to get lost in the numerous aspects of the types of WMD threats and causative agents. The key to student learning in this section is a combination of grouping the types of terrorism causes and agents and application of the information in the case studies. Use of adjuncts such as field operations guides and checklists are critical for field performance of EMS personnel due to the low probability of a terrorism incident actually occurring.

Distribute the Chapter 42 Objectives and give the students a few minutes to review the list. Lead a brief discussion of the objectives and start the lesson with a short story involving a WMD response.

LECTURE

The following suggested lecture outline is based on the Department of Transportation's EMT-Basic National Standard Curriculum. In some places, the DOT curriculum has been rearranged or expanded upon so that it is more complete or easier for the student to understand. The page numbers in parentheses refer to pages in the textbook. The parenthetical references in dark, heavy type are to figures, tables, and scans in the textbook.

EMS RESPONSE TO WEAPONS OF MASS DESTRUCTION

 I. Weapons of mass destruction (pp. 1161–1163) **(Fig. 42-1, p. 1162)**
   A. Weapons of mass destruction (pp. 1161–1163)
   1. Weapons intended to cause widespread and indiscriminate death and destruction.
   2. Mnemonics
      a. CBRNE
         (1) Chemical, Biological, Radiological, Nuclear, Explosive
   3. General prehospital approach to an incident involving weapons of mass destruction is similar to that for any disaster involving mass casualties.
   4. General method of dealing with disasters and special situations is often termed the "all-hazards approach."
 II. Prehospital response to WMD (pp. 1163–1165) **(Fig. 42-2, p. 1163)**

Handout 42-1
Chapter 42 Objectives Checklist

Lecture Master
You may wish to display Lecture Master 42 when presenting the lecture to the class.

Reading/Reference
Enrich, J., "The Expert Take: Assessing the Terrorism Issue Facing EMS," *Emergency Medical Services,* Jan. 2002.

On the Net
U.S. Federal Emergency Management Agency. www.fema.gov

Reading/Reference
Christen, Hank T., & Maniscalco, Paul M., *EMS Incident Management System: The Operations for Mass Casualty and High Impact Incidents.* Brady, 2002.

A. Supplies and equipment (p. 1163)
  1. Each type of WMD incident requires different types of specially trained personnel, equipment, and supplies.
      a. Nerve agents may require large amounts of certain drugs along with a massive number of ventilators.
      b. Chemical incidents may require special personal protective equipment such as breathing apparatus or hazardous materials suits.
      c. Large explosions with structural collapse may require heavy rescue equipment, specially trained search and rescue teams, electronic detection devices, and trained search dogs.
  2. A plan must be in place that will allow the communications center immediate access to the individuals who are capable of deploying the equipment, supplies, and personnel.
B. Medical direction (p. 1163)
  1. A plan should address how medical direction will be provided to EMS personnel at the scene as well as the credentials of EMS personnel.
  2. Since online medical direction is expected to be overloaded, one possibility is to make all protocols standing orders in a case involving weapons of mass destruction.
C. Provider preparation (p. 1164)
  1. EMS providers must be aware of the personal risks and dangers associated with responding to a weapons of mass destruction incident.
  2. Regarding patient care, EMS providers must be aware of various agents that can be used as weapons of mass destruction and the signs and symptoms of the conditions that result from exposure.
D. Responding to the scene (p. 1164)
  1. One of the most important aspects of a weapons of mass destruction incident is recognition.
  2. These incidents employ the same incident command system as does any multiple-casualty incident.
  3. Be wary of the possibility of secondary explosions when conventional weapons are used.
E. Issues of scene safety (pp. 1164–1165)
  1. There are significant differences between the effects of conventional, chemical, and most biological weapons as compared to the death, injury, and mass destruction of the nuclear weapon.
  2. Conventional, chemical, and most biological weapons place an extreme strain on the EMS system and medical care.
  3. The mass physical destruction of a nuclear weapon severely limits access to the scene.
  4. Chemical and biological weapons present a danger that is much more difficult to recognize and identify as compared to the nuclear or conventional blast.
F. Role of the EMT at the WMD incident (p. 1165)
III. Conventional weapons and incendiary devices (pp. 1165–1166)
  A. Explosives (p. 1165)
  1. Explosives create a blast wave or shock that moves out in all directions at sonic speed.
  2. If blast occurs in a closed room or space, the effects of the blast are amplified.

On the Net
www.citizencorp.gov

This site assists in preparing community volunteers to aid emergency response agencies during disaster or terrorism affecting communities.

On the Net
www.dhs.gov

The Department of Homeland Security is the government entity charged with preparing first responders, including EMTs, for response to domestic terrorism.

Reading/Reference
Emergency Response to Terrorism Self-Study Course. U.S. Fire Administration, 2000. www.usfa.fema.gov/ dhtml/fire-service/c-terror-pubs.cfm

Point of Interest
(1) There have been over 6,000 acts of domestic terrorism in the United States since 1900.
(2) Ninety-eight percent of all terrorism incidents involve incendiary or explosive devices.
(3) One ounce of radioactive power can contaminate an entire city when used in a dirty bomb.

Teaching Tip
Contact your local FBI office and ask for the WMD Special Agent in charge to provide an overview of the counterterrorism efforts in your area.

B. Primary, secondary, and tertiary effects (p. 1165) (Fig. 42-3, p. 1166)

  1. The blast of an explosion is considered to be the primary effect.

  2. Flying debris, shrapnel, and other projectiles cause secondary effects.

  3. The injuries produced when the patient is propelled by a blast or shock wave is referred to as tertiary effects.

C. Body position (p. 1165)

  1. Body position plays a role in determining the extent of the blast injury.

  2. Shrapnel and blast injuries can be reduced by dropping to a prone position facing away from the detonation.

D. Types of injuries (pp. 1165–1166)

  1. Lungs

    a. Lung injuries may occur from primary blast effects.

    b. Look for evidence of lung injury, such as altered mental status, dyspnea, blood-tinged sputum, respiratory distress, chest pain, and stroke-like signs and symptoms.

  2. Abdomen

    a. Blast injury may cause bleeding to the bowel or may allow a lacerated bowel to leak its content into the abdominal cavity.

    b. A victim who is close to the detonation may suffer an evisceration.

  3. Ears

    a. The eardrum may rupture from a blast.

    b. Patient may experience a temporary or permanent hearing loss.

  4. Crush injuries

    a. May occur as a result of structural collapse

    b. Crush syndrome is associated with entrapment for 4 hours or more.

  5. Shrapnel injuries

    a. Shrapnel may cause penetrating injury to the solid organs, hollow organs, connective tissue, and bone.

    b. Each may experience a different effect from the missile.

E. Incendiary devices (p. 1166)

  1. Create different injury patterns from conventional explosives

  2. Include napalm, thermite, magnesium, and white phosphorus

IV. Chemical agents (pp. 1166–1170)

  A. Chemical weapons (pp. 1166–1167)

    1. Among the most feared weapons of mass destruction

    2. It is imperative that EMS providers be familiar with the chemicals that are likely to be used and the necessary patient management.

  B. Properties of chemical weapons (p. 1167)

    1. Most chemicals for military use are stored in munitions (shells, rockets, bombs) as a liquid.

    2. Some riot-control agents are stored as solids, but become an aerosol once deployed.

    3. Some chemical agents, such as hydrogen cyanide, chlorine, and phosgene may be in the form of a gas in warm weather.

    4. Volatility

      a. Tendency of a chemical agent to evaporate

5. Persistence

    a. Characteristic of agents that do not evaporate quickly and tend to remain as a puddle for long periods of time

C. Types of chemical agents (pp. 1167–1170)

    1. Nerve agents (**Tables 42-1, p. 1167 and 42-2, p. 1168**)

        a. These are among the most deadly known chemicals

    2. Vesicants

        a. Group of chemical agents that result in damage to exposed skin, lungs, and eyes

    3. Cyanide

        a. Rapid-acting agent that disrupts the ability of the cell to use oxygen, leading to severe cellular hypoxia and eventually death

    4. Pulmonary agents

        a. Act primarily to cause lung injury and are commonly referred to as "choking" agents

        b. Include phosgene (CG), other halogen compounds, and nitrogen–oxygen compounds

    5. Riot-control agents

        a. Some are solids that become an aerosol when deployed

        b. Most recent type of riot-control agent is derived from the capsicum family of peppers.

    6. Industrial chemicals

V. Biological agents (pp. 1170–1172)

A. Biological agents (pp. 1170–1171)

    1. Made up of living organisms or the toxins produced by the living organisms and are used to cause disease in a target population

    2. To be effective as a WMD, the biological agent must reach the intended target.

    3. Respiratory tract is the most common and efficient portal of entry for most biological agents.

    4. Key to recognition of a biological attack is to distinguish a number of cases and timing of cases from the isolated case of an expected illness.

B. Specific biological agents (pp. 1171–1172)

    1. Pneumonia-like agents

        a. Presenting with fever and rapidly progressing dyspnea

        b. Anthrax

        c. Plague

        d. Tuleremia

    2. Encephalitis-like agents

        a. Presenting with fever and altered mental status

        b. Smallpox

        c. Venezuelan equine encephalitis

    3. Biological toxins

        a. Botulinum

        b. Ricin

        c. Staphylococcus enterotixin 13 (SEB)

        d. Epsilon toxin

        e. Trichothecene mycotoxins (T2)

    4. Other agents

        a. Cholera

        b. Viral hemorrhagic fevers (VHFs)

        c. Brucellosis

On the Net

www.btresponse.org

Centers for Disease Control sponsor this site and provide valuable information concerning preparing for and responding to bioterrorism.

Reading/Reference

Sachs, E.M., "The Bubonic Man: Lessons from a Bioterrorism Incident," *Emergency Medical Services,* Aug. 2000.

Slides/Videos

Oak Ridge Associated Universities. www.orau .gov/.../Instructor % 20PPT%20Slides/ Terrorism-Bioterrorism %20Communication.pdf

Slides/Videos

Northwest Center for Public Health Practice. http:// healthlinks. washington .edu/nwcphp/bt/

C. Emergency medical care for biological agents (p. 1172)
        1. Care for biological toxins is primarily supportive
        2. Only a few biological agents, such as smallpox, plague, and ebola, are highly contagious.
        3. Priorities in patient care include securing an adequate airway and ensuring that the patient is breathing adequately.
        4. The use of antibiotics and antitoxins is imperative in the management of patients exposed to biological agents.
        5. The best protection against biological weapons is prevention.

VI. Nuclear weapons and radiation (pp. 1173–1175)
    A. Nuclear weapons and radiation (p. 1173)
        1. Nuclear weapons can cause extensive death by a variety of mechanisms.
        2. There are three primary mechanisms of death associated with nuclear detonation: radiation, blast, and thermal burns.
    B. Radiation (p. 1173)
        1. X-ray radiation and gamma radiation—this powerful type of radiation is the most penetrating type and can travel far distances.
        2. Neutron radiation
            a. Powerful and very damaging particle that penetrates several hundred meters of air and easily passes through the body
        3. Beta radiation
            a. Low-speed, low-energy particle that is easily stopped by 6–10 feet of air, clothing, or the first few millimeters of skin
        4. Alpha radiation
            a. Very heavy and slow-moving particle that travels only in the air and is stopped by clothing or the outer layer of the skin
        5. Radiation Exposure
            a. Primary
            b. Exposure fallout
    C. Blast injuries (p. 1173)
        1. Nuclear detonation causes a rapid heating of air surrounding the nuclear ignition and an explosively expanding gas cloud.
        2. The shock wave and wind blast produce typical injuries as found in conventional weapons.
    D. Thermal burns (p. 1174)
        1. The thermal burn is the mechanism that causes most deaths and injury associated with nuclear detonation.
        2. Flame burns may result from ignition of clothing and building materials.
        3. Eye injuries may be associated with the brilliant light flash.
    E. Radiological Dispersal Devices (p. 1174)
        1. Also called a "dirty bomb," it is a conventional explosive attached to radioactive materials.
        2. It gains its destructive power first by the blast of the conventional explosive, and second by the spread of radioactive material all around the blast site.
    F. Assessment and care for nuclear detonation and radiation injuries (pp. 1174–1175)
        1. Assessment
            a. The closer the patient is to the detonation, the more severe the injuries expected.

b. Signs and symptoms
  (1) Nausea
  (2) Fatigue
  (3) Malaise
  (4) Dehydration
  (5) Reddening of the skin
  (6) Rapid onset of incapacitation
  (7) Cardiovascular collapse
  (8) Confusion
  (9) Burning or "on-fire" sensation with high doses
2. Emergency medical care
  a. Primary concern is for your own and the patient's protection.
  b. Primary concern is to manage the airway and ventilatory status of the patient.
  c. Manage burns as you would normally manage a thermal burn.
  d. In an area of nuclear fallout or radioactive contamination, taking iodine tablets before or immediately following exposure can reduce future thyroid cancer risk.

VII. Personal protection and patient decontamination (p. 1175) **(Fig. 42-4, p. 1175)**

CASE STUDY FOLLOW-UP

Ask a student to volunteer to read the Case Study that begins on page 1161 of the textbook. You may wish to use the following questions to engage students in a discussion of the Case Study Follow-up that begins on page 1176 of the textbook. Provide missing information and clarify ideas as needed.

Q1. As the first-arriving EMS unit, what are your initial responsibilities?

A1. One crew member must make contact with the fire department officer in charge; advise of your arrival, the location of staging for medical personnel, and find out if they suspect any hazardous conditions that would require decontamination or isolation of those involved in the incident. Begin an initial scene size-up and request additional resources for a large-scale MCI. The other crewmember can begin the triage of patients.

Q2. All available ambulances are needed to transport critical patients to appropriate facilities. Are there any options available to transport noncritical patients to appropriate facilities? If so, what are they?

A2. Because the incident occurred at a college football game, there will probably be plenty of buses that can be utilized for the transport of the "walking wounded." By controlling the transportation of these patients, they can be taken to appropriate facilities, and not overwhelm the resources of the closest facility.

Q3. What is the responsibility of the transportation officer?

A3. The transportation officer is responsible for tracking all patients that leave the scene, whether by ambulance, personal vehicle, or other means. The transportation officer must maintain records of each patient's name, identifying information, destination, and condition. The transportation officer arranges for transport and notifies the receiving facility of the patient and his or her condition.

Q4. Whose responsibility is it to release information to the media?

A4. *Individual departments/agencies should have a public information officer (PIO). It is the responsibility of this person to release any necessary information to the media. This person is trained to know what information can and cannot be released to the media without violating the patient's right to privacy. All other personnel should avoid contact with the media or respond "No comment."*

IN REVIEW

Assess students' ability to apply what they have learned by discussing the Review Questions on page 1177 of the textbook.

Q1. Name the types of weapons of mass destruction.

A1. *Weapons of mass destruction include biological, nuclear, incendiary, chemical, explosive, and radiological. (p. 1161)*

Q2. Describe the safety issues to EMS providers when responding to a scene where weapons of mass destruction have been used.

A2. *There are many safety issues that must be addressed by EMS providers. They include positioning of the vehicle and responders uphill, upwind, and at a safe distance to prevent responders from becoming victims. Responders must also be aware of the potential for secondary devices. Responders must be wearing appropriate personal protective equipment (PPE) for the type of potential exposure to prevent contamination. Responders should also be prepared to recognize the signs and symptoms associated with WMD to ensure appropriate treatment and transport of all victims. (pp. 1164–1165)*

Q3. Define a conventional weapon and incendiary device.

A3. *A conventional weapon is an explosive used to create massive destruction through the explosion; this includes the primary, secondary, and tertiary effects of the blast. An incendiary device is used to create a large amount of fire volume meant to burn persons and property. While there may be an explosion, it is not the primary objective. (pp. 1165–1166)*

Q4. Describe the injuries expected from detonation of an explosive.

A4. *The primary effect of the explosion will cause a shock wave that is especially harmful to hollow organs like the lungs, causing a pneumothorax. The secondary effect of the explosion causes penetrating and blunt force trauma to all parts of the body from projectiles, both large and small. Injury patterns from the secondary effect of the blast are dependent upon the victim's proximity to and position at the time of the blast. The tertiary effects of the explosion cause further blunt force trauma, as the body itself becomes a projectile. Other objects can also come to rest on the victim, causing additional injury. Expect penetrating trauma and crush injuries in this patient. (p. 1165)*

Q5. Explain the difference between a primary, secondary, and tertiary blast effect associated with an explosion.

A5. *The primary effect from an explosion is the shock wave that immediately follows the blast. The secondary effect of the explosion is from the shrapnel and other projectiles contacting the victim. The tertiary effect of the explosion is from the victim being propelled by the blast and then striking an object or the ground. (p. 1165)*

Q6. List and describe the different types of chemical agents used as weapons of mass destruction.

A6. *Nerve agents block the action of acetylcholinesterase. This allows an accumulation of acetylcholine, which will then cause continued, uncontrolled, and uncoordinated contraction of muscle fibers that continue until the muscle fatigues and then begins to die. Volatile agents are both a liquid and a vapor hazard.*

Vesicants cause damage to any area of the body exposed to the chemical. The agents were previously known as "blister agents" because they cause blistering, burning, and tissue death on contact. These agents tend to be liquid hazards at low temperatures and vapor hazard at warmer temperatures.

Cyanide prevents the cells of the body from utilizing oxygen. This quickly affects the brain and heart. Cyanide is a high vapor hazard and can also be ingested through contaminated food products. Pulmonary agents cause damage to the lungs, especially the smaller airways and the alveoli. This damage causes pulmonary edema, leading to respiratory failure. Pulmonary agents tend to be liquids that rapidly convert to heavy gases.

Riot-control agents are aerosolized solids like pepper spray. These agents cause extreme irritation on contact, which can include the respiratory tract if inhaled.

Industrial chemicals can vary in the type of effects they may cause, but they are transported and stored throughout the country in large, highly concentrated amounts. These chemicals can act like pulmonary agents, cyanide, or even nerve agents. (pp. 1167–1170)

Q7. Describe the emergency care for the different types of chemical agents.

A7. *Nerve agents require supportive care. This includes maintaining an airway through intubation and suctioning. They also require an antidote to combat the nerve agent. There is potential for antiseizure medication. This patient also needs wounds dressed to prevent further contamination and absorption of the nerve agent.*

Vesicants require immediate and thorough irrigation of all contaminated surfaces with water or a chemical decontamination kit. After irrigation, burns should be dressed with dry sterile dressings.

Cyanide exposure requires early respiratory support to include positive-pressure ventilation and intubation. These patients may also require an antidote of amyl nitrite to reverse the effects of the cyanide. Pulmonary agents require respiratory support to include high-flow oxygen, suctioning, and possible intubation.

Riot-control agents care is primarily supportive and typically involves removing the patient from the environment and irrigating the eyes with water or saline. Patients may also need oxygen therapy if suffering respiratory distress.

Industrial chemicals require a variety of medical interventions based on the presenting signs and symptoms. (pp. 1167–1170)

Q8. List and describe the various biological agents that are used as weapons of mass destruction.

A8. *Pneumonia-like agents include anthrax, plague, and tularemia. These agents cause shortness of breath, fever, and malaise. Encephalitis-like agents include smallpox and Venezuelan equine encephalitis. These agents cause headaches, fever, malaise, and altered mental status.*

Biological toxins include botulinum, ricin, and other toxins. While these toxins cannot be transmitted from one person to another, they are still some of the most dangerous compounds. These are not living organisms as the others, but are instead the products of living organisms.

Other agents include cholera, viral hemorrhagic fevers, and brucellosis. These viruses are very deadly and are still seen in epidemic proportions in developing nations. (pp. 1171–1172)

Q9. List the general principles of treatment of biological agent exposure.

A9. *The care of patients exposed to biological agents is primarily supportive. This includes maintaining an adequate airway with the potential for intubation. Respiratory support may be necessary with supplemental oxygen and positive-pressure ventilation, if needed. These patients also need antibiotic and fluid therapy, so appropriate medical treatment must be sought. (p. 1172)*

Q10. List and describe the different types of radiation.

A10. *Gamma and X-ray radiation are the same. This is a powerful type of radiation that is the most penetrating type and can travel long distances. This radiation is the major external hazard associated with nuclear detonation and reactor accidents.*

Neutron radiation is very damaging and easily passes through the body. It typically occurs in a nuclear chain reaction. The threat is greatest near a nuclear reactor or bomb explosion.

Beta radiation is low-speed, low-energy radiation. It is common in fallout decay and is a serious threat from ingestion of contaminated food and from inhalation of airborne particles.

Alpha radiation is very heavy and slow moving. It is a very serious internal hazard because it causes a great amount of damage over its short course of travel. (p. 1173)

Q11. List the injuries that are most likely to occur with detonation of a nuclear device.

A11. *The detonation of a nuclear device can cause three types of injuries. The first is from the radiation. There is the primary exposure for those in the vicinity of the explosion. This is of limited danger to persons not near the site of the detonation. There is also fallout. Fallout is radioactive dust and particles that travel through the air and can be distributed far from the site of the detonation. This causes radiation injuries to the cells of the body.*

A nuclear device also creates blast injuries similar to conventional weapons, only much more severe. The shock wave created can include windblasts of 160 mph, collapsing structures, leading to entrapment and crush injuries.

The nuclear device also causes thermal burns. These burns are caused by the intense amount of thermal energy released during the detonation. Close to the detonation site, many things are incinerated; however, a victim far from the site may only suffer superficial burns. (pp. 1173–1174)

Q12. Describe the general emergency care of a radiation exposure victim.

A12. *A radiation exposure victim requires maintenance of the airway and ventilatory status. Ensure a patent airway, which may necessitate tracheal intubation. Respiratory support may include oxygen therapy* *as well as positive-pressure ventilation. Manage burns with dry sterile dressings and sterile burn sheets, as with normal thermal burns. Irrigate and dress wounds with sterile dressings to minimize the risk of infection. (pp. 1174–1175)*

CRITICAL THINKING

Assess students' ability to respond to real-life emergency situations by discussing the Critical Thinking questions on page 1177 in the textbook.

Q1. What is the first action you would take?

A1. *The first action should be to have law enforcement and the hazardous materials team evaluate scene safety in order to prevent responder exposure and to protect against the possibility of a secondary device. Also, any others remaining in the immediate exposure area must be evacuated.*

Q2. How would you initially manage the patients?

A2. *Confer with the hazardous material team as to whether the patients require decontamination prior to assessment and treatment. The patients would first be removed from the toxic environment. An initial assessment would then be conducted. Patients displaying these signs and symptoms would be treated by ensuring their airway is open, suctioning any excessive secretions, initiating high-concentration oxygen therapy via a nonrebreather mask at 15 lpm for those with an adequate tidal volume and respiratory rate, and providing positive pressure ventilation by bag-valve-mask for any patients with an inadequate respiratory rate or tidal volume.*

Q3. What do you suspect they are suffering from?

A3. *Based on the patient descriptions of the event coupled with the signs and symptoms, the EMTs should assume that a terrorist attack has occurred utilizing an explosive device to disperse a chemical pulmonary agent. Pulmonary agents irritate the mucous membranes of the mouth, eyes, nose, and throat. Pulmonary edema may take several hours to develop. Continuously assess for signs of worsening respiratory distress and hypoxia. Exertion may worsen the condition; thus, do not allow the patients to exert themselves.*

CLASS EXERCISE

The following exercise uses a training device that is called a "tabletop" exercise, because it is conducted around a table. Actions and events are simulated. Tabletop exercises are commonly used to prepare local officials for how specific events may affect a community. The exercise simulates various aspects of dealing with the events of a WMD attack. The stage is a state and includes local, regional governmental, and federal governmental jurisdictions. The players are the key personnel who are involved in mitigating the effects of the event. The event occurs on Day 7 of the scenario and players are asked to use their own discretion in creating the scenario of the WMD event.

Scenario

Day 1: It is a cool winter evening and you are relaxing at home, watching TV. You are cheering for your favorite football team as they play against a bitter rival. You have no notion that unseen events, occurring while you are watching the game, could have such widespread consequences in your community.

On that tragic evening, a small truck about a quarter of a mile from the football stadium releases a spray of a liquid biological agent. The one-minute release creates an odorless and colorless cloud that is more than a half mile across. A light wind blows the aerosol across crowded parking lots, into and across the stadium crowd of 65,342 cheering fans, and continues toward the downtown metropolitan area. Following the release of the agent, the truck continues on its way and is out of the state by the time the game ends. Your team wins and you head to bed, happy and unsuspecting of the upcoming events.

About 15,000 of the fans are infected by the unseen cloud, and another 3,000 residents and business owners in the surrounding area are infected as well. The fans disperse quickly following the game. Most return to areas within 200 miles of the game site, while others return to distant states.

Day 2: The day is uneventful. The perpetrators of the silent attack leave the country by commercial airliner, completely undetected.

Day 3: You are on shift for the day. It begins with a mysterious rush of people seeking medical care at doctors' offices, medical clinics, and emergency departments throughout the region. Infected individuals are complaining of fever and cough. Others complain of more serious symptoms, including shortness of breath and chest pains. You are busy transporting patients with similar symptoms to a local emergency department and conducting interhospital transfers. The influx of patients results in only a few hospital admissions. Most patients are diagnosed with common flu and are treated by advising them to rest and drink lots of fluids.

Day 4: By now it is becoming obvious to local health officials that the increased volume of what seems to be upper respiratory infections is a serious matter. Regional health officials are contacted for support and guidance. By the evening of day 4, young, healthy adults are beginning to die. These unexplained deaths force regional and local health officials to contact the Centers for Disease Control (CDC) for support. Ninety-eight have died by midnight and another 1,200 are sick.

Day 5: You are forced to work an extra shift. Media outlets are focusing on the deaths of so many young and healthy individuals. Rumors are circulating that it might be a terrorist action, but health officials are reluctant to make such judgments before they have clear evidence. Blood and tissue specimens are sent to the CDC for analysis. An emergency meeting with the mayor and local medical experts is held to discuss the events and to determine how to handle the situation. Isolation of all patients with fever and cough is instituted. You have the busiest shift that you have ever experienced. A temporary morgue is set up by the local hospital to handle the increasing number of bodies.

Day 6: Once again you are needed to work an extra shift so that additional units can be placed in service to meet the increasing demand for transport services. You are constantly transporting critical patients to distant hospitals. EMS coworkers are being placed into service at the hospital to try and assist with the overwhelming number of patients. EMS staff, hospital staff, and clinical personnel are confused and desperate because of the increasing number of deaths. Late in the day a report comes in from the CDC that the blood culture of a young man who died was positive for a certain biological agent. The FBI is notified and they begin an investigation.

The mayor and the governor of the state are notified. Medical personnel are told that antibiotics must be given as soon as symptoms appear. Patients with serious symptoms will die regardless of treatment. Local supplies of antibiotics are dwindling. The governor declares a state of emergency and requests additional antibiotics from the federal government. Local hospitals are warned to expect a growing flood of patients after a public announcement is made. The football game is suspected as the source of the outbreak. All individuals who attended the game will be advised to report to designated distribution centers to receive antibiotics.

Thousands of people rush to the distribution centers. Others go to their personal physicians, clinics, and hospital emergency departments. The process of distribution of the antibiotics is haphazard and uncoordinated among the various agencies. Local supplies of antibiotics are expended. By midnight of Day 6, 2,300 patients are ill and 330 people have died. Health care facilities are overwhelmed by the constant influx of patients.

Day 7: By the morning of the seventh day, shelters and schools are opened because hospitals can accept no additional patients. The National Guard, the Centers for Disease Control, and the U.S. Department of Homeland Security, which includes a number of formerly independent emergency agencies, are all providing support. Again, you must work an additional shift. This is the fourth extra shift in a row. Now, federal resources are beginning to have an effect. Instead of your needing to provide constant out-of-area transfers of critical patients, National Guard planes are transporting critical patients to hospitals across the nation. You are assigned to an aid station located in an outlying area of the city. However, additional supplies of antibiotics are delayed; 3,300 are sick and over 850 have died.

Day 8: Today finally brings the arrival of federal supplies of antibiotics and the establishment of 50 additional distribution areas. You grab a few hours of sleep on a cot and are back at work early in the morning at the aid station. The National Guard maintains order at the distribution centers. Handling the corpses becomes an ever-increasing problem. Refrigerated trucks are used for a makeshift morgue. By midnight of the eighth day, 4,300 patients are sick and 1,700 people have died.

Day 9: Large numbers of critical city workers are absent. Police, firefighters, transportation workers, sewer and water officials, and retail staff at key businesses are out. Of course, EMS services are also short-handed. Schools and universities are closed. Looting in the city's center has begun, held somewhat in check by the would-be looters' fear of being out where they might catch the disease. By midnight of the ninth day 5,000 persons are ill and 2,500 have died.

Day 10: A total of 20,000 persons have become ill and 4,000 have died. By the end of the day, some officials think that the number of new illnesses and deaths are beginning to decrease.

Players

The exercise takes an hour. During that time, players will simulate a conference call, in real time, that occurs at 6:00 P.M. on Day 6. The following players are assembled on the conference call to plan immediate actions.

Mayor
County Commission Chairperson
Local Health Department Director
Local Police Chief
Local Congressman
Local Hospital Official

Sheriff
EMS Chief
Fire Chief
State Emergency Management Director
Governor
State Health Department Director
National Guard Commandant
Federal Emergency Management Director
Director of Public Health Service
State Senate President
Regional FBI Chief
Director of CDC

Initiating the Exercise

The meeting is chaired by the Governor. Each player is asked to carefully read the scenario and take a few minutes to prepare a list of needs based on the scenario and the position he or she has assumed. The Governor is asked to develop an agenda for the one-hour meeting based on the information supplied and to control and guide the conversation.

There is no one best solution to this scenario; rather, there are multiple solutions. Solutions that are reached by doing this exercise demands conversation, debate, and compromise. Set the clock for one hour and let the conversation begin.

ASSIGNMENTS

Assign students to read Chapter 43, "Advanced Airway Management," before the next class. Also ask them to complete Chapter 42 of the Workbook.

EVALUATION

Chapter Quiz Distribute copies of the Chapter Quiz provided in Handout 42-2 to evaluate student understanding of this chapter. Remind students not to refer to their textbooks or notes while taking the quiz.

Test Manager You may wish to create a custom-tailored test using Prentice Hall *TestGen for Prehospital Emergency Care, Eighth Edition* to evaluate student understanding of this chapter.

Online Test Preparation (for students and instructors) Additional test preparation is available through *EMT Achieve: Basic Test Preparation* at http://www.prenhall.com/EMTAchieve. Instructors can also monitor student mastery online.

REINFORCEMENT

Handouts If classroom discussions or performance on the quiz indicates that some students have not fully mastered the chapter content, you may wish to assign some or all of the Reinforcement Handouts for this chapter.

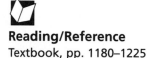

Reading/Reference
Textbook, pp. 1180–1225

Workbook
Chapter 42 Activities

Chapter Quiz
Handout 42-2

TestGen
Chapter 42 Test

Online Test Preparation
Send your students to
http://www.prenhall.com/
EMTAchieve

Handouts 42-3 to 42-5
Reinforcement Activities

TECH EXTRAS

Brady Skills Series EMT-B Videos/CD Have your students watch the skills come to life on either VHS or CD-ROM.

PowerPoint Presentation (for instructors) The PowerPoint material developed for this chapter offers useful reinforcement of chapter content.

Student CD A wide variety of material on this CD-ROM will reinforce and also expand student knowledge and skills.

Companion Website (for students) Additional review quizzes and links to EMS resources will contribute to further reinforcement of this chapter. Please visit http://www.prenhall.com/mistovich.

Brady Skills Series EMT-B Videos/CD
Visual Reinforcement

PowerPoint Presentation
Chapter 42

Student CD
Chapter 42

Companion Website
http://www.prenhall.com/mistovich

OBJECTIVES

OBJECTIVES CHECKLIST

Cognitive	Date Mastered
* Define weapons of mass destruction.	
* Discuss the role of EMS, particularly the role of the EMT-Basic, in response to a weapons of mass destruction attack.	
* Describe the primary, secondary, and tertiary effects of an explosive detonation.	
* Describe the characteristics of and the signs and symptoms and emergency medical care for the following chemical agents: nerve agents, vesicants, cyanide, pulmonary agents, riot-control agents, and industrial chemicals.	
* List agents and specific findings for the following types of biological agents and emergency medical care for biological agents: pneumonia-like agents, encephalitis-like agents, biological toxins, and other biological agents.	
* Discuss the types of radiation (x-ray and gamma, neutron, beta, and alpha), types of radiation exposure (primary and fallout), types of radiation injuries, assessment, and medical care for radiation injuries.	
* Describe appropriate personal protection and patient decontamination for chemical, biological, and nuclear weapons exposure.	

©2008 by Pearson Education, Inc.
Prehospital Emergency Care, 8th ed.

CHAPTER 42 QUIZ

Write the letter of the best answer in the space provided.

_____ **1.** A simple way to remember the types of WMD is to
  A. memorize the many types.   **C.** carry the CDC guide with you.
  B. use a mnemonic such as CBRNE.   **D.** call medical direction.

_____ **2.** Responding to a WMD incident requires
  A. special response strategies.
  B. special protective equipment.
  C. the same strategy and tactics used on other calls.
  D. permission from law enforcement officials.

_____ **3.** An example of a secondary injury from a WMD event would be
  A. being hit by flying debris.
  B. the blast from a bomb.
  C. hitting an object after being blown into the air.
  D. the psychological effect of the event.

_____ **4.** When responding to a WMD event which is most important?
  A. removing the patient first
  B. putting on protective equipment
  C. calling dispatch
  D. identifying the type and cause of the event

_____ **5.** Which is the most acceptable method of protecting yourself from respiratory exposure?
  A. Stay away from the exposure.   **C.** Use a HEPA or N-95 mask.
  B. Put a mask on all patients.   **D.** Use SCBA.

_____ **6.** Which is *not* one of the three initial roles of an EMT at a WMD incident?
  A. Establish and EMS Incident Command.
  B. Assume a triage leader position.
  C. Take a unit position.
  D. Become the staging officer.

_____ **7.** Nerve agents work by
  A. disrupting an enzyme at the nerve endings.
  B. killing the nerve cells.
  C. causing skin destruction.
  D. confusing the patient.

_____ **8.** A vesicant is an agent that affects the
  A. nerves.   **C.** skin, lungs, and eyes.
  B. gastrointestinal system.   **D.** brain.

_____ **9.** Cyanide causes deadly effects by
   A. paralyzing the victim.
   B. hyperthermia.

   C. removing Acth.
   D. disrupting cellular oxygen use.

_____ **10.** A radiation-enhanced weapon is one that
   A. contains only gamma radiation.
   B. uses biological material.

   C. is known as a "dirty bomb."
   D. poses no threat to the responder.

IN THE FIELD

Read the following real-life situation. Then answer the questions that follow.

You are dispatched to an incoming aircraft at the airport that has been diverted to your community after declaring an in-flight emergency. The only information from the flight crew is "there are many people having difficulty breathing and vomiting." Upon arrival you determine there are 123 passengers and 6 flight crew.

1. Your first actions (after protecting yourself) should include establishing a scene management system. How would you accomplish this?

2. You suspect a biological agent of some type. What public agencies could help you identify the causative agent?

3. This is an international flight and you gain information on a pandemic flu virus raging in the country where the flight originated. What action might you consider in isolating the plane and passengers?

4. What personal protective measures could you employ in this event?

CHAPTER 42 REVIEW

Write the word or words that best complete each sentence in the space provided.

1. As always your personal safety is your _____ when responding to a WMD incident.

2. A thorough knowledge of the _____ system will assist a responder with organizing the scene of a WMD event.

3. The effects from an explosion include primary, _____, and tertiary injuries.

4. Agents such as sulfur and nitrogen mustards, lewisite, and phosgene oxime are examples of _____.

5. Pulmonary agents act primarily to cause _____ injury and are commonly referred to as "choking" agents.

6. Anthrax is an example of a _____-like agent.

7. Botulinum toxin exposure leads to progressive paralysis eventually leading to _____ failure and death.

8. The three primary mechanisms of death associated with nuclear detonation are _____, _____, and _____.

9. Alpha radiation can be stopped by _____ and the outer layer of skin.

10. When approaching a WMD incident always approach from _____.

EMS RESPONSE TO WEAPONS
OF MASS DESTRUCTION: LISTING

1. List the types of WMD events in the mnemonic CBRNE.

2. List the three possible roles of the EMT at a WMD incident.

3. List six types of chemical WMD agents.

4. List the five types of nuclear radiation.

EMS Response to Weapons of Mass Destruction

Weapons of Mass Destruction (WMD)

Prehospital Response to WMD

Supplies and Equipment

Medical Direction

Provider Preparation

Responding to the Scene

Issues of Scene Safety

Role of the EMT at the WMD Incident

Conventional Weapons and Incendiary Devices

Explosives

Primary, Secondary, and Tertiary Effects

Body Position

Types of Injuries

Incendiary Devices

Chemical Agents

Properties of Chemical Weapons

Types of Chemical Agents

- Nerve agents
- Vesicants
- Cyanide
- Pulmonary agents
- Riot-control agents
- Industrial chemicals

Biological Agents

Specific Biological Agents

- Pneumonia-like agents
- Encephalitis-like agents
- Biological toxins
- Other agents

Emergency Medical Care
for Biological Agents

Nuclear Weapons and Radiation

Radiation

- Radiation exposure

Blast Injuries

Thermal Burns

Radiation-Enhanced Weapons

Assessment and Care for Nuclear
Detonation and Radiation
Injuries

- Assessment
- Emergency medical care

Personal Protection and Patient Decontamination

HANDOUT 42-2: Chapter 42 Quiz

1. B	4. D	7. A	9. D
2. C	5. C	8. C	10. C
3. A	6. D		

HANDOUT 42-3: In the Field

1. First-in crews establish the Incident Command System (ICS) by declaring the event, setting up a command post, and directing resources to accomplish the mission. Additional training in ICS is recommended, and you should check with your local response agencies to determine response procedures established under mutual aid.

2. The local health department, law enforcement, fire rescue, and the local hospital will assist initially and bring in other more regional groups such as the CDC, the Coast Guard, FEMA, and the FBI.

3. Isolate the aircraft and passengers by creating a "hot zone" with marking tape. Use law enforcement to assist in crowd control and wait until public health can evaluate the situation. If you were to allow the passengers to disperse or be transported to ill-equipped facilities, spread of the disease could be catastrophic.

4. Use of standard protective equipment such as gloves, masks, and distance from the victims will be the most effective. Do not expose yourself or other response personnel needlessly to this situation. Distance and shielding is the most effective way to manage this event.

HANDOUT 42-4: Chapter 42 Review

1. primary responsibility
2. Incident Command
3. secondary
4. vesicants
5. lung
6. pneumonia
7. respiratory
8. radiation, blast, thermal
9. clothing
10. upwind

HANDOUT 42-5: EMS Response to Weapons of Mass Destruction: Listing

1. Biological, nuclear, incendiary, chemical, and explosive
2. Establish Incident Command, Unit leader, Care provider
3. Nerve agents, vesicants, cyanide, pulmonary agents, riot-control agents, industrial chemicals
4. X-ray, neutron, gamma, beta, alpha

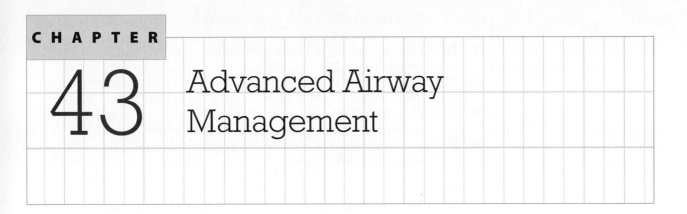

CHAPTER

43 | Advanced Airway Management

This chapter covers Lesson 8-1 and 8-2 of the U.S. Department of Transportation's EMT-Basic National Standard Curriculum.

OBJECTIVES

Numbered objectives are from the U.S. Department of Transportation's EMT-Basic National Standard Curriculum. Asterisked objectives, if any, pertain to material that is supplemental to the DOT curriculum. Page numbers refer to pages in the textbook.

Cognitive

8-1.1 Identify and describe the airway anatomy in the infant, child, and adult. (pp. 1182–1185)

8-1.2 Differentiate between the anatomy in the infant, child, and adult. (pp. 1184–1185)

8-1.3 Explain the pathophysiology of airway compromise. (pp. 1182–1186)

8-1.4 Describe the proper use of airway adjuncts. (p. 1186)

8-1.5 Review the use of oxygen therapy in airway management. (pp. 1185, 1186, 1187, 1192, 1198, 1199, 1202, 1203, 1207, 1215, 1218, 1220)

8-1.6 Describe the indications, contraindications, and technique for insertion of nasal gastric tubes. (pp. 1204–1206)

8-1.7 Describe how to perform the Sellick maneuver (cricoid pressure). (pp. 1191–1192)

8-1.8 Describe the indications for advanced airway management. (pp. 1186–1187)

8-1.9 List the equipment required for orotracheal intubation. (pp. 1187–1191)

8-1.10 Describe the proper use of the curved blade for orotracheal intubation. (p. 1188)

8-1.11 Describe the proper use of the straight blade for orotracheal intubation. (p. 1188)

8-1.12 State the reasons for and proper use of the stylet in orotracheal intubation. (pp. 1190–1191)

8-1.13 Describe the methods of choosing the appropriate size endotracheal tube in an adult patient. (pp. 1189–1190)

8-1.14 State the formula for sizing an infant or a child endotracheal tube. (pp. 1200–1201)

8-1.15 List complications associated with advanced airway management. (pp. 1198–1199)

8-1.16 Define the various alternative methods for sizing the infant and child endotracheal tube. (pp. 1201–1202)

Total Teaching Time
360 minutes

Resources Needed
- Scored Chapter 42 Quizzes
- Adult intubation model
- Laryngoscopes with a complete set of curved and straight blades of all sizes
- Tracheal tubes of all sizes
- Infant intubation model
- Two health professionals skilled in intubation to serve as teaching assistants

Additional Resources
Larmon/Davis, *Basic Life Support Skills*

Elling, *EMT Achieve: Basic Test Preparation*

Limmer/Mistovich/O'Keefe, *Audio Lecture & Study Guide: EMT*

Mistovich/Kuvlesky, *SUCCESS! for the EMT, Second Edition*

8-1.17 Describe the skill of orotracheal intubation in the adult patient. (pp. 1192–1198)

8-1.18 Describe the skill of orotracheal intubation in the infant and child patient. (pp. 1202–1203)

8-1.19 Describe the skill of confirming endotracheal tube placement in the adult, infant, and child patient. (pp. 1196–1198, 1202–1203)

8-1.20 State the consequence of and the need to recognize unintentional esophageal intubation. (pp. 1186, 1196, 1199)

8-1.21 Describe the skill of securing the endotracheal tube in the adult, infant, and child patient. (pp. 1198, 1203)

Affective

8-1.22 Recognize and respect the feelings of the patient and family during advanced airway procedures. (p. 1186)

8-1.23 Explain the value of performing advanced airway procedures. (pp. 1180, 1182, 1187, 1199)

8-1.24 Defend the need for the EMT-Basic to perform advanced airway procedures. (p. 1180)

8-1.25 Explain the rationale for the use of a stylet. (pp. 1180–1181)

8-1.26 Explain the rationale for having a suction unit immediately available during intubation attempts. (pp. 1191, 1199)

8-1.27 Explain the rationale for confirming breath sounds. (pp. 1196, 1203)

8-1.28 Explain the rationale for securing the endotracheal tube. (pp. 1198, 1203)

Psychomotor

8-1.29 Demonstrate how to perform the Sellick maneuver (cricoid pressure).

8-1.30 Demonstrate the skill of orotracheal intubation in the adult patient.

8-1.31 Demonstrate the skill of orotracheal intubation in the infant and child patient.

8-1.32 Demonstrate the skill of confirming endotracheal tube placement in the adult patient.

8-1.33 Demonstrate the skill of confirming endotracheal tube placement in the infant and child patient.

8-1.34 Demonstrate the skill of securing the endotracheal tube in the adult patient.

8-1.35 Demonstrate the skill of securing the endotracheal tube in the infant and child patient.

REVIEW

In the last lesson, "EMS Response to Weapons of Mass Destruction," students learned about the role of EMS in response to a weapons of mass destruction attack. They were introduced to the most widely used WMD, the effects of the various devices, and necessary treatments. They also learned that they should know and practice the "all-hazards approach" developed by their own area's disaster agencies. Distribute the quizzes from the last class. Go over each question on the quiz and handle any concerns students may have about the answers.

IINTRODUCTION TO MODULE 8/CHAPTER 43

Remind students that in Module 2 they learned that the airway is the first priority in treating every patient. Of all the skills students will learn in this course, and subsequently use on real patients in the field, airway management is the most important. Simply stated, patients without an

©2008 by Pearson Education, Inc.
Prehospital Emergency Care, 8th ed.

adequate airway die. No matter how good the care the EMT may render to a critically ill or injured patient, if the EMT cannot adequately clear and maintain that patient's airway, everything else he or she has done will be wasted because the patient will not be able to survive. In Module 2, students learned basic airway management skills. Module 8, Chapter 43, "Advanced Airway Management," goes beyond those basic skills. There are some situations in which manual maneuvers and basic airway adjuncts are not adequate to maintain or possibly even to establish an airway. In those situations, the use of advanced airway adjuncts is necessary. In the past, performance of advanced airway procedures was reserved for ALS personnel. However, it is the EMT who is usually first on the scene, and the time required for ALS backup to arrive and initiate advanced airway care could often spell the difference between life and death for the patient. For this reason, advanced airway skills are now included as an elective in the EMT curriculum—to be required of EMTs at the discretion of the medical director. If required in the students' jurisdictions, they will find learning and maintaining these skills to be challenging but, because learning the skills unquestionably offers the opportunity to save lives, well worth the effort.

Distribute the Chapter 43 Objectives Checklist, and give students a few minutes to look it over. Then briefly paraphrase the objectives for this lesson in your own words.

Handout 43-1
Chapter 43 Objectives
Checklist

Lecture Master
You may wish to display Lecture Master 43 when presenting the lecture to the class.

LECTURE

The following suggested lecture outline is based on the Department of Transportation's EMT-Basic National Standard Curriculum. In some places, the DOT curriculum has been rearranged or expanded upon so that it is more complete or easier for the student to understand. The page numbers in parentheses refer to pages in the textbook. The parenthetical references in dark, heavy type are to figures, tables, and scans in the textbook.

ADVANCED AIRWAY MANAGEMENT

I. **Airway and respiratory anatomy and physiology** (pp. 1182–1185) (You may also wish to have students review material on airway anatomy and physiology in Chapter 4, "The Human Body"; Chapter 7, "Airway Management, Ventilation, and Oxygen Therapy"; and Chapter 13, "Respiratory Emergencies.")
   A. Airway anatomy (pp. 1182–1184)
      1. Nose, mouth, and pharynx
         a. Oropharynx
         b. Nasopharynx
      2. Larynx (voice box)
         a. Contains the vocal cords
         b. Thyroid cartilage
            (1) Bulky, shield-like structure (Adam's apple) in anterior portion of neck
         c. Cricoid cartilage
            (1) Firm circle of cartilage below thyroid cartilage
         d. Epiglottis
            (1) Leaf-shaped cartilaginous structure that covers opening of larynx during swallowing (**Fig. 43-1, p. 1183**)
         e. Vallecula
            (1) Depression between base of tongue and epiglottis
         f. Glossoepiglottic ligament

            (1) Ligament in center of vallecula that helps support and suspend epiglottis
        g. True vocal cords
            (1) Can close the glottic opening, preventing air and foreign bodies from entering trachea
        h. Glottis (glottic opening)
            (1) Space between true vocal cords and glottis **(Fig. 43-2, p. 1183)**
        i. False vocal cords
            (1) Can close the glottic opening, preventing air and foreign bodies from entering trachea; lie above true vocal cords
        j. Arytenoids
            (1) Irregular pyramid-shaped paired cartilages located on top of posterior aspect of cricoid ring
        k. Corniculates
            (1) Cone-shaped paired cartilages attached to top of arytenoids
        l. Cuneiforms
            (1) Elongated paired cartilages attached to posterior arytenoids
    3. Trachea and bronchi
        a. Trachea
            (1) Extends from lower portion of larynx to the bronchi
        b. Trachealis muscle
            (1) Muscular wall that closes the trachea's C-shaped cartilage rings
        c. Mainstem bronchi
            (1) Main bronchi that split right and left from the trachea at fifth thoracic vertebra
        d. Carina
            (1) Point where the mainstem bronchi split from the trachea and enter the lungs
        e. Bronchioles
            (1) Small bronchial passages
    4. Lungs (To review the mechanics and physiology of respiration, refer to Chapter 4, "The Human Body" and Chapter 7, "Airway Management, Ventilation, and Oxygen Therapy.")
B. Airway anatomy in infants and children (pp. 1184–1185)
    1. Head
        a. Child's head is larger in proportion to body than an adult's.
        b. Placing padding under the head of children younger than 9 years old may cause airflow obstruction.
        c. Place small folded towel under shoulders of infants and young children to keep airway aligned and ensure airflow.
    2. Mouth, nose, and pharynx
        a. All these structures smaller and more pliable than adult's
        b. Infant basically a nose breather during much of first year
        c. Most common cause of airway obstruction is tongue falling back and blocking pharynx

3. Larynx (cricoid cartilage)
  a. Cricoid cartilage narrowest area in infants and children
  b. Cricoid cartilage less developed and less rigid than adult's
  c. Pressure on cricoid and overextension or overflexion of neck can cause obstruction.
  d. Endotracheal tube should be one-half size larger and smaller than the one estimated as correctly sized.
4. Trachea (windpipe) and bronchi
  a. These are narrower and shorter in infants and children.
  b. Trachea is softer and more flexible, so airway is more easily occluded by swelling or other obstruction.
  c. Small movements of head and neck may cause endotracheal tube to advance into right mainstem bronchus or out of glottis.
5. Chest wall and diaphragm
  a. Chest wall is softer; infants and children rely more heavily than adults on diaphragm for breathing.

II. Basic airway management (pp. 1185–1186)
  A. Assessing for adequate and inadequate breathing (To review assessment methods and basic methods of establishing and maintaining an airway, refer to Chapter 7, "Airway Management, Ventilation, and Oxygen Therapy.") (p. 1185)
  B. Establishing and maintaining an airway (pp. 1185–1186)
  C. Conditions where immediate use of advanced airway technique is necessary (p. 1186)
    1. Upper airway burns
    2. Anaphylaxis
  D. Reasons for using advanced airway management (p. 1186)
    1. Protecting patient from aspirating secretions, blood, or vomitus.
    2. Need for prolonged ventilation
    3. Basic airway techniques inadequate
  E. Oropharyngeal suctioning (p. 1186) (To review oropharyngeal suctioning, refer to Chapter 7, "Airway Management, Ventilation, and Oxygen Therapy.")

III. Orotracheal intubation (pp. 1186–1199)
  A. Orotracheal intubation (p. 1186)
    1. Insertion of tube through mouth and along oropharynx and larynx directly into trachea
  B. Tracheal (or endotracheal) tube (p. 1186)
    1. Tube used for orotracheal intubation
    2. Named because distal end is designed to be placed in trachea
  C. Laryngoscope (p. 186)
    1. Lighted device that allows visualization of the endotracheal tube as it enters and passes through the vocal cords
  D. Advantages (pp. 1186–1187)
    1. Provides complete control of airway
    2. Eliminates the risk of aspiration of material into lower airways and lungs
    3. Permits better ventilation and oxygen delivery
    4. Allows the passage of a suction catheter
    5. With positive-pressure ventilation, can overcome both mechanical and physiological problems that compromise normal ventilation

On the Net
Emergency airway management. http://www.rashad university.com/airandemairm.html

Slides/Videos
Brady Skill Series: EMT-B, "Suctioning through an Endotracheal Tube" "Nasogastric (NG) Tube" "Ventilatory Management—Assist with Endotracheal Intubation" "Ventilatory Management—Combitube" "Using a Pulse Oximeter"

Teaching Tip
Have students practice manual airway maneuvers on each other to get the feel of opening a human airway. Have them practice stabilizing the head and neck, and using the jaw thrust to simultaneously open the airway.

On the Net
Endotracheal intubation. http://www.capanes.com/General/intubation.htm

E. Indications (p. 1187)
  1. Inability to ventilate the apneic patient effectively with standard methods
  2. Patient cannot protect his or her own airway.
    a. Is unresponsive to any type of stimulus
    b. Has no gag reflex or loses the cough reflex
F. Body substance isolation (p. 1187)
G. Equipment (pp. 1187–1191)
  1. Laryngoscope
    a. Straight blade (**Figs. 43-3 and 43-4a, pp. 1188–1189**)
    b. Curved blade (**Figs. 43-3 and 43-4b, pp. 1188–1189**)
    c. Alternative blades
    d. Assembly
  2. Tracheal tubes (**Figs. 43-5 and 43-6, pp. 1189–1190**)
    a. Sizes
      (1) Adult male
        (a) 8.0–8.5 mm i.d.
      (2) Adult female
        (a) 7.0–8.00 mm i.d.
      (3) Emergency rule
        (a) 7.5 fits an adult in an emergency
      (4) Helpful to have one tube larger and one tube smaller than estimated available
    b. Components
      (1) 15 mm adapter
      (2) Pilot balloon
      (3) Cuff
      (4) Murphy eye
      (5) Length of tube for adults—33 cm
  3. Stylet (**Fig. 43-7, p. 1190**)
  4. Other intubation equipment
    a. Water-soluble lubricant (not petroleum-based lubricant)
    b. 10 cc syringe for cuff inflation
    c. Devices to secure properly positioned tube
    d. Oral airway or bite block
    e. Suction unit
    f. Large-bore and flexible French catheters
    g. Towels
H. Sellick's maneuver (cricoid pressure) (pp. 1191–1192) (**Fig. 43-8, p. 1192**)
  1. Advantages of maneuver
  2. Locating the cricoid cartilage
  3. Performing the maneuver
  4. Cautions
I. Tracheal tube insertion in an adult (pp. 1192–1198) (**Fig. 43-9, p. 1192**)
  1. Body substance isolation precautions
  2. Prior to any intubation attempt, the patient must be adequately ventilated with a bag-valve-mask device and supplemental oxygen
  3. Hyperoxygenate the patient for at least 1–2 minutes before the intubation attempt
  4. Gather the necessary equipment
  5. Position yourself at the patient's head
  6. Have a suction unit ready
  7. Position the patient's head

©2008 by Pearson Education, Inc.
Prehospital Emergency Care, 8th ed.

8. Stop ventilation and remove the oropharyngeal airway if one has been used.
   a. Ventilation must not be interrupted for more than 30 seconds while intubating
   b. If you cannot intubate within 30 seconds, stop the procedure and immediately resume hyperventilating the patient
   c. After a few minutes of hyperventilation, try again to intubate
9. Can use Sellick's maneuver (cricoid pressure) or BURP maneuver (thyroid pressure) to aid in visualization and prevent regurgitation
10. Hold the laryngoscope in your left hand and insert the blade into the right corner of the mouth, sweeping the tongue
11. Identify the glottic opening
12. Insert the tracheal tube through the right side of the mouth and guide through the vocal cords until the proximal end of the cuff is advanced about one-half to one inch beyond the vocal cords. Typically, the tube marker will be at about 19–23 cm at the level of the teeth.
13. Remove the laryngoscope blade and fold the blade down so that it is parallel with the handle
14. Hold the tube firmly at all times until it is properly secured in place
15. If a stylet was used, remove it gently by pulling it out in the direction it was inserted
16. With the syringe attached to the inflation port, inflate the cuff by injecting 10 cc of air. Remove the syringe when you have completed inflation so that the cuff does not deflate.
17. Have your partner attach the bag-valve device to the tracheal tube and begin to deliver positive-pressure ventilation.
18. Confirm correct tube placement
    a. Auscultate over the epigastrium
    b. Auscultate breath sounds
    c. End-tidal carbon dioxide detector (ETCO$_2$) (**Fig. 43-10, p. 1197**)
    d. Esophageal detection device (EDD) (**Fig. 43-11, p. 1197**)
    e. Exhaled condensation
19. Indications of improperly placed tube
    a. Inability to visualize the tracheal tube passing into the glottic opening
    b. Presence of air passing into the stomach with ventilation, as heard upon auscultation
    c. Lack of carbon dioxide when an end-tidal carbon dioxide tester is used
    d. Inability to rapidly aspirate air when using an esophageal detector device
    e. Absence of bilateral breath sounds upon auscultation, or unilateral breath sounds.
20. Indications of displaced tube
    a. A sudden drop in pulse oximeter reading
    b. Patient deteriorates rapidly, becomes combative, or begins to exhibit cyanosis
21. Secure with a commercial securing device that has been approved by medical direction

Point to Emphasize
Unrecognized placement of the tube in the esophagus rather than the trachea will rapidly result in death.

Point to Emphasize
The EMT should make only two attempts at orotracheal intubation. If both attempts fail, insert an oral airway, continue to ventilate the patient with high-concentration oxygen via the bag-valve mask, and aggressively suction the airway.

Point to Emphasize
Due to the seriousness of complications, if you are in doubt of proper tube placement, immediately withdraw the tube and manage the airway with basic airway adjuncts.

22. Once the tube has been secured, you should
   a. Ventilate the patient at the appropriate rate based on his age.
   b. Note the centimeter marking on the tracheal tube at the level of the teeth. This should be included in your written documentation.
   c. Insert an oral airway or other appropriate device to serve as a bite block.
23. Reassess breath sounds as often as possible

J. Complications (pp. 1198–1199)
   1. Adult patient not in cardiac arrest
      a. Hypertension, tachycardia, dysrhythmias
   2. Infants and children and some adults
      a. Bradycardia, hypotension
   3. Trauma to lips, tongue, gums, teeth, and airway
   4. Prolonged attempts at intubation
      a. Inadequate oxygenation and severe hypoxia
   5. Right mainstem intubation
      a. Hypoxia
   6. Misplacement of tracheal tube in esophagus
      a. Absence of ventilation or oxygenation
      b. Assessing proper placement with end-tidal carbon dioxide detector (**Fig 43-10a, p. 1197**)
      c. Assessing proper placement with syringe-type esophageal intubation (**Fig. 43-11, p. 1197**)
   7. Stimulation of gag reflex
      a. Vomiting
   8. Stimulation of epiglottis or vocal cords
      a. Laryngospasm
   9. Leaking cuff
   10. Accidental extubation
   11. Patient may extubate self

IV. **Orotracheal intubation in infants and children** (pp. 1199–1203)
   A. Indications in infants and children (p. 1199)
      1. Prolonged positive-pressure ventilation is required.
      2. Artificial ventilation cannot be delivered adequately.
      3. Clearly apneic patient
      4. Unresponsive patient with no gag reflex or cough
   B. Anatomical considerations (pp. 1199–1200)
      1. Smaller nose, mouth, and disproportionately larger tongue (make visualization of glottic opening and vocal cords difficult)
      2. Narrow cricoid cartilage (sizing based on internal diameter of cricoid cartilage, not glottic opening)
      3. Vocal cords and glottic opening more anterior and cephalad (make visualization difficult)
      4. Extreme sensitivity to hypoxia (stimulation of airway may cause bradycardia)
   C. Equipment for infants and children (pp. 1200–1202) (**Fig. 43-12, p. 1200**)
      1. Laryngoscope handles and blades
         a. Straight blade
         b. Curved blade
      2. Tracheal tubes (**Fig 43-13, p. 1201; Tables 43-1 and 43-2, pp. 1201–1202**)

Teaching Tip
Bring in a Broselow™ tape to demonstrate how to estimate tube size based on the height of a pediatric patient.

©2008 by Pearson Education, Inc.
Prehospital Emergency Care, 8th ed.

D. Tracheal tube insertion in an infant or a child
    1. Refer to procedure for adults.
    2. Plus follow special considerations:
        a. Hyperventilate at age-appropriate rate.
        b. Continuously monitor heart.
        c. Align axes of mouth, pharynx, and trachea to achieve better visualization of glottic opening.
        d. Be very gentle; never use force.
        e. Know that epiglottis may obstruct your view when using a straight blade.
        f. Apply Sellick's maneuver during intubation to reduce risk of vomiting.
        g. Insert uncuffed tube until glottic marker is at level of vocal cords.
        h. Insert cuffed tube until proximal end of cuff is about one-half inch beyond vocal cords.
        i. Hold tracheal tube in place until properly secured.
        j. Insert oropharyngeal airway as bite block.
        k. Confirm tube placement using methods described for adults.
        l. Know that heart rate and skin color should improve after proper tube placement.
        m. Note centimeter marker at level of patient's teeth or gums when tube is properly positioned.
        n. Immobilize patient's head after placement is confirmed and tube is secured.
        o. If tube is properly placed but inadequate lung expansion or tidal volume is noted, assess for one of the following causes:
            (1) Tube too small and there is an air leak around cricoid cartilage
            (2) Pop-off valve on bag-valve device is not deactivated, and air is escaping with ventilation.
            (3) Bag-valve device has leak or is not functioning properly.
            (4) EMT delivering ventilation not delivering adequate volume with each squeeze
            (5) Tube has become blocked with secretions or has kinked.
        p. Excessive ventilation force and/or volume can cause lung rupture and pneumothorax; as soon as chest rises adequately, cease ventilation

V. Nasogastric intubation in infants and children (pp. 1204–1206)
    A. Indications (p. 1204)
        1. Inability to artificially ventilate due to gastric distension
        2. Unresponsive patient
    B. Contraindications (p. 1204)
        1. Major facial, head, or spinal trauma
        2. Suspected airway disease such as epiglottitis or croup
        3. Patient has ingested certain caustic substances (alkalis) and some hydrocarbons.
    C. Equipment (p. 1204)
        1. NG tubes, assorted sizes **(Fig. 43-14, p. 1204)**
            a. Newborn/infant—8.0 French
            b. Toddler/preschooler—10.0 French
            c. School age—12 French
            d. Adolescent—14–16 French

Point to Emphasize
Because of the risk of cranial intubation with the NG tube, the presence of major facial trauma or head trauma is considered a contraindication for the nasogastric tube.

    2. 20 cc syringe to check tube placement

    3. Water-soluble lubricant

    4. Emesis basin

    5. Tape to secure tube

    6. Stethoscope

    7. Suction unit and suction catheters

  D. Insertion (pp. 1204–1206) **(Fig. 43-15, pp. 1205–1206)**

    1. Prepare and assemble equipment.

    2. Measure tube from tip of nose, around ear, to below xiphoid process.

    3. Lubricate distal end of tube.

    4. If trauma not suspected, place patient supine, with head turned to left side

    5. Pass tube along nasal floor.

    6. Check placement of tube.

      a. Aspirating stomach contents

      b. Auscultation over epigastrum while injecting 10–20 cc's of air into tube.

    7. Aspirate stomach contents and irrigate, if needed.

    8. Secure tube in place.

  E. Complications (p. 1206)

    1. Tracheal intubation

    2. Nasal trauma

    3. Vomiting

    4. Passage of tube into cranium if basilar skull fracture exists (very rare)

    5. Tube becoming curled in nose, mouth, or trachea

    6. Perforation of esophagus

VI. Orotracheal suctioning (pp. 1206–1209)

  A. Orotracheal suctioning (p. 1206)

    1. Process in which long, soft suction catheter is inserted through tracheal tube to clear secretions

  B. Indications (p. 1206)

    1. Obvious secretions

    2. Poor compliance with bag-valve device

  C. Suctioning technique (pp. 1207–1207) **(Fig. 43-16, pp. 1207–1208)**

    1. Preoxygenate patient.

    2. Hyperventilate patient.

    3. Check equipment; use sterile technique.

    4. Insert catheter without suction.

    5. Advance catheter to desired location.

    6. Apply suction and withdraw catheter in twisting motion.

  D. Complications (pp. 1208–1209)

    1. Hypoxia

    2. Cardiac dysrhythmias

    3. Coughing

    4. Mucosa damage leading to tracheal infections

    5. Bronchospasms

ENRICHMENT (OPTIONAL)

The following sections contain information that is valuable as background for the EMT, but that goes substantially beyond the U.S. Department of Transportation's EMT-Basic National Standard Curriculum.

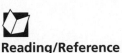

Reading/Reference
Anderson, R., "Digital and Nasal Endotracheal Intubation," *EMS Magazine,* Aug. 2002.

Reading/Reference
Fowler, "King LT-D to the Rescue," *JEMS,* July 2005.

CASE STUDY FOLLOW-UP

Ask a student volunteer to read the Case Study that begins on page 1182 of the textbook. You may wish to use the following questions to engage the students in a discussion of the Case Study Follow-up that begins on page 1222 of the textbook. Provide missing information and clarify ideas as needed.

Q1. Why do you elect to perform tracheal intubation?

A1. *Because of the evidence of an upper airway burn and your partner is having difficulty ventilating the patient with the BVM.*

Q2. What do you ask your partner to do while you prepare the equipment?

A2. *Hyperventilate the patient.*

Q3. Describe how you insert the tracheal tube.

A3. *The laryngoscopy is performed and the swelling to the upper airway is noted. When the glottic opening is visualized, the tracheal tube is inserted between the vocal cords. The cuff is inflated with 10 cc of air and the tube held securely as the bag-valve device is attached to the 15 mm adapter on the proximal end of the tracheal tube.*

Q4. After the tube is inserted, what do you do?

A4. *One EMT ventilates as the other inspects the chest for equal rise and fall and listens for gurgling over the epigastrium. There is no gurgling, so ventilation continues as an EMT auscultates over the apices and bases of both lungs. The breath sounds are equal bilaterally. An end-tidal CO_2 detector is attached and indicates adequate CO_2 levels after six ventilations. The tube is then taped securely in place, noting that the 22 cm marker is at the level of the teeth.*

Q5. Prior to transport, as you reassess the patient, you notice the tube has moved to the 26 cm marker at the level of the teeth. What do you do?

A5. *Auscultate the breath sounds and note that the sounds on the left are significantly diminished compared to the right. The tape securing the tube is removed and the cuff deflated using the 10 cc syringe. The tube is drawn back while auscultating breath sounds on the left until good breath sounds are heard. Pulling on the tube is stopped and breath sounds assessed on both sides. They are now equal bilaterally. The cuff is reinflated with 10 cc of air and the tube resecured with tape.*

IN REVIEW

Assess students' ability to apply what they have just learned by discussing the Review Questions on page 1225 in the textbook.

Q1. List the indications for performing tracheal intubation in the adult.

A1. *The indications for performing tracheal intubation in the adult include inability to ventilate the apneic patient; patient who is unresponsive to any stimuli; patient who has no gag or cough reflex. (p. 1187)*

Q2. Describe and contrast the use of straight and curved laryngoscope blades in tracheal intubation.

A2. *The straight laryngoscope blade is inserted under the epiglottis and directly lifts it to expose the vocal cords and the glottic opening. The curved blade is inserted into the vallecula and indirectly lifts the epiglottis. (pp. 1188–1189)*

Q3. Explain the following: (a) how to locate the cricoid cartilage, (b) how to perform Sellick's maneuver, and (c) reasons for using Sellick's maneuver.

A3. *(a) To locate the cricoid cartilage, palpate the thyroid cartilage with the tip of a finger until you find a depression at the inferior edge. Immediately inferior to the depression is the bulky cricoid cartilage. (b) For Sellick's maneuver (cricoid pressure), place an index finger and thumb on the anterior aspect just lateral to the midline of the cricoid cartilage and apply pressure straight back. (c) Sellick's maneuver is used to occlude the esophagus to help prevent air from going into the stomach and stomach contents from rising up the*

©2008 by Pearson Education, Inc.
Prehospital Emergency Care, 8th ed.

esophagus and being aspirated; also Sellick's maneuver can help in
visualizing the vocal cords and glottic opening. (pp. 1191–1192)

Q4. Explain the methods used to assess tracheal tube placement.

A4. *To assess tracheal tube placement, auscultate the epigastrium for*
presence of gurgling, which indicates an esophageal intubation; watch
for even chest rise and fall; and auscultate for breath sounds that are
equal bilaterally, signs that the tube has not entered a mainstem
bronchus. (pp. 1196–1198)

Q5. Name the laryngoscope blades preferred for intubating infants and
for intubating older children.

A5. *The straight laryngoscope blade is preferred with infants and the*
curved blade is preferred in older children. (p. 1200)

Q6. Regarding determining appropriate tracheal tube size in infants and
children: (a) describe techniques that may be used to determine
appropriate tube size, and (b) based on the sizing formula, state the
size tracheal tube you would use to intubate a 6-year-old child.

A6. *Regarding determining appropriate tracheal tube size in infants and*
children, (a) the techniques used include a commercial resuscitation
measuring tape, a sizing formula (4 + age in years/4); the size of the
patient's little finger; or the internal diameter of the nares. (b) Based
on the sizing formula, the tracheal tube used for a 6-year-old child
would be 5.5 mm i.d. (Both a 5 mm i.d. and a 6 mm i.d. should also
be available.) (pp. 1200–1202)

Q7. Describe the method of measuring the nasogastric tube in the infant
and child.

A7. *The nasogastric tube is measured from the tip of the nose, around the*
ear, and to the level of the xiphoid process. The most proximal hole
should be just below the process. (p. 1205)

Q8. List (a) indications and (b) contraindications for insertion of a
nasogastric tube in an infant or a child.

A8. *(a) Indications for insertion of the nasogastric tube in an infant or a*
child are if you are unable to ventilate because of gastric distension or
if the patient is unresponsive and at risk of vomiting gastric contents or
developing gastric distension. Contraindications for nasogastric tube
insertion are cases of major facial, head, or spinal trauma; suspected
airway disease such as epiglottitis or croup; if patient ingested certain
caustic substances (alkalis) and some hydrocarbons. (p. 1204)

Q9. List the complications associated with orotracheal suctioning.

A9. *Complications associated with orotracheal suctioning include cardiac*
arrhythmias, hypoxia, coughing, mucosa damage, and bronchospasm.
(pp. 1208–1209)

CRITICAL THINKING

Assess students' ability to respond to real-life emergency situations by discussing the Critical Thinking questions on page 1225 in the textbook.

Q1. As long as the patient has a carotid pulse, what is the most important intervention the EMT should now provide?

A1. *The most important intervention is to ensure a patent airway and to continue assisted ventilations with supplemental oxygen. The patient will be ventilated at a rate of 10 to 12 per minute with each ventilation delivered over a 1-second period.*

Q2. How could cricoid pressure, if it had been previously applied, have prevented the current airway obstruction?

A2. *Cricoid pressure, when properly applied, can prevent vomitus from entering the airway. When the cricoid ring is displaced posteriorly, it compresses the esophagus between the posterior cricoid ring and the vertebrae causing the esophagus to collapse. This prevents vomitus from moving up past the collapsed esophagus and entering the hypopharynx and entering the trachea. Also, the cricoid pressure prevents air from going down passed the compressed esophagus and entering the stomach reducing the incidence of gastric distention and regurgitation.*

Q3. What is the BURP technique, and why would it be an appropriate intervention for this patient during the laryngoscopy procedure?

A3. *The BURP technique (which stands for Backward, Upward, Rightward Pressure) is a method of applying external pressure in order to bring the glottic opening into better view during intubation. It would have helped in this situation by bringing the patient's anterior glottic opening into better view.*

Q4. In patients with an anterior glottic opening, what are some additional intubation adjuncts that could help with the intubation procedure?

A4. *Alternative laryngoscope blades such as the Grandview or Viewmax may provide for better visualization. Also, the use of the gum elastic bougie device may be used to introduce the endotracheal tube. Other alternative techniques for endotracheal tube insertion include digital and transillumination. If these fail, an alternative airway device may be necessary such as a Pharyngeo-tracheal Lumen (PtL®) airway, an esophageal tracheal Combitube® airway or a laryngeal mask airway (LMA).*

Q5. Following successful intubation, what are some clinical indications that would demonstrate that the tracheal tube is properly placed?

A5. *There are several ways to determine a properly placed tracheal tube, which include the absence of gurgling sounds while auscultating over the epigastrium during ventilation; watching for equal chest rise and fall during ventilation; confirming equal, bilateral breath sounds by auscultating the lungs during ventilation; the presence of carbon dioxide when using an end-tidal carbon dioxide detector; and obtaining the proper resistance when using a bulb- or syringe-type esophageal intubation detection device.*

SKILLS DEMONSTRATION AND PRACTICE

Write the following on a blackboard, a flipchart, or an overhead transparency:

1. Adult intubation
2. Infant intubation

Divide the class into teams of two. (If there is an odd number of students, one team of three is acceptable.) Explain to the students that each team is to visit both listed stations. At each station, a health professional will demonstrate the listed skills and then help each team member practice.

Provide students with the location of each demonstration and practice station.

Help students rotate through the stations. Visit each station to monitor progress of practice. Make sure that each team visits both practice stations.

When each team has completed each station, make sure that students return to the main classroom.

EVALUATION

Chapter Quiz Distribute copies of the Chapter Quiz provided in Handout 43-2 to evaluate student understanding of this chapter. Remind students not to refer to their textbooks or notes while taking the quiz.

Test Manager You may wish to create a custom-tailored test using Prentice Hall *TestGen for Prehospital Emergency Care, Eighth Edition* to evaluate student understanding of this chapter.

Online Test Preparation (for students and instructors) Additional test preparation is available through *EMT Achieve: Basic Test Preparation* at http://www.prenhall.com/EMTAchieve. Instructors can also monitor student mastery online.

CLOSING (OPTIONAL)

If this is the last lesson of the course, describe the next steps that must be taken by successful students to achieve licensure or certification as an EMT in your state and locality.

You may at this point choose to discuss and review the National Registry of Emergency Medical Technicians certification examination, which many state EMS systems use as the basis for their own certification exams.

Thank students for their participation in this course, and wish them every success with their EMS careers.

REINFORCEMENT

Handouts If classroom discussions or performance on the quiz indicates that some students have not fully mastered the chapter content, you may wish to assign some or all of the Reinforcement Handouts for this chapter.

Chapter Quiz
Handout 43-2

TestGen
Chapter 43 Test

Online Test Preparation
Send your students to
http://www.prenhall.com/
EMTAchieve

Handouts 43-3 to 43-6
Reinforcement Activities

**Brady Skills Series
EMT-B Videos/CD**
Visual Reinforcement

**PowerPoint
Presentation**
Chapter 43

Student CD
Chapter 43

Companion Website
http://www.prenhall.com/
mistovich

TECH EXTRAS

Brady Skills Series EMT-B Videos/CD Have your students watch the skills come to life on either VHS or CD-ROM.

PowerPoint Presentation (for instructors) The PowerPoint material developed for this chapter offers useful reinforcement of chapter content.

Student CD A wide variety of material on this CD-ROM will reinforce and also expand student knowledge and skills.

Companion Website (for students) Additional review quizzes and links to EMS resources will contribute to further reinforcement of this chapter. Please visit http://www.prenhall.com/mistovich.

Objectives Checklist

Cognitive		Date Mastered
8-1.1	Identify and describe the airway anatomy in the infant, child, and adult.	
8-1.2	Differentiate between the anatomy in the infant, child, and adult.	
8-1.3	Explain the pathophysiology of airway compromise.	
8-1.4	Describe the proper use of airway adjuncts.	
8-1.5	Review the use of oxygen therapy in airway management.	
8-1.6	Describe the indications, contraindications, and technique for insertion of nasal gastric tubes.	
8-1.7	Describe how to perform the Sellick maneuver (cricoid pressure).	
8-1.8	Describe the indications for advanced airway management.	
8-1.9	List the equipment required for orotracheal intubation.	
8-1.10	Describe the proper use of the curved blade for orotracheal intubation.	
8-1.11	Describe the proper use of the straight blade for orotracheal intubation.	
8-1.12	State the reasons for and proper use of the stylet in orotracheal intubation.	
8-1.13	Describe the methods of choosing the appropriate size endotracheal tube in an adult patient.	
8-1.14	State the formula for sizing an infant or a child endotracheal tube.	
8-1.15	List complications associated with advanced airway management.	
8-1.16	Define the various alternative methods for sizing the infant and child endotracheal tube.	
8-1.17	Describe the skill of orotracheal intubation in the adult patient.	
8-1.18	Describe the skill of orotracheal intubation in the infant and child patient.	
8-1.19	Describe the skill of confirming endotracheal tube placement in the adult, infant, and child patient.	
8-1.20	State the consequence of and the need to recognize unintentional esophageal intubation.	
8-1.21	Describe the skill of securing the endotracheal tube in the adult, infant, and child patient.	

OBJECTIVES

Affective		Date Mastered
8-1.22	Recognize and respect the feelings of the patient and family during advanced airway procedures.	
8-1.23	Explain the value of performing advanced airway procedures.	
8-1.24	Defend the need for the EMT-Basic to perform advanced airway procedures.	
8-1.25	Explain the rationale for the use of a stylet.	
8-1.26	Explain the rationale for having a suction unit immediately available during intubation attempts.	
8-1.27	Explain the rationale for confirming breath sounds.	
8-1.28	Explain the rationale for securing the endotracheal tube.	

Psychomotor		Date Mastered
8-1.29	Demonstrate how to perform the Sellick maneuver (cricoid pressure).	
8-1.30	Demonstrate the skill of orotracheal intubation in the adult patient.	
8-1.31	Demonstrate the skill of orotracheal intubation in the infant and child patient.	
8-1.32	Demonstrate the skill of confirming endotracheal tube placement in the adult patient.	
8-1.33	Demonstrate the skill of confirming endotracheal tube placement in the infant and child patient.	
8-1.34	Demonstrate the skill of securing the endotracheal tube in the adult patient.	
8-1.35	Demonstrate the skill of securing the endotracheal tube in the infant and child patient.	

CHAPTER 43 QUIZ

Write the letter of the best answer in the space provided.

_____ 1. The portion of the airway closest to the trachea is the
   A. hypopharynx.   C. oropharynx.
   B. nasopharynx.   D. nares.

_____ 2. The device used to shape and stiffen the tracheal tube is the
   A. Murphy eye.   C. bite block.
   B. stylet.   D. Sellick tube.

_____ 3. For tracheal intubation, the head of a patient with no suspected spinal injury should be placed in the _____ position.
   A. Fowler's   C. tripod
   B. sniffing   D. comfort

_____ 4. All of the following are true of the pediatric airway as compared to the adult airway *except*
   A. the tongue is larger.   C. the trachea is wider.
   B. the trachea is softer.   D. airways are smaller overall.

_____ 5. Before tracheal intubation is attempted, the patient should be hyperventilated at a rate of _____ breaths per minute.
   A. 16   C. 30
   B. 24   D. 36

_____ 6. A potentially lethal complication associated with orotracheal intubation is
   A. slowing of the heartbeat.   C. cuff leakage.
   B. soft tissue trauma.   D. esophageal intubation.

_____ 7. Which one of the following is *not* mandatory personal protective equipment during an intubation?
   A. mask   C. goggles
   B. gloves   D. gown

_____ 8. The laryngoscope blade that directly lifts the epiglottis is
   A. curved.   C. round.
   B. straight.   D. angulated.

_____ 9. The laryngoscope blade that is preferred for intubations in older children is
   A. curved.   C. round.
   B. straight.   D. angulated.

_____ 10. The tracheal tube without a cuff is for use with what type of patient?
   A. adult   C. anesthesia
   B. trauma   D. pediatric

_____ 11. In an adult, a properly placed tracheal tube will be inserted to a depth of about _____ centimeters as indicated by the tube marker at the teeth.
   A. 15–16   C. 19–23
   B. 20–35   D. 35–45

_____ **12.** Which one of the following is a contraindication for nasogastric intubation?
    A. bardycardia   **C.** tachycardia
    B. croup   **D.** hypoglycemia

_____ **13.** All of the following are indications for orotracheal intubation _except_
    A. cardiac arrest.
    B. an unconscious and unresponsive patient.
    C. a patient with partial airway obstruction.
    D. inability to ventilate an apneic patient.

_____ **14.** Sellick's maneuver involves applying direct pressure to the _____ cartilage.
    A. vallecula   **C.** tracheal
    B. cricoid   **D.** thyroid

_____ **15.** The laryngoscope blade should be used to sweep the tongue
    A. downwards and right.   **C.** downwards and left.
    B. upwards and left.   **D.** upwards and right.

_____ **16.** When intubating, the EMT should look for and visualize the
    A. vallecula.   **C.** trachea.
    B. vocal cords.   **D.** esophagus.

_____ **17.** Objective measures of proper tracheal tube placement include all of the following _except_
    A. use of pulse oximetry.
    B. auscultation.
    C. use of an esophageal intubation detection device (EIDD).
    D. use of an end tidal carbon dioxide detector.

_____ **18.** Which one of the following is an indication of correct tube placement in an orotracheal intubation?
    A. Breath sounds are present in the epigastrium.
    B. The abdomen rises with ventilations.
    C. Equal breath sounds are heard over the apices.
    D. Cyanosis develops.

_____ **19.** Breath sounds should be assessed after
    A. intubation.
    B. clinical changes in the patient.
    C. every major movement of the patient.
    D. all of these.

_____ **20.** Never apply orotracheal suctioning for longer than _____ seconds.
    A. 5   **C.** 20
    B. 15   **D.** 30

IN THE FIELD

Read the following real-life situation. Then answer the questions that follow.

"We arrived and found the patient in cardiac arrest with bystander CPR in progress. My partner began reassessment of the patient. He then proceeded to defibrillate the patient. The AED advised no shock, so he started CPR again while I intubated the patient.

"The patient was a middle-aged man who looked like he was the center for the Green Bay Packers. With his short neck and a large chest, I was having serious trouble intubating him. In fact, I missed the first time and knowing I had one shot left, I pulled out all the plugs and tried to get the tube in.

"After a minute of CPR without change in the patient's condition and having him intubated, we elected to package the patient and meet up with a Paramedic unit. That's when the trouble began. As we transferred the patient, he started turning blue. Then his stomach started getting bigger. The next thing you know, the patient erupted with vomitus. "After vigorous suctioning, we elected to extubate the patient and continue to ventilate him with a bag-valve mask. I was pretty discouraged because I thought I had gotten the tube into the trachea."

1. What other techniques could have made this intubation easier?

2. What other methods could have been used to confirm tracheal tube placement?

3. What deadly complication resulted and what was the EMT's error?

REINFORCEMENT

CHAPTER 43 REVIEW

Write the word or words that best complete each sentence in the space provided.

1. The leaf-shaped structure that covers the opening of the larynx during swallowing is the

   _____.

2. The chest wall in infants and children is _____ and more

   _____ than in adults.

3. The cartilage in the airway to which pressure is applied during Sellick's maneuver is the

   _____.

4. The trachea divides into the left and right bronchi at the _____.

5. Aspirated food and misplaced tracheal tubes usually end up going into the

   _____ mainstem bronchus.

6. When comparing airways of adults and children, the _____ is

   proportionally larger in a child than in an adult.

7. The narrowest portion of the pediatric airway is at the _____ cartilage.

8. Indications for tracheal intubation include the inability to ventilate the apneic patient and the

   inability of a patient to _____ his or her own airway.

9. The tracheal tube is placed into the trachea via direct _____ of the tube as

   it passes through the vocal cords.

10. Stimulation of the vagus nerve in the airway can lead to _____ heart rates.

11. Prolonged efforts at intubation can lead to _____.

12. A potentially lethal mistake that can be made while intubating is _____

    intubation.

13. Because of the typical placement of the lightbulb in the laryngoscope blade, the handle must be held

    in the _____ hand.

14. A(n) _____ laryngoscope blade is preferred for intubations in younger

    pediatric patients.

15. All blades are designed to bring the _____ _____

    into view.

16. The tip of a curved blade is placed into the _____

_____.

17. When checking the tracheal tube prior to intubation, if the pilot balloon fails, that means the

_____ also fails.

18. Generally, a properly placed tracheal tube will display the _____ cm mark at

the teeth of an adult.

19. With the stylet in place, the tracheal tube should be placed into a(n) _____ -

_____ shape.

20. The end of the stylet should *not* go past the _____

_____.

21. Prior to any intubation attempt, it is imperative that the patient be _____.

22. Application of pressure to the _____ cartilage will help with visualization of

the vocal cords.

23. The most dependable method of indirectly confirming tracheal tube placement is

_____.

24. A suspected basilar skull fracture is a contraindication for _____ intubation.

25. When there is any doubt about a tracheal tube's position, the EMT should

_____ the tube.

REINFORCEMENT

ADVANCED AIRWAY: LISTING

Complete the following lists.

1. List four advantages of controlling an airway through tracheal intubation.

2. List five possible complications of tracheal intubation.

3. List three pieces of personal protective equipment that are mandatory during a tracheal intubation.

4. List two indications for nasogastric intubation.

5. List three complications associated with orotracheal suctioning.

ORGANIZING A TRACHEAL INTUBATION

Demonstrate your understanding of tracheal intubation by putting the following steps in the process in proper order. Write 1 next to the step you would perform first, 2 next to the step that would come next, and so on.

_____ Attach bag-valve device to the tracheal tube.

_____ Lubricate distal end of tracheal tube.

_____ Apply Sellick's maneuver.

_____ Assemble the laryngoscope blade and handle.

_____ Inflate the tube cuff with 5–10 cc of air.

_____ Check suction unit.

_____ Insert laryngoscope blade and lift patient's tongue.

_____ Remove oropharyngeal airway.

_____ Take appropriate BSI precautions.

_____ Test the tracheal tube cuff.

_____ Remove stylet from tracheal tube.

_____ Hyperventilate the patient.

_____ Remove the laryngoscope blade.

_____ Secure tube in place.

_____ Insert the tracheal tube and guide it through the vocal cords.

_____ Place head of patient with no suspected spinal injury in sniffing position.

_____ Lubricate stylet and insert into tube.

_____ Position yourself at patient's head.

_____ Identify the glottic opening and vocal cords.

_____ Confirm tube placement.

_____ Reassess breath sounds as often as possible.

Advanced Airway Management

Airway and Respiratory Anatomy and Physiology Review

Airway Anatomy

Airway Anatomy in Infants and Children

Basic Airway Management Review

Oropharyngeal Suctioning

Orotracheal Intubation

Advantages

Indications

BSI Precautions

Equipment

- Laryngoscope
  - Straight blade
  - Curved blade
- Tracheal tubes
- Stylet
- Other equipment

Sellick's Maneuver

Procedure for Tracheal Tube Insertion in Adults

Complications

Orotracheal Intubation in Infants and Children

Indications in Infants and Children

Anatomical Considerations

©2008 by Pearson Education, Inc.
Prehospital Emergency Care, 8th ed.

HANDOUT 43-2: Chapter 43 Quiz

1. A	**6.** D	**11.** C	**16.** B
2. B	**7.** D	**12.** B	**17.** B
3. B	**8.** B	**13.** C	**18.** C
4. C	**9.** A	**14.** B	**19.** D
5. B	**10.** D	**15.** B	**20.** B

HANDOUT 43-3: In the Field

1. Placing the patient's head in the sniffing position; use of cricoid pressure (the Sellick maneuver).
2. Use of pulse oximetry, an end tidal carbon dioxide detector, or an esophageal intubation detection device (EIDD).
3. Extubation and esophageal intubation resulted. The EMT did not recheck tube placement after moving the patient.

HANDOUT 43-4: Chapter 43 Review

1. epiglottis
2. softer, flexible
3. cricoid
4. carina
5. right
6. tongue
7. cricoid
8. protect
9. visualization
10. slowed
11. hypoxia
12. esophageal
13. left
14. straight
15. glottic opening (vocal cords)
16. vallecula
17. cuff
18. 19–23
19. hockey-stick
20. Murphy eye
21. hyperventilated
22. cricoid
23. auscultation
24. nasogastric
25. remove

HANDOUT 43-5: Advanced Airway: Listing

1. Any four of the following: It allows complete airway control; it minimizes risk of aspiration; it permits better oxygen delivery; it provides the ability to perform deep tracheal suctioning; it can overcome mechanical and physiological problems that compromise normal ventilations.
2. Any five of the following: bradycardia and hypotension; tachycardia and hypertension; soft tissue trauma; hypoxia; vomiting; right mainstem intubation; esophageal intubation; accidental extubation; stimulation of the vagus nerve leading to laryngospasm.
3. Gloves, mask, goggles
4. Inability to provide effective positive-pressure ventilation due to gastric distension; unresponsive patient at risk of vomiting or developing gastric distension.
5. Any three of the following: hypoxia; cardiac dysrhythmias; coughing leading to increased pressure within the skull; soft tissue damage caused by the catheter; bronchospasm.

HANDOUT 43-6: Organizing a Tracheal Intubation

Reading down the column the order of steps is as follows: 18, 6, 11, 4, 17, 7, 12, 10, 1, 3, 16, 2, 15, 20, 14, 9, 5, 8, 13, 19, 21

Minor variations in step order may be acceptable; the instructor should decide.

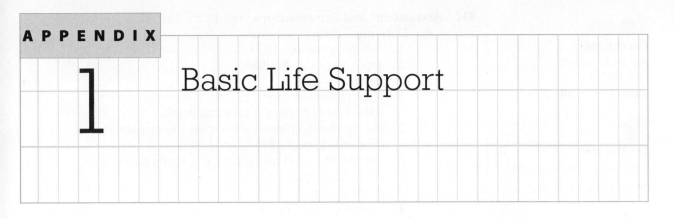

Basic Life Support

Before students can learn how to be EMTs, they must have completed a course in cardiopulmonary resuscitation (CPR). This lecture provides a review of the information that should have been acquired in that course. Students may wish to consult the American Heart Association, Healthcare Provider curriculum.

Present the review information in your own words, following the outline below. Page numbers in parentheses refer to pages in the textbook. References in dark, heavy type are to figures and tables in the textbook.

LECTURE

The following suggested lecture outline is based on the 2005 American Heart Association Guidelines for CPR and Emergency Cardiovascular Care. The page numbers in parentheses refer to pages in the textbook The parenthetical references in dark, heavy type are to figures, tables, and scans in the textbook.

BASIC LIFE SUPPORT

I. **Introduction** (p. 1226)
   A. Clinical death
      1. Cessation of breathing and heartbeat
   B. Biological death
      1. Irreversible brain damage
         a. Begins within 4-6 minutes after clinical death
   C. Stopping CPR
      1. Return of spontaneous breathing and circulation
      2. Advanced life support is begun
      3. Physician or advanced life support unit orders CPR discontinued.

II. **Age Delineation in CPR** (p. 1226)
   A. Infant
      1. Less than 1 year of age
   B. Child
      1. 1 year to onset of puberty
         a. Approximately 12-14 years of age
         b. Development of secondary sex characteristics
   C. Adult
      1. Onset of puberty (approximately 12–14 years of age) and older.

Total Teaching Time
8 hours

Resources Needed
American Heart Association CPR Curriculum

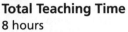

Additional Resources
Pocket Reference for the EMT-B and First Responder, Second Edition

BTLS: Basic Trauma Life Support for the EMT-B and First Responder

Instructional Methods in Emergency Services, Second Edition

EMT-Basic Self-Assessment Exam Prep

Point of Interest
Over-eager EMTs have initiated CPR on sleeping patients! Remind students that determining unresponsiveness usually involves more than a tap on the shoulder.

Point of Interest
The recovery position used to be known as the "coma" position.

III. Assessment and interventions (pp. 1226–1231)
 A. Determine unresponsiveness.
  1. Ask questions loudly.
  2. Tap patient on shoulder.
 B. Open the airway.
  1. Place patient in supine position, providing spinal stabilization if spinal injury suspected.
  2. Use head-tilt, chin-lift if no spine injury suspected. **(Fig. A1-1, p. 1227)**
  3. Use jaw-thrust maneuver if spine injury suspected. **(Fig. A1-2, p. 1227)**
 C. Check breathing.
  1. Look for chest rise and fall.
  2. Listen for escaping air during exhalation.
  3. Feel for air flow against your cheek.
  4. If patient is breathing adequately and no spine injury is suspected, place in recovery position. **(Fig. A1-3, p. 1228)**
 D. Ventilate.
  1. Use barrier device if possible. **(Fig. A1-4, p. 1228)**
  2. Administer 2 ventilations over 1 second each.
  3. If chest does not rise
   a. Reposition patient's head and try again.
  4. If chest still does not rise
   a. Use foreign body airway obstruction procedures.
  5. Only enough tidal volume for chest rise.
 E. Check for a pulse.
  1. Assess carotid pulse in adult or child.
  2. Assess brachial pulse in infant.
  3. Feel for pulse for at least 5 seconds and no more than 10 seconds (30–45 seconds if patient has been submerged in cool or cold water or suspected of being hypothermic).
 F. Deliver chest compressions.
  1. Position hands properly. **(Fig. A1-5, p. 1230)**
  2. Deliver compressions.
   a. Push hard and push fast

IV. Adult CPR performed by one rescuer (pp. 1231–1232) **(Fig. A1-6, p. 1231)**
 A. Rate.
  1. 100 compressions per minute
 B. Ratio
  1. 30 compressions to 2 ventilations (artificial)
 C. Ventilations
  1. 10-12 breaths per minute

V. Adult CPR performed by two rescuers (p. 1232) **(Fig. A1-6, p. 1231)**
 A. Rate
  1. 100 compressions per minute
 B. Ratio
  1. 30 compressions to 2 ventilations (artificial)
 C. Ventilations (no advanced airway)
  1. 10-12 breaths per minute
 D. Ventilations (advanced airway)
  1. 8-10 breaths per minute

VI. Performing CPR on infants (p. 1232) **(Fig. A1-7, p. 1233)**
 A. No signs of circulation or heart rate less than 60 beats per minutes with signs of poor perfusion
 B. Determine pulselessness

   1. Brachial pulse
  C. Hand position
   1. Two fingers just below the level of the nipples
   2. Two thumbs with hands encircling
  D. Chest depth
   1. 1/3 to 1/2 depth of the chest
  E. Rate
   1. 100 compressions per minute
  F. Ratio
   1. One rescuer
    a. 30 compressions to 2 ventilations (artificial)
   2. Two rescuer
    a. 15 compressions to 2 ventilations
VII. Performing CPR on children (p. 1232) **(Fig. A1-8, p. 1233)**
  A. No signs of circulation or heart rate less than 60 beats per minutes with signs of poor perfusion
  B. Determine pulselessness
   1. Carotid pulse
  C. Hand position
   1. Heel of one hand between the nipples
   2. Two hands as in adult, if needed for proper compression depth
  D. Chest depth
   1. 1/3 to 1/2 depth of the chest
  E. Rate
   1. 100 compressions per minute
  F. Ratio
   1. One rescuer
    a. 30 compressions to 2 ventilations (artificial)
   2. Two rescuer
    a. 15 compressions to 2 ventilations

OBSTRUCTED AIRWAY

I. Causes of foreign body airway obstruction (p. 1232)
  A. Tongue
  B. Foreign body
  C. Secretions
  D. Blood clots
  E. Cancerous condition of the mouth or throat
  F. Tonsil enlargement
  G. Injury to the face or jaw
  H. Acute epiglottitis
  I. Aspirated vomitus
  J. Broken dental bridges
II. Mild foreign body airway obstruction (p. 1233)
  A. Able to move air, breathe, or cough
  B. Don't interfere with the patient's attempts to expel the foreign object
  C. Watch for signs of reduced air passage
   1. Silent cough
   2. Inability to speak
   3. Inability to move air
   4. Cyanosis
  D. Transport rapidly
III. Severe foreign body airway obstruction (pp. 1233–1236)
  A. Signs and symptoms

1. Clutching the neck with the hands
2. Ability to nod but inability to speak
3. Silent cough
4. Inability to breathe
5. Labored use of muscles required in an attempt to breathe
6. Cyanosis
7. Unresponsiveness

IV. **Emergency care for a conscious severe foreign body airway obstruction patient** (pp. 1234–1235)
   A. Conscious adult or child with severe foreign body airway obstruction
      1. If the patient is standing or sitting
         a. Stand behind the patient
         b. Wrap your arms around the waist
            (1) Keep your elbows out, away from the patient's ribs
            (2) Make a fist with one hand, and place the thumb side on the midline of the abdomen slightly above the navel and well below the xiphoid process
         c. Grasp your fist with your other hand, thumbs toward the patient (**Fig. A1-9, p. 1234**).
         d. Press your fist into the patient's abdomen with a quick inward and upward thrust.
            (1) Deliver a series of up to 5 thrusts.
            (2) Make each thrust separate and distinct.
            (3) If obstruction not relieved, continue series of 5 thrusts until the object is released or the patient becomes unresponsive.
   B. Unresponsive adult or child with severe foreign body airway obstruction
      1. Place the patient in a supine position.
      2. Inspect inside the mouth.
         a. Only perform a finger sweep if the foreign object can be seen.
         b. Do not perform a blind finger sweep
      3. Perform a head-tilt, chin-lift maneuver
      4. Attempt to deliver 2 ventilations
      5. Deliver chest compressions
         a. 30 compressions in the adult
         b. 30 compressions in the child with one rescuer
         c. 15 compressions in the child with two rescuers
      6. Inspect inside the mouth.
         a. Only perform a finger sweep if the foreign object can be seen.
         b. Do not perform a blind finger sweep
      7. Perform a head-tilt, chin-lift maneuver
      8. Deliver 2 ventilations.
      9. Repeat the cycle of compressions and ventilations until the obstruction is removed or relieved by ALS or arrival at the medical facility.
   C. Severe foreign body airway obstruction in the obese or in late pregnancy
      1. Patient standing or sitting
         a. Stand behind the patient with your arms directly under the armpits
         b. Wrap your arms around the chest

   2. Position the thumb side of your fist on the midline of the sternum
      a. If you are near the margins of the rib cage, you are too low **(Fig. A1-10a, p. 1235)**
   3. Seize your fist firmly with your other hand and thrust backward sharply **(Fig. A1-10b, p. 1235)**
   4. Repeat until the object is expelled or the patient becomes unconscious
   5. If the obese or late stage pregnancy patient with a foreign body airway obstruction becomes unconscious, proceed with the same steps as for the unresponsive adult or child with severe foreign body airway obstruction

V. Severe foreign body airway obstruction in infants (pp. 1235–1236)
  A. Conscious choking but still responsive
   1. Transport rapidly
   2. Let the infant try to expel the foreign object by coughing
  B. Conscious infant with severe foreign body airway obstruction
   1. Straddle the infant over one of your arms **(Fig. A1-11, p. 1236)**
      a. Face down and the head lower than the trunk
      b. Support the infant's head by firmly holding the jaw
      c. Rest your forearm on your thigh for support
   2. With the heel of your other hand, deliver five back blows (slaps) rapidly and forcefully between the infant's shoulder blades
   3. If the foreign body has not been expelled
      a. Support the infant's head
      b. Sandwich the infant's body between your hands and turn the infant on his back
      c. Keep the head lower than the trunk
      d. Lay the infant on your thigh or over your lap with the head supported
      e. Deliver five quick, firm thrusts in the midsternal region with the same finger placement as for CPR chest compressions
   4. Repeat steps until the obstruction is expelled or the infant becomes unresponsive.
  C. Unconsious infant with severe foreign body airway obstruction
   1. Open the mouth and inspect inside the airway for the foreign body
      a. If it is seen, attempt to remove it with a finger sweep.
      b. Do not perform a blind finger sweep
   2. Perform a head-tilt, chin-lift maneuver and attempt to ventilate twice
   3. Deliver chest compressions
      a. 30 compressions with one rescuer
      b. 15 compressions with two rescuers
   4. Deliver 2 ventilations
   5. Continue compressions
   6. Repeat the cycle of compressions and ventilations until the obstruction is removed or relieved by ALS or arrival at the medical facility

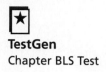

Chapter Quiz
Handout BLS-1

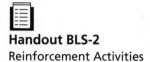

TestGen
Chapter BLS Test

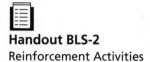

Handout BLS-2
Reinforcement Activities

EVALUATION

Chapter Quiz Distribute copies of the Chapter Quiz provided in Handout BLS-1 to evaluate student understanding of basic life support. Remind students not to refer to their textbooks or notes while taking the quiz.

Test Manager You may wish to create a custom-tailored test using Prentice Hall *TestGen for Prehospital Emergency Care,* Eighth Edition to evaluate student understanding of this chapter.

REINFORCEMENT

Handouts If classroom discussions or performance on the quiz indicates that some students have not fully mastered the chapter content, you may wish to assign some or all of the Reinforcement Handouts for this chapter.

BASIC LIFE SUPPORT QUIZ

Write the letter of the best answer in the space provided.

_____ 1. With the cessation of breathing and heartbeat, the patient is _____ dead.
   A. clinically
   B. biologically
   C. physiologically
   D. legally

_____ 2. After breathing and heartbeat stops, Irreversible brain damage occurs within:
   A. 1-2 minutes.
   B. 2-4 minutes.
   C. 4-6 minutes.
   D. 6-8 minutes.

_____ 3. Pulses are checked at the carotid artery for all of the following patients EXCEPT:
   A. infants.
   B. children.
   C. adults
   D. the elderly.

_____ 4. Unless a patient has been submerged in cool or cold water or has hypothermia, assessment for a pulse should take no longer than _____ seconds.
   A. 10
   B. 15
   C. 20
   D. 30

_____ 5. CPR procedures are different in infants than in adults EXCEPT for the:
   A. location of pulse checks.
   B. activation of EMS.
   C. determination of breathlessness.
   D. depth of compressions.

_____ 6. All of the following are correct procedures for a trauma patient needing resuscitation EXCEPT:
   A. rolling the patient onto his back with spinal stabilization.
   B. maintaining manual in-line cervical spine stabilization.
   C. opening the airway with the head-tilt, chin-lift.
   D. ventilating the breathless patient twice.

_____ 7. Most airway problems are caused by:
   A. loose dentures.
   B. vomitus.
   C. broken teeth.
   D. the tongue.

_____ 8. In rescue breathing, the first two breaths should be:
   A. delivered over 6 seconds.
   B. given as rapidly as possible.
   C. delivered slowly over 1 second.
   D. delivered over 4 seconds.

_____ 9. Which one of the following is NOT a valid reason for discontinuing artificial ventilation and CPR once begun?
   A. recovery of spontaneous breathing by the patient
   B. commencement of advanced life support measures
   C. a physician's directive
   D. a request by the patient's family to cease

_____10. The patient who is breathing adequately and who is NOT suspected of having a spine injury should be placed in the _____ position.
   A. recovery
   B. prone
   C. resuscitation
   D. stupor

_____ **11.** Chest compressions should be delivered at a rate of _____/minute.
    A. 100   **C.** 120
    B. 60–80   **D.** 55–75

_____ **12.** Which one of the following statements about delivering chest compressions is CORRECT?
    A. Lift the hand off the chest after each compression.
    B. Bend the elbows when delivering compressions.
    C. Deliver the compressions straight down with elbows locked.
    D. Deliver compressions over the superior sternum.

_____ **13.** The proper ratio of compressions to breaths in one-rescuer CPR for adults is:
    A. 5 to 1.   **C.** 20 to 2.
    B. 10 to 1.   **D.** 30 to 2.

_____ **14.** The proper ratio of compressions to breaths in one-rescuer CPR for infants and children is:
    A. 5 to 1.   **C.** 20 to 2.
    B. 10 to 1.   **D.** 30 to 2.

_____ **15.** Chest compressions in a child patient should be delivered at a rate of _____/minute.
    A. 80   **C.** 110
    B. 100   **D.** 120

_____ **16.** Check the pulse of an infant using the _____ artery.
    A. femoral   **C.** carotid
    B. brachial   **D.** radial

_____ **17.** In two-rescuer healthcare provider CPR on adult patients, the proper ratio of compressions to breaths is:
    A. 5 to 1.   **C.** 15 to 2.
    B. 10 to 1.   **D.** 20 to 2.

_____ **18.** If an initial series of 5 back slaps fails to dislodge a foreign object in an unresponsive infant who is not breathing, the EMT should:
    A. perform a blind finger sweep.   **C.** deliver 5 more back blows.
    B. deliver 5 chest thrusts.   **D.** perform a jaw-thrust maneuver.

_____ **19.** After an initial series of back splats and chest thrusts for an unresponsive infant who has a foreign body airway obstruction and is not breathing, the EMT should:
    A. perform a blind finger sweep.   **C.** deliver 5 back blows.
    B. deliver 5 more chest thrusts.   **D.** perform a jaw-thrust maneuver.

_____ **20.** The EMT should begin maneuvers to clear an airway obstruction only if the patient:
    A. starts to cough vigorously.   **C.** turns blue or gray.
    B. speaks at a high pitch.   **D.** requests assistance.

OBJECTIVES

BASIC LIFE SUPPORT REVIEW

Write the word or words that best complete each sentence in the space provided.

1. When the heart stops, _____ death occurs.

2. The objective of CPR is to prevent _____ death.

3. The first step in the assessment of the patient is to _____

_____ .

4. The best method of determining breathlessness is to _____ ,

_____ , and _____ for breathing.

5. If you are alone, EMS should be activated after it has been determined that the adult patient is

_____ .

6. Most airway problems are caused by the _____ .

7. When the patient is suspected of having a spine injury, the preferred method of opening the airway

is the _____ -_____ maneuver.

8. In artificial ventilation, if the first breath delivered is unsuccessful, then the rescuer should

_____ _____ _____ .

9. In CPR, chest compressions should be delivered over the center of the

_____ between the _____ .

10. When delivering chest compressions, the rescuer should keep his or her elbows

_____ .

11. The depth of chest compressions for adult CPR should be about _____ to

_____ inches.

12. In two-rescuer CPR for an infant or child, the ratio of compressions to breaths should be

_____ to _____ .

13. In one-rescuer CPR on an adult patient, the EMT should perform _____

cycles of compressions/ventilations before a pulse check.

14. When performing CPR on an infant under 1 year of age, deliver compressions using the

_____ _____ .

15. Elderly people are at a greater risk of choking because they have a slower

_____ _____ .

16. Any patient under age _____ is considered an infant for purposes of CPR.

17. The pulse of a child is checked at the _____

_____.

18. With infants and children, the EMT should perform CPR for _____

minute(s) before activating the EMS system.

19. For an unresponsive adult in whom you suspect a foreign body airway obstruction, the EMT

perform a(n) _____ _____ only when you can see

the obstruction.

20. After a foreign body is removed from the airway of any patient, always

_____ the patient.

APPENDIX 1 ANSWER KEY

HANDOUT BLS-1: Appendix 1 Quiz

1. A	**6.** C	**11.** A	**16.** B
2. C	**7.** D	**12.** C	**17.** C
3. A	**8.** C	**13.** D	**18.** B
4. A	**9.** D	**14.** D	**19.** D
5. C	**10.** A	**15.** B	**20.** C

HANDOUT BLS-2: Basic Life Support Review

1. clinical
2. biological
3. determine unresponsiveness
4. look, listen, feel
5. unresponsive
6. tongue
7. jaw-thrust
8. reposition the head
9. chest, nipples
10. locked
11. 1 1/2, 2
12. 30, 2
13. five
14. two fingers
15. gag reflex
16. one
17. carotid artery
18. 2
19. finger sweep
20. transport

2 ALS Assist Skills

At times, the Advanced EMT or Paramedic may ask the EMT to assist in setting up equipment so they can perform an advanced skill. Two of the most common advanced skills that EMTs may assist with are intravenous therapy and ECG monitoring. Be sure to follow your local protocol when assisting with ALS skills.

Total Teaching Time
1 hour

Additional Resources
Essentials of Paramedic Care, Second Edition

Paramedic Care, Principles & Practice, Second Edition

LECTURE

The following suggested lecture outline is based on materials covered in Appendix 2. The page numbers in parentheses refer to pages in the textbook. The parenthetical references in bold type are to figures, tables, and scans in the textbook.

ASSISTING IN INTRAVENOUS THERAPY

I. Used to administer fluids or medications (p. 1237)
II. Intravenous therapy equipment components (pp. 1237–1238)
  A. Catheter
    1. Catheters are sized according to diameter and length
      a. The diameter is identified by the gauge
        (1) The higher the gauge number, the smaller the diameter
      b. The length is in inches.
  B. Intravenous tubing
    1. Identified by the number of drops per minute it takes to deliver 1 ml of fluid
      a. Macro-drip tubing
        (1) 10-drop/ml
        (2) 15-drop/ml
        (3) 20-drop/ml
      b. Mini-drip tubing
        (1) 60-drop/ml
      c. The lower-drop tubings are able to deliver fluid at a faster rate
      d. The higher-drop tubings deliver fluid at a more controlled and slower rate
      e. Drops/ml may also be referred to as gtts/ml.
    2. Five major tubing components
      a. Spike
      b. Drip chamber
      c. Flow control or regulator valve
      d. Drug or needle injection port
      e. Hub connector

Point of Interest

Do not use any IV fluid after it's expiration date has passed; any fluid that appears cloudy, discolored, or laced with particulate; or any fluid whose sealed packaging has been opened or tampered with.

    C. Bag of fluid
        1. Identification
            a. Type of solution
            b. Amount of solution
            c. Expiration date
        2. Two pigtail devices
            a. Pull-type cover
            b. Injection port

III. Preparing the intravenous setup ("spiking the bag") (p. 1238)
    A. Remove the protective wrap (**Fig. A2-1a, p. 1238**)
    B. Check for impurities, particulate matter, and discoloration. Check the expiration date (**Fig. A2-1b, p. 1238**)
    C. Select the proper administration set based on the instructions from the Advanced EMT or Paramedic.
    D. Tear open the packaging of the solution set and uncoil the tubing
        1. Be careful not to let the ends of the tubing touch the ground.
    E. Close the flow regulator, if it is oepen, by rolling the stopcock valve away from the bag.
    F. Remove the protective covering from the intravenous bag pigtail port.
    G. Remove the protective cap or covering from the spike (**Fig. A2-1c, p. 1239**)
    H. Insert the spike into the intravenous bag pigtail port (**Fig. A2-1d, p. 1239**)
    I. Holding the bag higher than the drip chamber, squeeze the drip chamber once or twice to fill it to the marker line, which is about one-third full (**Fig. A2-1e, p. 1239**).
    J. Open the flow regulator to "flush" the tubing of all of the air (**Fig. A2-1f, p. 1239**).
    K. At this point, the intravenous bag is "spiked" and prepared for insertion into the hub of the catheter.

IV. Saline lock or heparin lock (pp. 1238–1239)
    A. Device that is attached to the hub of the catheter
    B. Filled with approximately 2ml of saline to keep the vein open and the intravenous site active (**Fig. A2-2, p. 1240**)
    C. There is no intravenous tubing.
    D. The saline remains in the lock device and keeps the vein from clotting.

ECG LEAD PLACEMENT

I. An electrocardiogram (ECG) is a device that provides information about the electrical activity of the heart. (p. 1239)

II. 3- or 4-lead electrode placement (limb leads) (pp. 1240–1241)
    A. Cleanse the skin (**Fig. A2-3a, p. 1240**)
        1. Use alcohol or an abrasive pad to remove dirt, body oil, and other substances.
        2. If there is a significant amount of chest hair, shave it quickly.
        3. Dry the skin if there is a large amount of diaphoresis (sweat).
        4. Some systems will use antiperspirant or tincture of Benzoin to keep the skin dry to allow for effective adhesion of the electrode.
    B. Apply the electrodes to the skin (**Fig. A2-3b, p. 1240**)
        1. One electrode is placed to the right side of the anterior chest just under the clavicle at the midclavicular line
            a. Negative lead
            b. White; labeled "RA"

2. The second electrode is applied to the left anterior chest just under the clavicle at the midclavicular line
   a. Ground lead
   b. Black, brown, or green; labeled "LA"
3. The third electrode is applied to the left lower chest at about the seventh intercostal space on the anterior axillary line
   a. Positive lead
   b. Red; labeled "RL"
4. If a fourth lead is to be used, the electrode is applied to the right lower lateral chest wall
   a. Green, labeled "LL"

III. 12-lead electrode placement (precordial leads) (pp. 1241–1243)
   A. Cleanse the skin (**Fig. A2-3a, p. 1240**)
   1. Use alcohol or an abrasive pad to remove dirt, body oil, and other substances.
   2. If there is a significant amount of chest hair, shave it quickly.
   3. Dry the skin if there is a large amount of diaphoresis (sweat).
   4. Some systems will use antiperspirant or tincture of Benzoin to keep the skin dry to allow for effective adhesion of the electrode.
   B. Place the four limb leads according to the manufacturer's recommendation. These are the right arm, right leg, left arm, and left leg electrodes and leads (**Fig. A2-4a, p. 1241**)
   C. The precordial leads are V_1, V_2, V_3, V_4, V_5, and V_6
   1. Placed on the anterior chest
   2. The electrode heads are imprinted with the respective lead numbers
   3. Place lead V_1 to the immediate right of the sternum at the fourth intercostal space (**Fig. A2-4b, p. 1241**)
   4. Place lead V_2 to the immediate left of the sternum at the fourth intercostal space (**Fig. A2-4c, p. 1241**)
   5. Out of order, next place lead V_4 to the left midclavicular line at the fifth intercostal space (**Fig. A2-4d, p. 1241**)
   6. Place lead V_3 midway between lead V_2 and V_4 on the left anterior chest (**Fig. A2-4e, p. 1242**)
   7. Place lead V_5 to the left anterior axillary line at the same level as V_4 (**Fig. A2-4f, p. 1242**)
   8. Place lead V_6 to the left midaxillary line at the same level as V_4 and V_5 (**Fig. A2-4g, p. 1242**).
   9. Check to ensure that all leads are properly placed, especially the precordial leads (**Fig. A2-5, p. 1243**) and that all of the leads are properly adhering and making good contact with the skin.

EVALUATION

EMTs assisting with advanced level skills would be regulated by the specific EMS system the EMT functions in and under the supervision of the medical director. An evaluation component is not included with this topic due to the EMT's normal scope of practice.

REINFORCEMENT

EMTs assisting with advanced level skills would be regulated by the specific EMS system the EMT functions in and under the supervision of the medical director. A reinforcement component is not included with this topic due to the EMT's normal scope of practice.